AF572636

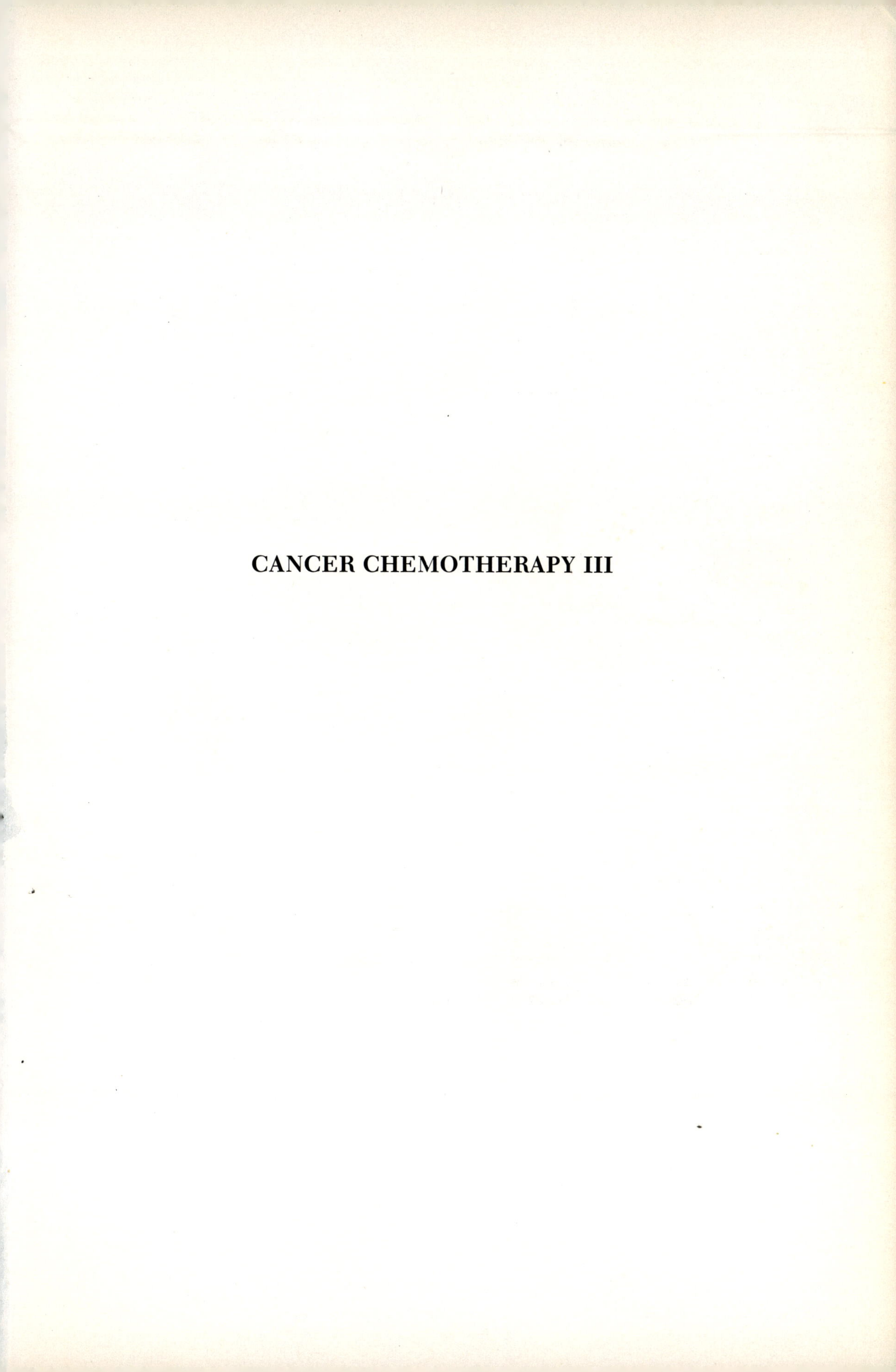

CANCER CHEMOTHERAPY III

CANCER CHEMOTHERAPY III

THE FORTY-SIXTH HAHNEMANN SYMPOSIUM

Edited by

ISADORE BRODSKY, M.D.
Herbert L. Orlowitz Professor of Medical Oncology and Hematology
Chairman, Department of Medical Oncology and Hematology
Herbert L. Orlowitz Institute
Hahnemann Medical College and Hospital
Philadelphia, Pennsylvania

SIGMUND BENHAM KAHN, M.D.
Professor and Vice Chairman, Department of Medical Oncology and Hematology
Herbert L. Orlowitz Institute
Hahnemann Medical College and Hospital
Philadelphia, Pennsylvania

JAMES F. CONROY, D.O.
Associate Professor
Department of Medical Oncology and Hematology
Herbert L. Orlowitz Institute
Hahnemann Medical College and Hospital
Philadelphia, Pennsylvania

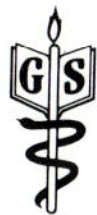

GRUNE & STRATTON
A Subsidiary of Harcourt Brace Jovanovich, Publishers
New York San Francisco London

Library of Congress Cataloging in Publication Data

Main entry under title:

Cancer chemotherapy III.

Includes bibliographies and index.

1. Cancer—Chemotherapy—Congresses. I. Brodsky, Isadore. II. Kahn, Sigmund Benham, 1933–
III. Conroy, James F. IV. Hahnemann Medical College and Hospital of Philadelphia. [DNLM: 1. Antineoplastic Agents—Pharmacodynamics—Congresses. 2. Neoplasms—Drug therapy—Congresses. W3 C1164]
RC271.C5C322 616.9'94'061 78-13554
ISBN 0-8089-1086-8

Grune & Stratton, Inc.
111 Fifth Avenue
New York, New York 10003

Distributed in the United Kingdom by
Academic Press, Inc. (London) Ltd.
24/28 Oval Road, London NW 1

Library of Congress Catalog Number 78-13554
International Standard Book Number 0-8089-1086-8
Printed in the United States of America

Dedicated to the memory of our
patients and friends

Barry Ashbee, beloved player and coach of the Philadelphia Flyers Hockey Club, who at age 37, in the prime of his life, died of leukemia. "It took an incurable blood disorder to quell a spirit that the loss of sight in one eye, a spinal fusion, torn ligaments in his knee, and a pinched nerve in his neck could not dampen."—Bob Clarke, Captain, Philadelphia Flyers

Valerie Reale, whose greatest dream was to help medical science conquer leukemia. With determination and hope she endured the first bone-marrow transplantation in Philadelphia, at Hahnemann Medical College and Hospital, but died eight months later at the age of 19.

Their unconquerable courage taught us the true values in life.

CONTENTS

III. Bone Marrow Physiology and Supportive Care

IV. Hematologic Neoplasms

Acknowledgment

We wish to thank Mr. Robert Schaefer, Ms. Edith Schwager, Mrs. Barbara Rubin, Mrs. Donna West, Miss Melanie Hughes, Ms. Jane Krumrine, Mrs. Leslie Costello, Mrs. Hilda Navarro, Evelyn Ross, and Mrs. Fay Zelle who helped so much in the preparation of this symposium and this volume.

Grants from the U.S. Public Health Service and Adria Laboratories contributed to the financial support of this symposium, and we gratefully acknowledge their assistance.

Once again we extend our heartfelt thanks and appreciation to the authors and to others who participated in the program. We hope this book will give you, the reader, as much help and enjoyment as these people have given us.

THE EDITORS

Preface

During the five years since the publication of the second volume of *Cancer Chemotherapy,* both our methods of treatment and our philosophy of managing the patient with cancer have changed. In 1972 many clinicians considered cancer chemotherapy generally useful only for patients with hematologic neoplasms or with widely metastatic disease. Except for women with choriocarcinoma, the patient with a solid tumor was not considered a candidate for chemotherapy at initial diagnosis.

The multidisciplinary approach to decision-making for patients with cancer virtually excluded the newly recognized subspecialist, the medical oncologist, and the value of cancer chemotherapy was often questioned. The concept that cancer is a systemic disease was not accepted by many because it was widely believed that if the tumor could not be locally excised or eradicated, there was little hope for a cure with drugs.

Many of these pessimistic views have changed in the last five years, and so have our approaches to the patient with cancer. Medical oncology is a rapidly expanding medical subspecialty. Occasionally, if the physician does not offer drug treatment for cancer, the patient will demand it. The success of the adjuvant programs provided further evidence for the systemic nature of most cancers, even though staging studies suggested that many tumors were localized or, at worst, had spread to circumscribed regions. In many institutions the surgeon, the radiotherapist, and the medical oncologist are now recognized as the team that must make the decision regarding treatment when the disease is first recognized. Oncologists acknowledge that an understanding of tumor cell kinetics and tumor biology is important in designing and applying cancer chemotherapy programs.

Though this symposium is directed primarily toward the specialist in medicine, surgery, radiology, gynecology, or pediatrics, it will also serve as an update and overview for the subspecialist in oncology. Physicians who deal with cancer patients will find the goals and limitations of therapy outlined. Because of the rapidly changing nature of the field, most of the contributors to this book have not written cookbook formulae for managing any particular disease, although they have described proven programs. Our methods in his volume have been somewhat altered because our philosophical approach to patients with neoplasms has changed. We have asked the participants to outline the state of the art in terms of management rather than restricting their analyses to chemotherapy alone.

The chapters are grouped into four areas: The first covers the mechanisms of action of chemotherapeutic agents in detail. This section also includes chapters on immunotherapy and anticoagulation as it relates to therapy and one chapter dealing with tumor cell kinetics and tumor biology that stresses those concepts that relate to chemotherapy and to adjuvant programs.

The clinical management of various solid tumors is presented in the second section. The issues stressed are those that are important in making therapeutic decisions not only from the viewpoint of chemotherapy but also from the perspectives of the surgeon and radiotherapist. The main emphasis, however, is on chemotherapy. A significant change in this section is the emphasis placed in many of the chapters on adjuvant chemotherapy; chapters on bone tumors and breast cancer emphasize this concept particularly well.

Because hematology and medical oncology are so closely related, in the third section, we continue our precedent of including material on bone marrow function and the supportive care of patients undergoing cancer therapy. We also include a chapter on marrow transplantation and expand the chapters on transfusion, especially the new methods of white-cell transfusion.

Lastly, the section on hematologic neoplasms has been updated and expanded. Included in this section are chapters on mycosis fungoides and related disease, the value of cytogenetics in diagnosis and follow-up, and more recent research dealing with the relation of viruses to hematologic neoplasia.

We have not included a section on regional chemotherapeutic techniques. These areas were reviewed in *Cancer Chemotherapy II*, and the methods, goals, and limitations have not changed appreciably in the last five years. We refer readers who desire an overview to that volume.

In the preface to *Cancer Chemotherapy II*, we pointed out deficiencies in the chemotherapeutic management of such common neoplasms as those of the lung, breast, colon, and cervix. We emphasized the success of chemotherapy in hematologic neoplasia. Today it is evident that adjuvant programs have increased the survival of patients with breast cancer and osteogenic sarcoma and that various combinations of cancer chemotherapy have achieved good responses in patients with metastatic oat-cell carcinoma. Recent evidence suggests that certain patients with diffuse histiocytic lymphoma ("reticulum cell sarcoma") may be cured with multidrug chemotherapy; but even if long-term cure is not assured, these patients certainly enjoy longer disease-free survival. In the next edition we hope to report the long-term control of such diseases as colon cancer and squamous-cell carcinoma of the lung.

We continue to stress that cancer is not a single disease and that no therapeutic program should be considered standardized or immutable for individual patients until such time as all patients with that tumor are cured. The most favorable outcome of cancer research would be the prevention of cancer; then there would be no need for treatises on drug therapy. This goal, however, may not be as easy to achieve as the development of effective cancer chemotherapeutic agents.

THE EDITORS

Contributors

NEIL ABRAMSON, M.D.
University of Florida at Jacksonville, and Baptist Medical Center, Jacksonville, FL

CLARA M. AMBRUS, M.D., PH.D.
The Roswell Park Memorial Institute, State of New York Department of Health, and Departments of Pediatrics and Pharmacology, State University of New York at Buffalo, Buffalo, NY

JULIAN L. AMBRUS, M.D., PH.D.
The Roswell Park Memorial Institute, State of New York Department of Health, and Departments of Internal Medicine and Experimental Pathology, State University of New York at Buffalo, Buffalo, NY

ROBERT E. BELLET, M.D., F.A.C.P.
Clinical Assistant Professor of Medicine, Temple University School of Medicine, and Research Physician, Melanoma Unit, Fox Chase Cancer Center, Philadelphia, PA

JOHN M. BENNETT, M.D.
Professor of Oncology in Medicine, Division of Clinical Services, University of Rochester Cancer Center, and Medical Oncology Unit, Department of Medicine, University of Rochester School of Medicine and Dentistry, Rochester, NY

DAVID BERD, M.D.
Clinical Instructor of Medicine, University of Pennsylvania School of Medicine, and Research Physician, Melanoma Unit, Fox Chase Cancer Center, Philadelphia, PA

DANE R. BOGGS, M.D.
Department of Medicine, University of Pittsburgh School of Medicine, Pittsburgh, PA

L. E. BOYLE, M.D.
Assistant Internist, Instructor in Medicine, Department of Medicine, Section of General Medicine and Clinical Oncology, The University of Texas System Cancer Center, M.D. Anderson Hospital and Tumor Institute, Houston, TX

LUTHER W. BRADY, M.D.
American Cancer Society Professor of Clinical Oncology, Hahnemann Medical College and Hospital, Philadelphia, PA

ADA BROOKS, M.D.
Clinical Pharmacology Branch National Cancer Institute, Bethesda, MD

C. DEAN BUCKNER, M.D.
Associate Professor of Medicine, University of Washington School of Medicine, and Associate Member, Division of Oncology, The Seattle Marrow Transplant Team, Fred Hutchinson Cancer Research Center, Seattle, WA

STEPHEN I. BULOVA, M.D.
Associate Professor, Department of Hematology and Medical Oncology, Director, Blood Bank, Hahnemann Medical College and Hospital, Philadelphia, PA

ELAINE M. BUNICK, M.D.
Division of Endocrinology and Metabolism, Department of Medicine, Hahnemann Medical College and Hospital, Philadelphia, PA

JOSEPH HOLLAND BURCHENAL, M.D.
Professor of Medicine, Cornell University Medical College, and Attending Physician, Memorial Sloan-Kettering Cancer Center, New York, NY

BRUCE CHABNER, M.D.
Clinical Pharmacology Branch, National Cancer Institute, Bethesda, MD

MARTIN H. COHEN, M.D.
NCI-VA Medical Oncology, Verterans Administration Hospital, Washington, D.C.

GERALD W. CRABTREE, PH.D.
Associate Professor of Biochemical Pharmacology (Research), Division of Biology and Medicine, Brown University, Providence, RI

WILLIAM A. CREASEY, PH.D.
Professor of Pharmacology and Pediatrics, University of Pennsylvania School of Medicine (Oncology), Children's Hospital of Philadelphia, Philadelphia, PA

MILTON H. DONALDSON, M.D.
Vice President for Cancer Control, Training and Education, The Fox Chase Cancer Center, and Associate Medical Director, American Oncologic Hospital, and Associate Professor of Pediatrics, University of Pennsylvania, and Associate Oncologist and Senior Physician, Children's Hospital of Philadelphia, Philadelphia, PA

BARRY J. ERLICK, PH.D.
Assistant Professor of Medical Oncology-Hematology and Biochemistry, Herbert L. Orlowitz Institute for Cancer and Blood Diseases, Hahnemann Medical College and Hospital, Philadelphia, PA

ALLAN J. ERSLEV, M.D.
Cardeza Research Professor of Medicine, Director, Cardeza Foundation, Thomas Jefferson University, Philadelphia, PA

H. HUGH FUDENBERG, M.D.
Department of Basic and Clinical Immunology and Microbiology, Medical University of South Carolina, Charleston, SC

ANTHONY A. FUSCALDO, PH.D.
Herbert L. Orlowitz Institute for Cancer and Blood Diseases, Hahnemann Medical College and Hospital, Philadelphia, PA

KATHRYN E. FUSCALDO, PH.D.
Professor, Department of Medical Oncology and Hematology, Herbert L. Orlowitz Institute for Cancer and Blood Diseases, Hahnemann Medical College and Hospital, Philadelphia, PA

DOV GORSHEIN, M.D.
Professor of Medicine, Director, Hematology and Oncology, Wright State University School of Medicine, and Associate Chief of Staff for Research and Development, Veterans Administration Center, Dayton, OH

EZRA M. GREENSPAN, M.D., F.A.C.P.
Clinical Professor of Medicine and Oncology, Mount Sinai School of Medicine, New York, NY

LINDA A. HAEGELE, M.D.
Instructor in Medical Oncology and Hematology, Herbert L. Orlowitz Institute for Cancer and Blood Diseases, Hahnemann Medical College and Hospital, Philadelphia, PA

PAUL Y. HOLOYE, M.D.
Assistant Internist and Professor of Medicine, Department of Medicine, Section of General Medicine and Clinical Oncology, The University of Texas System

Cancer Center, M.D. Anderson Hospital and Tumor Institute, Houston, TX

CHARLES M. HUGULEY, JR., M.D.
Professor of Medicine, Director, Emory University Cancer Center, Director, Division of Hematology and Oncology, Emory University School of Medicine, Atlanta, GA

NORMAN JAFFE, M.B., B.CH., DIP, PAED
Sidney Farber Cancer Institute, Children's Hospital Medical Center, and Harvard Medical School, Boston, MA

DOUGLAS E. JOHNSON, M.D.
Professor of Surgery, Chief, Section of Urology, The University of Texas System Cancer Center, M.D. Anderson Hospital and Tumor Institute, Houston, TX

ROBERT A. JOYCE, M.D.
Department of Medicine, University of Pittsburgh School of Medicine, Pittsburgh, PA

MORTIMER J. LACHER, M.D., F.A.C.P.
Associate Attending Physician, Memorial Hospital, and Clinician, Sloan-Kettering Institute, and Clinical Associate Professor of Medicine, Cornell University College of Medicine, New York, NY

VICTOR J. LANZOTTI, M.D.
Assistant Internist and Professor of Medicine, Department of Medicine, Section of General Medicine and Clinical Oncology, The University of Texas System Cancer Center, M.D. Anderson Hospital and Tumor Institute, Houston, TX

JACK LEVIN, M.D.
Professor of Medicine, Hematology Division, The Johns Hopkins University School of Medicine and Hospital, Baltimore, MD

DAVID B. LUDLUM, PH.D., M.D.
Professor and Chairman, Department of Pharmacology and Experimental Therapeutics, Albany Medical College, Albany, NY

EDWARD LUSTBADER, PH.D.
Biostatistician, The Institute for Cancer Research, Fox Chase Cancer Center, Philadelphia, PA

MICHAEL J. MASTRANGELO, M.D., F.A.C.P.
Clinical Associate Professor of Medicine, Temple University School of Medicine, and Research Physician, Melanoma Unit, Fox Chase Cancer Center, Philadelphia, PA

BENEDICTA MENESES, M.D.
Instructor in Medicine, Georgetown University School of Medicine, and Assistant Chief, Oncology Service, D.C. General Hospital, Washington, D.C.

FRANCO M. MUGGIA, M.D.
National Cancer Institute, Division of Cancer Treatment, Bethesda, MD

GERALD P. MURPHY, M.D., D.SC.
Director, Roswell Park Memorial Institute, Buffalo, NY

CHARLES MYERS, M.D.
Clinical Pharmacology Branch, National Cancer Institute, Bethesda, MD

DONALD PINKEL, M.D.
Professor, Department of Pediatrics, The Medical College of Wisconsin, and Director, The Midwest Children's Cancer Center, Milwaukee Children's Hospital, Milwaukee, WI

VICTORIO RODRIGUEZ, M.D.
Department of Developmental Therapeutics, The University of Texas System Cancer Center,

M.D. Anderson Hospital and Tumor Institute, Houston, TX, Southwest Oncology Associates, P.A., San Antonio, TX

LESLIE I. ROSE, M.D.
Division of Endocrinology and Metabolism, Department of Medicine, Hahnemann Medical College and Hospital, Philadelphia, PA

JEFFREY G. ROSENSTOCK, M.D.
Assistant Professor of Pediatrics, Hahnemann Medical College and Hospital, Philadelphia, PA

MARCEL ROZENCWEIG, M.D.
National Cancer Institute, Division of Cancer Treatment, Bethesda, MD

MELVIN L. SAMUELS, M.D.
Professor of Medicine, Chief, Section of General Medicine and Clinical Oncology, Department of Medicine, The University of Texas System Cancer Center, M.D. Anderson Hospital and Tumor Institute, Houston, TX

ALLAN J. SCHUTT, M.D.
Associate Professor of Medicine, Mayo Medical School, Consultant in Gastrointestinal Oncology, Mayo Clinic Department of Medical Oncology, Rochester, MN

THOMAS V. SEDLACEK, M.D.
Professor and Chairman, Director, Gynecologic Oncology, Department of Obstetrics and Gynecology, Hahnemann Medical College and Hospital, Philadelphia, PA

BRUCE I. SHNIDER, M.D.
Professor of Medicine, Director, Division of Medical Oncology, Department of Medicine, Georgetown University School of Medicine, and Chief, Oncology Service, D.C. General Hospital, Washington, D.C.

JOSEPH E. SOKAL, M.D.
Chief Cancer Research Clinician, Roswell Park Memorial Institute, and Research Professor of Medicine, State University of New York at Buffalo, Buffalo, NY

DAVID J. STRAUS, M.D.
Assistant Professor, Department of Medicine, Cornell University Medical College, and Assistant Attending Physician, Memorial Sloan-Kettering Cancer Center, New York, NY

GABRIEL VIRELLA, M.D., PH.D.
Department of Basic and Clinical Immunology and Microbiology, Medical University of South Carolina, Charleston, SC

ERIC C. VONDERHEID, M.D.
Associate professor of Dermatology, Skin and Cancer Hospital, Temple University Health Sciences Center, Philadelphia, PA

DANIEL D. VON HOFF, M.D.
National Cancer Institute, Division of Cancer Treatment, Bethesda, MD

PAUL E. WALLNER, D.O.
Associate Professor, Department of Radiation Therapy and Nuclear Medicine, Hahnemann Medical College and Hospital, Philadelphia, PA

Part I

The Pharmacology of Chemotherapeutic Drugs

Sigmund Benham Kahn

1

Tumor Biology and Its Implications for Cancer Chemotherapy

Cancer statistics for 1977 indicate that of the 690,000 new cancer patients diagnosed, 350,000 will be cured.[1] Because even ideally administered local therapy is curative in less than half of all patients with cancer, the only logical hope for increasing the patient salvage rate is some form of systemic chemotherapy.

While it is recognized that many of the drugs and their congeners described in the chapters of this text are not curative and will be replaced by newer agents in the future, the decision-making processes underlying the timing and selection of chemotherapy are fairly well defined and will remain constant even when current drug information is long outdated.

Most of the knowledge upon which these decisions are based rests upon an understanding of the biology of tumor. The purpose of this paper is to demonstrate that an understanding of cancer biology may be as important in reaching therapeutic decisions about chemotherapy as is the selection and development of new agents. The clinician should understand why adherence to dosage scheduling is important in any drug program, why debulking is necessary, and when therapy should be discontinued and then restarted. It is assumed that the type of agent chosen, the route of administration, the dosage of the agent and the various host factors such as nutrition and immune status are well-recognized variables influencing chemotherapy, and these issues will not be discussed in detail.

Supported by Hahnemann Cancer Center Program in Clinical Education, Grant number CA17963-03, National Institutes of Health.

Composition of Tumor

Malignant neoplasms are composed of cells that have been transformed. Malignant transformation imparts to a cell the ability to proliferate in an unregulated fashion and the capacity to invade and metastasize.[2] On the molecular level cancer cells have altered cell membranes,[3] increased levels of some enzymes,[4] increased transcriptional activity,[5] altered chromatin,[5] unstable and abnormal chromosomal patterns[6] and a variety of other processes. The mechanisms underlying neoplastic transformation are not germane to this chapter, although these mechanisms, once unraveled, will ultimately yield a cure. What is important and not recognized by physicians is that the cells of solid tumors and hematologic neoplasms are not uniform in composition or activity.[7] For example, it has been assumed that most cancers grow faster than their tissues of origin, that almost all tumor cells are growing and that very few tumor cells die a natural death. Not only are these concepts incorrect but the truth lies in the opposite direction.

There are three cellular compartments in any malignant neoplasm[8] (Fig. 1-1): (1) cells that are undergoing division and are said to be in the cell cycle; (2) cells that are capable of entering the cell cycle but that are not doing so—these cells are called resting or G_0 cells; (3) end-stage cells that have left the cell cycle never to return—these cells are destined to die a natural death.

Only cells in G_0 or in the cell cycle are capable of living forever. The only mechanism of immortality these cells have is to divide and start life anew. The number of cells in any single compartment shown in Figure 1-1 varies from tumor nodule to tumor nodule in a single patient and from patient to patient given any single kind of cancer. The proportion of the tumor that is in cell cycle is called the growth fraction (G_F). The G_F is the chief mechanism by which a tumor increases in size.[9] Growth fractions may be quite low in any malignant neoplasm. Cells of a neoplasm may increase in number by two other mechanisms; shortening the time in cycle or decreasing cell loss. Tumors may not be able to shorten the cell cycle time (indeed cycle times may be longer than normal),[5] and cells that die a natural death in any tumor nodule often exceed 50 per cent of tumor bulk.[10] In summary, malignant neoplasms are often slower growing than normal, have a large number of cells that are destined to die a natural death and have rather low growth fractions. It is the recognition of these facts that underlies therapeutic decisions of drug selection and timing in cancer chemotherapy.

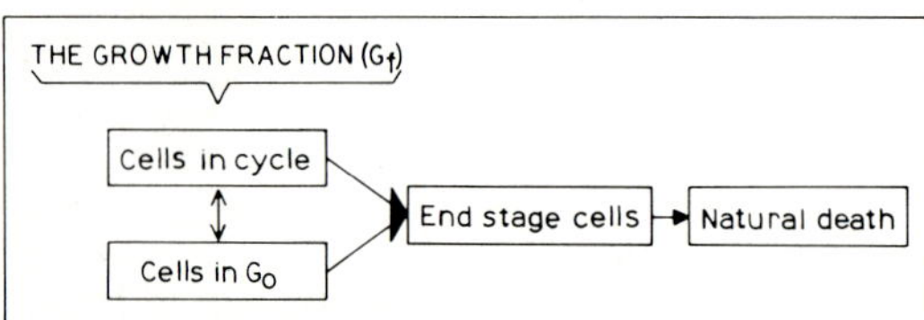

FIG. 1-1. The cellular compartments of a neoplasm (G_f = growth fraction; G_0—cells not in cycle but capable of entering the cycle given the appropriate stimulus.)

The Cell Cycle

Because almost all cancer chemotherapeutic drugs inhibit cellular division, an understanding of the cell cycle is imperative. Every cell that undergoes division, be it a normal cell or a cancer cell, must pass through the cell cycle. The cell cycle has been defined as the interval between the midpoint of mitosis in a cell and the midpoint of a subsequent mitosis in one or both daughter cells.[8] There is an orderly sequence of events that occurs between these points, and four phases have been demarcated (Fig. 1-2). The *S*-phase deals with the synthesis of nucleic acid, while the *M*-phase signifies the process of mitosis. The G_1 and G_2 phases (*G* stands for gap) are associated with metabolic activity, but the processes are less obvious morphologically than biochemically. The interface between S and G_1 or G_2 is called the S/G_1 or S/G_2 boundary. G_0 cells are capable of entering the cycle but at that moment are not in cycle. (For a complete review of all phases see ref. 5.)

In Figure 1-3, one can note the relationship of these concepts to the selection of the type and timing of cancer chemotherapy. For purposes of this discussion the cancer cells noted in Figure 1-3 are leukemic blasts as compared to normal hematopoietic tissue.[11]

A particular drug that exerts its effects on cancer cells no matter whether the cells are in G_0 or are in the cell cycle is called a noncycle-active drug, and it yields cell-killing curves shown in Figure 1-3A. In this figure cyclophosphamide, an alkylating agent, is

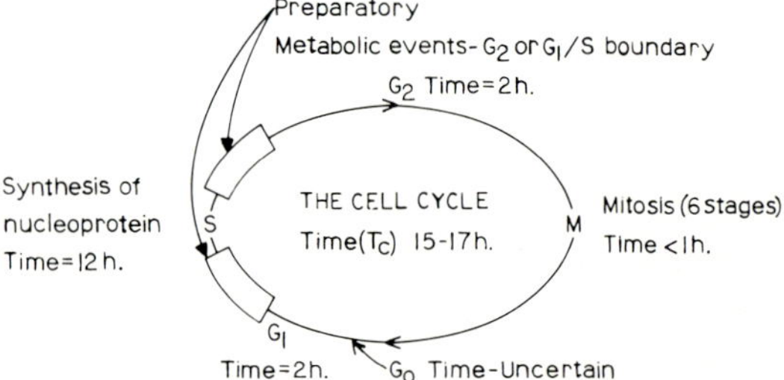

FIG. 1-2. The cell cycle (the steps required for cellular division) S = synthesis of nucleoprotein; M—mitosis; G_0—resting cells capable of entering cycle but not doing so; G_1 and G_2—intervals between S and M during which time various preparatory events occur. The times given vary from neoplasm to neoplasm and are not exact, but are relatively correct.

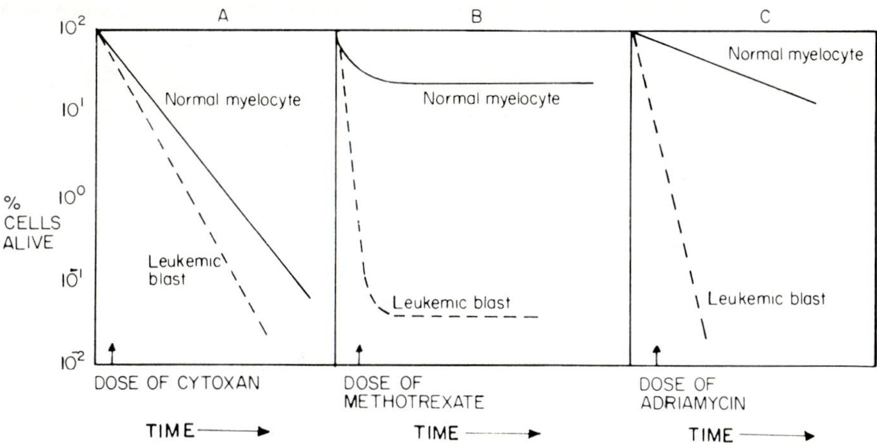

FIG. 1-3. Cell kills of cells of a neoplasm versus cell kills of normal hematopoietic tissues following administration of a non-cycle-active (A); phase-specific (B); cycle-active (C) agent.

given as an example of a non-cycle-active drug. A second class of drugs exerts an effect on cells only when the cells are in a particular phase of the cell cycle. Such drugs are called phase-specific agents. Their cell-killing curves are depicted in Figure 1-3B. Methotrexate (MTX), an antimetabolite that inhibits nucleic acid synthesis by interfering with folate metabolism, is an example of a phase-specific drug. The third class of chemotherapeutic agents is called cycle-specific. These drugs exert their lethal effects only when cells are in cycle and yield curves depicted in Figure 1-3C. An example of this type of agent is adriamycin, an antitumor antibiotic, which inhibits dividing cells at several points in the cell cycle.

The reader should note carefully that in these illustrations the same degree of cancer cell death is associated with different degrees of normal cell death. The greater the cancer cell kill is for a given degree of toxicity, the higher is the therapeutic index. The ultimate basis of the therapeutic index herein described is the fact that normal bone marrow cells are highly regulated and have limited and well-defined growth fractions. Cancer cells are unregulated and have different growth fractions, and the various cellular compartments fail to interact properly. Thus, cell kill may be increased, provided the timing of treatment allows normal cells to recover.

Table 1-1 gives a classification of antitumor drugs based upon these mechanisms of action. Knowledge of the mechanism of action enables the physician to modify dosage scheduling to maximize total cell kill and minimize patient toxicity. For example, a non-cycle-specific agent has no differential toxicity against cancer cells (Fig. 1-3A), and it is the total dosage of this type of drug that predicts the toxic level. On the other hand, phase-specific and cycle-specific agents may be more or less toxic to tumor cells (Fig. 1-3B and 1-3C) when compared to normal cells depending upon the growth fraction, but increasing the dosage of the drug does not lead to increased toxicity to normal tissue. Indeed, higher dosages may increase tumor cell kill if the basis of tumor resistance is failure of the drug to penetrate the cancer cell. The mechanisms of action of particular drugs are outlined in subsequent chapters and also in reference 12.

The most appropriate method of increasing tumor cell kill while decreasing toxicity to normal tissues would be to induce the tumor cells to enter the cell cycle while at the same time inducing normal cells to remain out of cycle. Once all the tumor cells are in cycle, a phase- or cycle-specific agent might yield cure without appreciable toxicity to normal tissues. Unfortunately, there are no mechanisms which will induce all of the viable cells of a tumor to enter the cycle. Figure 1-4 indicates, however, that the smaller the cell number in any tumor nodule, the faster the

TABLE 1-1. *Functional Classification of Some Cancer Chemotherapeutic Drugs*

Group	Type	Dosage Limitation Depends upon	Some Common Examples	Area(s) of Cycle Affected
Alkylating agent	Non-cycle-specific	Total dosage administered	Nitrogen mustard Cyclophosphamide Chlorambucil	G_0, M, G_1
Antimetabolite	Phase-specific	Timing of dosage	Methotrexate 5-FU 6-MP Cytosine arabinoside	S, or (G_1/S boundary)
Antibiotic	Cycle-specific	Timing and to lesser extent total dosage	Actinomycin Adriamycin Bleomycin Daunorubicin Mitomycin	G_2, M (some G_1)
Steroid	Non-cycle-specific (but uncertain)	?	Prednisone Estrogens Androgens Progesterone	Uncertain
Plant Alkaloids	Phase-specific	Timing of dosage	Vincristine Vinblastine	M or M/G_1
Miscellaneous	Cycle-specific and non-cycle-specific	Timing or total dosage	DTIC Procarbazine Hydroxyurea L-asparaginase CCNU	S, G_1

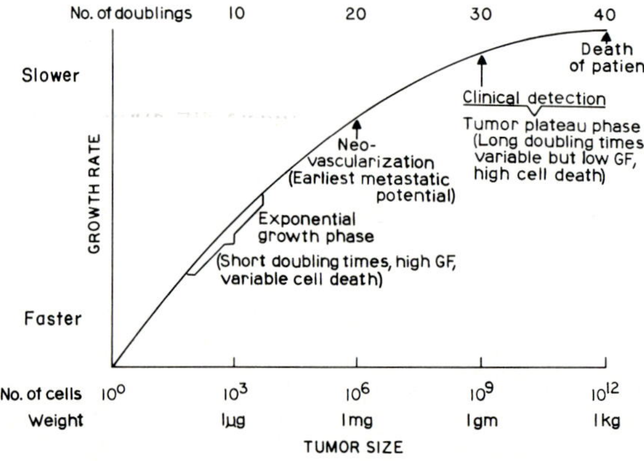

FIG. 1-4 Relationship of growth rate, number of doublings, cell number and tumor size (weight).

growth rate.[13] Since tumor growth rate depends upon growth fraction, it is obvious that smaller tumors are more likely to be sensitive to the effects of cancer chemotherapy than are larger tumors. Hence, increasing the therapeutic index of cancer chemotherapy involves reducing tumor bulk or tumor burden to as low a level as possible before some form of cancer chemotherapy is given. This principle underlies the concept of adjuvant chemotherapy.

Another method of increasing the therapeutic index of cancer chemotherapy is to synchronize tumor cells so that they are in one phase of the cycle while at the same time normal cells are in another phase. It is recognized that certain tumor cells have longer G_1 or G_2 phases than their cells of origin.[5] For example (Fig. 1-5), a leukemic blast cell may have a G_2 phase that is 4 hours longer than a normal myeloblast. If one administered an agent such as vincristine, both normal and tumor cells would be arrested in mitosis. At the end of the inhibitory effect of the vincristine, both cells complete the cell cycle. Normal cells will complete G_2 4 hours before their tumor counterparts. In Figure 1-5, MTX was administered 15 hours after vincristine. At this time normal tissue had completed the S-phase and was resistant to the growth-inhibiting effects of MTX, while the tumor tissue was in the midst of the S-phase and was highly susceptible to the effects of the drug. These concepts underlie the design of many protocols. Much of the evidence upon which these decisions are made, however, is based upon in vitro studies of transplanted animal tumors. The data may not always be applicable to individual patients with one particular form of cancer or another.

Doubling Times and Cell Turnover

One of the most important aspects of therapeutic decision making in cancer chemotherapy rests upon an understanding of the concepts of doubling time and cell turnover in malignant tumors. Doubling time is the net time it takes for a tumor to double its cell number.[13] Given a tumor consisting of 100 cells, for example, the doubling time would be the time that it would take the tumor to become 200 cells. It is important to distinguish between the cell cycle time and the doubling time. The cell cycle time (T_c) is the time it takes the cell to go through the cell cycle. Many normal and neoplastic tissues have in vitro cycle times that vary between 15 and 72 hours. (In Fig. 1-1, an in vitro T_c of 17 hours is presented.) With a growth fraction of 100 per cent the cell cycle time and doubling time are identical. Information based upon in vitro and in vivo studies of normal and cancer cells, however, yields mathematically derived data tabulated in Table 1-2. In this table the doubling time, the T_c and the growth fraction have been derived from experimental and clinical observations, and several combinations have been mathematically analyzed. Cell birth rate (arbitrarily given as 100 cells) and cell death rate have been derived by mathematics. These data show that most tumors, either with high or low growth fractions and doubling times varying between 1 and 13 weeks, have an appreciable natural cell death. These tumors, therefore, are slow-growing and are not likely to be eradicated by phase- or cycle-specific agents. Normal tissues such as the bone marrow or GI tract have high growth fractions, short cell cycle times and short doubling times. While normal tissues may be exquisitely sensitive to phase- or cycle-specific cancer chemotherapy, they have little natural cell death, and their rapid growth potential means rapid recovery of cell number following treatment with cytotoxic drugs.

Doubling times for many solid tumors are measured in terms of months rather than days.[13] It is not unusual to note clinically measured doubling times of 90 days in certain solid tumors. Doubling times of leukemic blasts are about 4 days.[11] The doubling time of a myelocyte of the bone marrow is about 60 hours.[14] The rather long doubling times of malignant neoplasms, a reflection of little understood internal metabolic processes, would suggest that large tumors are often in a stationary or slowly increasing growth phase, whereas normal tissues are often in an exponential growth phase. The relationship between cell number and growth rate is depicted in Figure 1-4.

The data in Figure 1-4 also demonstrate several other diagnostic and therapeutic prob-

TABLE 1-2. *Relationship of Birth and Death of Cells in Tumors with Various Growth Rates**

Doubling (Days)	Time (Wks)	T_c (Hours)	Growth Fraction (G_f) %	Cells Born #	Cells that Die/100 Born #
I Tumors with short T_c and high G_f					
7	(1)	30	50	100	76
14	(2)	30	50	100	89
21	(3)	30	50	100	93
28	(4)	30	50	100	95
56	(8)	30	50	100	97
90	(13)	30	50	100	98
II. Tumors with short T_c and low G_f					
7	(1)	30	10	not mathematically possible	
14	(2)	30	10	100	36
21	(3)	30	10	100	58
28	(4)	30	10	100	69
56	(8)	30	10	100	84
90	(13)	30	10	100	90
III. Tumors with long T_c and high G_f					
7	(1)	60	50	100	48
14	(2)	60	50	100	76
21	(3)	60	50	100	85
28	(4)	60	50	100	89
56	(8)	60	50	100	95
90	(13)	60	50	100	97
IV. Tumors with long T_c and low G_f					
7	(1)	60	10	not mathematically possible	
14	(2)	60	10	not mathematically possible	
21	(3)	60	10	100	14
28	(4)	60	10	100	36
56	(8)	60	10	100	69
90	(13)	60	10	100	81

(The author wishes to express his appreciation to Mr. Edward Pequignot, data process manager and statistician, Hahnemann Cancer Institute.)

*The data here derived from the formula:
$A = P(1 + i)^n$ where P is the number of cells to begin with, i is the rate (birth or death), n is the number of periods of cycles, and A is the final number of cells produced or dying.

lems posed by the cancer patient. Most cancers are not detected until a tumor burden of 1 g or 10^9 cells is reached. If there were no cell death, a single cell would be obligated to divide 30 times to reach 10^9 cells. (Because of cell death, tumor cells have to divide more than 30 times to reach a tumor burden of 10^9 cells.) Death of the patient usually occurs when 10^{12} cells or a 1000 g tumor burden is reached. This takes only another 10 doublings. Vascularization refers to the phenomenon whereby a tumor induces the formation of its own blood supply. This occurs at about the twentieth doubling. At this point tumor weight is 1 mg. The potential for metastasis may occur at about this time. Note well that hardly any patient with a tumor burden of 10^6 cells (weight of tumor—1 mg.) would have symptoms or signs of malignant neoplasm. Finally, as noted before, the smaller the num-

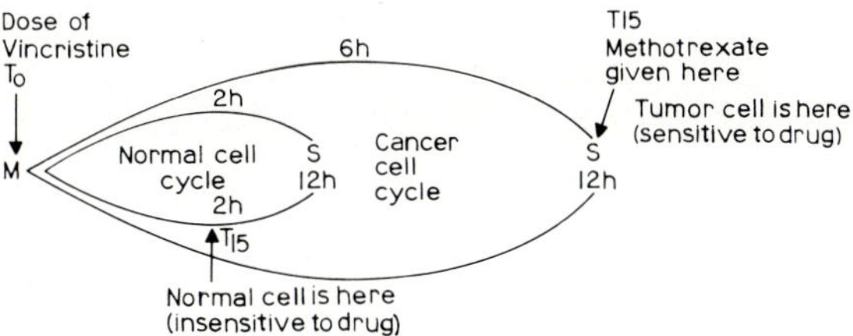

FIG. 1-5 A relative comparison of the normal cell cycle and the cell cycle of a cancer cell. Note that the G phases (see Fig. 2 for definition) are longer for the cancer cells than for normal, allowing for differential cytotoxicity of chemotherapy against normal and cancer cells.

ber of cells in the tumor nodule, the faster the rate of growth. (In Figure 1-4, growth rate decreases as tumor burden increases.)

Chemotherapy, to be curative, must reduce the tumor burden to zero or to such low levels that the body's own defenses can eradicate the remaining cells. Based upon the data in Figure 1-4, debulking by chemotherapy the patient who has a large tumor burden would probably demand a non-cycle-active agent in fairly high dosage. The toxicity of non-cycle-active agents is totally dosage dependent.[15] Continuous administration will, therefore, eventually lead to toxicity. Because very small tumor nodules have high growth fractions, phase- or cycle-specific agents would be the more logical choices in the maintenance or adjuvant chemotherapy programs. For practical purposes surgery or X-ray therapy (being local modalities of therapy) are used to debulk the primary tumor, and the adjuvant chemotherapy programs often utilize low doses of non-cycle-active drugs (to avoid cumulative toxicity) and moderate doses of phase- or cycle-specific agents. The non-cycle-active agents "debulk" the neoplastic nodules inducing a proliferative response which makes the cells sensitive to cycle-active drugs.

Following completion of chemotherapy, recovery rates of most cancer cells are somewhat slower than normal cells.[14] Thus, administration of cycle- or phase-specific agents

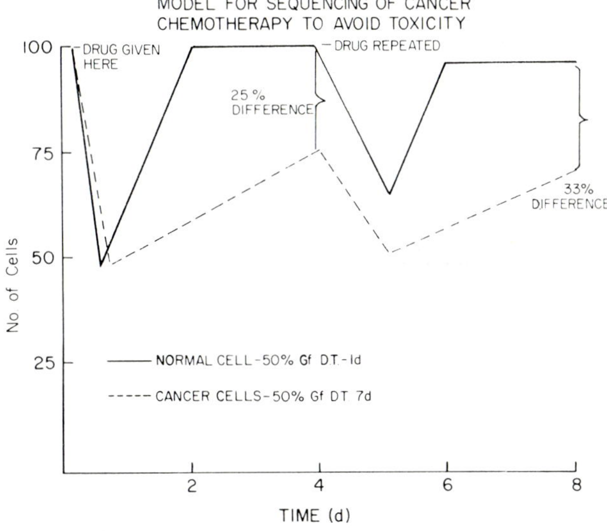

FIG. 1-6. Model illustrating differential cell reduction of normal versus 100 cancer cells based upon more rapid recovery of normal cells versus cancer cells.

over a period not to exceed two cell cycles of marrow or GI tissues (the dosage-limiting organs) will not given rise to much toxicity, while at the same time will yield maximum cancer cell kill.[8] For example, Figure 1-6 illustrates a patient with a low tumor burden of 100 cancer cells. In this figure the normal cells are 100 stem cells in the bone marrow. For the sake of discussion let us assume that the doubling time of the normal cell is 24 hours[14] and that the doubling time of the tumor is 7 days while the growth fraction of both normal and cancer cells is 50 per cent. If one delivered a dose of an anticancer drug by intravenous infusion over a 24 hour period, during that time period no normal cells and no cancer cells would grow. At the conclusion of treatment, 50 normal cells and 50 cancer cells would remain. When the effects of the chemotherapy have worn off, the normal and the tumor cells begin to grow. Because the normal cell doubling time is only one day, within a day or so almost all of the normal cells have reconstituted themselves. Because the doubling time of the cancer cells is 7 days, however, in a few days no more than 25 to 30 per cent of the cancer cells have regrown. If on the fourth day one repeated the injection of the drug, the second cycle of chemotherapy would begin with 100 normal cells but with only 75 cancer cells. This example shows that one has developed differential cell kill based, not so much upon differences in anticancer specificity of chemotherapy, but rather on the differences in the rate of recovery of normal tissues. These considerations underlie the maintenance programs so prevalent in the treatment of acute leukemia and Hodgkin's disease, and the adjuvant programs that follow the primary resection of breast or colon cancer.

Cancer Chemotherapeutic Drugs—Classification and Toxicity

Rather than commit to memory a long list of old and new cancer chemotherapeutic drugs, Table 1-1 classifies the drugs according to their mechanism of action in the cell cycle.[8]

Table 1-3 *Dosage Limitation and Toxicity of Cancer Chemotherapy*

Drug	Dosage Limited by	Other Effects (Not Uniformly Dosage Limiting)	Usual Schedule	Monitoring Tests
A. Alkylating agents				
Examples:				
Cyclophosphamide Nitrogen mustard Chlorambucil	Marrow function	Nausea, alopecia	Intermittent q 3-4 w (cont. low dose in selected instances)	Blood count Record of total dosage
B. Antimetabolites				
Examples:				
Methotrexate 5-FU Cytosine arabinoside 6-MP	Marrow function GI ulceration	Nausea Hepatic toxicity	Intermittent q 4-7 d	Record time frequency— Hepatic function

TABLE 1-3 (continued)

Drug	Dosage Limited by	Other Effects (Not Uniformly Dosage Limiting)	Usual Schedule	Monitoring Tests
C. Antibiotics				
Examples: Doxorubicin Bleomycin Actinomycin Mitomycin	Marrow function Cardiac & pulmonary impairment	Nausea Radiation sensitization Alopecia Slough if infiltrates (must be given I.V.)	Intermittent q 3-4 w usually	Record total dosage—(Doxorubicin & Bleomycin) EKG & chest X-ray Blood count
D. Plant alkaloids				
Examples: Vincristine Vinblastine	Neuropathy	Leukopenia (mild) Alopecia Slough if infiltrates (must be given I.V.) Constipation	Intermittent	Neurologic evaluation
E. Steroids				
Examples: Prednisone Conj. estrogens Testosterone Anabolic agents	Diabetes Fluid retention & hypertension	Acne Hirsuitism Vag. bleeding Hyperuricemia Liver dysfunction	Daily or intermittent	B.P. Blood sugar Electrolytes
F. Miscellaneous				
a. DTIC	a. ———	a. Nausea must be given I.V.	Intermittent	a. ———
b. Procarbazine	b. Marrow function (virtually limited to Hodgkin's disease)	b. Nausea Rash	Intermittent	b. Blood count
c. CCNU	c. Marrow function	c. Nausea	q 4-6 w	c. Blood count

Unless agents that will kill cancer cells independent of the cell cycle are developed, this table will remain valid and applicable to agents that will be developed in the future. All that need be known about any new agent is its chemical configuration (i.e., alkylating agent, antimetabolite, etc.), or its expected action in the cell cycle, in order to determine the appropriate dosage schedules and limitations.

Table 1-3 lists dosage limitations and toxicity of many commonly used agents. It should be emphasized that for non-cycle-active drugs the total dosage is more important than the timing of the doses, whereas the opposite is true for cycle- or phase-specific agents.[8] The maintenance programs using non-cycle-active agents may yield cumulative toxicity upon proliferative tissues such as the bone marrow and GI tract, while this is not the case for cycle- or phase-specific drugs. Nonproliferative toxicity, e.g., bleomycin pulmonary fibrosis, may be totally dose dependent, however. These nonproliferative toxicities cannot be predicted and must be determined empirically for each agent.

Therapeutic Decision Making

The data presented in Table 1-4 overviews the clinical effectiveness and future goals of cancer chemotherapy. Virtually all neoplasms are given a place in this table, and the purpose of this overview is to stress that when faced with therapeutic decisions, chemotherapy must be given a place equal to that of surgery or X-ray therapy.

The next decision concerns the timing of chemotherapy. When the diagnosis of cancer is first made, the patient may have a relatively high tumor burden. The histology of the tumor and the stage of the presenting lesion aid the clinician in the selection of the appropriate procedures for eradication of the primary tumor. In reference to chemotherapy, not only are the various agents selected based upon the histopathology of the primary tumor, but also the staging information indicates whether the patient has to be treated for grossly metastatic disease or for micrometastatic disease. If there is a great likelihood of micrometastatic disease, the use of adjuvant chemotherapy is indicated.

In general, the following principles govern the design of cancer chemotherapy programs.

1. Non-cycle-active agents are often selected initially when there is a large tumor burden. Macroscopic tumor nodules often have low growth fractions making them relatively resistant to cycle- and phase-specific drugs.
2. Adjuvant and maintenance programs often depend upon cycle- or phase-specific drugs, since micrometastatic tumor nodules have high growth fractions. If non-cycle-active drugs are also used, their dosage must be fairly low to avoid cumulative toxicity.
3. Even though a drug may not effect a great reduction in tumor cell number when the tumor burden is great, the same drug may actually be effective when the tumor burden is small.
4. Normal tissues "grow faster" than do cancerous tissues. Short bursts of phase-specific drugs followed by rest periods are less toxic to the bone marrow and to the GI tract and have better therapeutic indexes than the same drug delivered as a small dose on a continuous basis.
5. Cycle-specific agents should not be administered for periods of time that exceed more than 1 to 2 cycle times of normal hematopoietic or gastrointestinal tissue if one is to avoid toxicity.[8] A dosage of MTX of 2.5 mg. q 6 hours for 4 days will create maximum toxicity for a given tumor cell kill. A dosage of 40 mg. of MTX every fourth day will kill just as many tumor cells and will result in little clinically significant toxicity.
6. For any phase- or cycle-specific agent, a maximum dosage is achieved whereby normal tissues will not show increased toxicity, while tumor tissue may suffer dramatically increased cell death because of the phenomenon of increased penetration into the tumor.

The most recent advance in cancer chemotherapy has been the development of the adjuvant chemotherapy programs. Prior to a few years ago, the only patients given adjuvant chemotherapy (i.e., when tumor burden was hardly visible) were patients with acute leukemia,[16] Hodgkin's disease[17] or non-Hodg-

TABLE 1-4. *The Spectrum of Effectiveness of Cancer Chemotherapy*

A. Neoplasms Cured by Chemotherapy	% of Patients with Normal Survival
Disease	
Trophoblastic disease in women	>90
Acute leukemia childhood	25–50
Wilms' tumor (with surgery and X-ray therapy)	80
Hodgkin's disease (stage III & IV)	40–60
Testicular tumors (selected)	10

B. Metastatic Neoplasms with Chemotherapy Induced Prolongation in survival (some cures)	% of Responders
Disease	
Non-Hodgkin's lymphomas	60–80
Acute non-lymphoblastic leukemia	60
Chronic granulocytic leukemia	90
Multiple myeloma	50
Breast cancer	75

C. Metastatic neoplasms symptomatically palliated

Colon	Ovary	Thyroid, adrenal	Carcinoid	Melanoma
Stomach	Endometrium	Testis	Kaposi's sarcoma	Hepatoma
Head & neck	Female cervix	Lung		Chronic lymphatic leukemia
	Islet cell tumor			Soft tissue sarcomas

D. Neoplasms Treated Primarily for Cure Where Adjuvant Chemotherapy Proved Successful or Ought to be Tested

Breast *	Melanoma (Stage II)
Head & neck	Osteogenic sarcoma *
Colon (Dukes' C)	Female Cervix (Stage III)
Stomach (with negative nodes)	Ovarian (Stage II)
	Lung

E. Neoplasms Which Require Study to Determine Effectiveness of Palliation

Pancreas, brain tumors, kidney

*adjuvant programs successful

kin's lymphoma.[18] About 4 years ago the breast adjuvant study was begun.[19] It had been demonstrated about 10 years ago that patients with obvious metastatic disease from breast cancer would respond to multi-drug chemotherapy that usually utilized an alkylating agent and several antimetabolites like 5-FU and MTX.[20] There were no cures, however, despite a large number of complete responses.[21] It was then proposed that patients who were at high risk for recurrence of breast cancer in metastatic sites be treated before these metastases became clinically obvious. The rationale behind these suggestions has been described above, and Figure 1-4 summarizes the relationship between tumor burden, doubling time, growth rate and cell number. The goal of adjuvant chemotherapy was to reduce an approximate tumor burden of less than 10^9 cells to an amount less than 10^5 cells. It was suggested that the immune system could eradicate the remaining cells and the patient would be cured. At this Symposium on cancer chemotherapy, Dr. Ezra Greenspan reported the results of the adjuvant program and indicated that use of these programs may cure approximately one-third more patients than had been hitherto possible with the use of surgery, or surgery and X-ray therapy.[22] The most recent results of the Italian breast adjuvant program indicate that premenopausal breast patients with positive lymph nodes (stage II disease) show longer disease-free intervals after 4 years of adjuvant chemotherapy than do nontreated matched controls.[23] This breast adjuvant program chose a 1 year period of treatment utilizing a combination of cyclophosphamide, 5-fluorouracil, and MTX. The treatment time chosen was arbitrary and, since we cannot measure tumor burdens less than 10^9 cells, may not have been adequate. Future data will yield the answer to this problem and, undoubtedly, the length of time that the adjuvant is given will be modified once the results have been evaluated.

For the patient with macroscopic metastatic disease the same principles apply, although the length of time that the drugs are administered is often shorter. Once metastases are detected, it is senseless to wait until the tumor burden becomes so great that the patient has already developed many symptoms. By that time, most of the tumor nodules will be relatively large and will have poor blood supply and low growth fractions. In these instances large doses of "debulking" chemotherapy would be required but, because these patients are often debilitated, the toxicity of these programs becomes prohibitive.[24] Similarly, once it has been determined that the tumor burden is increasing despite the administration of cancer chemotherapy, it is senseless to continue such therapy. In short, chemotherapy for metastases should be given as early as possible at a time when the tumor burden is minimal. Chemotherapy ought to be stopped when, despite an appropriate trial of a given group of drugs, the tumor continues to advance.

Combination Chemotherapy

There are several reasons for the use of combinations of drugs as opposed to single drug therapy. First, because each drug in the combination has usually been shown to have some antitumor effect, the sum of these effects is likely to kill more cells than the kill obtained when each agent is used alone. Second, if each drug in the combination has a different dose limitation or toxicity, full dosages of each could be administered and the tumor, now exposed to multiple agents in full dosage, would receive the sum of several killing potentials. In brief, the therapeutic index may be increased dramatically. Finally, one or several of the drugs in the combinations may recruit cells into cycle or synchronize cells already in cycle, thus increasing the cytotoxicity of the other drugs in the combination without increasing the systematic toxicity.[25] The breast adjuvant program of cytoxan, 5-FU and MTX utilizes lower doses of cyclophosphamide, 5-FU and MTX than if each were used alone. Thus toxicity is reduced, but tumor cell kill reflecting the sum of the three agents is maximized. Even more important is the fact that in the breast protocol cyclophosphamide might debulk the tumor nodules, inducing many cells to enter the cell cycle where they would be more sensitive to the effects of MTX and 5-FU. Another example showing synchronization is the combination of vincristine and MTX that has been outlined in Figure 1-5.

End Results Analysis

The data presented in Figure 1-4 indicate that a patient with a tumor burden of less than 10^9 cells will have no clinically evident disease. Because about three doublings comprise a log*, the length of time to recurrence reflects the level to which the tumor burden was reduced by the therapy given. Since doubling times are variable, matched controls are necessary to evaluate the effects of any new drug program. Usually the end point is a disease-free interval or overall survival. If we were able to detect when tumor bulk was as

*The use of the word "log" refers to logarithm of the base 10. Thus, log 10^9 is 9. Reducing tumor burden from 10^9 to 10^8, reduces the cell count by one log.

low as a few cells, it would not be necessary to utilize survival or disease-free intervals as a measure of the effectiveness of cancer chemotherapy. Until such tests are developed, matched series will be required.

Future Prospects

Until a specific anticancer drug or group of drugs is developed, the following factors will be important in the design of cancer chemotherapy programs.

1. Type of agent: Does the agent have any efficacy at all in the animal screens? Unfortunately, in vitro methods for evaluating efficacy of potential anticancer agents utilizing human tissue have not been devised, but are sorely needed.
2. The mechanism of action of the agent in reference to the cell cycle must be recognized so that the agent can be matched to certain tumors and combined with other agents.
3. Dosage and scheduling of agents currently available, and those that are to be developed, must be carefully evaluated and reevaluated. It is probable that there are some tumors that could be controlled by drugs available today if the dosage and schedule of these drugs were altered. (Table 1-4, D and E)
4. The duration of exposure to, and the route of administration of, the drugs must be carefully evaluated.
5. Drugs must be developed which have selective action against malignant tissues to the exclusion of normal tissues. An evaluation of differences in enzyme content of tumor cells may lead to more specific antitumor drugs.
6. Analysis of the kinetics of tumor tissue compared to normal tissue must be made. Synchronization and recruitment are important elements in chemotherapy programs.
7. Drug distribution and tissue levels must be measured.
8. Drug metabolism and excretion patterns must be evaluated and incorporated into the program.
9. Methods to increase the penetration of the drug into tumor sites must be devised. In conjunction with this effort, the use of anticoagulants to increase the penetration of drugs into tumors has been suggested.[26]
10. The interactions of drugs with other agents must be recognized.
11. The action of drugs on the immune system and the role of the immune system in the eradication of small tumor burdens must be evaluated.

Summary

This chapter has outlined those principles which underlie therapeutic decision making in reference to cancer chemotherapy. A basic knowledge of tumor kinetics is essential for an understanding of cancer chemotherapy and has been outlined. Because all cancer chemotherapeutic drugs inhibit cell division, the cell cycle has been reviewed. An outline of the mechanisms of action of the various classes of drugs related to the cell cycle has been given. The rationale for adjuvant chemotherapy and combination chemotherapy has been outlined. The principles underlying the timing and scheduling of drugs and the successes and future goals of cancer chemotherapy have also been presented. The major goal of the chapter has been to teach the non-oncology specialist those principles which underlie cancer treatment decision making in reference to chemotherapy, thus helping the primary physician to support his patients during the treatment of their disease.

References

1. Cancer Facts and Figures. New York, American Cancer Society, 1977
2. Horsfall B L: Cancer and viruses. Bull NY Acad Med 42:167–181, 1966
3. Martinez-Palomo A: Intercellular junctions in normal and malignant cells. Pathobiol Annu 261–269, 1971
4. Weber G: Enzymology of cancer cells. N Engl J Med 296:486–493, 541–551, 1977
5. Baserga R: Multiplication and Division in Mammalian Cells. Biochemistry of Disease, Vol. 6. New York, Marcel Dekker, 1976, p 78–102
6. Sandberg A, Hossfeld D K: Chromosomes in the pathogenesis of human cancer and leukemia, in Holland J F, Frei E III (eds): Cancer Medicine. Philadelphia, Lea & Febiger, 1973, p 151
7. Tubiana M: The kinetics of tumor cell proliferation and radiotherapy. J. Radiol 44:325–347, 1971
8. Hill B T, Baserga R: The cell cycle and its significance for cancer treatment. Cancer Treatment Rev 2:159–175, 1975
9. Govosto F, Pileri A: The cell cycle and cancer in Baserga R (ed): New York, Marcel Dekker, 1971, p 99–138
10. Bresciani F: Cellular radiation biology. M D Anderson Hosp Symposium, Baltimore, Williams & Wilkins, 1965, p 547–557
11. Lampkin B C, McWilliams N B, Mauer A M: Cell kinetics and chemotherapy in acute leukemia. Semin Hematol 9:211–223, 1972
12. Brodsky I, Kahn S B, Moyer JH (eds): Cancer Chemotherapy II. New York, Grune & Stratton, 1972.
13. Steel G G: Cytokinetics of neoplasia, in Holland J F, Frei E III (eds): Cancer Medicine. Philadelphia, Lea & Febiger, 1973, p 125
14. Cronkite E P: Kinetics of leukemic cell proliferation, in Dameshek W, Dutcher R (eds): Perspectives in Leukemia. New York, Grune & Stratton, 1968, p 158–186
15. Van Duuren B L (ed): Biological effects of alkylating agents. Ann NY Acad Sci 163:589, 1969
16. Henderson E S: The treatment of acute leukemia. Semin Hematol 6:271–319, 1969
17. DeVita V T Jr. Serpick A, Carbone P P: Combination chemotherapy of advanced Hodgkin's disease. Ann Intern Med 73:881–895, 1970
18. Schein P S, DeVita V T Jr. Hubbard S. et al: Bleomycin, adriamycin, cyclophosphamide, vincristine and prednisone (BACOP) combination chemotherapy in the treatment of advanced histiocytic lymphoma. Ann Intern Med 85:417–422, 1976
19. Fisher B, Carbone P, Economou S G, et al: 1-phenylalanine mustard (L-PAM) in the management of primary breast cancer: A report of early findings. N Engl J Med 292:117–122, 1975
20. Cooper R: Combination chemotherapy of hormone resistant breast cancer. Proc Am Assoc Cancer Res 10:15, 1969
21. Greenspan E: Combination cytotoxic chemotherapy in advanced disseminated breast carcinoma. M Sinai J Med NY 33:1–27, 1966
22. Greenspan E: Chemotherapy of breast cancer, in Brodsky I, Conroy J F, Kahn S B (eds): Cancer Chemotherapy III. New York, Grune & Stratton, 1978, ch 11
23. Bonadonna G, Brusamolino E. Valagussa B S, et al: Combination chemotherapy as an adjuvant treatment in operable breast cancer. N Engl J Med 294:405–410, 1976
24. Livingston R B, Einhorn L H, Boddey G P, et al: COMB, (cyclophosphamide, oncovin, methyl CCNU, bleomycin), a four drug combination in solid tumors. Cancer 36:327–332, 1975
25. Costanzi J J, Lankas D, Gagliano R G, et al: Intravenous bleomycin as a potential synchronizing agent in human disseminated malignancies. Cancer 38:1503–1506, 1976
26. Brodsky I: Leukemia and the hypercoagulable state. Pathogenic and therapeutic implications. J Med 5:38–49, 1974

David B. Ludlum

2
The Alkylating Agents and Nitrosoureas

The introduction of alkylating agents to clinical medicine during World War II marked the beginning of modern cancer chemotherapy. Since then, careful studies of these agents have contributed to our basic understanding of cancer and its treatment. Accordingly, it seems appropriate to begin this discussion with a review of these important compounds.

Although the mechanism of action of the alkylating agents has not been completely elucidated, it is well known that they modify nucleic acids and interfere with deoxyribonucleic acid (DNA) synthesis in vivo. Since they can also be mutagenic, carcinogenic, or teratogenic under certain laboratory conditions, it appears that an attack on the genetic apparatus, most likely DNA, is basic to their action.

For these reasons we shall consider reactions of alkylating agents with nucleic acids and nucleic acid models only, omitting discussion of their effects on other cellular constituents. This will result in a chapter of manageable size, but even so, many careful investigations cannot be mentioned; fortunately, most of these are covered in other recent reviews and collected works.[1-11]

Although it has been assumed for many years that all of these agents act by a similar mechanism, it should probably be emphasized that important differences exist among them. For example, a lack of cross resistance is now recognized among the more classical alkylating agents as well as between the alkylating agents and nitrosoureas.[12] As might be expected, molecular explanations for these differences are being sought in several laboratories.

Structures of the Alkylating Agents and Nitrosoureas

Many of the common alkylating agents are related to mechlorethamine or nitrogen mustard. This compound, together with other nitrogen mustards, is shown in Figure 2-1. These agents contain two chloroethyl groups which can react separately with electron-rich sites in nucleic acids. Thus, they have a potential for crosslinking as described below.

Of the mustards listed in Figure 2-1, mechlorethamine, chlorambucil and melphalan are highly reactive compounds in the form in which they are administered. Cyclophosphamide, however, must be activated by the liver before it can alkylate. It was introduced with the hope that this activation would occur in the tumor itself and it is possible that such

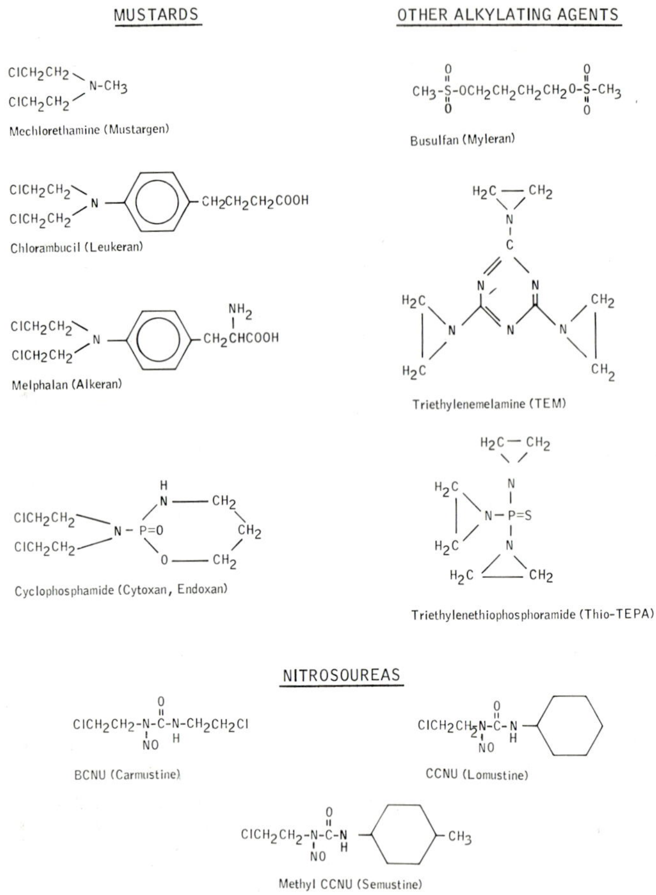

MUSTARDS

Mechlorethamine (Mustargen)

Chlorambucil (Leukeran)

Melphalan (Alkeran)

Cyclophosphamide (Cytoxan, Endoxan)

OTHER ALKYLATING AGENTS

Busulfan (Myleran)

Triethylenemelamine (TEM)

Triethylenethiophosphoramide (Thio-TEPA)

NITROSOUREAS

BCNU (Carmustine)

CCNU (Lomustine)

Methyl CCNU (Semustine)

FIG. 2-1. Representative alkylating agents and nitrosoureas.

tumor-specific activation may yet be achieved with other agents.

Many alkylating agents have been synthesized with functional groups other than the bis-chloroethyl amine grouping of nitrogen mustard. Three of these are included in Figure 2-1. The first, busulfan, alkylates by a displacement of the methanesulfonate group and can crosslink through a $-CH_2CH_2CH_2CH_2-$ bridge. It is an unusual compound that reacts with nucleic acids to form crosslinks[13,14] and with S-containing amino acids to form substituted thiophenes[15] in a reaction whose significance is still unknown.

The two ethylenimines, triethylenemelamine and triethylenethiophosphoramide, contain a characteristic imine grouping which resembles the cyclized imonium group of activated nitrogen mustard (see below). Since these compounds are quite basic and are protonated at tissue pH, they do not have the improved permeability characteristics originally envisioned.

The nitrosoureas shown at the bottom of Figure 2-1 are more lipid soluble than classical alkylating agents and can cross the blood-brain barrier. Consequently they have applications in the treatment of central nervous system (CNS) tumors. The nitrosoureas produce unique modifications of nucleic acids which may help to explain differences in their pharmacological behavior from the more classical agents.

GENERAL PHARMACOLOGY OF THE ALKYLATING AGENTS AND THE NITROSOUREAS

If we adopt a hypothesis that the alkylating agents and nitrosoureas produce their cytotoxic effects by altering DNA, then successful treatment with these agents must involve the steps shown in Table 2-1. After the agent is absorbed and distributed, it may be converted spontaneously or enzymatically to a different alkylating species. Unless this activation occurs in the region of DNA, the active species must presumably be transported to the cell nucleus. In this section, we shall discuss the steps involved in absorption, distribution and activation of the agent and consider the molecular pharmacology of DNA alteration in the next section.

The more reactive, or less reliably absorbed, agents are given intravenously. Thus, of the agents in Figure 2-1, mechlorethamine, triethylenethiophosphoramide, and carmustine (BCNU) are customarily given intravenously. Cyclophosphamide may be given by either the intravenous or oral route and the rest of the agents are usually given orally. Most of the classical agents are rather polar and do not penetrate the blood-brain barrier, but the nitrosoureas have relatively good lipid solubility and are very useful for treating CNS tumors. Lipid soluble compounds of this sort that decompose slowly may also prove to be useful in penetrating and treating solid tumors.

As administered, the agent must usually be activated before it can react with DNA. Three rather different examples of this are shown in Figure 2-2. Many nitrogen mustards, including mechlorethamine, cyclize spontaneously in neutral aqueous solution to produce an imonium form which is presumed to be the active alkylating species.

TABLE 2-1. *Steps Involved in the Alkylation of DNA Bases*

1. Absorption and distribution of the agent.
2. Formation of an active alkylating species in one or more intermediate steps.
3. Transportation of the active species to the DNA template.
4. Chemical modification of the DNA.

The activation of cyclophosphamide, however, is much more complex. The first step involves a ring hydroxylation by liver mixed-function oxidases. The resulting 4-hydroxycyclophosphamide is apparently released from the liver and picked up by individual tumor cells. Spontaneous decomposition of 4-hydroxycyclophosphamide within the tumor cell releases acrolein and phosphoramide mustard which is presumed to be the active species.[16] The intermediate 4-hydroxycyclophosphamide, instead of decomposing spontaneously to the active phosphoramide mustard, can also be enzymatically oxidized and inactivated. Increased activity of these enzymes could easily explain the development of resistance.[17]

The nitrosoureas evidently decompose spontaneously in aqueous solution to generate chloroethyl carbonium ions.[18-20] Since this species is also generated from CCNU, it is evident that it arises from the nitroso end of the nitrosourea.

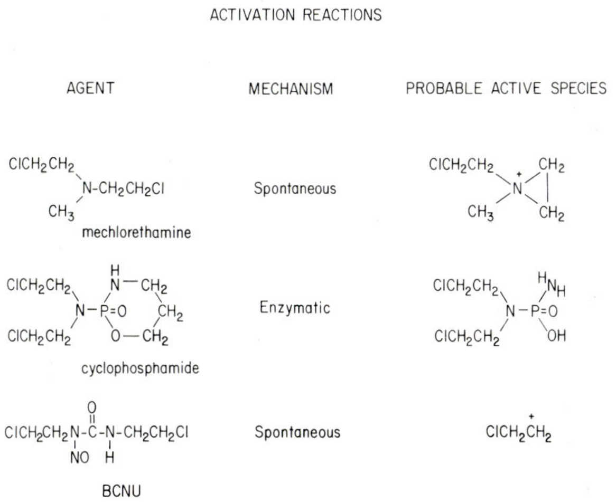

ACTIVATION REACTIONS

AGENT	MECHANISM	PROBABLE ACTIVE SPECIES
$ClCH_2CH_2N(CH_3)CH_2CH_2Cl$ mechlorethamine	Spontaneous	$ClCH_2CH_2(CH_3)N^{+}$ (aziridinium ring with CH_2–CH_2)
$(ClCH_2CH_2)_2N$–P(=O) in ring with N(H)–CH_2–CH_2–CH_2–O; cyclophosphamide	Enzymatic	$(ClCH_2CH_2)_2N$–P(=O)(NH_2)(OH)
$ClCH_2CH_2N(NO)$–C(=O)–N(H)–CH_2CH_2Cl BCNU	Spontaneous	$ClCH_2\overset{+}{C}H_2$

FIG. 2-2. Activation of alkylating agents and nitrosoureas.

It is not always clear which form of a particular agent enters the tumor cells. The nitrosoureas probably enter by passive diffusion to generate the active species intracellularly. There is considerable evidence, however, that nitrogen mustard is transported by a carrier mechanism.[21,22] This carrier system is saturable at high levels of mustard and is blocked by choline and hemicholinium, suggesting that it is the same system which normally transports choline. Clearly, cells could become resistant to nitrogen mustard by losing the ability to transport this compound.

The development of resistance is, of course, a problem with the alkylating agents as with most other antitumor agents. In addition to the mechanisms mentioned above, cells may become resistant by inactivating the agents or by repairing damage that has been done to cellular DNA by them. A detailed account of these mechanisms has been published by Connors.[23]

Another problem encountered with these agents is, of course, their toxicity. Bone marrow depression, which is generally limiting, follows a different time course for the alkylating agents and nitrosoureas; it may take 4 or 5 weeks for the nadir to appear with the latter. GI toxicity with nausea and vomiting is common with most of these agents. Cyclophosphamide has a tendency to cause alopecia and hemorrhagic cystitis which may reach serious proportions. Spermatogenesis may also be affected and, since the agents are teratogens, they should be strictly avoided in pregnancy.

Molecular Pharmacology of the Alkylating Agents and the Nitrosoureas

In this section we shall consider the chemistry of DNA alkylation and the biological consequences of these reactions. Studies in this area are directed towards identifying cytotoxic lesions and maximizing these effects on the tumor while minimizing possible side effects including mutagenesis and chemical carcinogenesis.

Although it took many years to establish the fact with certainty, physical and chemical measurements have shown that phosphate groups in nucleic acids are extensively alkylated.[24-26] Because the genetic information contained in a nucleic acid is imparted by the sequence of bases, however, much more attention has been paid to alterations in their structure.

The pioneering work of Brookes and Lawley[13,27] established substitution in the 7-position of guanine as the most prevalent base modification. Since that time, one or more investigators have shown that all of the free oxygens and nitrogens in the pyrimidines and purines can be substituted under certain conditions.[28-32] Because of the unique importance of DNA and the fact that alterations in its structure can be magnified, the importance of minor alkylation sites cannot be dismissed. In fact, there is a growing realization that differences among different alkylating agents may result from differences in the pattern of alkylation. Indeed, certain lesions may be associated more with the toxic effects of mutagenesis and carcinogenesis than with the desired antitumor activity.

It has been a general observation that monofunctional agents have less therapeutic value than compounds with two or more alkylating groups. These compounds can form crosslinks within a single molecule or bind two macromolecules together with a covalent bond. The existence of such crosslinks between the two strands of DNA may be demonstrated by the reversible denaturation of double-stranded DNA molecules.[33,34]

Apparent exceptions to the rule that clinically useful agents contain two or more alkylating groups are two nitrosoureas shown in Figure 2-1: CCNU or chloroethylcyclohexyl nitrosourea and methyl-CCNU or methylcyclohexyl chloroethyl nitrosourea. As suggested in the last edition of this book, however, and now experimentally evident,[35] haloethyl groups can be transferred from the nitrosoureas to nucleosides, thus converting them into alkylating agents. If the nucleoside that accepts the haloethyl group is contained in a DNA molecule, crosslinks can be formed between two DNA strands.

Although the main chemical features of alkylation have been elucidated, specific details of the process may be very important. Lawley and Brookes[27] have shown that the secondary structure of DNA influences the site of alkylation, and studies with polynucleotides[36] have shown that this influence is very marked indeed. Changes in secondary structure during replication may well explain the increased sensitivity of tumor or rapidly dividing normal cells to these agents.

Once the original base modification has occurred, there are several additional possibilities which are listed in Table 2-2. Since alkylation of a purine generally weakens the sugar-base bond, alkylation can be followed by depurination leading to spontaneous scission of the sugar phosphate backbone. Alternately, the modified base may be recognized by endonucleases which remove it. This may be followed by further enzymatic breakdown or repair of the damage using the information contained in the opposite strand of DNA. Finally, as discussed below, the altered base may remain in the DNA template leading to inactivation of the template, or to the transmission of inaccurate information. The last possibility could, of course, lead to either cytotoxicity or mutagenesis.

The cytotoxic effects of alkylation can be evaluated at a molecular level with the use of microorganisms. Bacteriophage which contain double-stranded nucleic acids are more sensitive to the action of difunctional agents than those that contain single-stranded material.[3,37,38] This suggests that interstrand crosslinks are important in producing a lethal effect. Even bacteriophage which contain single-stranded nucleic acids, however, are more sensitive to difunctional agents than to monofunctional ones which indicates that intrastrand links are also important in explaining lethality. The studies described below suggest that somewhat different factors govern the lethality of different compounds; however, the cytotoxic action of clinically useful agents probably depends on crosslinking.

Lawley and coworkers[34] have published a detailed study of the action of sulphur mustard and half mustard on the T7 coliphage, a virus which contains double-stranded DNA. At the mean lethal dose for immediate inactivation by mustard gas, there were 1.3 moles of di-(guanin-7-yl-ethyl) sulfide and 7 moles of monoalkylation products per mole of DNA polymer, whereas at the mean lethal dose for half mustard there were 280 moles of monoalkylation products. These data indicate that formation of the crosslinked diguaninyl product is a particularly damaging event. Approximately one-quarter of the diguaninyl molecules are associated with interstrand crosslinks and the remainder with intrastrand links.

TABLE 2-2. *Consequences of Base Alkylation*

1. Spontaneous depurination.
2. Enzymatic excision without repair. Damage may be magnified.
3. Enzymatic excision with repair and recovery of function.
4. Continued presence in DNA. Template may be inactivated or replicated inaccurately.

A relatively large number of alkylations were required for immediate inactivation by the monofunctional half mustard. Subsequent depurination and hydrolysis of DNA at alkylated base positions caused more extensive inactivation than alkylation itself.

Verly and Brakier have studied the action of nitrogen mustard, ethyl methanesulfonate, busulfan, and diepoxybutane on the same T7 phage.[39] Crosslinks were again associated with lethality for nitrogen mustard; when survival was followed after treatment with this agent, bonds between DNA strands first increased in number and then decreased.

On the other hand, treatment of T7 with ethyl methanesulfonate resulted in lethality which increased steadily after exposure, presumably due to depurination and hydrolysis. Surprisingly, when T7 was treated with the difunctional agent, busulfan, there was no evidence for interstrand crosslinking. Intrastrand crosslinks were not ruled out, but the concentrations of busulfan and ethyl methanesulfonate required for equal lethality were similar. It thus appears that ethyl methanesulfonate and busulfan have a very similar action on T7 phage; some additional factor must operate to explain the difference between these two agents in higher organisms. Diepoxybutane, also studied by Verly and Brakier, had a combined difunctional and monofunctional action.

When the effects of alkylating agents are studied in growing bacteria or mammalian cells, intracellular enzymes become extremely important in modifying the initial damage to DNA. These enzymes evidently recognize the alkylated base and remove it, an action which can either magnify the damage or open the way for subsequent repair.

Papirmeister and Davison[40] first demonstrated the loss of sulphur mustard alkylation products from the DNA of *Escherichia coli*. Bacteria which were treated with this agent and then incubated gradually regained their ability to synthesize DNA and to reproduce after an initial lag. Since sulphur mustard products were eliminated during this period, it was assumed that growth returned only after repair of damaged DNA.

Magnification of the original damage may occur if the alkylated DNA is subject to endonuclease attack without subsequent repair. Work by Papirmeister and coworkers has suggested that DNA of T1 bacteriophage is sensitized to endonuclease attack by adenine rather than guanine alkylation.[41]

The effects of alkylating agents on mammalian cells have been studied by many different groups including Roberts and coworkers, who published the results of a detailed study of HeLa cells.[42] Here again, the difunctional agent, sulphur mustard, is much more toxic than the monofunctional derivative; DNA synthesis again appears to be the cellular process most sensitive to alkylation. By using synchronous cultures, it was shown that cells in the late G_1 (postmitotic) or early S (DNA synthetic) phases are particularly sensitive to the effects of alkylation.

When cells are treated during these phases, there is an immediate inhibition of DNA synthesis and a delay in division and onset of the next (second) DNA synthetic cycle. It is evident, however, that some recovery has occurred by the third synthetic cycle. This is attributed to repair of alkylated DNA, a process that is accompanied by release of alkylated products. Thus, the same general features of cytotoxicity appear to be present in both mammalian and bacterial cells.

The experiments described above are concerned with the lethal action of alkylating agents and with modifications in lethality which may be imposed by cellular metabolism. The problem of relating a particular alteration in nucleic acid structure to a specific biological effect can be approached by incorporating the modified base in a synthetic polynucleotide template.[43] These polymers can be prepared with a known composition and used in model biochemical studies to obtain direct information on the biological effects of alkylation.

TABLE 2-3. *Informational Content of Methylated Bases*

7 Methylguanine	Pairs Normally	(45)
0–6 Methylguanine	Miscodes	(46)
3 Methylcytosine	Miscodes	(47-49)
0–4 Methylthymine	Miscodes	(50)

Focusing on the substituted base found most frequently after treatment with methylating agents, Wilhelm and Ludlum studied the ability of copolymers which contained 7-methylguanine to promote polypeptide synthesis.[44] The experiments were designed to detect the incorporation of amino acids which would have been polymerized if 7-methylguanine mispaired like adenine. No evidence for such misincorporation was obtained; instead, the overall ability of the 7-methylguanine-containing templates to promote polypeptide synthesis was diminished.

More extensive studies have been performed using DNA or RNA polymerase to copy polydeoxynucleotides or polyribonucleotides which contain alkylated bases. Results of these experiments are shown in Table 2-3 together with the appropriate references. It is evident, first of all, that 7-methylguanine retains the base-pairing properties of guanine. Other methylated bases which appear as minor alkylation products have been found to convey misinformation, probably because the structural alterations are at sites involved in base pairing. More elaborate base modifications such as those resulting from their reactions with BCNU[51] are still being investigated. As this information becomes available, it may be possible to classify agents according to the number of cytotoxic and potentially mutagenic modifications which they produce and to avoid long-term complications of therapy.

CONCLUSIONS

The wide range of clinical applications of the alkylating agents and nitrosoureas will become apparent in the following chapters.

Future developments, based on current research, can be predicted in several areas. Recognizing the differences in base modifications which are produced by the nitrosoureas and classical alkylating agents, we may anticipate that new DNA-modifying agents will be discovered. As with other antitumor agents, it appears likely that improvements in dose scheduling will also be made with the alkylating agents. Finally, more sophisticated use will probably be made of combinations of alkylating agents and other compounds which augment their activity by, for example, inhibiting the action of repair enzymes.

References

1. Lawley P D: Effects of some chemical mutagens and carcinogens on nucleic acids. Progr Nucleic Acid Res Mol Biol 5:89, 1966
2. Ross W C J: Biological Alkylating Agents. London, Butterworth, 1962
3. Loveless A: Genetic and Allied Effects of Alkylating Agents. University Park & London, Pennsylvania State University Press, 1966
4. Van Duuren B L (ed): Biological effects of alkylating agents. Ann NY Acad Sci 163:589, 1969
5. Connors T A: Mechanism of action of 2-chloroethylamine derivatives, sulfur mustards, expoxides, and aziridines, in Sartorelli A C, Johns D G (eds): Handbook of Experimental Pharmacology, vol. 38, part 2. Berlin, Springer-Verlag, 1975, pp 18–34
6. Fox B W: Mechanism of action of methanesulfonates, in Sartorelli A C, Johns D G (eds): Handbook of Experimental Pharmacology, vol. 38, part 2. Berlin, Springer-Verlag, 1975, pp 35–46
7. Ludlum D B: Molecular biology of alkylation: An overview, in Sartorelli A C, Johns D G (eds): Handbook of Experimental Pharmacology, vol. 38, part 2. Berlin, Springer-Verlag, 1975, pp 6–17
8. Price C C: Chemistry of alkylation, in Sartorelli A C, Johns D G (eds): Handbook of Experimental Pharmacology, vol. 38, part 2. Berlin, Springer-Verlag, 1975, pp 1–5
9. Ross W C J: Rational design of alkylating agents, in Sartorelli A C, Johns D G (eds): Handbook of Experimental Pharmacology, vol. 38, part 1. Berlin, Springer-Verlag, 1975, pp 33–51
10. Singer B: The chemical effects of nucleic acid alkylation and their relation to mutagenesis and carcinogenesis. Progr Nucleic Acid Res Mol Biol 15:219, 1975
11. Wheeler G P: Mechanism of action of nitrosoureas, in Sartorelli A C, Johns D G (eds): Handbook of Experimental Pharmacology, vol. 38, part 2. Berlin, Springer-Verlag, 1975, pp 65–84
12. Schabel F M Jr: Synergism and antagonism among antitumor agents, in Univ of Texas Grad Sch of Biomed Sci at Houston (eds): Pharmacological Basis of Cancer Chemotherapy. M D Anderson Hospital and Tumor Institute at Houston. Baltimore, Williams & Wilkins, 1975, pp 595–623
13. Brookes P, Lawley P D: The reaction of mono- and di-functional alkylating agents with nucleic acids. Biochem J 80:496, 1961
14. Brakier L, Verly W G: The lethal action of ethyl methanesulfonate, nitrogen mustard, and myleran on the T7 coliphage. Biochim Biophys Acta 213:296, 1970
15. Roberts J J, Warwick G P: The mode of action of tumor growth-inhibiting alkylating agents. II. Studies of the metabolism of myleran. The reaction of myleran with some naturally occurring thiols in vitro. Biochem Pharmacol 6:217–227, 1961
16. Colvin M, Brundrett R B, Kan M N, et al: Alkylating properties of phosphoramide mustard. Cancer Res 36:1121, 1976
17. Connors T A: Alkylating agents. Topics in Current Chemistry 52:141, 1975
18. Colvin M, Cowens J W, Brundrett R B, et al: Decomposition of BCNU (1,3-bis (2-chloroethyl)-1-nitrosourea) in aqueous solution. Biochem Biophys Res Commun 60:515, 1974
19. Reed D J, May H E, Boose R B, et al: 2-chloroethanol formation as evidence for a 2-chloroethyl alkylating intermediate during chemical degradations of 1-(2-chloroethyl)-3-cyclohexyl-1-nitrosourea and 1-(2-chloroethyl)-3-(trans-4-methylcyclohexyl)-1-nitrosourea. Cancer Res 35:568, 1975
20. Montgomery J A, James R, McCaleb G S, et al: Decomposition of N-(2-chloroethyl)-N-nitrosoureas in aqueous media. J Med Chem 18:568, 1975
21. Goldenberg G J, Vanstone C L, Israels L G, et al: Evidence for a transport carrier of nitrogen mustard in nitrogen mustard-sensitive and -resistant L5178 Y lymphoblasts. Cancer Res 30:2285, 1970
22. Goldenberg G J: The role of drug transport in resistance to nitrogen mustard and other alkylating agents in L5178 Y lymphoblasts. Cancer Res 35:1687, 1975

23. Connors T A: Mechanisms of clinical drug resistance to alkylating agents. Biochem Pharmacol 23: 89, (Suppl 2), 1974
24. Ludlum D B: Reaction of nitrogen mustard with synthetic polynucleotides. Biochim Biophys Acta 142:282, 1967
25. Rhaese H J, Freese E: Chemical analysis of DNA alterations. IV. Reactions of oligodeoxynucleotides with monofunctional alkylating agents leading to backbone breakage. Biochim Biophys Acta 190:418, 1969
26. Bannon P, Verly W: Alkylation of phosphates and stability of phosphate triesters in DNA. Eur J Biochem 31:103, 1972
27. Lawley P D, Brookes P: Further studies on the alkylation of nucleic acids and their constituent nucleotides. Biochem J 89:127, 1963
28. Loveless A: Possible relevance of 0-6 alkylation of deoxyguanosine to the mutagenicity and carcinogenicity of nitrosamines and nitrosamides. Nature 223:206, 1969
29. Lawley P D, Orr D J, Shah S A: Reaction of alkylating mutagens and carcinogens with nucleic acids: N-3 of guanine as a site of alkylation by N-methyl-N-nitrosourea and dimethyl sulphate. Chem-Biol Interactions 4:431, 1971/72
30. Lawley P D, Orr D J, Shah S A, et al: Reaction products from N-methyl-N-nitrosourea and deoxyribonucleic acid containing thymidine residues. Synthesis and identification of a new methylation product 0^4-methylthymidine. Biochem J 135:193, 1973
31. Kusmierek J T, Singer B: Sites of alkylation of poly U by agents of varying carcinogenicity and stability of products. Biochim Biophys Acta 442:420, 1976
32. Singer B: All oxygens in nucleic acids react with carcinogenic ethylating agents. Nature 264:333, 1976
33. Kohn K W, Spears C L, Doty P: Inter-strand crosslinking of DNA by nitrogen mustard. J Molec Biol 19:266, 1966
34. Lawley P D, Lethbridge J H, Edwards P A, et al: Inactivation of bacteriophage T7 by mono- and difunctional sulphur mustards in relation to cross-linking and depurination of bacteriophage DNA. J Molec Biol 39:181, 1969
35. Tong W P, Ludlum D B: Mechanism of action of the nitrosoureas I. Role of fluoroethyl cytidine in the reaction of BFNU with nucleic acids. Biochem Pharmacol, 27:77, 1978
36. Ludlum D B: Alkylation of polynucleotide complexes. Biochim Biophys Acta 95:674: 1965
37. Yamamoto N, Naito T: Inactivation by nitrogen mustard of single- and double-stranded DNA and RNA bacteriophages. Science 150:1603, 1965
38. Yamamoto N, Naito T, Shimkin M B: Mechanism of inactivation of DNA and RNA bacteriophages by alkylating agents in vitro. Cancer Res 26:2301, 1966
39. Verly W G, Brakier L: The lethal action of monofunctional and bifunctional alkylating agents on T7 coliphage. Biochim Biophys Acta 174:674, 1969
40. Papirmeister B, Davison C L: Elimination of sulfur mustard-induced products from DNA of *Escherichia coli*. Biochem Biophys Res Commun 17:608, 1964
41. Papirmeister B, Dorsey J K, Davison C L, et al: Sensitization of DNA to endonuclease by adenine alkylation and its biological significance. Fed Proc 29:726, 1970
42. Roberts J J, Brent T P, Crathorn A R: The mechanism of the cytotoxic action of alkylating agents on mammalian cells, in Campbell P N (ed): The Interaction of Drugs and Subcellular Components in Animal Cells. London, Churchill, 1968, pp 5–27
43. Ludlum D B, Warner R C, Wahba A J: Alkylation of synthetic polynucleotides. Science 145:397, 1964
44. Wilhelm R C, Ludlum D B: Coding properties of 7-methylguanine. Science 153:1403, 1966
45. Ludlum D B: The properties of 7-methylguanine-containing templates for ribonucleic acid polymerase. J Biol Chem 245:477, 1970
46. Gerchman L L, Ludlum D B: The properties of 0-6 methylguanine in templates for RNA polymerase. Biochim Biophys Acta 308:310, 1973
47. Ludlum D B, Wilhelm R C: Ribonucleic acid polymerase reactions with methylated polycytidylic acid templates. J Biol Chem 243: 2750, 1968
48. Ludlum D B: Alkylated polycytidylic acid templates for RNA polymerase. Biochim Biophys Acta 213:142, 1970
49. Singer B, Fraenkel-Conrat H: Messenger and template activities of chemically modified polynucleotides. Biochemistry 9:3694, 1970
50. Abbott P J, Saffhill R: DNA synthesis with methylated poly (dA-dT) templates: Possible role of O^4-methylthymine as a promutagenic base. Nucl Acids Res 4:761, 1977
51. Ludlum D B, Kramer B S, Wang J, et al: Reaction of 1,3-Bis(2-chloroethyl)-1-nitrosourea with synthetic polynucleotides. Biochemistry 14:5480, 1975

Charles Myers
Ada Brooks
Bruce Chabner

3

The Value of Monitoring Plasma Methotrexate Concentrations During Antineoplastic Therapy

Introduction

While routine drug level monitoring has become a practical and rewarding adjunct to therapy for infectious and cardiovascular diseases, such efforts have not been a common practice in antineoplastic chemotherapy. The reasons for the slow development of drug level monitoring with antineoplastic drugs are several, but the primary obstacle has been the lack of sufficiently sensitive and specific assays for the active principal. The sole exception to this situation has been the rapid growth of research interest in the clinical pharmacology of antifolate compounds, principally MTX.

Clinical monitoring of MTX pharmacokinetics has been greatly expedited by the development of several highly sensitive (less than 10^{-8}M levels in plasma), and specific, assay methods. Two of these, enzyme inhibition[1] and competitive enzyme binding[2,3], take advantage of the drug's high affinity to bind to dihydrofolate reductase, and give comparable clinical determinations with the same samples. It should be noted that the present enzyme-based methods for MTX assay are also applicable to the assay of other tight-binding antifolates of current clinical interest, including aminopterin, Baker's antifol and others.[4] The third widely used method, a radioimmunoassay developed with antisera to a MTX-albumin complex, has similar sensitivity but less well defined specificity.[5] The cross-reactivity of these assays with possible MTX metabolites will require further elucidation in view of mounting evidence that significant metabolism of this drug may occur particularly during high-dose infusion therapy. Metabolites may become the predominant compounds present in plasma at later time points due to their slower excretion relative to the parent compound.[6,7] A fourth assay, based on the inhibition of growth of *S. faecium* in vitro, has also been used, but has undefined specificity.[8]

While the availability of reliable assay methods has been a great advantage in the monitoring of antifolate chemotherapy, two other factors, unique to antifolate pharmacol-

The following chapter dealing with the antifols is presented in a fashion different than other chapters in this segment. Rather than review the clinical pharmacology of all antifols, the utility and methods of high-dose MTX therapy are presented. In reality the use of this drug in this fashion makes MTX a different type of agent than in its use in lower dosages. The reader should keep this in mind. The clinical efficacy of MTX infusions is especially emphasized in Chapter 22 by N. Jaffe.

ogy, have provided the impetus for recent clinical investigations: (1) the rapidly evolving understanding of the relationship between extracellular drug level and cytotoxicity for normal and malignant tissues, and (2) the use of MTX in a wide variety of schedules and routes of administration, each possessing its own spectrum of clinical toxicities and a unique pharmacokinetic profile. Thus, the routine use of MTX assays has grown out of a desire to design schedules of administration with clearly defined objectives in terms of drug distribution and drug concentrations in plasma, central nervous system (CNS) and other fluid compartments.

Prior to considering individual applications of drug monitoring, it would be helpful to outline certain principles regarding cellular toxicity of antifolate. It is now clear that MTX produces its cytotoxic effect by tightly binding to its target enzyme, dihydrofolate reductase, thus preventing the repletion of intracellular pools of tetrahydrofolates. Maintenance of this block, however, requires the presence of quantities of free drug in excess of the intracellular concentration of enzyme.[9] Furthermore, a specific threshold of extracellular drug concentration exists for each tissue, above which DNA synthesis is effectively blocked.[10] Proliferation of mouse bone marrow (and probably human marrow as well) is inhibited by drug concentrations above 1×10^{-8}M, while DNA synthesis in gastrointestinal epithelium is effectively blocked by concentrations above 5×10^{-9}M. Studies with mouse bone marrow in vitro and in vivo indicate that an increase in the efficiency (rate) of cell kill occurs with progressively high drug concentrations above the threshold value.[11] In addition to drug concentration, the duration of exposure appears to be a second important determinant of cytotoxicity.[12] Thus, higher drug concentrations are tolerated with minimal myelosuppression for up to 42 hours[13] if leucovorin rescue is instituted at that time. Somewhat longer periods of exposure are well tolerated for plasma levels less than 1×10^{-6}M, although tolerable concentration and time parameters have not been established for other regimens. With this information in mind, it will be possible to understand the interpretation and use of plasma drug level monitoring.

In the following discussion we will describe the specific uses of routine monitoring to aid antifolate therapy.

High Dose Methotrexate Therapy

The wide range of use of MTX in clinical chemotherapy has been extended by the demonstration that high doses, otherwise lethal to the patient, can be given if followed by the rescue agent, 5-formyl tetrahydrofolic acid (leucovorin). The rationale underlying this regimen is that high extracellular concentrations of drug may lead to enhanced drug penetration into poorly perfused or transport-defective tumor cells. High-dose infusion regimens are currently under investigation in numerous disease states, including osteogenic sarcoma (for both established disease and in the adjuvant setting), breast cancer, histiocytic lymphoma and head and neck cancer. While improved therapeutic results, as compared to conventional regimens, have been demonstrated only for osteogenic sarcoma[14] and head and neck cancer, the attractive rationale of this type of therapy has led to its growing use. High dose regimens, however, employing doses of 50 mg/kg or greater, have led to occasional serious toxicities and death.[15] This toxicity was particularly troublesome since it occasionally occurred in patients treated in the adjuvant situation with no known residual disease, and was difficult to predict or anticipate. Recent work has implicated renal precipitation of MTX, or its metabolite 7OH-MTX, as a likely initial event leading to renal failure, delayed drug excretion, ineffective leucovorin rescue and severe myelosuppression and mucositis. It appears that urinary alkalinization and a high urine volume during drug infusion can lower the incidence of toxic episodes by preventing MTX precipitation.[16,17] Such measures, however, are not uniformly effective, and monitoring of plasma drug concentration has become the primary measure utilized to detect patients at high risk of toxicity. Two studies, one from Memorial Sloan-Kettering[18] and the second from our laboratory at the National Cancer Institute,[19] have shown that: (1) patients who later become toxic invariably have elevated drug levels at 24 or 48 hours after drug infusion; (2) on the bases of early detection, certain therapeutic maneuvers, such as increased doses of leucovorin or forced diuresis, can be instituted to prevent the development of toxicity in patients with high plasma drug concentrations.

An example of the importance of drug concentration monitoring is provided by the case of patient 7 (Fig. 3-1). This patient, a 54-year-old male with soft tissue sarcoma, received a 6-hour infusion of 50 mg/kg, followed by leucovorin, 15 mg/m^2 every 6 hours for 7 doses. Forty-eight hours after beginning drug infusion he was found to have an elevated plasma concentration of MTX (0.96 μM versus 0.25 μM in nontoxic patients). On the basis of this abnormal value, increased leucovorin, 75 mg/m^2, was continued for an additional 11 days until plasma MTX concentration finally fell below the cytotoxic threshold of 1×10^{-8}M. Clinical toxicity was minimal with a white blood count nadir of 3200 on day 7 and a normal platelet count throughout this course. In our experience with over 400 treatment cycles of high-dose MTX, persistently elevated drug levels at 48 and 72 hours are invariably associated with severe myelosuppression unless supportive measures such as increased and extended leucovorin rescue (as used in this patient) are instituted promptly.[19]

The specific guidelines for normal or "safe" plasma concentration of MTX at specific time points after drug infusion have been described for two high-dose regimens (Table 3-1) in two separate studies, and these studies show surprisingly close correlation despite the differences in duration of infusion, and in the methods used to monitor drug concentration. A 24-hour value greater than 1×10^{-5}M, a 48-hour greater than 1×10^{-6}M, or a 72 hour value greater than 1×10^{-7}M, all carried a high likelihood of subsequent toxicity. We have chosen to monitor drug disappearance at 48 hours since the range in normal or "nontoxic" values is somewhat narrower at this point and the rate of decline of plasma values is slower than at earlier time points, minimizing the effect of deviations in the time of sample collection. It is likely that the "safe" value will differ for schedules with longer or shorter durations of drug infusion or major changes in dose, and will also depend on the

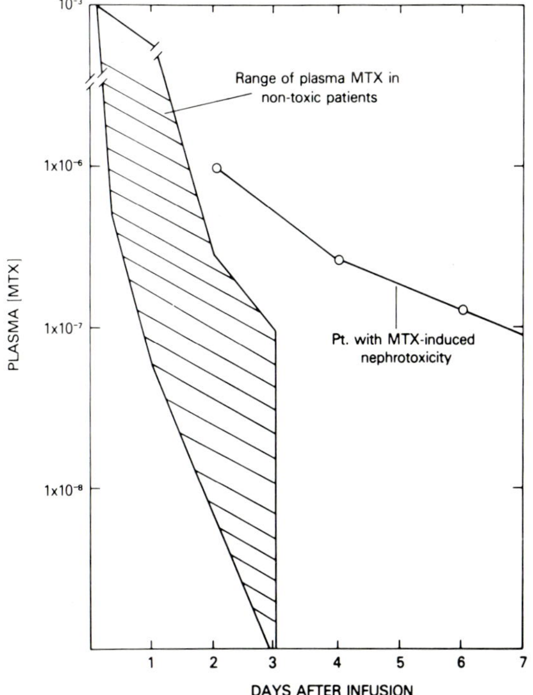

FIG. 3-1. Pharmacokinetic decay of methotrexate in plasma of nontoxic patients, and in toxic patient as described in text. Hatched area indicates the range of values in nontoxic patients who received 50 to 250 mg per kg, given as a six-hour infusion, beginning at time 0.

TABLE 3-1. *Plasma Methotrexate Guidelines in Monitoring High Dose Methotrexate Infusions*

	Ref.	Schedule of Infusion	Duration	Leucovorin Dose	Rescue Frequency	Toxic Methotrexate Level
1.	(19)	50–250 mg/kg	6 hrs.	15 mg/m²	q6h × 7	>0.96 μM at 48 hrs.
2.	(18)	8 gm/m²	4 hrs.	9–15 mg/m²	q6h × 12	>10 μM at 24 hrs. >1 μM at 48 hrs. >0.1 μM at 72 hrs.
3.	(16)	1.0 gm/m²	push	10 mg/m²	q6h × 11	>1.0 μM at 24 hrs.

dose and duration of leucovorin rescue. Thus, safe limits will have to be established for each new regimen which incorporates any major changes.

In the patient who develops acute renal failure during high-dose MTX therapy, drug level monitoring becomes an indispensable asset in determining the duration and magnitude of supplemental leucovorin rescue. Because of the toxicity to bone marrow of drug concentrations above 1×10^{-8}M, we have empirically chosen to continue rescue until plasma levels fall below this point. There are only approximations to guide dosage of leucovorin, since the pharmacokinetics of this compound are not completely understood. On the basis of in vitro studies, it is believed that a competitive relationship exists between MTX and leucovorin, and leucovorin levels must approach those of the antifolate in order to effect rescue. As a rough approximation, it is estimated that leucovorin doses of 15 mg/m² provide peak plasma levels of 1 μM; in the presence of higher concentrations of MTX, leucovorin dosage should be increased accordingly. Thus, the plasma MTX determination is central to the decision regarding leucovorin dosage.

Plasma MTX assays have made possible an analysis of the effectiveness of measures designed to accelerate MTX clearance in patients with renal failure. Recent work[20] has shown that peritoneal dialysis is virtually useless in promoting MTX clearance, while hemodialysis is capable of clearing 35 to 50 ml of plasma per minute, a figure well below that of normal renal clearance and, in one reported case, less than the renal clearance in a patient with mild renal failure (serum creatinine 2.5 mg/100 ml).

Enzymatic cleavage with carboxypeptidase G_1 has successfully removed circulating MTX in animals,[21] and in one clinical case,[22] but is not as yet available clinically on a routine basis. Other measures, including charcoal hemofiltration, are also undergoing analysis.

METHOTREXATE MONITORING IN PATIENTS WITH HEPATIC OR RENAL DYSFUNCTION

Present knowledge is incomplete with respect to the effect of renal or hepatic dysfunction on MTX disposition in humans. It is known that the bulk of conventional or high doses is excreted in the urine within 24 hours through a process that likely includes both tubular reabsorption of filtered drug and then tubular secretion. Renal failure leads to an altered clearance of MTX in proportion to the decrease in creatinine clearance[23] although the individual variability in renal excretion in patients with "normal" serum creatinine and BUN may be as great as might be anticipated in cases of mild renal dysfunction. At the present time, the best recommendation that can be made is to alter initial doses in proportion to the decrease in creatinine clearance and to further adjust therapy on the basis of monitored plasma values and toxicity.

Hepatic dysfunction has no known effect on MTX pharmacokinetics in humans. The drug undergoes enterohepatic circulation in animals, but controversy exists as to the extent and importance of biliary excretion in humans.[24] Little of the parent drug exits in the stool, and it is possible that significant metabolism of MTX takes place in liver, generating 7-OH-methotrexate,[25] and perhaps in the bowel where gut flora metabolism may yield the glutamate cleavage product, 2-4 diamino-N-10 methyl pteroic acid.[26] As mentioned previously, there is evidence in humans, monkeys and rodents of the presence of significant plasma concentrations of metabolite, equal to or greater than parent drug levels at late time points following both conventional and high doses. This evidence consists mainly of an excess of radioactivity present in plasma, as compared to reductase-inhibiting or binding activity, implying the presence of a non-inhibitory metabolite. The prospects for isolation and identification of metabolites in plasma have improved with development of high pressure liquid chromatographic techniques for separation of folate derivatives,[27] and structural identification of the plasma metabolites is currently under way in several laboratories.

Chemotherapy of Malignancies of the Central Nervous System

In no area of clinical chemotherapy has pharmacokinetic information had greater influence on the design of therapeutic regimens than in the therapy of CNS malignancies. This subject has been reviewed in detail in the recent "Workshop on Antimetabolites and the Central Nervous System";[28] only the major applications of drug level monitoring in the central nervous system will be discussed in this paper.

The primary uses of MTX assays in CSF have been: (1) to define pharmacokinetics and distribution in normal and disease states, (2) to provide guidelines for altering schedules and routes of administration, and (3) to aid in the differential diagnosis of MTX neurotoxicity versus progression of meningeal malignancy. The impetus for elucidation of the pharmacokinetics of MTX in CSF came from the studies of Bleyer et al, who detected marked delay in the disappearance of methotrexate from CSF in patients with drug-induced neurotoxicity as compared to nontoxic patients.[29] These studies defined a normal biphasic disappearance curve with half-lives ($\tau \frac{1}{2}$) of 4.5 and 14 hr, and indicated for the first time the practicality of routine pharmacological monitoring of CSF therapy.[30] Subsequent work by Shapiro and co-workers[31] showed a limited movement of drug between the lumbar and ventricular fluid compartments, a finding of considerable importance because of the reliance of chemotherapists on lumbar routes of administration for treating meningeal leukemia. Experimental protocols are now under study to compare the efficacy of MTX injected directly into the ventricular system via an Ommaya reservoir as compared to lumbar injection in the treatment of leukemic meningitis. Preliminary results indicate at least equivalent therapeutic efficacy for injections via the direct intraventricular route.[32] Bleyer has proposed the use of small frequent intraventricular injections as opposed to conventional lumbar therapy as a means of reducing neurotoxicity and has demonstrated the feasibility of selecting and achieving specific intraventricular levels based on pharmacokinetic models of drug disposition.[30] It is likely that intraventricular reservoir injection will become the preferred approach to therapy of established malignant disease of the leptomeninges.

The study of drug transit between plasma and CSF has been most rewarding, offering insight into the systemic toxicity of intrathecal therapy and suggesting high-dose systemic therapy as an alternative to intrathecal injection. Jacobs et al showed that, after intrathecal administration, methotrexate crosses slowly into the systemic circulation, moving primarily by bulk flow of CSF with a clearance approximating 20 ml per hour.[33] The levels achieved in plasma following lumbar injection, however, remained at toxic concentrations of greater than 1×10^{-8}M for up to 36 hours, a duration which may produce bone marrow suppression unless systemic leucovorin is used. The prolonged presence of plasma MTX after lumbar, intrathecal or intraventricular injections contrasts with the rapid disappearance and minimal toxicity of the same doses of drug given via the intravenous route.[33] While transport between the plasma and CSF compartments is limited, sufficient transit takes place to allow exploration of high-dose systemic therapy of leukemic meningitis as an alternative to direct CSF injection. The results of ongoing trials are too preliminary to allow conclusion regarding the relative efficacy of these routes, but it is clear that cytotoxic ($>10^{-8}$M) levels can be achieved and maintained for at least 48 hours.[16,34,35] CSF levels were, in general, 10 per cent or less of simultaneous plasma concentrations, although the plasma-CFS ratio varies with different schedules and changes with time following drug administration.[16,35,36,37]

Third Space Pharmacokinetics and Monitoring

In addition to insights provided for systemic and intrathecal chemotherapy by drug level monitoring, studies from Huffman et al,[38] and our own work,[39] explained the pharmacokinetics of transfer of drug from plasma to third space fluid compartments.

The presence of fluid accumulations in either pleural or peritoneal cavities causes characteristic delays in the elimination of MTX from the peripheral circulation due to an apparent hangup or depot effect of such compartments. An example of such an effect is illustrated in Figure 3-2, which shows the delayed elimination of MTX from plasma and ascites fluid of a patient with ovarian cancer and approximately a three-liter volume of ascites fluid. From this curve, it is apparent that there is an initial net movement of MTX from the systemic circulation into the ascites fluid with equilibration achieved at about 12 hours. As the plasma level falls with time, a period is entered in which the drug concentration in ascites fluid exceeds that of the plasma. During this latter period, the MTX in ascites fluid acts as a depot for the release of drug into the plasma compartment, resulting in an exaggerated delay in the MTX disappearance curve with a terminal $\tau 1/2$ of 36 hours as compared to a normal terminal $\tau 1/2$ of 12 hours. This propensity of either pleural or peritoneal effusions to act as a depot is dependent upon two characteristics: (1) the permeability of either the peritoneal or pleural membrane, which restricts flow of MTX into and out of that cavity, and (2) the volume of fluid in that cavity.*[40] Since the permeability of third compartment membranes is probably relatively constant in most clinical situations, the major variable determining the rate of clearance from this third space will be the volume of fluid. With large peritoneal and pleural effusions, the magnitude of this effect can be great enough to cause a markedly increased exposure of the patient's normal tissues to toxic levels of the drug. The practical management of this problem involves either of two approaches. Where possible, the fluid may be drained from either the pleural or peritoneal cavity prior to the administration of MTX. The alternate approach would be to very carefully

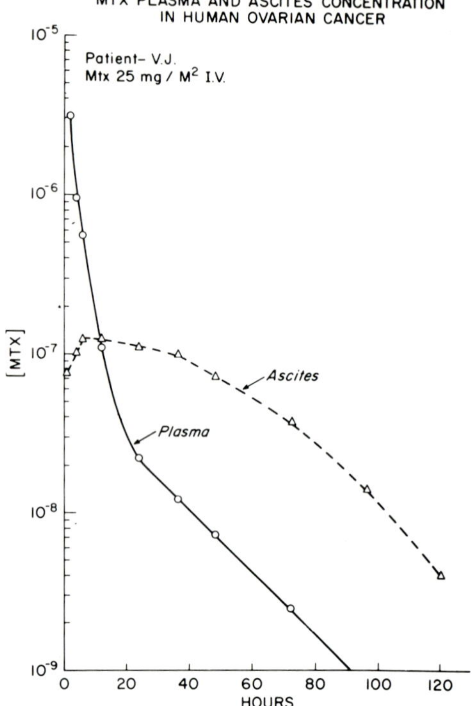

FIG. 3-2. Disappearance of methotrexate from plasma (solid line) and ascites (dashed line) following intravenous injection of 25 mg per m² dose in patient with ovarian carcinoma.

*The clearance of MTX from the third space compartment can be expressed by the formula:

$$Q = PA/V$$

where P is the permeability of a given compartment surface for a given drug, A is the surface area of the compartment, and V is the volume of fluid in the compartment.

monitor plasma MTX levels and begin leucovorin rescue if, at 24 to 36 hours, the plasma levels remain elevated.

The pharmacokinetics of this third space effect can be formalized according to the model illustrated in Figure 3-3. This simple diagrammatic model includes only two compartments, one for the third space and the other for the rest of the body. Each compartment is characterized by a volume and a drug concentration. Movement of drugs between the two compartments, as stated previously, is dependent on surface area and a permeability constant, resulting in a simple clearance value stated in milliliters per minute (ml/min), in the same fashion as renal clearance is calculated. In addition, the systemic compartment includes a pathway or pathways for drug elimination, again characterized by a clearance constant resulting from renal, hepatic or other mechanisms of drug elimination. Based on this model, it is possible to visualize utilization of third space sequestration in a way which may be of greater therapeutic importance than the depot accumulation in third spaces after systemic administration. In an increasing number of clinical situations, direct administration of drugs into a third space is being used as therapy because of certain characteristics which become readily apparent from this model. The first and most widely recognized situation where such an approach is utilized is in the therapy of meningeal involvement with either carcinoma or leukemia as previously discussed. Similarly, nitrogen mustard injection into the pleural space and ^{32}P injection into ascites have been utilized for many years to deal with malignant effusion.

In these situations, with limited diffusion of drug into the systemic circulation, the total concentration × time exposure in the third compartment vastly exceeds that in the plasma space. The results of direct intraperitoneal or intrapleural administration of MTX have not been previously studied but might be expected to behave in a fashion similar to that of the intrathecal installation, resulting in a significant concentration differential between the third space and the plasma. Predictions based on the therapeutic potential of such a route of administration have never been fully explored. Certainly there are clinical conditions where the ability to achieve very high local levels of MTX in the absence of significant systemic toxicity might be of value, as in the treatment of ovarian carcinoma.

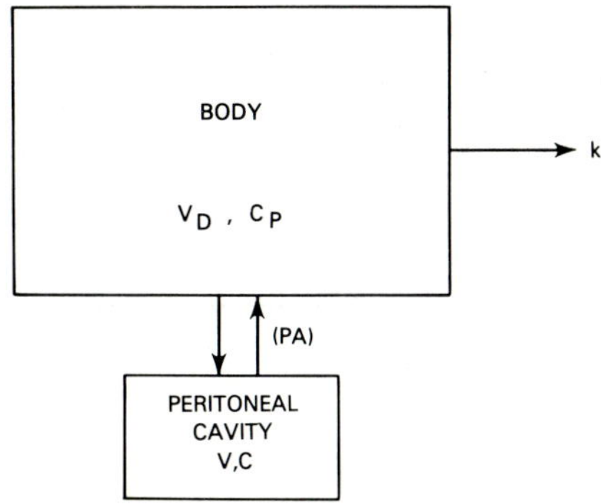

FIG. 3-3. Two-compartment representation of drug distribution between peritoneal cavity and the remainder of body space. V_D is the volume of distribution in the total body compartment, excluding ascites, and C_p is the drug concentration in this compartment. V and C are corresponding volume and concentration in the ascites compartment. P is the permeability and A the area of the peritoneal compartment, and k is the elimination rate constant from the total body compartment

Drug Interactions and Monitoring

After conventional doses of MTX, or in high-dose protocol, the major route of elimination of MTX is via both filtration and tu-

TABLE 3-2. *Drugs Which May Compete with Methotrexate for the Proximal Tubular Weak Acid Transport System*

1. Sulfonamide
2. Thiazides
3. Penicillin and its semisynthetic derivatives
4. Phenylbutazone
5. Cephalosporins
6. Probenecid
7. Uric Acid
8. Salicylates
9. Barbiturates
10. Nalidixic Acid
11. Nitrofurantoin

bular secretion. Normal MTX renal clearance has been estimated to be 200 ml/minute.[20] For this reason, any factor which impairs glomerular filtration or tubular secretion can lead to prolonged plasma levels of MTX and, therefore, severe toxicity. Certainly co-administration of MTX with potential renal toxins must be accompanied by careful monitoring of the plasma methotrexate levels, so that leucovorin rescue may be begun in a timely fashion if needed. Because tubular secretion is also involved in elimination of MTX from plasma, co-administration of other weak acids may conceivably delay the secretion or the elimination of MTX (see Table 3-2). At present this drug interaction is largely theoretical as there are no studies of the effect of such common agents as aspirin or carbenicillin on the excretion of methotrexate. In the absence of firm guidelines, it would seem prudent to monitor plasma MTX levels in those patients who are receiving any of the drugs listed in Table 3-2 along with MTX, particularly in a high-dose MTX regimen.

References

1. Bertino J R, and Fischer G A: Techniques for study of resistance to folic acid antagonists. Methods Med Res 10:297–307, 1964
2. Myers C E, Lippman M E, Eliot H M, Chabner B A: Competitor protein binding assay for methotrexate. Proc Natl Acad Sci USA 72:3683–3686, 1975
3. Arons E, Rothenberg S P, DaCosta M, et al: A direct ligand binding radioassay for the measurement of methotrexate in tissues and biological fluids. Cancer Res 35:1407–1410, 1975
4. Myers C E, Eliot H M, Chabner B A: Competitor dihydrofolate reductase binding assay for triaginate, methasquin, and aminopterin. Cancer Treat Rep 60:615–616, 1976
5. Levine L, Powers E: A radioimmunoassay for methotrexate. Res Commun Chem Pathol Pharmacol 9:543–554, 1974
6. Kimelberg H K, Biddlecombe S M, Bourke R S: Distribution and degradation of [^{3}H] methotrexate after intravenous and cerebral intraventricular injection in primates. Cancer Res 37:157–165, 1977
7. Huffman D H, Wan S H, Azarnoff D L, et al: Pharmacokinetics of methotrexate. Clin Pharmacol Ther 14:572–579, 1973
8. Mehta B M, Hutchison D J: Microbiologic assays of cancer chemotherapeutic agents. Cancer Treat Rep 61:597–602, 1977
9. Goldman I D: Analysis of the cytotoxic determinants for methotrexate (NSC-740): A role for "free" intracellular drug. Cancer Chemother Rep 6:51–61, 1975
10. Chabner B A, Young R C: Threshold methotrexate concentration for in vivo inhibition of DNA synthesis in normal and tumorous target tissues. J Clin Invest 52:1804–1811, 1973
11. Pinedo H M, Chabner B A: Role of drug concentration, duration of exposure and endogenous metabolites in determining methotrexate cytotoxicity. Cancer Treat Rep 61:709–715, 1977
12. Pinedo H M, Zaharko D S, Bull J M, et al: The relative contribution of drug concentration and duration of exposure to mouse bone marrow toxicity during continuous methotrexate infusion. Cancer Res 37:445–450, 1977
13. Levitt M, Mosher M B, DeConti R C, et al: Improved therapeutic index of methotrexate with "leucovorin rescue." Cancer Res 33: 1729–1734, 1973
14. Jaffe N, Paed D: Recent advances in the chemotherapy of metastatic osteogenic sarcoma. Cancer 30:1627–1631, 1972
15. Von Hoff D D, Penta J S, Helman L J, et al: The incidence of drug-related deaths secondary to high dose methotrexate and citrovorum administration. Cancer Treat Rep 61:745–748, 1977
16. Pittman S W, Frei E III: Weekly methotrexate-calcium leucovorin rescue: Effect of alkalinization on nephrotoxicity; pharmacokinetics in the CNS; and use in CNS non-Hodgkin's lymphoma. Cancer Treat Rep 61:691–694, 1977
17. Stoller R G, Jacobs S A, Drake J C, et al: Pharmacokinetics of high-dose methotrexate (NSC-740). Cancer Chemoth Rep 6:19–24, 1975
18. Nirenberg A, Mosende C, Mehta B, et al: High-dose methotrexate with citrovorum factor rescue: Predictive value of serum methotrexate concentrations and corrective measures to avert toxicity. Cancer Treat Rep 61:779–783, 1977
19. Stoller R G, Hande K R, Jacobs S A, et al: Use of plasma pharmacokinetics to predict and prevent methotrexate toxicity. N Engl J Med 297:630–633, 1977
20. Hande K R, Balow J E, Drake J C, et al: Clear-

ance of methotrexate by peritoneal and hemodialysis. Ann Intern Med, (in press)

21. Chabner B A, Johns D G, Bertino J R: Enzymatic cleavage of methotrexate provides a method for prevention of drug toxicity. Nature 239:395–397, 1972
22. Bertino J R, Skeel R, Makulu D, et al: Initial clinical studies with carboxypeptidase G_1 (CPG_1), a folate depleting enzyme. Clin Res 22:483 (abstr), 1974
23. Kristensen L O, Weismann K, Hutters L: Renal function and the rate of disappearance of methotrexate from serum. Eur J Clin Pharmacol 8:439–444, 1975
24. Leme P R, Creaven P J, Allen L M, et al: Kinetic model for the disposition and metabolism of moderate and high-dose methotrexate (NSC-740) in man. Cancer Chemother Rep 59:811–817, 1975
25. Jacobs S A, Stoller R G, Chabner B A, et al: 7-hydroxy methotrexate as a urinary metabolite in human subjects and rhesus monkeys receiving high-dose methotrexate. J Clin Invest 57:534–538, 1976
26. Valerino D M, Johns D G, Zaharko D S, et al: Studies of the metabolism of methotrexate by intestinal flora. I. Identification and study of biological properties of the metabolite 4-amino-4-deoxy-N^{10}-methyl-pteroic acid. Biochem Pharmacol 21:821–831, 1972
27. Watson L, Cohen J L, Chan K K: High pressure liquid chromatographic determination of methotrexate and its major metabolite 7-hydroxy methotrexate in human plasma. Cancer Treat Rep, (in press)
28. Shapiro W B, Mehta B M, Hutchison D J, (eds): Proceedings of the Workshop on Antimetabolites and the Central Nervous System. Cancer Treat Rep 61:505–757, 1977
29. Bleyer W A, Drake J C, Chabner B A: Neurotoxicity and elevated cerebrospinal-fluid methotrexate concentration in meningeal leukemia. N Engl J Med 289:770–773, 1973
30. Bleyer W A, Dedrick R L: Clinical pharmacology of intrathecal methotrexate. I. Pharmacokinetics in nontoxic patients after lumbar injection. Cancer Treat Rep 61:703–708, 1977
31. Shapiro W R, Young D F, Mehta B M: Methotrexate distribution in cerebrospinal fluid after intravenous, ventricular, and lumbar injections. N Engl J Med 293:161–166, 1975
32. Shapiro W R, Posner J B, Ushio Y, et al: Treatment of meningeal neoplasms. Cancer Treat Rep 61:733–744, 1977
33. Jacobs S A, Bleyer W A, Chabner B A, et al: Altered plasma pharmacokinetics of methotrexate administered intrathecally. Lancet 1:455–456, 1975
34. Rosen G, Ghavimi F, Nirenberg A, et al: High dose methotrexate with citrovorum factor rescue for the treatment of central nervous system tumors in children. Cancer Treat Rep 61:681–690, 1977
35. Freeman A I, Wang J J, Sinks L F: High Dose methotrexate in acute lymphocytic leukemia. Cancer Treat Rep 61:727–732, 1977
36. Berlinger N J, Mehta B M, Juhn S K, Hutchison D J: Perilymph penetration of methotrexate in cats. Cancer Treat Rep 61:613–616, 1977
37. Blasberg B G, Patlak C S, Shapiro W R: Distribution of methotrexate in the cerebrospinal fluid and brain after intraventricular administration. Cancer Treat Rep 61:633–642, 1977
38. Wan S H, Huffman D H, Azarnoff D L, et al: Effect of route of administration and effusions on methotrexate pharmacokinetics. Cancer Res 34:3487, 34–91, 1974
39. Dedrich R L, Meyers C E, Bungay P M, DeVita V T: Pharmacokinetic rationale for peritoneal drug administration in the treatment of ovarian cancer. Cancer Treat Rep 62:1–12, 1978
40. Zaharko D S, Dedrick R L: Antifolates: in vivo considerations. Cancer Treat Rep 61:513–518, 1977

Gerald W. Crabtree

4

Mechanisms of Action of Pyrimidine and Purine Analogues

The "mechanism of action" of a chemotherapeutic agent is the manner in which it exerts its effects (cytotoxic, cytolytic, etc.). For many purine and pyrimidine analogues used as anticancer agents, the mechanisms of action have not been definitely identified. Rather, possible mechanisms of action have been proposed and the identification of the particular event(s) responsible for their action remain to be elucidated.

The large number of pyrimidine and purine analogues developed and examined over the years makes the task of a comprehensive review of this field impossible within the limits of this review. Instead, specific examples of each of these classes of agents will be used to illustrate various possible sites of action which may be responsible for the cytotoxicities of many of these compounds. The analogues to be discussed here (arabinosylcytosine for the pyrimidines; 6-thioguanine, 6-selenoguanine, and some adenosine analogues for the purines) have not been chosen because they are the most useful compounds from a clinical point of view, nor because most information is available on them, but because they illustrate that, even though such compounds have been studied in depth, their sites of action are still equivocal. In addition, other, perhaps better known, representatives of these classes of agents have been discussed in previous volumes of this series.[1,2] In the discussion of these compounds which follows, many pertinent references will not be included—only specific references will be made to illustrate various points. This procedure should not be interpreted as a value judgment on the omitted material but as a concession to the limitations of space in this review.

Pyrimidines and purines are found as major constituents of cells both at the level of polymerized nucleotides (DNA, RNA) and as "free" nucleotides (ATP, GTP, etc.). Free nucleosides and bases usually represent only a very small percentage of the total pyrimidine and purine contents of cells. In addition to serving as precursors for nucleic acid synthesis, free nucleotides also play roles in energy metabolism, in group transfer reactions, as mediators of hormone action (e.g., 3′-5′-cyclic AMP) and as metabolic regulators. Pyrimidine and purine analogues, as a general rule, must also be converted to their respective nucleotides before they are active as chemotherapeutic agents. Therefore, a generalized scheme

Supported by grants CA 13943 and CA 07340 from the United States Public Health Service and CH-7R from the American Cancer Society.

of nucleotide metabolism will be presented below for each of the two major types of analogues under study.

Figure 4-1 presents a "backbone" scheme of the anabolic pathways involving pyrimidine nucleotides. Thus, pyrimidine nucleotides may be synthesized by a *de novo* pathway or from preformed pyrimidines (some of the nucleoside kinases are shown here). Uridine monophosphate (UMP), the useful end product of the *de novo* pathway, can be converted (at the level of UTP) into cytidine nucleotides and cytidine triphosphate (CTP) and UTP can be incorporated into RNA. For DNA synthesis, cytidine diphosphate (CDP) is reduced by ribonucleotide reductase to deoxycytidine diphosphate (dCDP) which can be converted readily into deoxycytidine triphosphate (dCTP). Uridine diphosphate (UDP) is reduced by this same enzyme to deoxyuridine diphosphate (dUDP), this is dephosphorylated and deoxythymidine monophosphate (dTMP) is formed from deoxyuridine monophosphate (dUMP) in a reaction catalyzed by thymidylate synthetase. Deoxythymidine triphosphate (dTTP) is synthesized from dTMP, and dTTP together with dCTP can be incorporated into DNA.

Pyrimidine Analogues (1-β-D-arabinofuranosylcytosine)

Arabinosylcytosine (1-β-D-arabinofuranosylcytosine; cytosine arabinoside, cytarabine; cytosar; araC) is viewed biologically as an analogue of 2′-deoxycytidine (see Fig. 4-2) rather than cytidine, even though the sugar moiety does contain a 2′-hydroxyl group. AraC must be phosphorylated to inhibit cellular proliferation.[3] The enzyme responsible for this conversion, deoxycytidine kinase (reaction 1, Fig. 4-1), has been isolated and partially purified from various mammalian sources, including L1210 cells[4] and calf thymus cells.[5] 2′-Deoxycytidine appears to have more affinity for the enzyme than does araC which may explain, in part, reversal of araC effects by 2′-deoxycytidine.[6,7] Further support for the role of deoxycytidine kinase in the phosphorylation of araC is that one of the major mechanisms of resistance to araC appears to be diminished deoxycytidine kinase activity.[6-8]

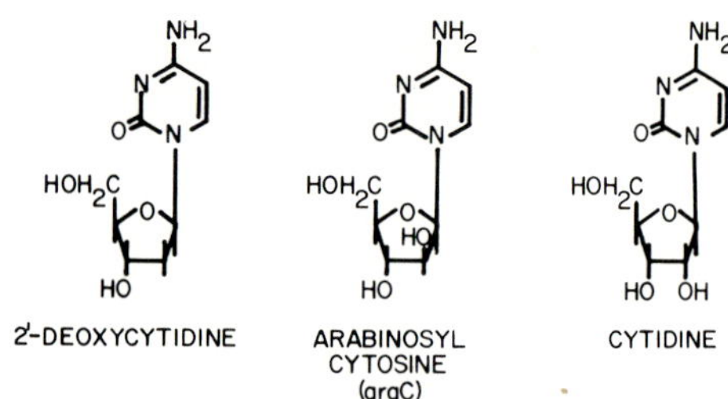

FIG. 4-2 Structural formulae of 2′-deoxycytidine, arabinosylcytosine and cytidine.

AraCMP appears to be converted readily to araCDP and araCTP by the same nucleotide kinases which convert the respective deoxycytidine nucleotides (Fig. 4-1). In fact, the predominant form of araC in cells appears to be araCTP.[8,9]

Much evidence has accumulated over the years which shows that araC inhibits the syn-

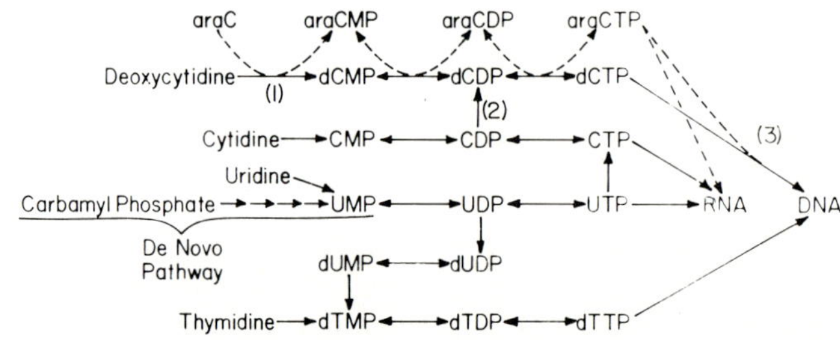

FIG. 4-1 Simplified metabolic scheme of pyrimidine nucleotide metabolism. Dashed arrows indicate reactions in which arabinosylcytosine or its nucleotides participate. Numbers in parentheses refer to the following enzymic reactions: (1) deoxycytidine kinase, (2) ribonucleoside diphosphate reductase, (3) DNA polymerase.

thesis of DNA in various types of mammalian cells.[3,10-16] The actual "site" of this inhibitory effect, however, has been the subject of controversy. The three major "sites" which have been investigated most intensively are: (1) the ribonucleoside diphosphate reductase reaction (reaction 2, Fig. 4-1); (2) the DNA polymerase step (reaction 3, Fig. 4-1); and (3) incorporation of araC into nucleic acids.

Early studies by Chu and Fischer pointed to inhibition of ribonucleoside diphosphate reductase by a phosphorylated metabolite of araC as being a primary site of action of this analogue.[3,6] They showed that the incorporation of [^{3}H]uridine into deoxycytidine nucleotides and DNA was reduced by treatment of cells with araC, whereas incorporation into RNA was unaffected. Further evidence to support this hypothesis was obtained when they showed that 2′-deoxycytidine could reverse the effects of araC, presumably because the 2′-deoxycytidine could be converted directly to dCTP and this would circumvent the block at the CDP → dCDP step by the araC nucleotide. AraC was also shown to inhibit the uptake of other precursors such as cytidine into DNA. [10,13,15,16] Support for the hypothesis that inhibition of the reduction of CDP to dCDP is the primary factor in the cytotoxic action of araC has, however, diminished within the last few years.

AraC treatment can result in irreversible damage to cells and simple competitive inhibition by an araC nucleotide cannot account for this observation. Furthermore, ribonucleoside diphosphate reductase partially purified from Novikoff hepatoma is only moderately inhibited by araCDP and araCTP to about the same degree as is shown with dCTP.[17] Finally, recent data on the changes in the sizes of intracellular pools of deoxyribonucleotides after exposure of cells to araC, reveal that only transient decreases in dCTP pools are seen in mouse embryo cells, whereas the levels of deoxyadenosine triphophate (dATP), dTTP and deoxyguanosine triphosphate (dGTP) increased.[18] AraC treatment has no effect on the pools of deoxycytidine phosphates in human leukemic leukocytes.[19]

In 1964, when much of the work on the mechanism of action of araC was focused on ribonucleoside diphosphate reductase, Cardeilhac and Cohen reported that DNA polymerase from *E. coli* was not inhibited by araCTP.[20] With crude DNA polymerase preparations from mammalian cells, however, araCTP was shown to be inhibitory and competed with dCTP.[19,21,22] These findings were extended by studies with DNA polymerases from calf thymus[23] and L-cells[24] which revealed that araCTP had inhibition constant (K_i) values of the same order of magnitude as the Michaelis constant (K_m) values for dCTP. Recent studies by Momparler[25] verified that inhibition by araCTP depends on competition with dCTP when he showed that with calf thymus DNA polymerase and poly (dA-dT) as template, araCTP did not inhibit the incorporation of dTTP into acid-insoluble material. As an interesting sidelight to the studies discussed above, work with viral RNA-directed DNA polymerase has revealed that this enzyme is more potently inhibited by araCTP than is the DNA-dependent enzyme.[26] This result may explain, in part, the ability of araC to interfere with replication of, and transformation by, oncogenic RNA viruses.

The third possibility that araC may exert lethality by its incorporation into DNA has also been examined in detail. Furth and Cohen were unable to detect significant incorporation of araCTP into DNA using the DNA polymerases from calf thymus or bovine lymphosarcoma.[23] Chu and Fischer,[6,10] however, reported the incorporation of radioactivity into the DNA and RNA of L5178Y cells incubated with [^{3}H]araC. Subsequently, they were able to isolate labelled araCMP after degrading the nucleic acids of such treated cells.[11] These studies have been confirmed by other workers using various types of cells.[13,16,27] It should be noted, however, that in all of these studies, the amount of araCTP incorporation into DNA appeared to be quite small.

Studies similar to these with intact cells have also been performed at the isolated enzyme level. AraCTP can partially substitute for dCTP in DNA synthesis catalyzed by the DNA was observed with L-cell DNA polymerase.[24] No evidence was obtained in either of these reports for the incorporation of the analogue into a terminal position of the polynucleotide chain. Momparler found that calf thymus DNA polymerase catalyzed the incorporation of [^{3}H]araCTP into poly dC:poly dG but not into poly (dA:dT).[25] In contrast to previous reports, however, when DNA containing [α-^{32}P]-araCMP was synthesized enzymatically using denatured DNA as template, and the labelled DNA was digested enzymatically, data were obtained which suggested that incorporation of araCTP into the DNA resulted in the termination of polynucleotide chain growth.

The importance of araC incorporation into DNA as being a major factor in the cytotoxic action of this drug is open to question. With mouse L-cells, no correlation could be established between cell death and incorporation of araC into DNA.[24] In L5178Y cells, at high levels of araC, acute cell death appeared to correlate with incorporation of the drug into RNA rather than into DNA.[10,11] Chu[29] confirmed these results and extended this work by showing that incorporation of [^{3}H]araC into the DNA of L5178Y cells ceased after 1 hour of incubation, whereas incorporation into RNA was linear and correlated with cell death. Incorporation of araCTP into DNA was reduced by pretreatment of cells with MTX, although much more cell death occurred. Furthermore, analysis of time course studies with labelled RNA on sucrose gradients revealed that [^{3}H]araC was incorporated mostly into RNA in the 2-16S region. Further fractionation of the 2-16S material showed that label appeared first in 1-2S RNA, then in 2-4S RNA, and then in heavier RNA. Chu also reported that pretreatment of cells with araC caused marked inhibition of the incorporation of [^{3}H]uridine into 2-7S RNA but did not inhibit incorporation into other RNA fractions.[29]

From the studies outlined above, it appears that araC can be incorporated into all polynucleotides but that only incorporation into small molecular weight RNA may be important for acute cytotoxicity. Incorporation into DNA may play a role in delayed effects (chromosome damage, etc.) seen with this analogue. Inhibition of ribonucleoside diphosphate reductase may play a role under certain special conditions (e.g., high dose therapy). At the present time, however, the metabolic effect of araC that is most implicated as responsible for its antitumor action is inhibition of DNA polymerase.

Purine Analogs

6-Thioguanine and 6-Selenoguanine

Some of the reactions involving purine nucleotides are given in Figure 4-3. Thus, purine nucleotides may be synthesized via *de novo* and preformed pathways. In many types of cells, adenine and guanine nucleotides are interconvertible, the common nucleotide being IMP (inosine 5′-monophosphate).

6-Thioguanine (6-TG) is identical in structure to the natural purine base guanine with the exception that the oxygen atom on the 6-position of the purine ring is replaced by a sulfur atom (Fig. 4-4). The initial step in the "activation" of 6-TG is its conversion to 6-thioGMP in a reaction (reaction 1, Fig. 4-3) catalyzed by hypoxanthine-guanine phosphoribosyltransferase (HGPRTase). This conversion is necessary for the cytotoxic action of

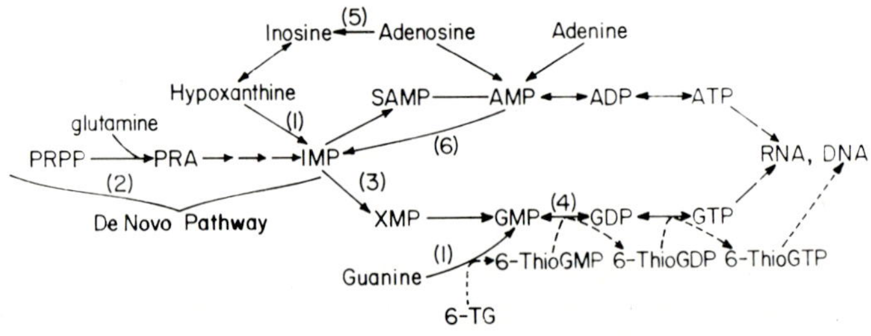

FIG. 4-3 Simplified metabolic scheme of purine nucleotide metabolism. Dashed arrows indicate reactions in which 6-thioguanine or its nucleotides participate. Numbers in parentheses refer to the following enzymic reactions: (1) hypoxanthine-guanine phosphoribosyltransferase, (2) PRPP-amidotransferase, (3) IMP dehydrogenase, (4) GMP kinase, (5) adenosine deaminase, (6) 5′-AMP deaminase.

6-TG.[30] Although 6-thioGMP is a major metabolite of 6-TG in many types of cells, 6-thioGDP and 6-thioGTP have also been detected.[31-38] Three major areas have been investigated in efforts to relate effects of 6-TG metabolites to cytotoxicity: (1) purine biosynthesis *de novo*, (2) interconversions of purine nucleotides, and (3) incorporation into DNA.

The first committed step of the *de novo* pathway of purine biosynthesis is catalyzed by the enzyme PRPP-amidotransferase (reaction 2, Fig. 4-3) which is subject to pseudofeedback inhibition by 6-thioGMP.[39-43] The enzyme from pigeon liver is inhibited by 6-thioGMP with a K_i value of 0.1 mM.[40] With the enzyme from mouse tumor cells, 50 per cent inhibition was achieved at a 6-thioGMP concentration of 0.27 mM.[43] Thus, inhibition of this enzyme by 6-thioGMP may be manifested in some types of 6-TG-treated cells since concentrations of 6-thioGMP of 0.1 mM or greater may be achieved in such cells.[31,32,36] These data with isolated PRPP-amidotransferases have been corroborated in experiments which show that the incorporation of [^{14}C]glycine into purines is inhibited in cells pretreated with 6-TG.[36,44] Possible metabolites of 6-TG other than 6-thioGMP, such as 6-methylthioGMP, do not appear to play a role in the inhibition of purine biosynthesis *de novo* by 6-TG.[43]

One of the enzymes involved in purine nucleotide interconversions which has been reported to be inhibited by 6-thioGMP is IMP dehydrogenase[45-47] (reaction 3, Fig. 4-3), which catalyzes the first of two steps in the conversion of IMP to GMP. Since the inhibition is reversed by sulfhydryl reagents,[32,46] the formation of disulfide bonds between the active site of the enzyme and 6-thioGMP appears to play a role in the inhibition. GMP kinase (reaction 4, Fig. 4-3) has also been the subject of much interest in the past. The enzyme from hog brain and Sarcoma 180 cells was shown to be inhibited competitively by 6-thioGMP ($K_i = 6 \times 10^{-5}$M; K_m for GMP $= 1 \times 10^{-5}$ M) and although 6-thioGMP appeared to be a substrate for the enzyme, the maximal velocity was low.[48]

As a consequence of the studies discussed above, Miech et al postulated that the presence of 6-thioGMP in cells, by inhibiting reactions catalyzed by PRPP-amidotransferase, IMP dehydrogenase and GMP kinase, might result in a general depletion of guanine nucleotides within the cells and this depletion could have serious, possibly lethal, consequences.[32,48] In the light of recent data, however, this hypothesis must be reevaluated. Miller et al[49] have shown that previous data obtained by Meich and coworkers[32,48] concerning the inhibition of GMP kinase by 6-thioGMP were in error due to the presence of an artifact in the spectrophotometric assay system used for their experiments. The recent studies showed that the weak inhibition by 6-thioGMP (K_i about 2.3 mM) is related to the alternative substrate activity of this compound (K_m = 2.1 mM; V_{max} about 3 per cent of that with GMP as substrate).[49] Thus, at concentrations of 6-thioGMP achieved in cells treated with 6-TG, inhibition of GMP kinase per se does not appear to be the site of action of this analogue. This conclusion has been supported by studies with intact cells which indicate that pretreatment of cells with 6-TG has little or no effect on the conversion of guanine to GTP.[36,50,51] In view of the other metabolic inhibitions seen with 6-thioGMP (see above), however, the slow reactivity of 6-thioGMP with GMP kinase and the resultant transient accumulation of 6-thioGMP may be responsible for certain of the cytolytic manifestations of 6-TG.[36]

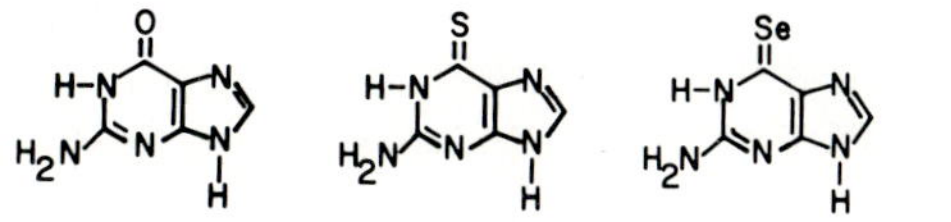

GUANINE 6-THIOGUANINE 6-SELENOGUANINE

FIG. 4-4 Structural formulae of guanine, 6-thioguanine and 6-selenoguanine.

The third possible mode of action of 6-TG is via incorporation into DNA. LePage and coworkers, in intensive studies, have concluded that the incorporation of 6-TG into DNA and cellular toxicity are related.[44,52-55] Their results showed that, whereas *de novo* purine biosynthesis was inhibited to the same extent in both 6-TG-sensitive and insensitive lymphomas,[44] incorporation of 6-TG into DNA was much lower in the 6-TG-insensitive tumor than in the sensitive cells.[44,54] In apparent support of the DNA incorporation theory, β-2′-deoxythioguanosine was shown to have antitumor activity against 6-TG-resistant tumor lines and to the 6-TG-insensitive Mecca lymphosarcoma[56] and was found to be incorporated into the DNA of Mecca cells much more rapidly than 6-TG.[55] Presumably, β-2′-deoxythioguanosine has an advantage over 6-TG as a chemotherapeutic agent because fewer steps would be required for its incorporation into DNA. As noted by Nelson et al,[51] however, the results with β-2′-deoxythioguanosine and Mecca lymphosarcoma appear to be inconclusive since this tumor has poor chemotherapeutic response to this analogue nucleoside and, in fact, seems to be resistant to both 6-TG and β-2′-deoxythioguanosine. In this regard, sublines of human epidermoid carcinoma (H. Ep. #2) and L1210 cells resistant to 6-mercaptopurine by virtue of a loss in hypoxanthine-guanine phosphoribosytransferase (HGPRTase) activity, are clearly cross-resistant to both 6-TG and β-2′-deoxythioguanosine.[57]

In spite of the inconclusive nature of some of the work with β-2′-deoxythioguanosine discussed above, much additional support has accumulated for the "6-TG incorporation into DNA" theory as an explanation of cytotoxicity to 6-TG. Thus, araC, a well-established inhibitor of DNA synthesis (see above), protected mice against 6-TG toxicity.[58-60] Nelson et al reported that inhibition of DNA synthesis in H. Ep. #2 cells in culture by 1 mM thymidine protected cells against 6-TG, whereas inhibition of RNA synthesis by a combination of 6-azauridine and deoxycytidine did not protect cells against this analogue.[51] In the same study, 6-TG toxicity was not reversed by aminoimidazolecarboxamide (bypasses the blockage of PRPP-amidotransferase) suggesting that inhibition of purine biosynthesis *de novo* was not responsible for 6-TG effects and incorporation of labelled hypoxanthine or guanine into GTP was not affected by 6-TG treatment. Accordingly, these workers concluded that 6-TG was toxic due to its incorporation into cellular DNA. Consistent with this conclusion are data obtained by Barranco and Humphrey.[61] Using synchronized Chinese hamster ovarian cells, these workers showed that exposure of cells to β-2′-deoxythioguanosine for short intervals during various phases of the cell cycle did not prevent further progression of these cells through the cycle and into mitosis even though 90 per cent of the cells were ultimately destined to die; that is, lethality of the treatment was not expressed immediately and cells completed the cycle during which they were exposed to the drug. Similar investigations by Tidd and coworkers revealed that exposure of L5178Y cells in culture to 6-mercaptopurine, 6-TG or β-2′-deoxythioguanosine, for a 13-hour-period did not result in immediate cellular death and in fact, cellular multiplication continued for one or more divisions before death occurred.[62,64] Therefore, the delayed cytotoxicity seen in cells treated with 6-thiopurines was attributed to the time necessary for incorporation of the drug into DNA. Interestingly, 6-mercaptopurine appeared to be incorporated into cellular DNA in the form of 6-TG.[64]

The significance of "delayed cytotoxicity" as unequivocal evidence for the incorporation of purine analogues into cellular DNA as being a mechanism of drug action is questionable, however, in the light of recent data obtained with 6-selenoguanine (Fig. 4-4) and its derivatives. 6-Selenoguanine (6-SeG) and its ribonucleoside (6-SeGR) and deoxyribonucleoside derivatives are known to be comparable in antitumor activities to the corresponding 6-thio compounds.[65-71] Biochemical studies have shown that 6-TG and 6-SeG are similar in substrate activity for several enzymes of purine metabolism.[69,72] As noted above, 6-TG or its ribonucleoside, 6-TGR, can form significant amounts of 6-thioGDP and 6-thioGTP when incubated with intact cells.[34-38] Similar experiments with 6-SeG or 6-SeGR have revealed that primarily the 5′-monophosphate nucleotide, 6-SeGMP, accumulates intracellularly with the formation of only small amounts of di- and triphosphate nucleotides even after prolonged exposure to the drugs.[34,35,69,73] Thus, if the 6-selenoguanine compounds are not converted intracellularly into polyphosphate nucleotides in substantial quantities, they should not be incorporated into cellular DNA at toxic levels. In support of this hypothesis, LePage has reported that the incorporation of radioactivity from [^{75}Se]-labelled 6-SeGR (or its α- and β-deoxyribonucleoside counterparts) into the DNA of 6C3HED lymphosarcoma cells (susceptible to treatment with 6-selenoguanine nucleosides but not 6-TGR) is below detectable levels.[71] Recent work by Robison et al, however, has revealed that virtually identical "delayed cytotoxicities" are manifested when L5178Y cells are treated with either 6-TGR or 6-SeGR.[37] Under conditions in which delayed cytotoxic effects were seen, 6-TGR was shown to be converted into 6-thioGMP, 6-thioGDP and 6-thioGTP whereas 6-SeGR accumulated primarily at the 6-SeGMP level with the formation of only small amounts of the di- and triphosphate nucleotides.

In summary, no single mechanism of action of 6-TG can be singled out for all types of cells at the present time. DNA incorporation may play a role in some cells but this may not be true for all types of cells.[51] On the other hand, effects of accumulation of the 5′-monophosphate nucleotide derivatives of such analogues cannot be ruled out as a viable mechanism to explain the cytotoxicity of 6-TG and related compounds.[36,37]

An important corollary to the material discussed above is the potential usefulness of the 6-selenoguanine compounds as chemotherapeutic agents. Although the seleno analogues appear to be as effective as their thio counterparts as antitimor agents, they do not appear, from evidence presently at hand, to be capable of being incorporated into the DNA. Thus, all of the undesirable consequences of such incorporation, for example, carcinogenesis, mutagenesis and teratogenesis, should be avoided through the use of 6-seleno compounds for chemotherapy.

Adenosine Analogues and Adenosine Deaminase Inhibitors

Adenosine analogues are receiving much interest as potential chemotherapeutic agents (for recent reviews, see references 74–79). The usefulness of these analogues is limited by their reactivity with the enzyme adenosine deaminase (ADA) (reaction 5, Fig. 4-4) which is responsible for the inactivation of many of these compounds[74-76,80,81] before they can be converted into their respective nucleotides (a prerequisite for cytotoxicity). Two mechanisms for circumventing the ADA reaction while maintaining the chemotherapeutic potential of adenosine analogues are: (1) the development of analogues which are resistent to deamination by ADA but which may be converted into analogue nucleotides, and (2) the identification of potent inhibitors of ADA which may be co-administered with analogues which are subject to inactivation by ADA. The latter mechanism will be discussed below.

A series of ADA inhibitors (see Fig. 4-5) which vary greatly in potency has been identified. Included in this series are coformycin (3 - β - D - ribofuranosyl - 6,7,8 - trihydroimidazo[3,4-d][1,3]diazepin-8-(R)-ol),[82] 2′-deoxycoformycin ((R)-3-(2-deoxy-β-D-erythropentofuranosyl)-3,6,7,8-tetrahydroimidazo[4,5-d][1,3]diazepin-8-ol, Covidarabine),[83] EHNA (erythro-9-(2-hydroxy-3-nonyl)adenine),[84] and DHMPR (1,6-dihydro-6-hydroxymethylpurine ribonucleoside).[85]

Initial studies with partially purified human erythrocytic ADA which employed classical methods of enzyme inhibition analysis revealed that the natural products of the ADA reaction, inosine and 2′-deoxyinosine, had K_i values of 1.2×10^{-4} M and 0.60×10^{-4} M, respectively, whereas coformycin appeared to be a very potent competitive inhibitor with a K_i value of about 1×10^{-8} M.[80] In the light of more recent investigations[86] which utilized new methodology for the study of tight-binding enzyme inhibitors,[87] however, the K_i value for coformycin was revised to about 1×10^{-10} M. Agarwal et al have compared the effectiveness of various inhibitors of ADA using these new theoretical approaches.[88] The K_i values determined by these workers were: 2′-deoxycoformycin, 2.5×10^{-12} M; coformycin, 1.2×10^{-10} to 1×10^{-11} M; EHNA, 1.6×10^{-9} M; DHMPR, 1.3×10^{-6} M.

Recently, several reports have appeared which illustrate the usefulness of ADA inhibitors in potentiating the chemotherapeutic activity of adenosine analogues (see Fig. 4-5). Most of these studies have been performed with 9-β-D-arabinofuranosyladenine (araA, adenine arabinoside). This analogue has been shown to have antitumor[89,90] and antiviral[91,92] activity. Although its exact mechanism of action has not been completely elucidated, inhibition of DNA synthesis appears to be mainly responsible for its activity.[23,75,93,94] The antitumor effectiveness of araA has been shown to be limited by its rapid deamination (by ADA) to the nontoxic compound, ara-

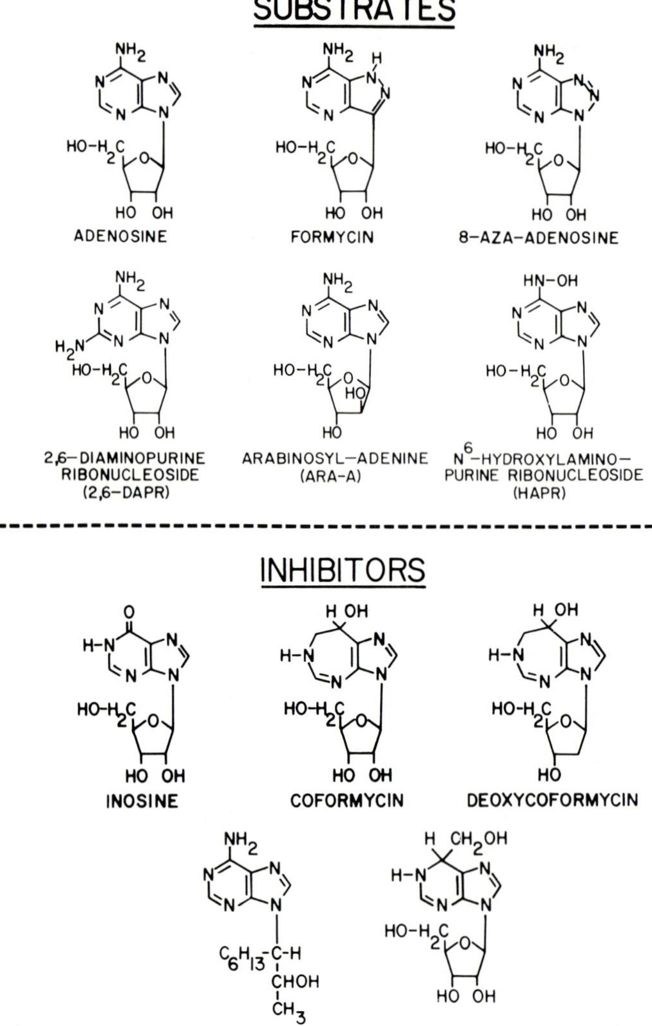

FIG. 4-5 Structural formulae of some substrates and inhibitors of adenosine deaminase.

binosyl-hypoxanthine.[89,90,95,96] Plunkett and Cohen have reviewed the subject of ADA inhibition as a means of increasing the activity of adenosine analogues including araA.[97]

AraA, in combination with the ADA inhibitor EHNA, gave increased survival times of mice bearing Ehrlich ascites carcinoma in comparison to treatment with araA alone.[97] Similarly, 2′-deoxycoformycin significantly enhanced the cytostatic and cytotoxic properties of araA against L1210 cells in vivo[98-100] and in vitro,[99] against P388 cells in vivo,[100] and against 6C3HED lymphosarcoma in vivo.[98] AraA alone is completely inactive against L1210 cells, apparently because this tumor has high levels of ADA.[95,101]

2′-Deoxycoformycin has also been used to potentiate the antitumor activities of adenosine analogs other than araA. Thus, the activity of cordycepin (3′-deoxyadenosine) against murine leukemias L1210 and P388 and human lymphoblastic leukemia CEM in vitro and against P388 in vivo was markedly enhanced by cotreatment with 2′-deoxycoformycin.[101] Replacement of 2′-deoxycoformycin with EHNA also gave enhancement of the cytotoxic effects of cordycepin in vitro.[97] The antitumor effects of several other adenosine analogues against P388 in vitro and in vivo have been reported to be enhanced by prior treatment with 2′-deoxycoformycin.[102] Of the 7 analogues examined in that study, only the activity of tubercidin (7-deazaadenosine), a compound which is not a substrate for ADA, was unaffected by 2′-deoxycoformycin pretreatment.

At the biochemical level, studies have been performed which illustrate that cotreatment of cells with an ADA inhibitor drastically modifies the metabolism of adenosine and adenosine analogues by such cells. Rose and Brockman showed that when L1210 cells were removed from mice 1 hour after treatment with araA alone, araATP levels were near the lower limits of detection.[103] When araA and 2′-deoxycoformycin were co-administered, araATP levels increased fourfold. Similarly, human erythrocytes which normally rapidly deaminate adenosine and its analogues have been shown to be capable of incorporating substantial amounts of adenosine into ATP and of formycin (7-amino-3-β-D-ribofuranosyl-pyrazolo[4,3-d]pyrimidine) into formycin 5′-triphosphate when pretreated with coformycin.[104-106] Other adenosine analogues including araA, 8-azaadenosine, N^6-hydroxylaminopurine ribonucleoside, 2,6-diaminopurine ribonucleoside (see Fig. 4-5) and various N-methyl derivatives of formycin have also been examined with the human erythrocyte system.[106,107] In each case, when analogues that were substrates for ADA were incubated alone, little or no synthesis of analogue nucleotides was seen. When cells were pretreated with coformycin, however, large amounts of analogue nucleotides accumulated.

From the work described above, it appears that combinations of adenosine and analogues and ADA inhibitors provide possible potent new tools for chemotherapy. One of the questions which must be answered, is however, "Do the ADA inhibitors affect enzymes of purine nucleoside and nucleotide metabolism other than ADA?" In this regard, Agarwal and Parks have recently reported that whereas the ADA inhibitors DHMPR and EHNA had no effect on the activity of rabbit muscle 5′-AMP deaminase, both coformycin and 2′-deoxycoformycin were inhibitory.[108] Interestingly, although 2′-deoxycoformycin was shown to be about fourfold more inhibitory to ADA than was coformycin,[88] 2′-deoxycoformycin was 30- to 70-fold less inhibitory than coformycin for 5′-AMP deaminase. In view of the key role played by 5′-AMP deaminase (reaction 6, Fig. 4-4) in the regulation of purine nucleotide interconversions and in the deamination of amino acids in some tissues,[109] inhibition of this activity may result in severe toxicity. As indicated by Agarwal and Parks, one might predict that toxicity resulting from inhibition of 5′-AMP deaminase would be much greater with coformycin than with 2′-deoxycoformycin and would be negligible with compounds such as EHNA or DHMPR.[108]

References

1. Hitchings G H, Elion G B: Mechanisms of action of purine and pyrimidine analogues, in Brodsky I, Kahn S B (eds): Cancer Chemotherapy I. New York, Grune & Stratton, 1967, p 26
2. Hitchings G H, Elion G B: Mechanisms of action of purine and pyrimidine analogues, in Brodsky I, Kahn S B, Moyer J H (eds): Cancer Chemotherapy II. New York, Grune & Stratton, 1972. p 23
3. Chu M Y, Fischer G A: A proposed mechanism of action of 1-β-D-arabinofuranosylcytosine as an inhibitor of the growth of leukemic cells. Biochem Pharmacol 11:423, 1962
4. Kessel D: Some observations on the phosphorylation of cytosine arabinoside. Mol Pharmacol 4:402, 1968
5. Momparler R L, Fischer G A: Mammalian deoxynucleoside kinases. I. Deoxycytidine kinase: Purification, properties and kinetic studies with cytosine arabinoside. J. Biol Chem 243:4298, 1968

6. Chu M Y, Fischer G A: Comparative studies of leukemic cells sensitive and resistant to cytosine arabinoside. Biochem Pharmacol 14:333, 1965
7. Schrecker A W, Urshel M J: Metabolism of 1-β-D-arabinofuranosylcytosine in leukemia L1210: Studies with intact cells. Cancer Res 28:793, 1968
8. Schrecker A W: Metabolism of 1-β-D-arabinofuranosylcytosine in leukemia L1210: Nucleoside and nucleotide kinases in cell free extracts. Cancer Res 30:632, 1970
9. Momparler R L, Chu M Y, Fischer G A: Studies on a new mechanism of resistance of L5178Y murine leukemia cells to cytosine arabinoside. Biochim Biophys Acta 161:481, 1968
10. Chu M Y, Fischer G A: Effects of cytosine arabinoside on the cell viability and uptake of deoxypyrimidine nucleosides in L5178Y cells. Biochem Pharmacol 17:741, 1968
11. Chu M Y, Fischer G A: The incorporation of ^{3}H-cytosine arabinoside and its effect on murine leukemic cells (L5178Y). Biochem Pharmacol 17:753, 1968
12. Young C W, Hodas S: Acute effects of cytotoxic compounds on incorporation of precursors in DNA, RNA, and protein of HeLa cell monolayers. Biochem Pharmacol 14:205, 1965
13. Silagi S: Metabolism of 1-β-D-arabinofuranosylcytosine in L cells. Cancer Res 25:1446, 1965
14. Karon M, Henry P, Weissman S, et al: The effect of 1-β-D-arabinofuranosylcytosine in the cell cycle. Cancer Res 26:166, 1966
15. Kaplan A S, Brown McK, Ben-Porat T: Effect of 1-β-D-arabinofuranosylcytosine on DNA synthesis. I. In normal rabbit kidney cell cultures. Mol Pharmacol 4:131, 1968
16. Creasey W A, DeConti R C, Kaplan S R: Biochemical studies with 1-β-D-arabinofuranosylcytosine in human leukemic leukocytes and normal bone marrow cells. Cancer Res 28:1074, 1968
17. Moore E C, Cohen S S: Effects of arabinonucleotides on ribonucleotide reduction by an enzyme system from rat tumor. J Biol Chem 242:2116, 1967
18. Skoog L, Nordenskjold B: Effects of hydroxyurea and 1-β-D-arabinofuranosylcytosine on deoxynucleotide pools in mouse embryo cells. Eur J Biochem 19:81, 1971
19. Inagaki T, Nakamura T, Wakisaka G: Studies on the mechanism of action of 1-β-D-arabinofuranosylcytosine as an inhibitor of DNA synthesis in human leukemic leukocytes. Cancer Res 29:2169, 1969
20. Cardeilhac P T, Cohen S S: Some metabolic properties of nucleotides of 1-β-D-arabinofuranosylcytosine. Cancer Res 24:1595, 1964
21. Kimball A P, Wilson M J: Inhibition of DNA polymerase by 1-β-D-arabinosylcytosine and reversal of inhibition by deoxycytidine-5′-triphosphate. Proc Soc Exp Biol Med 127:429, 1968
22. Momparler R L: Effect of cytosine arabinoside-5′-triphosphate on mammalian DNA polymerase. Biochem Biophys Res Commun 34:465, 1969
23. Furth J J, Cohen S S: Inhibition of mammalian DNA polymerase by the 5′-triphosphate of 1-β-D-arabinofuranosylcytosine and the 5′-triphosphate of 9-β-D-arabinofuranosyladenine. Cancer Res 28:2061, 1968
24. Graham F L, Whitmore G F: Studies in mouse L-cells on the incorporation of 1-β-D-arabinofuranosylcytosine into DNA and on inhibition of DNA polymerase by 1-β-D-arabinofuranosylcytosine-5′-triphosphate. Cancer Res 30:2636, 1970
25. Momparler R L: Kinetic and template studies with 1-β-D-arabinofuranosylcytosine 5′-triphosphate and mammalian deoxyribonucleic acid polymerase. Mol Pharmacol 8:362, 1972
26. Tuominen F W, Kenney F T: Inhibition of RNA-directed DNA polymerase from Rauscher leukemia virus by the 5′-triphosphate of cytosine arabinoside. Biochem Biophys Res Commun 48:1469, 1972
27. Creasey W A, Papac R J, Markin M E. et al: Biochemical and pharmacological studies with 1-β-D-arabinofuranosylcytosine in man. Biochem Pharmacol 15:1417, 1966
28. Furlong N B, Gresham C: Inhibition of DNA synthesis but not of poly-dAT synthesis by the arabinose analogue of cytidine in vitro. Nature 233:212, 1971
29. Chu M Y: Incorporation of arabinosylcytosine into 2-7S ribonucleic acid and cell death. Biochem Pharmacol 20:2057, 1971
30. Brockman R W: Mechanisms of resistance to anticancer agents, in Haddow A, Weinhouse S (eds.): Advances in Cancer Research, vol. 7. New York, Academic Press, 1963, p 129
31. Moore E C, LePage G A: The metabolism of 6-thioguanine in normal and neoplastic tissues. Cancer Res 18:1075, 1958
32. Miech R P, Parks R E Jr, Anderson J H, et al: An hypothesis on the mechanism of action of 6-thioguanine. Biochem Pharmacol 16:2222, 1967
33. LePage G A: The metabolism of α-2′-deoxythioguanosine in murine tumor cells. Can J. Biochem 46:655, 1968
34. Kong C M, Parks R E Jr: Incorporation of the purine moieties of guanosine and inosine an-

alogs into nucleotide pools of human erythrocytes. Biochem Pharmacol 24:807, 1975
35. Parks R E Jr, Crabtree G W, Kong C M, et al: Incorporation of analog purine nucleosides into formed elements of human blood: Erythrocytes, platelets, and lymphocytes. Ann N Y Acad Sci 255:412, 1975
36. Crabtree G W, Nelson J A, Parks R E Jr: Failure of 6-thioGMP to inhibit guanylate kinase in intact cells. Biochem Pharmacol, 26:1577, 1977
37. Robison B, Chu M Y, Parks R E Jr: Similar delayed cytotoxicity produced by 6-thioguanosine and 6-selenoguanosine. Cancer Res, (in press)
38. Nelson J A, Parks R E Jr: Biochemical mechanisms for the synergism between 6-thioguanine and 6-(methylmercapto) purine ribonucleoside in sarcoma 180 cells. Cancer Res 32:2034, 1972
39. Henderson J F: Feedback inhibition of purine biosynthesis in ascites tumor cells by purine analogs. Biochem Pharmacol 12:551, 1963
40. McCollister R J, Gilbert W R Jr, Ashton D M, et al: Pseudofeedback inhibition of purine synthesis by 6-mercaptopurine ribonucleotide and other purine analogues. J Biol Chem 239:1560, 1964
41. Henderson J F, Caldwell I C, Paterson A R P: Decreased feedback inhibition in a 6-(methylmercapto)purine ribonucleoside-resistant tumor. Cancer Res 27:1773, 1967
42. Hill, D L, Bennett L L Jr: Purification and properties of 5-phosphoribosylpyrophosphate amidotransferase from adenocarcinoma 755 cells. Biochemistry 8:122, 1969
43. Allan P W, Bennett L L Jr: 6-Methylthioguanylic acid, a metabolite of 6-thioguanine. Biochem Pharmacol 20:847, 1971
44. LePage G A, Jones M: Purine thiols as feedback inhibitors of purine synthesis in ascites tumor cells. Cancer Res 21:642, 1961
45. Atkinson M R, Morton R K, Murray A W: Inhibition of inosine 5′-phosphate dehydrogenase from Ehrlich ascites-tumour cells by 6-thioinosine 5′-phosphate. Biochem J 89:167, 1963
46. Hampton A: Reactions of ribonucleotide derivatives of purine analogs at the catalytic site of inosine 5′-phosphate dehydrogenase. J Biol Chem 238:3068, 1963
47. Anderson J H, Sartorelli A C: Inhibition of inosinic acid (IMP) dehydrogenase by purine nucleotide analogs. Fed Proc 26:730, 1967
48. Miech R P, York R, Parks R E Jr: Adenosine triphosphate-guanosine 5′-phosphate phosphotransferase. II. Inhibition by 6-thioguanosine 5′-phosphate of the enzyme isolated from hog brain and sarcoma 180 ascites cells. Mol Pharmacol 5:30, 1969
49. Miller R L, Adamczyk D L, Spector T, et al: Reassessment of the interactions of guanylate kinase and 6-thioguanosine 5′-phosphate. Biochem Pharmacol, 26:1573, 1977
50. Lau K F, Henderson J F: Inhibitors of purine metabolism in Ehrlich ascites tumor cells in vitro. Cancer Chemother Rep 3:95, 1972
51. Nelson J A, Carpenter J W, Rose L M, et al: Mechanism of action of 6-thioguanine, 6-mercaptopurine, and 8-azaguanine. Cancer Res 35:2872, 1975
52. Sartorelli A C, LePage G A: Metabolic effects of 6-thioguanine. II. Biosynthesis of nucleic acid purines in vivo and in vitro. Cancer Res 18:1329, 1958
53. LePage G A: Incorporation of 6-thioguanine into nucleic acids. Cancer Res 20:403, 1960
54. LePage G A: Basic biochemical effects and mechanism of action of 6-thioguanine. Cancer Res 23:1202, 1963
55. LePage G A, Junga I G: The utilization of α-2′-deoxythioguanosine by murine tumor cells. Mol Pharmacol 3:37, 1967
56. LePage G A, Junga I G, Bowman B: Biochemical and carcinostatic effects of 2′-deoxythioguanosine. Cancer Res 24:835, 1964
57. Nelson J A, Kuhns J N, Carpenter J W: Lack of activity of β-2′-deoxythioguanosine against two tumors resistant to 6-thioguanine. Cancer Res 35:1372, 1975
58. Schmidt L H, Montgomery J A, Laster W R Jr, et al: Combination therapy with arabinosylcytosine and thioguanine. Proc Am Assoc Cancer Res 11:70, 1970
59. Skipper H E: Combination Therapy: Some concepts and results. Cancer Chemother Rep 4:137, 1974
60. Schabel F M Jr: Synergism and antagonism among antitumor agents, in Univ of Texas Grad Sch of Biomed Sci at Houston (eds): Pharmacological Basis of Cancer Chemotherapy. M D Anderson Anderson Hospital and Tumor Institute at Houston. Baltimore, Williams & Wilkins, 1975, p 595
61. Barranco S M, Humphrey R M: The effects of β-2′-deoxythioguanosine on survival and progression in mammalian cells. Cancer Res 31:583, 1971
62. Tidd D M, Kim S C, Horakova K, et al: A delayed cytotoxic reaction for 6-mercaptopurine. Cancer Res 32:317, 1972
63. Tidd D M, Paterson A R P: Distinction between inhibition of purine nucleotide synthesis and the delayed cytotoxic reaction of 6-mercaptopurine. Cancer Res 34:733, 1974

64. Tidd D M, Paterson A R P: A biochemical mechnism for the delayed cytotoxic reaction of 6-mercaptopurine. Cancer Res 34:738, 1974
65. Mautner H G, Jaffe J J: 6-Selenoguanine (2-amino-6-selenopurine). Synthesis and biological studies. Biochem Pharmacol 5:343, 1961
66. Mautner H G, Chu S H, Jaffe J J, et al: The synthesis and antineoplastic properties of selenoguanine, selenocytosine and related compounds. J Med Chem 6:36, 1963
67. Chu S H: Potential antitumor agents. Selenoguanosine and related compounds. J Med Chem 14:254, 1971
68. Chu S H, Davidson D D: Potential antitumor agents. 2. α- and β-2′-deoxy-6-selenoguanosine and related compounds. J Med Chem 15:1088, 1972
69. Ross A F, Agarwal K C, Chu S H, et al: Studies on the biochemical actions of 6-selenoguanine and 6-selenoguanosine. Biochem Pharmacol 22:141, 1973
70. Milne G H, Townsend L B: Synthesis and antitumor activity of α- and β-2′-deoxy-6-selenoguanosine and certain related derivatives. J Med Chem 17:263, 1974
71. LePage G A: New purine analogs, in Buculoss P, Veronisi V, Cascinelli N (eds): Proceedings of the Eleventh Cancer Congress, vol. 3. Florence, Italy, 1974, (abstr) Amsterdam, Excerpta Medica, 1975, p 248
72. Kong C M, Parks R E Jr: Human erythrocytic hypoxanthine-guanine phosphoribosyltransferase: Effect of pH on the enzymatic reaction. Mol Pharmacol 10:648, 1974
73. Parks R E Jr, Brown P R, Kong C M: Incorporation of purine analogs into the nucleotide pools of human erythrocytes, in, Sperling O, DeVries A, Wyngaarden J B (eds): Purine Metabolism in Man, Vol. 41A. New York, Plenum, 1974, p 117
74. Bloch A (ed): Chemistry, biology and clinical uses of nucleoside analogs. Ann N Y Acad Sci, vol 255. New York, N Y Acad Sci 1975
75. LePage, G A: Purine arabinosides, xylosides, and lyxosides, in Sartorelli A C, Johns D G (eds): Antineoplastic and Immunosuppressive Agents. II. Handbook of Experimental Pharmacology, vol. 37/2. New York, Springer-Verlag, 1975, p 426
76. Nichol C A: Antibiotics resembling adenosine: Tubercidin, toyocamycin, sangivamycin, formycin, psicofuranine, and decoyinine, in Sartorelli A C, Johns D G (eds): Antineoplastic and Immunosuppressive Agents. II. Handbook of Experimental Pharmacology, vol. 37/2. New York, Springer-Verlag, 1975, p. 434
77. Crabtree G W, Senft A W: Pathways of nucleotide metabolism in *Schistosoma mansoni* - V. Adenosine cleavage enzyme and effects of purine analogs on adenosine metabolism in vitro. Biochem Pharmacol 23:649, 1974
78. Agarwal K C, Parks R E Jr: Adenosine analogs and human platelets. Effects on nucleotide pools and the aggregation phenomenon. Biochem Pharmacol 24:2239, 1975
79. Senft A W, Crabtree G W: Pathways of nucleotide metabolism in *Schistosoma mansoni* - VII. Inhibition of adenine and guanine nucleotide synthesis by purine analogs in intact worms. Biochem Pharmacol, 26:1847, 1977
80. Agarwal R P, Sagar S M, Parks R E Jr: Adenosine deaminase from human erythrocytes: Purification and effects of adenosine analogs. Biochem Pharmacol 24:693, 1975
81. Suhadolnik R J: Nucleoside Antibiotics. New York, Wiley Interscience, 1970
82. Sawa T, Fukugawa Y, Homma I, et al: Mode of inhibition of coformycin on adenosine deaminase. J Antibiot 20:227, 1967
83. Woo P W K, Dion H W, Lange S M, et al: A novel adenosine deaminase and araA deaminase inhibitor, (R)-3-(2-deoxy-β-D-erythropentofuranosyl)-3,6,7,8-tetrahydroimidazo [4,5-d] [1,3]diazepin-8-ol. J Hetero Chem 11:641, 1974
84. Schaeffer H J, Schwender C F: Enzyme inhibitors 26. Bridging hydrophobic and hydrophilic regions on adenosine deaminase with some 9-2(hydroxy-3-alkyl)adenines. J Med Chem 17:6, 1974
85. Evans B, Wolfenden R: A potential transition state analog for adenosine deaminase. J Am Chem Soc 92:4751, 1970
86. Cha S, Agarwal R P, Parks R E Jr: Tight-binding inhibitors—II. Non-steady state nature of inhibition of milk xanthine oxidase by allopurinol and alloxanthine and of human erythrocytic adenosine deaminase by coformycin. Biochem Pharmacol 24:2187, 1975
87. Cha S: Tight-binding inhibitors—I. Kinetic behavior. Biochem Pharmacol 24:2177, 1975
88. Agarwal R P, Spector T, Parks R E Jr: Tight-binding inhibitors—IV. Inhibition of adenosine deaminases by various inhibitors. Biochem Pharmacol 26:359, 1977
89. Brink, J J, LePage G A: Metabolic effects of 9-β-D-arabinofuranosylpurines in ascites tumor cells. Cancer Res 24:312, 1964
90. Brink J J, LePage G A: Metabolism and distribution of 9-β-D-arabinofuranosyladenine in mouse tissues. Cancer Res 24:1042, 1964
91. Schabel F M Jr: The anti-viral activity of 9-β-D-arabinofuranosyladenine (ara-A). Chemotherapy 13:321, 1968

92. Pavan-Langston D, Buchanan R A, Alford C A Jr (eds): Adenine Arabinoside: An Antiviral Agent. New York, Raven, 1975
93. York J L. LePage G A: A proposed mechanism for the action of 9-β-D-arabinofuranosyladenine as an inhibitor of the growth of some ascites cells. Can J Biochem 44:19, 1966
94. Furth J J, Cohen S S: Inhibition of mammalian DNA polymerase by the 5′-triphosphate of 9-β-D-arabinofuranosyladenine. Cancer Res 27:1528, 1967
95. Brink J J, LePage G A: 9-β-D-arabinofuranosyladenine as an inhibitor of metabolism in normal and neoplastic cells. Can J Biochem 43:1, 1965
96. Plunkett W, Cohen S S: Metabolism of 9-β-D-arabinofuranosyladenine by mouse fibroblasts. Cancer Res 35:412, 1975
97. Plunkett W, Cohen S S: Two approaches that increase the activity of analogs of adenine nucleosides in animal cells. Cancer Res 35:1547, 1975
98. LePage G A, Worth L S, Kimball A P: Enhancement of the antitumor activity of arabinofuranosyladenine by 2′-deoxycoformycin. Cancer Res 36:1481, 1976
99. Cass C E, Au-Yeung T H: Enhancement of 9-β-D-arabinofuranosyladenine cytotoxicity to mouse leukemia L1210 in vitro by 2′-deoxycoformycin. Cancer Res 36:1486, 1976
100. Schabel F M Jr, Trader M W, Laster W R Jr: Increased therapeutic activity of 9-β-D-arabinofuranosyladenine against leukemia P388 and L1210 by an adenosine deaminase inhibitor. Proc Am Assoc Cancer Res 17:46, 1976
101. Johns D G, Adamson R H: Enhancement of the biological activity of cordycepin (3′-deoxyadenosine) by the adenosine deaminase inhibitor 2′-deoxycoformycin. Biochem Pharmacol 25:1441, 1976
102. Adamson R H, Zaharevitz D W, Johns D G: Enhancement of the biological activity of adenosine analogs by the adenosine deaminase inhibitor 2′-deoxycoformycin. Pharmacology 15:84, 1977
103. Rose L M, Brockman R W: Analysis by high-pressure liquid chromatography of 9-β-D-arabinofuranosyladenine 5′-triphosphate (AraATP) levels in murine leukemia cells. J Chromatogr 133:335, 1977
104. Agarwal R P, Crabtree G W, Parks R E Jr, et al: Purine nucleoside metabolism in the erythrocytes of patients with adenosine deaminase deficiency and severe combined immunodeficiency. J Clin Invest 57:1025, 1976
105. Parks R E Jr, Agarwal R P, Crabtree G W: Role of adenosine deaminase (ADA) in the incorporation of adenosine analogs into the nucleotide pools of human erythrocytes and other blood elements. Pharmacologist 18:156, 1976
106. Agarwal R P, Cha S, Crabtree G W, et al: Coformycin and deoxycoformycin: Tight-binding inhibitors of adenosine deaminase, in Robins R K, Townsend L B, Harmon R E (eds): Symposium on Chemistry and Biology of Nucleosides and Nucleotides (American Chemical Society Advances in Chemistry Series). New York, Academic Press, (in press)
107. Dollinger M R, Krakoff I H: Hemolysis induced by 6-N-hydroxylaminopurine riboside, an adenosine analogue. Clin Pharmacol Ther 17:57, 1975
108. Agarwal R P, Parks R E Jr: Potent inhibition of muscle 5′-AMP deaminase by the nucleoside antibiotics coformycin and deoxycoformycin. Biochem Pharmacol 26:663, 1977
109. Lowenstein J M: Ammonia production in muscle and other tissues: The purine nucleotide cycle. Physiol Rev 52:382, 1972

William A. Creasey

5
Vinca Alkaloids

The vinca alkaloids are dimeric indole derivatives composed of vindoline and catharanthine structures (Fig. 5-1). These alkaloids are obtained from the Madagascan periwinkle plant, *Catharanthus roseus* G. Don, usually known as *Vinca rosea* Linn. Antitumor activity was first identified during screening of the plant for the antidiabetic properties traditionally ascribed to it. Various aspects of the botany, chemistry and biological activity of these agents have been collected in one volume.[1] A large number of alkaloids have been isolated from the periwinkle plant, but the only ones that have been shown to possess anticancer activity are vinblastine, vincristine, vinleurosine, vinrosidine, rovidine and leurosivine. The latter two are minor components that have not been studied adequately. Vinleurosine and vinrosidine have reached clinical trial but do not appear to offer any advantage over the widely-used alkaloids vinblastine and vincristine. Most of the semisynthetic derivatives that have been prepared have proved less active than the naturally-occurring drugs, examples being 6,7-dihydrovinblastine[2] and vinglycinate, the 4-N,N-dimethylaminoacetyl derivative of desacetylvinblastine.[3] An exception to this is desacetylvinblastine amide or vindesine, which is now undergoing extensive clinical trials.[4,5]

Structure-activity Relationships

The general structural requirements for antitumor activity have been listed.[6] They include retention of the free hydroxyl functions and of the basic nature of the indole nitrogen in the catharanthine moiety. Furthermore, reduction leads to partial or complete loss of activity depending on the portion of the molecule that is reduced. 6,7-Dihydrovinblastine, for example, is only one-tenth as active as the parent drug. Removal of the 4-acetyl group may modify the spectrum of activity, but does not cause complete loss of potency as once was thought to be the case.

Biological Activity

A wide variety of biological effects have been ascribed to the *Vinca* alkaloids (Table 5-1). Not all members of this class exhibit all these actions at tolerated therapeutic dose levels, however. Apart from their antitumor action, the most characteristic effect of the group is the arrest of cell division in metaphase. This C-mitotic arrest, which resembles that produced by colchicine, results from dissolution of the mitotic spindle rather than

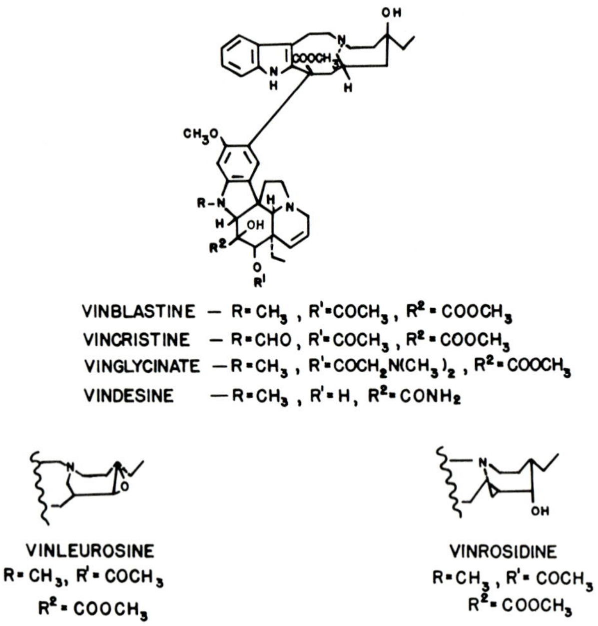

VINBLASTINE — R = CH_3, R' = $COCH_3$, R^2 = $COOCH_3$
VINCRISTINE — R = CHO, R' = $COCH_3$, R^2 = $COOCH_3$
VINGLYCINATE — R = CH_3, R' = $COCH_2N(CH_3)_2$, R^2 = $COOCH_3$
VINDESINE — R = CH_3, R' = H, R^2 = $CONH_2$

VINLEUROSINE
R = CH_3, R' = $COCH_3$
R^2 = $COOCH_3$

VINROSIDINE
R = CH_3, R' = $COCH_3$
R^2 = $COOCH_3$

FIG. 5-1. Structural formulas of the *Vinca* alkaloids.

from major damage to chromosomes. Although mitotic arrest may be a factor in cytotoxicity, this is not completely certain. What is known is that the most sensitive phase of the cell cycle from the point of view of a lethal effect is not mitosis but the S phase.[7] Interestingly, this is also the phase during which most antimetabolites are maximally lethal. Vincristine is characterized by neurological toxicity of the form of a polyneuritis; there also appears to be a component of muscle spindle and end plate damage. Vinblastine only produces such effects at doses that give prohibitive hematopoietic depression. Such depression is not encountered with normal doses of vincristine. Vindesine resembles both vinblastine and vincristine in the spectrum of side effects that it elicits. Vinleurosine is distinctive in that it produces a shock-like syndrome with severe hypotension when injected rapidly; otherwise it resembles vinblastine in both toxicity and spectrum of activity. The anti-inflammatory effect, which is manifested only in acute gouty episodes and has only been demonstrated for vinblastine, may be a function of disturbances in the phagocytotic, saltatory and metabolic activities of polymorphonuclear leukocytes that infiltrate the inflamed joint, as is the case with colchicine.[8] These effects, as well as changes in shape and movement, dissolution of microtubules and some aspects of neurological toxicity, all appear to have a common basis in interaction of drug with the microtubule system. Secretion of certain hormones, such as

TABLE 5-1. *Biological Actions of the Vinca Alkaloids*

1. Cytotoxicity — antitumor effect, action on normal tissues
2. Mitotic Arrest — block in metaphase
3. Anti-inflammatory Action — gout only
4. Neuromuscular Actions — neurotoxicity, muscle spindle and end plate damage
5. Autonomic Actions
6. Cytological Changes — microtubule loss, change in cell shape, autophagy, ribosome clumping
7. Immunosuppression
8. Actions on Secretion and Phagocytosis — altered hormone secretion, changes in plasma lipoproteins and lysosome function
9. Teratogenesis

insulin, thyroid hormones and corticosteroids, is affected in various ways by *Vinca* alkaloids. In these cases, necessary steps in secretion, such as pinocytosis of thyroglobulin, movement and elimination of secretory granules and mobilization of lysosomes appear to be the critically sensitive processes. Production of plasma lipoproteins involves some of the same microtubule-dependent steps. Immunosuppression and teratogenesis are biological lesions produced by most agents that interfere with growth and cell division. The *Vinca* alkaloids also exert these actions but not to as marked a degree as many other anticancer drugs.

Microtubule Interactions

The microtubule system consists of tubules about 250 Å in diameter that may occur singly, but are most frequently found either as loose aggregates or highly ordered assemblies that are associated with, or actual compenents of, organelles such as the mitotic spindle, cilia, flagella or membranes.[9,10] These tubules are themselves derived from protofibrils, commonly 13 but occasionally 11 or 12, which are composed of tubulin, a protein that normally exists as a heterodimer of molecular weight 110,000. Tubulin has been considered to be a rather conservative protein from an evolutionary point of view, and has a similar structure in all eukaryote organisms; it is now becoming clear that considerable heterogeneity in fact exists. Even within one cell, tubulin may exist in the form of both a soluble component of sedimentation coefficient 6S, and 36S ring, spiral and/or hoop structures that may represent nucleation centers for assembly of microtubules.[11] These components comprise a pool of precursors that is in equilibrium with formed microtubular structures (Fig. 5-2). The kinetics of the equilibrium may vary widely for different structures—the tubules of the cilia and flagella, for example, being rather stable.[12] Structures derived from the microtubules are involved either in move-

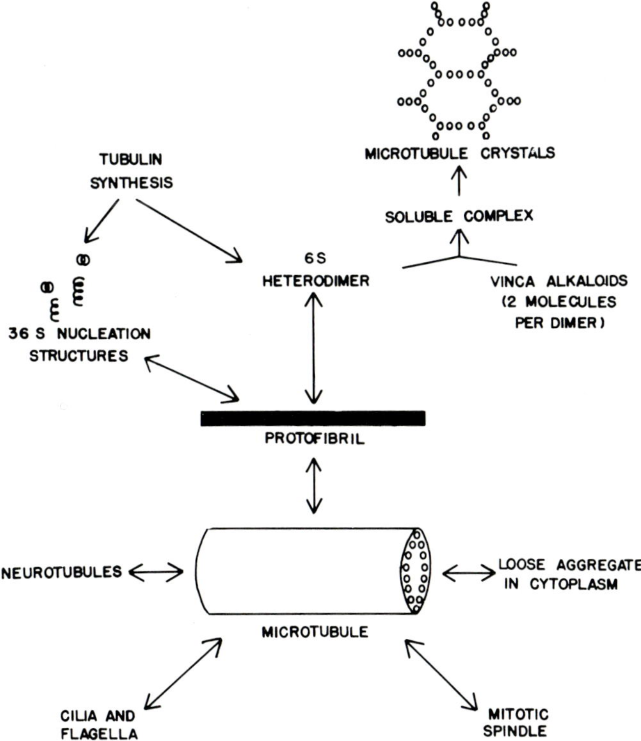

Fig. 5-2. Schematic representation of the microtubule system with indication of the mode of intervention of *Vinca* alkaloids.

ment or in maintaining shape and rigidity. The mitotic spindle, which is associated with rapid movements during anaphase, and the neurotubules, which are involved in axonal transport, are good examples. The type of motion that is involved in mitosis could take the form of microtubules sliding over each other, although physical loss of subunits leading to shortening of the tubules is also possible.[13]

The *Vinca* alkaloids, like colchicine, interact with tubulin dimer to form a complex; this process has been reviewed quite extensively,[14,15] and will be only briefly summarized here. There are three classes of high-affinity binding sites on the tubulin dimer molecule. Two sites (one very poorly exchanging) are occupied by GTP, one is specific for colchicine, and two associate with vinblastine on each molecule of dimer.[16] Kinetic constants for binding appear to vary markedly with the source of the tubulin. High-affinity binding of vinblastine is sensitive to high concentrations of sodium chloride but not urea, is stabilized by colchicine, griseofulvin and podophyllotoxin, and is inhibited by other *Vinca* alkaloids. Binding is most complete between pH6 and 8. There are, in addition, 10 to 20 sites of lower affinity per tubulin molecule, at which *Vinca* alkaloids may interact. They are involved in the precipitation of the protein and in the formation of microtubule crystals. The latter are pseudocrystalline aggregates that are formed specifically by the *Vinca* alkaloids, and not by colchicine. They are formed in a wide variety of cells, from starfish oocytes to human leukocytes, and consist of structurally-modified tubules of altered dimensions arranged in hexagonal fashion to produce structures up to several microns in length.[17]

These binding interactions, whether giving rise to soluble complex or microtubule crystals, will deplete the pool of unpolymerized tubulin. As a result, those structures in rapid equilibrium, such as the spindle, will dissociate readily. Neurotubules are somewhat less labile, while the tubules in cilia are relatively resistant. Many of the effects of these drugs on biological processes that are dependent on microtubule function thus become explicable on the basis of this depletion as the underlying mechanism. Binding by microtubule protein also may account for the high intracellular levels of vinblastine that have been described in such cells as leukocytes[18] and platelets.[19] Since in vitro vinblastine, vincristine and vindesine all appear to bind to microtubule protein and prevent its polymerization with about the same efficacy,[20] it is evident that other factors must be involved in order to bring about the very different spectra of activity and side effects of these drugs. In addition, cytotoxicity may not be completely explicable on the basis of what has proven to be a reversible phenomenon, as reflected by spindle dissolution.[21] Early studies showed a lack of correlation between mitotic arrest in the bone marrow and subsequent development of leukopenia in patients receiving vinblastine or vincristine.[22] The most plausible factor that might intervene to bring about cell death is inhibition of biosynthetic processes and damage to macromolecules, which are known to result from exposure to the *Vinca* alkaloids (Fig. 5-3); this would also be consistent with S-phase lethality of these alkaloids.

Nucleic Acid Biosynthesis

Inhibition of nucleic acid biosynthesis has been reported for all the vinca alkaloids that have been screened for this activity. The relative reductions in RNA and DNA synthesis vary with both the drug and the experimental or clinical tumor or normal tissue system examined. Vinblastine and vincristine inhibit the synthesis of both DNA and RNA in Ehrlich ascites carcinoma cells,[23] rat spleen and bone marrow[24] and thymus cells,[25] mouse brain,[26] human leukemic leukocytes,[27] cultured rat embryos[28] and HEp-2 cells.[29] Among the minor alkaloids, vinleurosine[30] and vinrosidine[31] are inhibitors of nucleic acid synthesis in Sarcoma 180 and rat thymus cells, respectively. The mechanisms involved in these inhibitory effects are unknown. Cline has reported[27] a direct inhibition of preparations of RNA polymerase by vincristine, while in nucleated erythrocytes stimulated with erythropoietin, vinblastine prevented the increase in activity of high molecular weight cytoplasmic DNA polymerase.[32] Whether there is inhibition of enzyme activity per se, or whether association of drug occurs with nu-

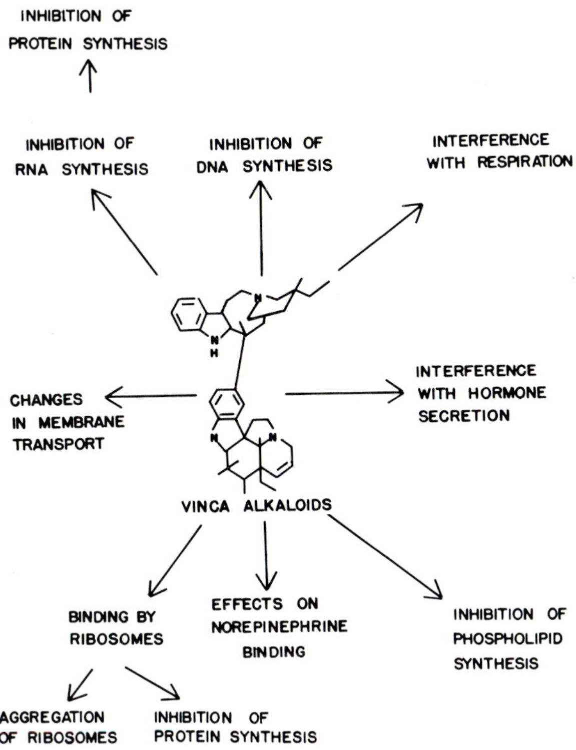

FIG. 5-3. Biochemical sites of action of the *Vinca* alkaloids.

cleic acid to reduce template activity, has not been determined at present. The latter is possible in view of the complex formation between colchicine and DNA that has only been detected by changes in optical rotation.[33] Colchicine acts like the *Vinca* alkaloids in so many ways that an analogy in this area seems very possible. Altered mucleoside transport, seen after exposure to vinleurosine[30] also offers a possible mechanism, at least for a portion of the effect seen in whole cells.

PROTEIN SYNTHESIS

In view of the effects of *Vinca* alkaloids on the synthesis of nucleic acids, it might be anticipated that protein synthesis would be affected as a result. Inhibition of protein synthesis has been reported after treatment with *Vinca* alkaloids in Ehrlich ascites carcinoma cells,[34,35] human leukemic leukocytes[27] and rat embryos in culture in vivo.[28] This type of inhibition can be seen, however, under conditions in which RNA synthesis is not inhibited, as in normal human leukocytes exposed to vinblastine or vincristine in vitro.[36] Thus, effects on RNA synthesis cannot be the only source of reduced protein fabrication. The uptake of amino acids by cells may be inhibited by *Vinca* alkaloids. In the only example that has been studied in detail, there exists a competitive relationship between the transport of vinblastine and glutamic acid.[36] Such effects could contribute to depression of protein synthesis. More likely to exert significant effects, however, is the interaction of these drugs with ribosomes. Vinblastine causes the precipitation or formation of aggregates of ribosomes in *Escherichia coli,* which lacks microtubules,[37] human leukemic lymphoblasts and mouse fibroblasts,[38] and in suspensions of ribosomes.[39] This aggregation phenomenon is likely to be related to the binding of vinblastine by ribosomes, especially by the lighter subunits (Fig. 5-4). As a result of this interaction, synthesis of protein by a cell-free system containing ribosomes is inhibited by vinblastine to the extent of 31 per cent at 10^{-5}M.[40]

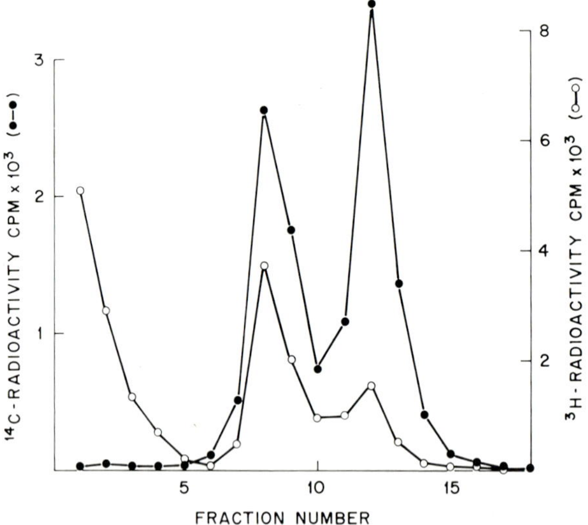

FIG. 5-4. The binding of tritium labeled vinblastine by ribosomes from S 180 cells. Sedimentation of ^{14}C-labeled ribosomal subunits (●—●) with bound tritiated vinblastine (○—○) through a 5-20% sucrose gradient. From Swerdlow B, Creasey W A: Binding of vinblastine in vitro to ribosomes of sarcoma 180 cells. Biochem Pharmacol 24:1243, 1975, with permission of the publisher.

LIPID SYNTHESIS

Demyelination of nerve fibers[41] is a process suggestive of a possible intervention by vincristine in lipid metabolism. Synthesis of total lipids is inhibited by vincristine in rat embryos.[28] Further detailed studies have shown that phospholipid synthesis is the more specific target in the gastrocnemius muscle of rats treated with vincristine,[42] and in Sarcoma 180 cells incubated with vinleurosine[30] or vincristine.[43]

MISCELLANEOUS EFFECTS

Interference with respiratory processes has been ascribed to the *Vinca* alkaloids and colchicine in such systems as tumor cells[44] and leukocytes during phagocytosis.[45] A variety of effects of antimitotic agents on hormone secretion have been described. They include inhibition of thyroid hormone mobilization[46] and insulin secretion,[47] and increased release of adrenal steroids.[48] Hyponatremia, secondary to inappropriate secretion of antidiuretic hormone, has been described.[49] The syndrome was prevented by rigorous fluid restriction.[50] Microtubule interactions may form the basis for many of these effects. An interesting membrane effect of vincristine is its ability to promote accumulation of MTX intracellularly through inhibiting efflux;[51] this has received clinical application. Finally, there is evidence that vinblastine is able to inhibit the uptake of norepinephrine by adrenergic fibers[52] and of 5-hydroxytryptamine by rat brain synaptosomes,[53] as well as to sensitize the myocardium to norepinephrine.[54] These autonomic effects also may stem, at least in part, from microtubule interactions. It is also worth noting that these alkaloids are indole derivatives, and some other compounds of this class, such as reserpine, are active autonomic agents.

DISTRIBUTION AND METABOLISM

Difficulties in the preparation of radiolabeled vinblastine and vincristine delayed the acquisition of knowledge about their metabolic fate. Much more information has become available once relatively pure drugs could be obtained by catalytic exchange. In rats given tritiated vinblastine, intestinal excretion accounted for 25 per cent over a 24-hour period, whereas urinary output was only about 6 per cent. Of the radioactivity in the blood of this species, 60 per cent was in the platelets, 15 per cent in the leukocytes, 10 per cent in the red cells and 15 per cent in the plasma; 50 per cent of the plasma tritium and all the platelet radioactivity was present as unchanged drug.[19] In dogs, fecal excretion (30–36 per cent) exceeded urinary elimination (12–17 per cent; Fig. 5-5) of vinblastine over a 9-day period. Levels of tritium label in the leukocytes were 2 to 12 times those in the coincident plasma and were accounted for almost entirely as vinblastine. Half-lives for labeled vinblastine in these animals were 17 to 38 minutes and 3 to 5 hours (Fig. 5-6). Vinblastine was the major biliary component (47–81 per cent), and desacetylvinblastine the major metabolite.[18] Studies in humans indicate a biphasic plasma clearance with half-lives of about 4 and 190 minutes for vinblastine. Here also, platelets and leukocytes concentrated the drug. By 72 hours, 19 to 23 per cent had been excreted in the urine and 25 to 41 per cent in the stools; unchanged drug accounted for 17 to 50 per cent of urinary radioactivity but a very small fraction of fecal label.[56]

Early studies on the disposition of vincristine relied on bioassay with KB cells.[57,58] They indicated a rapid clearance of drug from the serum with overall half-lives of a little over 1 hour in dogs, monkeys and children. Using tritiated vincristine, a biphasic plasma clearance curve with a secondary half-life of 70 minutes was obtained. There were very high levels of tritium in the spleen, adrenal, small intestine, thyroid and heart.[59] A carrier-mediated transport system is involved in the uptake of vincristine by many tumor cells;[60] the operation of such a mechanism could be related to the glutamate antagonism mentioned above.[36] Like vinblastine and colchicine, vincristine undergoes significant (up to 75 per cent) binding by serum proteins, most notably the α- and β-globulins.[61]

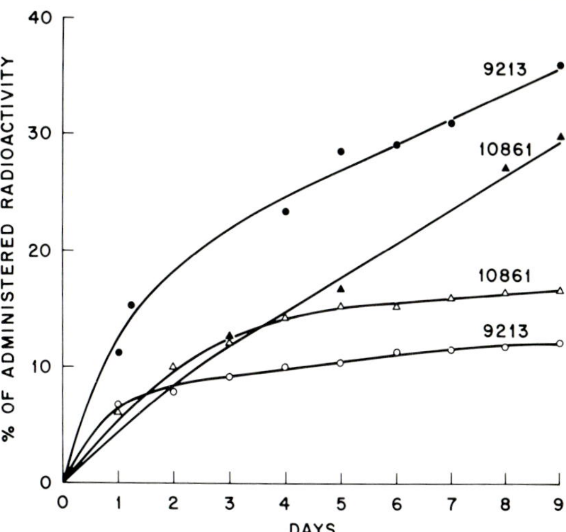

FIG. 5-5. Urinary (○—○, Δ—Δ) and fecal (●—●, ▲—▲) excretion of radioactivity derived from tritium labeled vinblastine (0.15 mg/kg) administered to 2 dogs. From Creasey W A, Scott A I, Wei C C, et al: Pharmacological studies with vinblastine in the dog. Cancer Res 35:1116, 1975 with permission of the publisher.

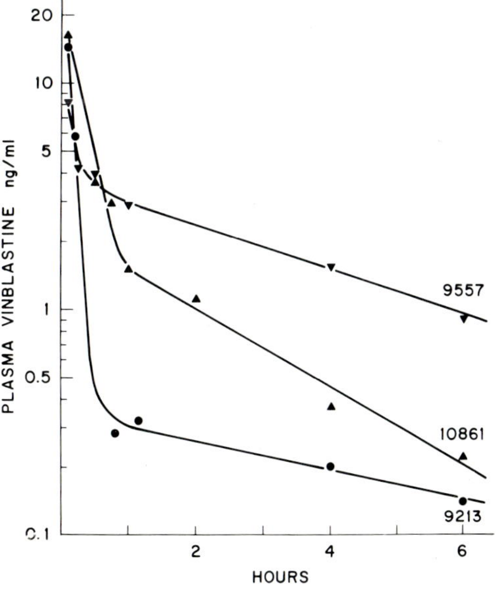

FIG. 5-6. Plasma clearance curves (early portion) of vinblastine in 3 dogs receiving 0.15 mg/kg of tritium-labeled drug. From Creasey W A, Scott A I, Wei C C, et al: Pharmacological studies with vinblastine in the dog. Cancer Res 35:1116, 1975 with permission of the publisher.

Clinical Implications of Pharmacological Data

The pattern of binding of plasma proteins, slow, primarily biliary excretion and concentration of these alkaloids in certain cells, are entirely consistent with the type of dosage schedule that has been found tolerable in the clinic. Early attempts to administer these drugs at more frequent intervals led to unacceptable escalation of toxicity.[6] Since the usefulness of the *Vinca* alkaloids lies in their integration into combination chemotherapy and multimodal protocols, mention of this aspect is in order. As agents that arrest cells in mitosis, the *Vinca* alkaloids should cause a modification of tumor cell population in the direction of increasing the proportion of cells with sensitivity to some alkylating agents that show greater lethal action in this phase of the cell cycle. Vincristine, because of its essential lack of toxicity to the bone marrow is a useful agent for inclusion in protocols that utilize myelosuppressive drugs. Finally, the ability of these agents to modify membrane function may be turned to use in combinations based on pharmacologic principles, as it has been in the case of combinations of MTX and vincristine.

Conclusion

The *Vinca* alkaloids exert a variety of biologic effects that can be ascribed firstly to their interaction with the subunit protein of the microtubule system, and secondly to inhibition of biosynthetic pathways. In their patterns of distribution and excretion, these alkaloids exhibit biphasic plasma clearance curves, concentration by cell types such as platelets and leukocytes and a primarily biliary route of excretion. These factors have cell cycle kinetic and toxicological implications for the use of these agents in combination chemotherapy.

References

1. Taylor W I, Farnsworth N R: The Catharanthus alkaloids, Botany, Chemistry, Pharmacology and Clinical Use. New York, Marcel Dekker, 1975
2. Noble R L, Beer C T, McIntyre R W: Biological effects of dihydrovinblastine. Cancer 20:885, 1967
3. Armstrong J G: New derivatives of the *vinca rosea* alkaloids. Acta Genet Med (Roma) 17:193, 1968
4. Sweeney M J, Cullinan G J, Poore G A, et al: Experimental antitumor activity of vinblastine amides. Proc Amer Assoc Cancer Res 15:37, 1974
5. Todd G C, Gibson W R, Griffing W J, et al: The preclinical study of desacetylvinblastine amide. Proc Amer Assoc Cancer Res 16:70, 1975
6. Johnson I S, Armstrong J G, Gorman M, et al: The vinca alkaloids: A new class of oncolytic agents. Cancer Res 23:1390, 1963
7. Madoc-Jones H, Mauro F: Interphase action of vinblastine and vincristine: Differences in their lethal action through the mitotic cycle of cultured mammalian cells. J Cell Physiol 72:185, 1968
8. Malawista S E: Colchicine: A common mechanism for its antiinflammatory and antimitotic effects. Arthritis Rheum 11:191, 1968
9. Olmsted J B, Borisy G G: Microtubules. Ann Rev Biochem 42:507, 1973
10. Burnside B: The form and arrangement of microtubules: An historical primarily morphological review. Ann N Y Acad Sci 253:14, 1975
11. Kirschner M W, Suter M, Weingarten M, et al: The role of rings in the assembly of microtubules in vitro. Ann N Y Acad Sci 253:90, 1975
12. Behnke O, Forer A: Evidence for four classes of microtubules in individual cells. J Cell Sci 2:169, 1967
13. McIntosh J R, Cande Z, Snyder J, et al: Studies on the mechanism of mitosis. Ann N Y Acad Sci 253:407, 1975
14. Wilson L: Action of drugs on microtubules. Life Sci 17:303, 1975
15. Creasey W A: Vinca alkaloids and colchicine, in Sartorelli A C, Johns D G (eds): Handbook of Experimental Pharmacology, vol. 38 part II. Berlin, Springer-Verlag, 1975, p 670
16. Bryan J: Definition of three classes of binding sites in isolated microtubule crystals. Biochemistry 11:2611, 1972
17. Bensch K G, Malawista S E: Microtubule crystals in mammalian cells. J Cell Biol 40:95, 1969
18. Creasey W A, Scott A I, Wei C C, et al: Pharmacological studies with vinblastine in the dog. Cancer Res 35:1116, 1975

19. Hebden H F, Hadfield J R, Beer C T: The binding of vinblastine by platelets in the rat. Cancer Res 30:1417, 1970
20. Himes R H, Kersey R N, Heller-Bettinger I, et al: Action of the vinca alkaloids vincristine, vinblastine and desacetyl vinblastine amide on microtubules in vitro. Cancer Res 36:3798, 1976
21. Malawista S E, Sato H, Bensch K G: Vinblastine and griseofulvin reversibly disrupt the living mitotic spindle. Science 160:770, 1968
22. Frei E III, Whang J, Scoggins R B et al: The stathmokinetic effect of vincristine. Cancer Res 24:1918, 1964
23. Creasey W A, Markiw M E: Biochemical effects of the vinca alkaloids II. A comparison of the effects of colchicine, vinblastine, and vincristine on the synthesis of ribonucleic acids in Ehrlich ascites carcinoma cells. Biochim Biophys Acta 87:601, 1964
24. Van Lancker J L, Flangas A L, Allen J: Metabolic effects of vinblastine. I The effect of vinblastine on nucleic acid synthesis in spleen and bone marrow. Lab Invest 15:1291, 1966
25. Jones R G W, Richards J F, Beer C T: Biochemical studies with the vinca alkaloids II. Effect of vinblastine on the biosynthesis of nucleic acids and their precursors in rat thymus cells. Cancer Res 26:882, 1966
26. Agustin B M, Creasey W A: Effects of vinca alkaloids on the synthesis of RNA in mouse brain. Nature 215:965, 1967
27. Cline M J: Effect of vincristine on synthesis of ribonucleic acid and protein in leukaemic leucocytes. Brit. J Haematol 14:21, 1968
28. Krowke R, Zimmerman B, Merker H J: Biochemical and electron microscopic studies of rat embryos in in vivo culture. Naunyn Schmiedebergs Arch Pharmakol 266:382, 1970
29. Wagner, E K, Roizman B: Effect of the vinca alkaloids on RNA synthesis in human cells in vitro. Science 162:569, 1968
30. Creasey W A: Biochemical effects of the vinca alkaloids—IV. Studies with vinleurosine. Biochem Pharmacol 18:227, 1969
31. Richards J F, Jones R G W, Beer C T: Biochemical studies with the vinca alkaloids I. Effect on nucleic acid formation by isolated cell suspensions. Cancer Res 26:876, 1966
32. Roodman G D, Hutton J J, Bollum F J: DNA polymerase activities during erythropoiesis. Effects of erythropoietin, vinblastine, colcemid, and daunomycin. Exp Cell Res 91:269, 1975
33. Ilan J, Quastel J H: Effect of colchicine on nucleic acid metabolism during metamorphosis of *Tenebrio molitor* L and in some mammalian tissues. Biochem J 100:449, 1966
34. Creasey W A, Markiw M E: Biochemical effects of the vinca alkaloids III. The synthesis of ribonucleic acid and the incorporation of amino acids in Ehrlich ascites cells in vitro. Biochim Biophsy Acta 103:635, 1965
35. Warnecke P, Seeber S: Agriffspunkte von vinca-alkaloiden im protein and Nucleinsäure Stoffwechsel. Z Krebsforsch 71:361, 1968
36. Creasey W A, Bensch K G, Malawista S E: Colchicine, vinblastine, and griseofulvin: Pharmacological studies with human leukocytes. Biochem Pharmacol 20:1579, 1971
37. Kingsbury E W, Voelz H: Induction of helical arrays of ribosomes by vinblastine sulfate in *Escherichia coli*. Science 166:768, 1969
38. Krishan A, Hsu D: Vinblastine-induced ribosomal complexes. Effect of some metabolic inhibitors on their formation and structure. J Cell Biol 49:927, 1971
39. Wilson L, Bryan J, Ruby A, et al: Precipitation of proteins by vinblastine and calcium ions. Proc Natl Acad Sci USA 66:807, 1970
40. Swerdlow B, Creasey W A: Binding of vinblastine in vitro to ribosomes of sarcoma 180 cells. Biochem Pharmacol 24:1243, 1975
41. Gottschalk P G, Dyck P J, Kiely J M: Vinca alkaloid neuropathy: Nerve biopsy studies in rats and in man. Neurology 18:875, 1968
42. Graff G L A, Guening C, Hildebrand J: Action du sulfate de vincristine sur le gastrocnémien de rat I. Mis en évidence de deux compartements, metaboliquement distincts, pour le phosphate inorganique: Effets sur les phosphates organiques acidosolubles et les phospholipides C R Soc Biol (Paris) 161:2645, 1967
43. Creasey W A: Biochemistry of dimeric *Catharanthus* alkaloids, in Taylor W I, Farnsworth N R (eds): The Catharanthus Alkaloids. Botany, Chemistry, Pharmacology and Clinical Use. New York, Marcel Dekker, 1975, p 209
44. Obrecht P, Fusenig N E: Die wirkung von vincaleukoblastin (velbe[R]) auf die glykolyse von tumor zellen. Europ J Cancer 2:109, 1966
45. Goldfinger S E, Howell R R, Seegmiller J E: Suppression of metabolic accompaniment of phagocytosis by colchicine. Arthritis Rheum 8:1112, 1965
46. Wolff J, Bhattacharyya B: Microtubules and thyroid hormone mobilization. Ann N Y Acad Sci 253:763, 1975
47. Lacy P E, Howell S L, Young D A, et al: New hypothesis on insulin secretion. Nature 219:1177, 1968
48. Chung L W K, Gabourel J D: Adrenal steroid release by vinblastine sulfate and its contribution to vinblastine sulfate effects on rat thymus. Biochem Pharmacol 20:1749, 1971

49. Slater L M, Wainer R A, Serpick A A: Vincristine neurotoxicity with hyponatremia. Cancer 23:122, 1969
50. Stuart M J, Cuaso C, Miler M, et al: Syndrome of recurrent increased secretion of antidiuretic hormone following multiple doses of vincristine. Blood 45:315, 1975
51. Bender R A, Bleyer W A, Frisby S A, et al: Alteration of methotrexate uptake in human leukemia cells by other agents. Cancer Res 35:1305, 1975
52. Costa M, Filogamo G: Effecti della colchicina nella fibre adrenergiche dei plessi nervosi intestinal. Boll Soc Ital Biol Sper 46:865, 1970
53. Nomura Y, Segawa T: Influences of colchicine and vinblastine on the uptake of 5-hydroxytryptamine and norepinephrine by rat brain synaptosomes and small vesicle fractions. J Neurochem 24:1257, 1975
54. Bennett, T, Gardiner S M: The effects of intravenous injections of vinblastine or vincristine on the responses of the rat heart to nerve stimulation and to drugs. Br J Pharmacol 53:444P, 1975
55. Beer C T, Richards J F: The metabolism of vinca alkaloids part II. The fate of tritiated vinblastine in rats. Lloydia 27:352, 1964
56. Owellen R J, Hartke C A: The pharmacokinetics of 4-acetyl tritium vinblastine in two patients. Cancer Res 35:975, 1975
57. Dixon, G J, Dulmadge E A, Mulligan L T, et al: Cell culture bioassay for vincristine sulfate in sera from mice, rats, dogs, and monkeys. Cancer Res 29:1810, 1969
58. Morasca L, Rainisio C, Masera G: Duration of cytotoxic activity of vincristine in the blood of leukemic children. Europ J Cancer 5:79, 1969
59. Owellen R J, Donigian D W: (^{3}H) Vincristine. Preparation and preliminary pharmacology. J Med Chem 15:894, 1972
60. Bleyer W A, Frisby S A, Oliverio V T: Uptake of vincristine by murine leukemia cells. Biochem Pharmacol 24:633, 1975
61. Donigian D W, Owellen R J: Interaction of vinblastine, vincristine and colchicine with serum proteins. Biochem Pharmacol 22:2113, 1973

Joseph Holland Burchenal
David J. Straus

6
Mechanisms of Action of Antitumor Antibiotics

During the past 25 years there has been large-scale screening of antibiotic filtrates for their activity against animal tumors, both in vivo and in vitro, and a large number of active materials have been found, but, because of duplication and difficulties in isolation, few have come to clinical trial; of these, only a small group have shown practical clinical activity. Because of the limitations of time and space, it is on this small select group that we would like to concentrate. The mechanisms of action of these clinically active compounds have been studied in isolated enzyme systems, in bacteria, in cell culture and in normal or neoplastic tissues in the intact animal.

The first antitumor antibiotics, on which mechanism of action studies were done, were the glutamine antagonists, azaserine (O-diazoacetyl-L-serine) and DON (6-diazo-5-oxo-L norleucine). These two naturally occurring diazo compounds were isolated from broth filtrates of *Streptomyces* and their chemical structures were determined in 1954 by Fusari and co-workers[1] and by Diom et al[2] in 1956. These compounds are closely related in structure to glutamine. They were shown by Stock et al[3] and Clarke et al[4] to have rather marked antitumor effect against Sarcoma 180, and later against various strains of mouse leukemia[5,6] and experimental tumors in mice.[7-9] Original clinical studies of these compounds in 1954 and 1957[10,11] showed very little beneficial effect but later studies by Karnofsky et al[12,13] demonstrated these compounds to be active and useful in the treatment of trophoblastic tumors. DON, particularly, appears to be practical in that it can be given by mouth, and dosages that are essentially nontoxic produce permanent remissions in women with relatively slow-growing trophoblastic tumors. It appears to be definitely inferior to methotrexate or actinomycin D, however, in the treatment of fulminating choriocarcinoma.[13]

In the metabolic pathway for the synthesis of purines, both azaserine and DON block the conversion of formylglycineamide ribotide (FGAR) to the corresponding formylglycineamidine ribotide (FGAM), a process involving glutamine and a phosphoribosylformyl glycineamidine synthetase. The antimetabolites are tightly bound to this enzyme so that, in an in vitro system, if they react with the enzyme prior to the addition of glutamine, they cannot be displaced.[14] The glutamine antagonists also act earlier in the metabolic pathway for the synthesis of the purine skel-

Supported by Grants NCI-05826, 07848, 18856, ACS Laurens Hammond Memorial CH-27S, and the Hearst Foundation.

eton to block the reaction of 5-phosphoribosyl-1-pyrophosphate with glutamine to form 5-phosphoribosylamine. This system is not as sensitive to the antimetabolites as the preceding one.[15] Because of this interference with de novo synthesis of purines, azaserine and 6-MP have been studied and found synergistic against Sarcoma 180 by Stock and others.[15a] DON also acts to prevent the transfer of the amide nitrogen of glutamine to uridylic acid to form cytidylic acid, and to xanthylic acid to form guanylic acid.[16]

Diazo-oxo-norvaline (DONV) was synthesized by Handschumacher et al[17] in the hope that it would be an antagonist of asparagine, and, therefore, be of value in combination with the enzyme asparaginase in the treatment of asparagine-dependent tumors and leukemias. Unfortunately, this compound binds irreversibly with asparaginase and thus prevents its deamination of asparagine.[18] It has not so far been shown to be of therapeutic value.[19]

A congener, 5-chloro-5-oxo-2-aminopentanoic acid, synthesized by Khedouri and co-workers,[20] and shown by them to be an inhibitor of asparagine synthetase,[21] has been shown by our group to potentiate the effects of asparaginase in sensitive mouse leukemias.[22]

Actinomycin, the first crystalline antibiotic obtained from a *Streptomyces* and the first antibiotic shown to have antitumor activity, was isolated by Waksman and Woodruff in 1940.[23] It was active against rodent tumors[24,25] and was shown by Schulte[26] to be the first antibiotic with activity against human tumors. The actinomycins have their greatest field of usefulness in Wilms' tumor in children, as shown by Farber et al[27,28] and Tan and co-workers,[29] in uterine choriocarcinomas by Ross et al,[30] in the lymphomas by Schulte[26] and in combination with methotrexate and chlorambucil in testicular tumors by Li et al.[31] A rather interesting finding is that, in children with Wilms' tumor, actinomycin D appears to protect against the development of second primary tumors in the irradiated area.[31]

The structures of some of the actinomycins have been elucidated and different derivatives separated out or specifically synthesized by Brockman et al.[32,33] Although they differ markedly in toxicity, there is no evidence showing any one of them definitely more effective in mouse leukemia than actinomycin D, or having a different mechanism of action.[34]

Actinomycin D inhibits DNA-dependent RNA synthesis[35-37] and this effect is reversed by the addition of an excess of native DNA.[38,39] A slower interference with DNA replication has been found in some in vitro cell systems.[39a] In vitro, actinomycin combines with DNA.[40-44] The DNA-actinomycin complexes are unafffected by ionic strength, are preferentially formed with native rather than denatured DNA and show absolute base specificity for guanine.[45] It is suggested that this specificity is mediated by the amino group located in the minor groove of the DNA helix. This binding results in intercalation of actinomycin D with DNA as shown by studies with "sheared" DNA preparation in its ability to unwind "supercoiled" virus DNA.[46] X-ray crystallography had elucidated the major features of actinomycin D-DNA binding: (1) intercalation of the phenoxazone ring of actinomycin between guanine-cytosine sequences in DNA, (2) hydrogen bonding between the polypeptide portion of the DNA molecule and deoxyguanosines on opposite DNA chains, and (3) the coincidence of the two-fold axis of symmetry of the three polypeptide rings of the actinomycin molecule with that of DNA[47-49] The binding is specific for double helical DNA, and will not occur with double helical RNA, DNA-RNA hybrids or single-stranded DNA or RNA.[50] Actinomycin in vitro inhibits RNA polymerase.[38,39] Studies in vivo with liver tissue[51-53] or ascites cells,[54] with cells in culture[35,40,55-57] or with isolated enzyme systems,[36,39,42,58-62] all indicate the inhibition of RNA polymerization by the complexing of actinomycin with the DNA templates.

Cell kinetic studies have shown a block of cells in G_2. Cytotoxicity seems to be maximum at, or near, early S-phase.[46,63,64] DNA strand-breaks also occur in tissue culture with Chinese hamster ovary, and mouse mammary, tumor cells.[63] Differential retention rather than differential uptake seems to be an important factor in specific tissue sensitivity to the drug.[65]

Mitomycin C, an antibiotic isolated from *Streptomyces caespitosus*,[66,67] has a wide range of antitumor activity against transplantable mouse and rat tumors.[68] Broad clinical trials in Japan and in the United States have shown its effect in lymphomas, chronic leukemias and some forms of solid tumors.[69-72] It appears to be a useful agent for the treatment of chronic granulocytic leukemia, and also for gastrointestinal and breast malignancies.[73] Studies on the structure of mitomycin C[74-77] have shown it to contain a quinone ring, a carbamate and an aziridine ring, and at one time or another, certain compounds containing any of these groups have been shown to have independent chemotherapeutic action in some animal tumors. Mitomycin C probably functions as a bifunctional or trifunctional alkylating agent when it is activated. Mitomycin binds to DNA by covalent and noncovalent bonds and, like other alkylating agents, causes cross-linking of DNA strands.[78,79] The site of covalent bonding is possibly the O_6 position of guanine.[79] Mitomycin selectively inhibits DNA synthesis in bacteria[80-82] and mammalian cells in cultuie.[83] The early inhibition of DNA synthesis by mitomycin C is probably the result of a failure in the synthesis or utilization of precursors, but not of a primary depolymerization of DNA.[84] The early inhibition of DNA synthesis precedes inhibition of RNA synthesis and is accompanied by lowered mitotic activity. The finding that RNA is not affected initially indicates that the inhibition of DNA synthesis is not caused by a disturbance in the metabolism of precursors common to both DNA and RNA. The simultaneous inhibition of thymidine incorporation, and of mitosis, suggests that the primary action is on the final assembly of DNA. Mitomycin C causes chromosome damage in many cell systems, including phytohemagglutinin-stimulated cultured human lymphocytes,[85,86] and has been shown to be carcinogenic in rats and mice.[73]

Mithramycin is closely related chemically to olivomycin and chromomycin. It was isolated from *Streptomyces* in 1962,[87] chromomycin from *S. griseus 7* in 1958[88] and olivomycin from *S. olivoreticuli 16749* in 1962.[89] All three are active against rodent tumors and have had beneficial effects in some human tumors as well; mithramycin is now recommended for actinomycin D-resistant testicular tumors and is also useful in the treatment of hypercalcemia associated with malignancy.[90] Olivomycin is considerably less toxic, and requires a larger dosage, than mithramycin or chromomycin.[91] In many spectrophotometric tests, the three drugs are indistinguishable but, by using a series of four solvent systems, Gause[91] has been able to separate the three. Chromomycin A_3 has been reported to selectively inhibit the biosynthesis of RNA in mammalian cells grown in cell culture, human bone marrow cells and human leukemic leukocytes, while the formation of DNA was not affected.[91,92] Olivomycin produces selective inhibition of the synthesis of RNA in the cells of Sarcoma 180 in the mouse.[93] Except for the Mg^{++} requirement, the properties of chromomycin, mithramycin and olivomycin, in respect to their binding to DNA in vitro, are similar to those of actinomycin. Their tumor-inhibiting properties and their toxicity differ somewhat from those of the actinomycins, however.[91]

The anthracyclines are among the most clinically useful antitumor antibiotics. Daunomycin (daunorubicin) was isolated by DiMarco et al. in 1963 and was shown to have activity against certain animal tumors.[94-98] It was originally studied clinically by Tan and co-workers[99,100] and Bernard et al,[101] and was shown to produce remissions in acute leukemias.

Adriamycin (hydroxyldaunomycin) was isolated from a mutant bacteria, *Streptomyces penucetius* var. *caesius*, and its antitumor activity was demonstrated in 1969 by DiMarco and colleagues.[102] Clinical trials were begun in Italy by Bonadonna in 1969,[103] and in the U.S.A. in 1970.[104] Unlike daunomycin, adriamycin has shown significant activity in a variety of solid tumors including sarcomas, breast carcinoma, lymphoma, neuroblastoma, bronchogenic carcinoma, germ cell testis tumors, bladder carcinoma and various epidermoid carcinomas.[104-106] Major limiting toxicity are myelosuppression and myocardial damage. The most common current dosage schedule for adriamycin as a single agent is 60-75 mg/M^2 intravenously every 21 days.[105]

Following the suggestions of De Duve[107] "lysosmotrophic" complexes of daunomycin[108] and adriamycin[109] were found to be more effective against L1210 leukemia, administered by some routes, than free drugs alone. According to this concept, a greater therapeutic index may be attained if the drug complex is taken up selectively by tumor cells with endocytic properties, and not by normal (cardiac) cells that lack this property.[107-108] Phase I studies of adriamycin-DNA complexes showed comparable acute toxicity with adriamycin alone.[109] Total cumulative doses and patient numbers were too small to permit evaluation of cardiac toxicity. Daunomycin-DNA, in combination with vincristine and cytosine arabinoside, gave complete responses in 11 of 19 patients (58 per cent) with nonlymphoblastic leukemia. This is comparable to regimens using daunomycin alone.[110]

Several analogues of daunomycin and adriamycin are currently under evaluation. Rubidizone (benzoylhydrazone daunorubicin), a semisynthetic derivative of daunomycin, was found to be less cardiotoxic than daunomycin or adriamycin in a rat model system.[111] Its antitumor effect and myelotoxicity were comparable to that of adriamycin in mouse spleen colonies of normal marrow (CFU-S) and P388 leukemia.[112] Cross-resistance with daunomycin, adriamycin, vincristine and vinblastine has been demonstrated in Ehrlich ascites tumor.[113] Rubidazone, as a single agent in previously untreated patients, resulted in complete remissions in 40 of 70 patients (57 per cent), with acute myelogenous leukemia, four out of five (80 per cent), with acute lymphocytic leukemia and 12 out of 14 (86 per cent), with acute monocytic leukemia.[114] A 39 per cent complete response rate was attained on previously treated adults with acute leukemia.[115] Rubidazone has some activity against lymphomas[114] but, as shown in a preliminary report, no activity was seen against solid tumors in adults.[116] Clinical trials of rubidazone in solid tumors are currently under way at Memorial Sloan-Kettering Cancer Center. N-Trifluoroacetyladriamycin-14-valerate (AD32), an adriamycin analogue, was more effective than adriamycin in L1210 and P388 mouse leukemias with less toxicity.[117,118] The antitumor effect of AD32 was superior to that of adriamycin in Ridgeway osteogenic sarcoma, and AD32 exhibited activity in a P388 leukemia resistant to adriamcyin.[119]

Adriamycin and daunomycin penetrate cells rapidly and locate in the nucleus.[121,122] Daunomycin causes damage to the nucleolus, and it has been suggested that its effect on ribosomal RNA synthesis is a consequence of this damage.[121] Both drugs cause chromatid and chromosome damage in animal cells and human fibroblasts and leukocytes.[121-126] Daunomycin has been found to be carcinogenic in rats.[127] Adriamycin and daunomycin both produce a unique fluorescence which can be localized to nuclear structures in exposed cells by fluorescent microscopy.[128] A large number of studies have shown that the drugs interfere with DNA-directed DNA and RNA synthesis in vitro, in vivo in tissue culture cell lines, in cells of tumor bearing animals[121,122,129] and in human lymphocytes.[125] An association of antibiotics and DNA cause alterations in the physicochemical properties of each, suggesting formation of a complex between the two.[121,122,129] Stable drug-DNA complexes are formed by intercalation of the aglycone ring of the drug between the base pairs of the DNA helix. DiMarco[121,122] has also suggested that electrostatic attractions between the protonated 3′-amino group of the daunosamine sugar and the phosphate groups of the helix and hydrogen bonds, and possibly between the 9-hydroxy of the aglycone ring and an adjacent phosphate of a DNA base, are also involved in the drug-DNA interaction. This suggestion is consistent with a stereochemical model of drug-DNA interaction constructed by Pigram and associates from X-ray diffraction studies in which the amino sugar moiety of the drug is located in the large groove of DNA and the hydrophobic portions of the base pairs of DNA and the hydrophobic aglycone ring of the antibiotic overlap.[130] Further evidence favoring intercalation was provided by experiments in which daunomycin caused the unwinding of supercoiled closed-circle viral DNA in a manner similar to actinomycin D.[46] Several studies suggest that the inhibition of DNA-directed DNA and RNA synthesis is due to interference with the DNA template rather than directly with the polymerase enzymes.[121,122,128] There has been some suggestion that adenine-thymine sequences and base pairs are the preferential sites of drug inhibition.[122,129,131]

Kinetic studies in animal and human tissue culture cell lines suggest that daunomycin and adriamycin cause delays in all phases of the cell cycle,[123] but that the delay is most pronounced by the G and S phases.[133,134] Cytotoxic effects of the drug were most pronounced in S-phase in most studies,[123,134,135] although synchronized Chinese hamster ovary cells were also sensitive in the M-phase.[132] In cell lines in which a "plateau" slow-growth phase is induced in a portion of cells in G1, both adriamycin and daunomycin exhibit cytotoxic effects, although this effect is greater in cells in an exponential growth phase.[132,134,136] The effects of the administration of daunomycin to leukemic patients on the kinetics of the leukemic cells have shown blocks of cells in G2 and G1 and maximum cytotoxicity in S-phase in some studies,[137,138] but these effects have not been found consistently in others.[139]

It is possible that cytotoxic effects may not be totally related to DNA synthesis by daunomycin and adriamycin as the cell kinetic studies suggest. Cell kill has also been seen in tissue culture studies at levels of the drugs which cause a minimal inhibition of 3H-thymidine uptake and the suggestion has been made that his may be related, even at these dosages to chromosome damage which results in lethal interference with other cell metabolism.[122,129,134]

Carminomycin, another anthracycline, was isolated from *Actinomadura carminata* and has been shown to be more effective in L1210 leukemia by the intravenous route than daunomycin at doses of equivalent toxicity.[120] Activity was also found in lymphosarcoma, esophageal and bronchogenic carcinoma in mice.[120] Myelotoxicity was its major acute side effect in dogs.[120] This drug is currently undergoing Phase I and Phase II trials in the U.S.S.R.

Other effects of the drugs may be unrelated to DNA binding. Gonsalves and coworkers found inhibitory effects of daunomycin and adriamycin on respiration in isolated mitochondria from normal tissues and in ascites Ehrlich tumor cells,[140] Folkers and associates have found in vitro inhibition of succinoxidase and NADH oxidase, respiratory chain enzymes requiring coenzyme Q10 as a cofactor, by adriamycin, daunomycin and carminomycin.[141]

An antimitotic effect of daunomycin was seen at doses that do not affect DNA synthesis.[122,132] N-acetyl-daunomycin, which is a weak inhibitor of nucleic acid synthesis, is able to block mitosis.[122] The work of Dano on the cross-resistance of daunomycin, adriamycin, vincristine and vinblastine in Ehrlich ascites tumors, also raises the possibility that some of the effects of the anthracyclines could be on the mitotic spindle, although common mechanisms of transport of the drugs into and out of the cells may also be an important factor in cross-resistance.[142]

At a cellular and molecular level, it is not possible to easily account for the differential clinical effects of daunomycin and adriamycin. In vivio and in vitro studies of the differential effects of the two antibiotics on DNA and RNA synthesis, as well as studies of differential uptake of the two drugs by intake cells, vary with the system used.[121,129,143]

Adriamycin has been shown to be less immunosuppressive than daunomycin. In mice infected with Moloney sarcoma virus, preinfection as postinfection treatment with daunomycin result in tumor progression and early recurrence, respectively. Preinfection treatment with adriamycin does not effect host-mediated tumor regression and postinfection treatment with adriamycin delays recurrence longer than treatment with daunomycin.[144] In skin allografts in mice[145] and in mice that were administered P388 leukemia after previous immunosuppressive whole body irradiation, adriamycin shows less of an immunosuppressive effect than daunomycin.[143] By contrast, however, adriamycin, blunted the primary oral antibody response to sheep red blood cells in mice, although daunomycin suppressed the secondary response more than adriamycin.[145]

Carminomycin seems to be unique among the anthracyclines in its preferential inhibition of DNA over RNA synthesis in cultured L1210 leukemic cells. Approximately equal levels of inhibition of both are seen with daunomycin and adriamycin.[129] Recent studies have shown a lack of DNA-binding by AD32, suggesting that this compound is either converted to a DNA-binding metabolite or that it has a different mechanism of action than the other anthracyclines.[146]

Since cardiotoxicity limits the long-term administration of adriamycin and daunomycin, the search for less cardiotoxic congeners is being pursued by Zbinder et al.[147] In addition, recent studies have suggested that α tocopherol protects mice against the lethal cardiotoxicity of adriamycin[148] and clinical studies with this combination are in progress. Folkers has suggested that coenzyme Q10 may also be effective in this respect.[149]

The bleomycins were isolated from *Streptomyces verticillus.* Myelosuppression was mild and the limiting toxicity was extensive damage to the skin[150] and the lung. The selectivity of therapeutic[151,152] and toxic effects upon epidermal tissues suggests preferential drug localization therein and this has been confirmed by drug distribution studies.[153,154] Since the first clinical trials conducted in Japan by Ichikawa and co-workers,[155] bleomycin has been extensively used in this country. Clinical responses have been seen in epidermoid carcinomas of the head and neck and uterine cervix, germ cell testis tumors and lymphomas.[156,157] A variety of schedules have been used in various chemotherapeutic combinations. Currently, at Memorial Sloan-Kettering Cancer Center, a 7-day continuous intravenous infusion is being used in protocols for germ cell testicular tumors[158] and head and neck carcinoma.[159] A low-dose daily subcutaneous schedule is used in the protocol for poor prognosis Hodgkin's Disease.[160]

A non-enzymatic reaction of the bleomycins with DNA causes single- and double-strand scissions.[161,162] Single-strand scission appears to be directly correlated with cytotoxicity in L1210 leukemia.[163] Binding to DNA seems to involve the B-aminoalanine amide and the carbamoyl moieties of the bleomycin molecule.[162] Thymine bases seem to be split from DNA.[164,165] It has been suggested that strand scission occurs when a critical amount of thymine has been liberated from DNA.[164] Morphologic studies have shown that bleomycin induced chromosome damage in animal tissue culture cell lines,[166] in vivo bone marrow preparations[167] and in human lymphocytes simulated with phytohemagglutinin.[168] In cell-free biochemical studies, bleomycin inhibited the action of DNA-dependent DNA and RNA polymerase, presumably by interfering with the DNA template, although DNA but not RNA synthesis was inhibited in intact cells. Protein synthesis was not affected.[164,165] DNA ligase, the enzyme which repairs DNA breaks, is also inhibited by bleomycin in rat hepatoma cells.[169] In rat hepatoma cells, DNA fragmentation is more marked in tumors sensitive to, than in tumors resistant to, bleomycin.[170] Another mechanism of resistance to bleomycin is suggested by studies of a bleomycin-inactivating enzyme which hydrolyzes the B-aminoalanine amide group from the molecule.[161,162] Levels of this enzyme were lower in epidermoid skin carcinoma than in sarcomas induced in mice by methylcholanthene.[171] Lower levels were also found in sensitive rather than in resistant rat hepatoma cells.[162] A third mechanism for resistance in rat hepatoma cells was suggested by studies which showed less binding of ^{14}C-bleomycin to DNA of resistant, than of sensitive, rat hepatoma cells.[172] Cell tissue culture kinetic studies have shown that cytotoxicity is most marked in the M and then the G2 phases of the cell cycle.[173,174] Bleomycin is also cytotoxic to tissue culture cells in which a "plateau" growth phase has been induced in which a portion of cells are resting in G1.[175,176,177] Effects of bleomycin on the immune system are unclear. No significant bleomycin effect was seen in humoral immunity or spleen cell-mediated tumor cytotoxicity in mice.[178] Inhibition was greater for B-lymphocyte cultures, however, than bone marrow cultures (CFU-C) in mice treated with bleomycin.[179]

Streptozotocin, a nitrosourea antibiotic isolated from *Streptomyces achromogenes,*[180] was shown by Schein and colleagues[181,182] to produce diabetes and to have an antitumor effect without significant bone marrow toxicity. Therapeutic effectiveness of this agent was demonstrated in patients with advanced lymphoma, islet cell tumors of the pancreas, malignant melanoma and sarcoma.[183] Streptozotocin differs from the synthetic chloroethyl nitrosourea, BCNU, by methyl and aminoglucose replacement of the two chloroethyl groups. Schein and co-workers[181,182] also showed that the diabetogenic property of streptozotocin seemed to be related to its ability to reduce levels of pyridine nucleotides in mouse liver and pancreatic islet cells. This ability seemed to be related to the substitution of a methyl for a chloroethyl group. The aminoglucose group appeared to facilitate entry of streptozotocin into the islet cells.[181,182,184,185] The marrow-sparing effect also seemed to be related to the animoglucose group.[181] With these observations in mind, two new derivatives combining aminoglucose and chloroethyl groups, tetraacetyl chlorozotocin and chlorozotocin, were synthesized by Johnston and co-workers.[186] The latter compound, which is water soluble, was found to be as effective as BCNU in L1210 leukemia with less marrow toxicity.[187,188] This decrease of marrow toxicity has also been found in human marrow cells.[189] Chlorozotocin and streptozotocin apparently alkylate DNA, but the mechanism of their marrow-sparing effect is unclear at present.[189] Cytotoxic effects were greater in non-cycling Chinese hamster ovary cells with chlorozotocin than with streptozotocin. Chlorozotocin caused an earlier and more marked pile-up of cells in G2. Both drugs caused non-disjunctive errors in mitosis and formation of polyploid cells. Thus, kinetic effects seemed to be greater on cell division than on DNA replication.[190] Chlorozotocin is currently undergoing Phase 1 clinical investigation in several institutions, including Memorial Sloan-Kettering Cancer Center.

Asparaginase has been shown to produce remissions in approximately 60 per cent of patients with ALL and 10 per cent of those with AML, and it has not had significant reproducible activity in other types of leukemia or solid tumors. The remissions in acute leukemia are of short duration, with a median duration of about three months, and resistance frequently develops rapidly. It is probable that asparaginase must be combined with other agents to realize its full therapeutic potential.[191-193] Fortunately, its antileukemic effects are potentiated by a large number of compounds of diverse mechanisms of action, such as actinomycin D, vincristine, daunomycin, adriamycin, arabinofuranosyl cytosine (Ara-C), thioguanine and 5-hydroxypicolinaldehyde thiosemicarbazone (5-HP). A clinical evaluation suggested that a sequential combination of vincristine, prednisone, daunomycin, Ara-C plus thioguanine and asparaginase might be of value.[194]

Asparaginase-sensitive leukemic cells in both mouse and man lack the enzyme, asparagine synthetase, and so must rely on an exogenous source of asparagine. The mechanism of action of asparaginase is the destruction of the plasma asparagine, thus depriving these cells of an amino acid essential for protein synthesis. DNA and RNA synthesis are also inhibited by asparaginase. Cells developing resistance to asparaginase contain large quantities of the enzyme, asparagine synthetase, and the mechanism of host resistance is presumably the induction of this enzyme into the resistant cell.

There have been several C-nucleoside antibiotics which have had some effect on experimental tumors. One of these is Pyrazomycin (pyrazofurin) which was isolated from a fermentation broth of S. *candidus*.[195] The structure has been elucidated as 3(5)ribosyl-4-hydroxypyrazolo-5(3)carboxamide.[196] It has a definite antiviral effect and inhibits the growth of Walker carcinoma 256 in rats.[196] It is a strong inhibitor of orotidylic acid decarboxylase.[197] Phase I and II studies in man have shown that it has an extremely long half-life and some minor effects on lymphomas, particularly mycosis fungoides, have been noted.[198] This has been more striking when pyrazofurin has been given in combination with F3TdR.[199] Several other C-nucleosides with antitumor effects have been isolated from antibiotic filtrates and tested for antitumor activity by various Japanese investigators. Formycin has been shown by Ishuzuka et al[200] to inhibit the growth of the Ehrlich ascites tumor and to increase the life span of mice with L1210 leukemia by 50 per cent when given intraperitoneally starting 2 hours after i.p. (intraperitoneal) inoculation of 10^6 cells. Similar antitumor effects have been shown for oxazinomycin[201] and showdomycin.[202] Most of these effects were achieved with drugs administered i.p. shortly after small i.p. tumor inoculations and were relatively minor. No clinical therapeutic effect for these other naturally occurring C-nucleosides has been reported.

A close analogue of these C-nucleoside antibiotics is 5-ribofuranosylisocytidine or pseudoisocytidine. This compound was synthesized by Chu et al[203] in hopes of obtaining a more stable analogue of 5-azacytidine which would have an equal or greater antitumor effect with less undesirable side-effects. Pseudoisocytidine, to the best of our knowledge, is the first synthetic pyrimidine C-nucleoside for which any antitumor effects have been demonstrated.[204] Pseudoisocytidine acts as an antagonist of cytidine. Its inhibitory effects in tissue culture and its toxic and therapeutic effects in mouse leukemia in vivo can be blocked by cytidine, but not by deoxycytidine or thymidine.[205] It is active in vitro and in vivo against lines of leukemic cells made resistant to ara-C, 6-mercaptopurine, platinum diammino dichloride and methotrexate. Similarly, lines of leukemia made resistant to pseudoisocytidine are still highly sensitive to ara-C, methotrexate, mercaptopurine, vincristine, actinomycin D, adriamycin and platinum diammino dichloride. It has been shown by Fox et al[205A] to be chemically stable at 7.4 for 6 days at 22°C and at least 3 days at 37°C. Preliminary studies by Kreis[207] have shown no deamination on incubation in vitro with cytidine deaminase from mouse kidneys. These data suggest that, in contrast to ara-C and azacytidine, pseudoisocytidine is stable against both enzymatic and chemical catabolism. Labeled pseudoisocytidine is incorporated into RNA and DNA and is excreted intact in the urine, over 90 per cent in the first 24 hours, as shown by Zedeck et al.[206] Preclinical toxicology and pharmacology has been done by Philips et al.[208] It is hoped that this compound will be active in patients with AML whose disease has become resistant to ara-C and 2,2′-anhydro-1-B-D-arabinofuranosyl-5-fluorocytosine (AAFC).

Therapeutic value of the antibiotics alone and particularly in combination with cancer chemotherapy is firmly established. Actinomycin D in trophoblastic disease, Wilms' tumor, embryonal rhabdomyosarcoma, Ewing's tumor and germ cell tumors; adriamycin in osteogenic sarcoma, breast, oat cell cancer of the lung, soft part sarcomas and acute leukemias; and bleomycin in head and neck tumors, lymphomas and germ cell tumors, to mention but a few, form an essential part of our armamentarium. It is to be hoped that the newer analogues at present under study will be even more beneficial.

References

1. Fusari, S A, Haskell, T H, Frohardt R B, Bartz Q R: Azaserine, a new tumor-inhibitory substance: Structural studies. J Amer Chem Soc 76:2881, 1954
2. Diom H W, Fusari S A, Jakubowski Z L, Zora J G, Bartz Q R: 6-Diazo-5-oxo-L-norleucine, a new tumor-inhibitory substance. II. Isolation and characterization. J Amer Chem Soc 78:3075, 1956
3. Stock C C, Reilly H C, Buckley S M, et al: Azaserine, a new tumor-inhibitory substance: Studies with Crocker mouse sarcoma 180. Nature 173:71, 1954
4. Clarke D A, Reilly H C, Stock C C: Comparative study of 6-diazo-5-oxo-L-norleucine and *O*-diazoacetyl-L-serine on sarcoma 180. Proc Amer Ass Cancer Res 2:100, 1956 (abstract)
5. Burchenal J H, Murphy M L, Yuceoglu M, Horsfall M: The effect of a new antimetabolite, *O*-diazoacetyl-L-serine, in mouse leukemia. Proc Amer Ass Cancer Res 1:7 (abstr), 1954
6. Burchenal J H, Dagg M K: Effects of 6-diazo-5-oxo-L-norleucine and 2-ethylamino-thiadiazole on strains of transplanted mouse leukemia. Proc Amer Ass Cancer Res 2:97 (abstr), 1956
7. Gellhorn A, Hirschberg E (eds): Investigation of diverse systems for cancer chemotherapy screening. Cancer Res 15, (Suppl 3), 1955
8. Sugiura K, Schmid M S: Effects of antibiotics on growth of variety of mouse and rat tumors. Proc Amer Ass Cancer Res 2:151 (abstr), 1956
9. Sugiura K, Stock C C: Effect of *O*-diazoacetyl-L-serine (azaserine) on growth of various mouse and rat tumors. Proc Soc Exp Biol Med 88:127, 1955
10. Ellison R R, Karnofsky D A, Sternberg S S, et al: Clinical trials of *O*-diazoacetyl-L-serine (azaserine) in neoplastic disease. Cancer 7:801, 1954
11. Magill G B, Myers W P L, Reilly H C, et al: Pharmacological and initial therapeutic observations on 6-diazo-5-oxo-L-norleucine (DON) in human neoplastic disease. Cancer 10:1138, 1957
12. Karnofsky D A, Golbey R B, Li M C: Remissions induced in trophoblastic tumors by 6-diazo-5-oxo-L-norleucine (DON). Proc Amer Ass Cancer Res 5:33, 1964
13. Karnofsky D A, Golbey R B, Li M C: Remissions induced in trophoblastic tumors by 6-diazo-5-oxo-L-norleucine (DON). *In* Holland J F, Hreshchyshyn M M (eds) Choriocarcinoma, vol. 3. (UICC Monograph, New York, Springer-Verlag, 1967, pp 126–134
14. Levenberg B, Melnick I, Buchanan J M: Bio-

synthesis of purines. XV. The effect of aza-L-serine and 6-diazo-5-oxo-L-norleucine on inosinic acid biosynthesis de novo. J Biol Chem 225:163, 1957

15. Goldthwait D A: 5-Phosphoribosylamine, a precursor of glycinamide ribotide. J Biol Chem 222:1051, 1956

15a. Tarnowski G S, Stock C C: Effects of combinations of azaserine and 6-diazo-5-oxo-L-norleucine with purine analogs and other antimetabolites on the growth of two mouse mammary carcinomas. Cancer Res 17:1033–1039, 1957

16. Anderson E P, Law L W: Biochemistry of cancer. Ann Rev Biochem 29:577, 1960

17. Handschumacher R E, Bates C J, Chang P K, et al: 5-Diazo-4-oxo-L-norvaline: Reactive asparagine analog with biological specificity. Science 161:62, 1968

18. Jackson R C, Handschumacher R E: *Escherichia coli* L-asparaginase. Catalytic activity and subunit structure. Biochemistry 9:3585, 1970

19. Handschumacher R E: Personal communication.

20. Khedouri E, Anderson P M, Meister A: Selective inactivation of the glutamine binding site to *Escherichia coli* carbamyl phosphate synthetase by 2-amino-4-oxo-5-chloropentanoic acid. Biochemistry 5:3552, 1966

21. Horowitz B, Meister A: Asparagine synthetase from RADAI leukemia cells, in Bernard J, Boiron M (eds): La L-asparaginase. International Symposium on L-asparaginase, Paris, 1970. Paris, Centre National de la Recherche Scientifique, 1971, pp 243–351

22. Burchenal J H, Clarkson B D, Dowling M D, Jr, et al: Experimental and clinical studies of L-asparaginase in combination therapy, in Bernard J, Boiron M (eds): La L-asparaginase. International Symposium on L-asparaginase, Paris, 1970. Paris, Centre National de la Recherche Scientifique, 1971, pp 243–351

23. Waksman S A, Woodruff H B: Bacteriostatic and bactericidal substances produced by a soil actinomyces. Proc Soc Exp Biol Med 45:609, 1940

24. Reilly H C, Stock C C, Buckley S M, Clarke D A: The effect of antibiotics upon the growth of sarcoma 180 in vivo. Cancer Res, 13:684, 1953

25. Hackmann C: Experimentelle untersuchungen über die wirkung von actinomycin C (HBF 386) bei bösartigen geschwülsten. Z Krebsforsch. 58:607, 1952

26. Schulte G: Erfahrungen mit neuen cytostatischen mitteln bei hämoblastosen und carcinomen und die abgrenzung ihrer wirkungen gegen roentgentherapie. Z Krebsforsch. 58:500, 1952

27. Farber S, D'Angio G, Evans A, Mitus A: Clinical studies on actinomycin D with special reference to Wilms' tumor in children. Ann N Y Acad Sci 89:421, 1960

28. Farber S: Current clinical and experimental studies in cancer chemotherapy. Cancer Chemother Rep 13:159, 1961

29. Tan C T C, Dargeon H W, Burchenal J H: The effects of actinomycin D on cancer in childhood. Pediatrics 24:544, 1959

30. Ross G, Stolbach L L, Hertz R: Actinomycin D in the treatment of methotrexate resistant trophoblastic disease in women. Cancer Res 22:1015, 1962

31. Li M C, Whitmore W F, Golbey R, Grabstalt H: Effects of combined drug therapy on metastatic cancer of testis. JAMA 174:1291, 1960

31a. D'Angio G J, Meadows A, Mike V, et al: Decreased risk of radiation-associated second malignant neoplasms in actinomycin D treated patients. Cancer 37:1177, 1976

32. Brockmann H, Bohnsack G, Franck B, et al: Zur konstitution der actinomycine. Angew Chem 68:70, 1956

33. Brockmann H: Structural differences of the actinomycins and their derivatives. Ann N Y Acad Sci 89:323, 1960

34. Burchenal J H, Oettgen H F, Reppert J A, Coley V: The effect of actinomycins and their derivatives on a spectrum of transplanted mouse leukemia. Ann N Y Acad Sci 89:399, 1960

35. Franklin R M: The inhibition of ribonucleic acid synthesis in mammalian cells by actinomycin D. Biochim Biophys Acta 72:555, 1963

36. Kahan E, Kahan F M, Hurwitz J: The role of deoxyribonucleic acid in ribonucleic acid synthesis. VI. Specificity of action of actinomycin D. J Biol Chem 238:2491, 1963

37. Reich E: Biochemistry of actinomycins. Cancer Res 23:1428, 1963

38. Goldberg I H, Rabinowitz M: Actinomycin D inhibition of deoxyribonucleic acid-dependent synthesis of ribonucleic acid. Science 136:315, 1962

39. Hurwitz J, Furth J J, Malamy M, Alexander M: The role of deoxyribonucleic acid in ribonucleic acid synthesis. III. The inhibition of the enzymatic synthesis of the ribonucleic acid and deoxyribonucleic acid by actinomycin D and proflavin. Proc Nat Acad Sci USA 48:1222, 1962

39a. Bacchetti S, Whitmore G F: Actinomycin D: Effects on mouse L-cells. Biophys J 9:1427, 1969

40. Kawamata J, Imanishi M: Interaction of actinomycin with deoxyribonucleic acid. Nature 187:1112, 1960
41. Kersten W: Interaction of actinomycin D with constituents of nucleic acids. Biochim Biophys Acta 47:610, 1961
42. Kersten W, Kersten H, Rauen H M: Action of nucleic acid on the inhibition of growth by actinomycin of *Neurospora crassa*. Nature 187:60, 1960
43. Kirk J M: The mode of action of actinomycin D. Biochim Biophys Acta 42:167, 1960
44. Rauen H M, Kersten H, Kersten W: Zur Wirkungsweise von Actinomycinen Hoppe Seyler Z Physiol Chem 321:139, 1960
45. Ward D C, Reich E, Goldberg I H: Base specificity in the interaction of polynucleotides with antibiotic drugs. Science 149:1259, 1965
46. Waring M: Variation of the supercoils in closed circular DNA by binding antibiotics and drugs: Evidence for molecular models involving intercalation. J Mol Biol 54:247, 1970
47. Sobell H M, Jain S C: Stereochemistry of actinomycin binding to DNA II. Detailed molecular model of actinomycin-DNA complex and its implications. J Mol Biol 68:21, 1972
48. Sobell H M: The stereochemistry of actinomycin binding to DNA and its implications in molecular biology. Prog Nucl Acid Res Mol Biol 13:153, 1973
49. Sobell H M: How actinomycin binds to DNA. Sci Amer 231:82, 1974
50. Reich E, Cerami A, Ward D C: Actinomycin, in Gottlieb D, Shaw P D (eds): Antibiotics, vol. I. Mechanism of action. New York, Springer-Verlag, 1967, p 714
51. Schwartz H S, Dodergren J E, Garofalo M, Sternberg S S: Actinomycin D: Effects on nucleic acid and protein metabolism in intact and regenerating liver of rats. Cancer Res 25:307, 1965
52. Merits I: Actinomycin inhibition of RNA synthesis in rat liver. Biochem Biophys Res Commun 10:254, 1963
53. Revel M, Hiatt H H: The stability of liver messenger RNA. Proc Nat Acad Sci USA 51:810, 1964
54. Harbers E, Müller W: On the inhibition of RNA synthesis by actinomycin. Biochem Biophys Res Commun 7:107, 1962
55. Baltimore D, Franklin R M: The effect of mengovirus infection on the activity of the DNA-dependent RNA polymerase of L-cells. Proc Nat Acad Sci USA 48:1383, 1962
56. Blum J J, Buctow D E: Effects of actinomycin D on acetate-starved and logarithmically growing *Euglena gracilis*. Biochim Biophys Acta 68:625, 1963
57. Levinthal C, Keynan A, Higa A: Messenger RNA turnover and protein synthesis in *B. subtilis* inhibited by actinomycin D. Proc Nat Acad Sci USA 48:1631, 1962
48. Cavalieri L F, Nemchin R G: The mode of action of actinomycin D with DNA. Biochim Biophys Acta 87:641, 1964
59. Goldberg I H, Rabinowitz M, Reich E: Basis of actinomycin action. I. DNA binding and inhibition of RNA-polymerase synthetic reactions by actinomycin. Proc Nat Acad Sci USA 48:2094, 1962
60. Hamilton L D, Fuller W, Reich E: X-ray diffraction and molecular model building studies of the interaction of actinomycin with nucleic acids. Nature 198:538, 1963
61. Haselkorn R: Actinomycin D as a probe for nucleic acid secondary structure. Science 143:682, 1964
62. Reich E: Actinomycin: Correlation of structure and function of its complexes with purines and DNA. Science 143:684, 1964
63. Roots R, Smith K C: Effects of actinomycin D on cell cycle kinetics and the DNA of Chinese hamster and mouse mammary tumor cells cultivated in vitro. Cancer Res 36:3654, 1976
64. Tokey R A, Petersen D F, Anderson E C, Puck T T: Life cycle analysis of mammalian cells. III. The inhibition of division in Chinese hamster cells by puromycin and adinomycin. Biophys J 6:567, 1966
65. Schwartz H S: Some determinants of the therapeutic efficacy of actinomcyin D (NSC-3053), Adriamycin (NSC-123127), and daunorubicin (NSC-83142). Cancer Chemother Rep 58:55, 1974
66. Wakaki S, Marumo H, Tomioka H, et al: Isolation of new fractions of antitumor mitomycins. Antibiot Chemother 8:228, 1958
67. Wakaki S: Recent advances in research on antitumor mitomycins. Cancer Chemother Rep. 13:79, 1961
68. Sugiura K: Antitumor activity of mitomycin C. Cancer Chemother Rep 13:51, 1961
69. Jones R Jr: Mitomycin D. A preliminary report of studies on human pharmacology and initial therapeutic trial. Cancer Chemother Rep 2:3, 1959
70. Frank W, Osterberg A E: Mitomycin C (NSC-26980)—An evaluation of the Japanese reports. Cancer Chemother Rep 9:114, 1960
71. Osamura S: Present state of chemotherapy of chronic leukemia in Japan. Cancer Chemother Rep 13:145, 1961
72. Evans A E: Mitomycin C. Cancer Chemother Rep 14:1, 1961
73. Crooke S T, Bradder W T: Mitomycin C: A review. Cancer Treatment Rep 3:121, 1976

74. Lefemine D V, Dann M, Barbatschi F, et al: Isolation and characterization of mitomycin and other antibiotics produced by *Streptomyces verticillatus.* J Amer Chem Soc 84:3184, 1962
75. Webb J S, Cosulich D B, Mowat J H, et al: Structures of mitomycins A, B and C and porfiromycin. J Amer Chem Soc 84:3185, 1962
76. Webb J S, Cosulich D B, Mowat J H, et al: Structures of mitomycins A, B and C, and porfiromycin. J Amer Chem Soc 84:3187, 1962
77. Tulinsky A: The structure of mitomycin A. J Amer Chem Soc 84:3188, 1962
78. Goldberg I H, Friedman P A: Antibiotics and nucleic acids. Ann Rev Biochem 40:775, 1971
79. Tomasz M, Mercade C M, Olsen J, Chatterjie N: The mode of interaction of mitomycin C with deoxyribonucleic acid and other polynucleotides in vitro. Biochemistry 13:4878, 1974
80. Shiba S, Terawaki A, Taguchi T, Kawamata J: studies on the effect of mitomycin C on nucleic acid metabolism in *Escherichia coli* strain B. Biken J 1:179, 1958
81. Shiba S, Terawaki A, Taguchi T, Kawamata J: Selective inhibition of formation of deoxyribonucleic acid in Escherichia coli by mitomycin C. Nature 183:1056, 1959
82. Reich E, Shatkin A J, Tatum E L: Bacteriocidal action of mitomycin C. Biochim Biophys Acta 53:132, 1961
83. Reich E, Franklin R M: Effect of mitomycin C on the growth of some animal viruses. Proc Nat Acad Sci USA 47:1212, 1961
84. Schwartz H S, Sternberg S S, Philips F S: Pharmacology of mitomycin C. IV. Effects in vivo on nucleic acid synthesis; comparison with actinomycin D. Cancer Res 23:1125, 1963
85. Howell P C: Mitotic inhibition and chromosome damage by mitomycin in human leukocyte cultures. Exp Cell Res 33:445, 1964
86. Morad M, Jonassen J, Lindstem J: Distribution of mitomycin C induced breaks in human chromosomes. Hereditas 74:273, 1973
87. Rao K V, Cullen W P, Sobin B A: A new antibiotic with antitumor properties. Antibiot Chemother 12:182, 1962
88. Tatsuoka S, Nakazawa K, Miyake A, et al: Isolation, anticancer activity and pharmacology of a new antibiotic chromomycin A_3. Gann Suppl 49:23, 1958
89. Gause G F, Ukholina R S, Sveshinikova M A: Olivomycin: A new antibiotic produced by *Actinomyces olivoreticuli.* Antibiotiki 7:34, 1962
90. Slayton R E, Snider B I, Elias E, et al: New approach to the treatment of hypercalcemia. The effect of short-term treatment with mithramycin. Clin Pharmacol Ther 12:833, 1971
91. Gause G F: Olivomycin, mithramycin, chromomycin: Three related cancerostatic antibiotics. In Goldin A, Hawking F, Schnitzer R J (eds): Advances in Chemotherapy, vol. 2. New York, Academic Press, 1965, pp 179–195
92. Wakisaka G, Uchino H, Nakamura T, et al: Selective inhibition of biosynthesis of ribonucleic acid in mammalian cells by chromomycin A_3. Nature 198:385, 1963
93. Layashenko V A: The effect of olivomycin on the content of nucleic acids in the transplantable mouse sarcoma 180. Antibiotiki 9:520, 1964
94. DiMarco A, Gaetani M, Dorigotti L, et al: Experimental studies on the antitumor activity of daunomycin: A new antibiotic with new antitumor activity. Tumori 49:203, 1963
95. DiMarco A, Soldati M, Fioretti A, Dasdia T: Studies on the activity of daunomycin, a new antitumor antibiotic, on normal and tumor cells growing "in vitro". Tumori 49:235, 1963
96. Grein A, Spalla C, DiMarco A, Canevazzi G: Descrizione e classificazione di un attinomicete *(Streptomyces peucetius sp. nova)* produttore di una sostanza ad attività antitumorale: La daunomicina. G. Microbiol 11:109, 1963
97. DiMarco A, Gaetani M, Orezzi P, et al: "Daunomycin," a new antibiotic of the rhodomycin group. Nature 201:706, 1964
98. Dorigotti L: An electron-microscopic study of the changes produced by daunomycin on HeLa cells. Tumori 50:117, 1964
99. Tan C, Tasaka H, DiMarco M: Clinical studies of daunomycin C. Proc Amer Assoc Cancer Res 6:64 (abstr), 1965
100. Tan C, Tasaka H, Yu K-P, et al: Daunomycin, an antitumor antibiotic, in the treatment of neoplastic disease: Clinical evaluation with special reference to childhood leukemia. Cancer 20:333, 1967
101. Bernard J, Jacquillat C L, Boiron M, et al: Essai de traitement des leucémies aigues lymphoblastiques et myeloblastiques par un antibiotique nouveau: La rubidomycine (13057 RP). Presse Med 75:19, 1967
102. DiMarco A, Gaetani M, Scarpinato B: Adriamycin (NSC-123,127): A new antibiotic with antitumor activity. Cancer Chemother Rep 53:33, 1969
103. Bonadonna G, Montardini S, DeLena M, Fossati-Bellanti F: Clinical evaluation of adriamycin, a new antitumor antibiotic. Br Med J 3:503, 1969
104. Tan C, Etcubanas E, Wollner N, et al: Adriamycin—An antitumor antibiotic in the treat-

ment of neoplastic diseases. Cancer 32:9, 1973
105. Blum R H, Carter S K: Adriamycin, A new anticancer drug with significant clinical activity. Ann Intern Med 80:249, 1974
106. O'Bryan R M, Lace J K, Talley R W, et al: Phase II evaluation of adriamycin in human neoplasia. Cancer 32:1, 1973
107. DeDuve C, De Barsky T, Poole B. et al: Commentary, Lysosomotrophic agents. Biochem Pharmacol 23:2495, 1974
108. Trouet A, Deprez-De Campeneere D, De Duve C: Chemotherapy through lysosomes with a DNA-Daunorubicin complex. Nature (New Biology) 239:110, 1972
109. Rozencweig M, Kenis Y, Atassi G, et al: DNA-adriamycin complex: Preliminary results in animals and man. Cancer Chemother Rep 6:131, 1975
110. Cornu G, Michaux J L, Sokal G, Trouet A: Daunorubicin-DNA: Further clinical trials in acute non-lymphoblastic leukemia. Europ J Cancer 10:695, 1974
111. Zbinden G, Brandle E: Toxicologic screening of daunorubicin (NSC 82151), adriamycin (NSC-123127) and their derivatives in rats. Cancer Chemother Rep 59:707, 1975
112. Alberts D S, Van Daden Weetters T: Rubidazone versus adriamcyin: An evaluation of their differential toxicity in the spleen assay system. Br J Cancer 34:64, 1976
113. Skovsgaard T: Development of resistance to rubidazone (NSC-164011) in Ehrlich ascites tumor in vivo. Cancer Chemother Rep 59:301, 1975
114. Jacquillat C, Weil M, Gemon-Auclerc M F, et al: Clinical study of rubidazone (22 050 R P), a new daunorubicin derived compound in 170 patients with acute leukemias and other malignancies. Cancer 37:653, 1976
115. Benjamin R S, Keating M J, McCredie K B: Reinduction chemotherapy of acute leukemia with rubidazone. Am Soc Hematol 19th Annual Meeting. Boston, 1976, p 76
116. Chauvergne J, Durand M: Essai de chimiotherapie de tumeur solides par la rubidazone. Etude preliminaire de 21 observations. Bordeaux Med 6:1757, 1973
117. Israel M, Pegg W J, Hirst M, et al: Significant antitumor activity of N-trifluoroacetyl-adriamycin-14-valerate (AD32), a new adriamycin analog. Proc Am Assoc Cancer Res 16:116, 1975
118. Israel M, Modest E J, Frei E: N-trifluoroacetyladriamycin-14-valerate, an analog with greater antitumor activity and less toxicity than adriamycin. Cancer Res 35:1365, 1975
119. Parker L M, Israel M, Hirst M, et al: Further in vivo studies with N-trifluoroacetyl-adriamycin-14-valerate (AD32). Proc Am Assoc Cancer Res 17:108, 1976
120. Gause G F, Brazhnikova M G, Shorin V A: A new antitumor antibiotic carminomycin (NSC-18024). Cancer Chemother Rep 58:255, 1974
121. DiMarco A, Arcamone F, Zunino F: Daunomycin (daunorubicin) and adriamycin and structural analogues: Biological activity and mechanism of action, in Corcoran J W, Hahn F E (eds): Antibiotics, vol. III: Mechanism of Action of Antimicrobial and Antitumor Agents. New York, Springer-Verlag 1975, p 101
122. DiMarco A: Adriamycin (NSC-123127): Mode and mechanism of action. Cancer Chemother Rep 6:91, 1975
123. Hittelman W N, Rao P N: The nature of adriamycin induced cytotoxicity in Chinese hamster cells as revealed by premature chromosome condensation. Cancer Res 35:3027, 1975
124. Vig B K: Chromosome aberrations induced in human leukocytes by the antileukemic antibiotic adriamycin. Cancer Res 31:32, 1971
125. Whang Peng J, Leventhal B G, Adamson J W, Perry S: The effects of daunomycin on human cells in vivo and in vitro. Cancer 23:113, 1969
126. Newsome Y L, Littlefield L G: Adriamycin induced chromosome aberrations in human fibroblasts. J Nat Cancer Inst 55:1061, 1975
127. Sternberg S, Phillips F S, Cronin A P: Renal tumors and other lesions in rats following a single intravenous injection of daunomycin. Cancer Res 32:1029, 1972
128. Egorin M J, Hildebrand R C, Cimino E F, Badrur N R: Cytofluoresence localization of adriamycin and daunorubicin. Cancer Res 34:2243, 1974
129. Henry D W: Adriamycin, in Santorelli A C (ed): Cancer Chemotherapy, A Symposium Sponsored by the Division of Medicinal Chemistry at the 169th Meeting of the American Chemical Society, Philadelphia, PA, April 7, 1975. Washington, D C, Am Chem Soc, 1976, p 15
130. Pigram W J, Fuller W, Hamilton L D: Stereochemistry of intercalation: Interaction of daunomycin with DNA. Nature (New Biol) 235:17, 1972
131. Chandra P: Role of chemical structure in biochemical activity of daunorubicin (NSC-82151), adriamycin (NSC-123129), and some structural analogs: Macromolecular interaction and their biologic consequences, Cancer Chemother Rep 6:115, 1975
132. Barranio S C: Review of the survival and cell

kinetics effects of adriamycin (NSC-123127) on mammalian cells. Cancer Chemother Rep 6:147, 1975

133. Tobey, R A: Effects of cytosine arabinoside, daunomycin, mithramycin, azacytidine, adriamycin and camptothecin on mammalian cell cycle transverse. Cancer Res 32:2720, 1972
134. Krishan A, Frei E: Effect of adriamycin on cell cycle traverse and kinetics of cultured human lymphoblasts. Cancer Res 36:143, 1976
135. Kin S H, Kim J H: Lethal effect of adriamycin on the division cycle of HeLa cells. Cancer Res 32:323, 1972
136. Barranco S C, Novak J K: Survival responses of dividing and non-dividing mammalian cells after treatment with hydroxy urea, arabinosylcytosine, or adriamycin. Cancer Res 34:1616, 1974
137. Ernst P: Perturbation of generation cycle of human leukemic blast cells in vivo by daunomycin. Scand J Haematol 11:13, 1973
138. Stryckmans P A, Manaster J, Lachapelle F, Socquet M: Mode of action of chemotherapy in vivo on human acute leukemia. I Daunomycin. J Clin Invest 52:126, 1973
139. Arlin Z, Fried J, Clarkson B: Effects of daunomycin on human leukemic cells in vivo as studied by flow microfluorimetry. Proc Am Assoc Cancer Res 16:180, 1975
140. Gonsalves M, Blanco U, Hunter J, et al: Effects of anticancer agents on the respiration of isolated mitochondria and tumor cells. Europ J Cancer 10:567, 1974
141. Iwamoto Y, Hansen I L, Porter T H, Folkers K: Inhibition of co-enzyme Q10 enzymes, succinoxidase and MADH-oxidase by adriamycin and other quinones having antitumor activity. Biochem Biophys Res Comm 58:633, 1974
142. Dano K: Experimentally developed cellular resistance to daunomycin. Acta Path Microbiol Scand 256:11–80 (Suppl), 1976
143. Schwartz H S, Kanter P M: Cell interactions: Determinants of selective toxicity of adriamycin. (NSC-123127) and daunorubicin (NSC-82156). Cancer Chemother Rep 6:107, 1975
144. Casazza A M, DiMarco A, DiCuonzo G: Interference of daunomycin and adriamycin on the growth and regression of murine sarcoma virus (Moloney) tumors in mice. Cancer Res 31:1971, 1971
145. Vecci A, Mantovani A, Tagliabue A, Spreafico F: A characterization of the immunosuppressive activity of adriamycin and daunomycin on humoral antibody production and tumor allograft rejection. Cancer Res 36:1222, 1976
146. Sengupto S K, Seshadri R, Modest E J, Israel M: Comparative DNA-binding studies with adriamycin (ADR), N-trifluoroacetyladriamycin-14-valerate (AD32) and related compounds. Proc Am Assoc Cancer Res 17:109, 1976
147. Zbinder G, Brandle E: Toxicologic screening of daunorubicin (NSC-82151), adriamycin (NSC-123127), and their derivatives in rats, Cancer Chemother Rep part 1, 59:707–715, 1975
148. Myers C E, McGuire W, Young R: Adriamycin: amelioration of toxicity by -Tocopherol, Cancer Treat Rep 60:961–962, 1976
149. Folker K: Personal Communication
150. Ishizuka M, Takayama H, Takeuchi T, Umezawa H: Activity and toxicity of bleomycin. J Antibiot (Tokyo) 20:15, 1967
151. Ichikawa T, Nakano I, Hirokawa F: Bleomycin treatment of the tumors of penis and scrotum. J Urol 102:699, 1969
152. Takeda K, Sagawa Y, Arakawa T: Therapeutic effect of bleomycin for skin tumors. Gann 61:207, 1970
153. Ishizuka M, Kimura K, Iwanaga J, et al: Biological studies on individual bleomycins. J Antibiot (Tokyo) 21:592, 1968
154. Umezawa H, Ishizuka M, Hori S, et al: The distribution of ^{3}H-bleomycin in mouse tissue. J Antibiot (Tokyo) 21:638, 1968
155. Ichikawa T: Discovery of clinical effects of bleomycin and its further development. Prog Biochem Pharmacol II:143, 1976
156. Yagoda A, Mubherzi B, Young C, et al: Bleomycin, an antitumor antibiotic. Clinical experience in 274 patients. Ann Intern Med 77:861, 1972
157. Carter S K, Blum R H: Current status of American studies with bleomycin. Prog. Biochem Pharmacol II:158, 1976
158. Cvitkovic E, Hayes D, Goldberg R: Primary combination chemotherapy (VAB III) for metastatic or unresectable germ cell tumors. Proc Am Assoc Cancer Res 17:296 (abstr), 1976
159. Randolph V, Vallejo A, Strong E W, Wittes R E: Combination treatment with chemotherapy and radiotherapy in head and neck cancer. Proc Am Soc Clin Oncol (abstr C-278), 1977, p 336
160. Case D C, Young C W, Nisce L, et al: Eight-drug combination chemotherapy (MOPP and ABDV) and local radiotherapy for advanced Hodgkin's disease. Cancer Treat Rep 60:1217, 1976
161. Umezawa H: Studies on bleomycin: Chemistry and the biological action. Biomedicine 18:459, 1973

162. Umezawa H: Structure and action of bleomycin. Prog Biochem Pharmacol 11:18, 1976
163. Kohn K W, Ewig R A G: Effect of pH on the bleomycin-induced DNA single strand scission in L1210 cells and the relation to cell survival. Cancer Res 36:3839, 1976
164. Muller W E G, Zahn R K: Effect of bleomycin on DNA, RNA, protein, chromatin and on cell transformation by oncogenic RNA viruses. Prog Biochem Pharmacol 11:28, 1976
165. Muller W E G, Totsuba C, Nusser I, et al: Bleomycin inhibition of DNA synthesis in isolated enzyme systems and in intact cell systems. Biochem Pharmacol 24:911, 1975
166. Daskal Y, Crooke S T, Smetana K, Busch H: Ultrastructural study of the effect of bleomycin A_2 on the nucleolus and its possibly related cytoplasmic constituents in N orikott hepatoma cells. Cancer Res 35:374, 1975
167. Kurten S, Obe G: Premature chromosome condensation in the bone marrow of Chinese hamsters after application of bleomycin in vivo. Mutat Res 27:285, 1975
168. Promchainant C: Cytogenic effect of bleomycin on human leukocytes in vitro. Mutat Res 28:107, 1975
169. Ono T, Miyaki M, Tuguchi T, Ohashi M: Actions of bleomycin on DNA ligase and polymerases. Prog Biochem Pharmacol 11:48, 1976
170. Miyaki M, Morohashi S, Ono T: Single strand scission and repair of DNA in bleomycin sensitive and resistant rat ascites hepatoma cells. J Antibiot 26:369, 1973
171. Umezawa H, Takeuchi T, Hori S, et al: Studies on the mechanism of antitumor effect of bleomycin on squamous cell carcinoma. J Antibiot 25:409, 1972
172. Miyaki M, Ono T, Hori S, Umezawa H: Binding of bleomycin to DNA in bleomycin-sensitive and resistant rat ascites hepatoma cells. Cancer Res 35:2015, 1975
173. Barranco S C, Humphrey R M: The effects of bleomycin on survival and cell progression in Chinese hamster cells in vitro. Cancer Res 31:1218, 1971
174. Clarkson J M, Humphrey R M: The significance of DNA damage in the cell cycle sensitivity of Chinese hamster ovary cells to bleomycin. Cancer Res 36:2345, 1976
175. Barranco S C, Novak J K, Humphrey R M: Response of mammalian cells following treatment with bleomycin and 1, 2-bis(2-chloroethyl)-1-nitrosourea during plateau phase. Cancer Res 33:691, 1973
176. Barranco S C, Humphrey R M: Response of mammalian cells to bleomycin induced potentially lethal and sublethal damage. Prog Biochem Pharmacol 2:78, 1976
177. Mauro F, Bright G, Elli R, et al: Plateau phase cultures as a system for studying the effects of bleomycin in view of its utilization in vivo. Prog Biochem Pharmacol 2:93, 1976
178. Drugli A M, Robie K M, Mitchell M S: Failure of bleomycin to affect humoral or cell-mediated immunity in the mouse. Cancer Res 34:2504, 1974
179. De Jager R L, Moore M A S: Effects of bleomycin on myeloid and lymphoid cell proliferation in the mouse. Proc Am Assoc Cancer Res 17:170 (abstr), 1976
180. Herr R R, Jahnke J K, Argondelis A D: The structure of streptozotocin. J Am Chem Soc 89:4808, 1967
181. Schein P S, Cooney D A, Vernon M L: The use of nicotinamide to modify the toxicity of streptozotocin diabetes without loss of antitumor activity. Cancer Res 27:2324, 1967
182. Schein P S: 1-Methyl-1-nitrosurea and dialkylnitrosamine depression of nicothamide adenine dinucleotide. Cancer Res 29:1226, 1969
183. Schein P S, O'Connell M J, Blom J, et al: Clinical antitumor activity and toxicity of streptozotocin (NSC-85998). Cancer 34:993, 1974
184. Schein P S, Cooney D A, McMenamin M G, Anderson T: Streptozotocin diabetes—further studies on the mechanism of depression of nicotinamide adenine dinucleotide concentrations in mouse pancreas and liver. Biochem Pharmacol 22:2625, 1973
185. Anderson T, Schein P S, McMenamin M G, Cooney D A: Streptozotocin diabetes. Correlation with extent of depression of pancreatic islet nicotinamide adenine dinucleotide. J Clin Invest 54:672, 1974
186. Johnston T P, McCaleb G S, Montgomer J A: Synthesis of chlorozotocin, the 2-chloroethyl analog of the anticancer antibiotic streptozotocin. J Med Chem 18:104, 1975
187. Anderson T, McMenamin M G, Schein P S: Chlorozotocin, 2 (3-(2-chloroethyl-)3-nitrosouried) D glucopyranose, an antitumor agent with modified bone marrow toxicity. Cancer Res 35:761, 1975
188. Schein P S, Pnaasci L, Woolley P V, Anderson T: Pharmacology of chlorozotocin (NSC-178248), a new nitrosourea antitumor agent. Cancer Treat Rep 60:801, 1976
189. Schein P, Bull J, McMenamin M, Macdonald J: DNA synthesis by human bone marrow after incubation with BCNU or chlorozotocin (DCNU, NSC-178248). Proc Amer Assoc Cancer Res 17:122, 1975
190. Tobey R A, Oka M S, Crissman H A: Differential effects of two chemotherapeutic agents, streptozotocin and chlorozotocin, on the

mammalian cell cycle. Eur J Cancer 11:433, 1975

191. Oettgen H F: Clinical evaluation of L-asparaginase, in Bernard J, Boiron M (eds): La L-asparaginase. International Symposium on L-asparaginase, Paris, 1970. Paris, Centre National de la Recherche Scientifique, 1971, pp 243–351
192. Burchenal J H: Clinical evaluation and future prospects of asparaginase. in Mathé G (ed): Recent Results in Cancer Research, vol. 30. Heidelberg, Springer-Verlag, 1970, pp 20–27
193. Burchenal J H, Clarkson B D, Dowling M D Jr, et al: Experimental and clinical studies of L-asparaginase in combination therapy, in Bernard J, Boiron M (eds): La L-asparaginase. International Symposium on L-asparaginase, Paris, 1970. Paris, Centre National de la Recherche Scientifique, 1971, pp 243–351
194. Oettgen H F, Tallal L, Tan C C, et al: Clinical experience with L-asparaginase. in Grundmann E, Oettgen H F (eds): Recent Results in Cancer Research, vol. 33. Heidelberg, Springer-Verlag, 1970, pp 219–235
195. Williams R H, Gerzon K, Hoehn M, DeLong D C: 158th National Meeting, American Chemical Society, New York, 1969, Abstract, Micr. 38
196. Gerzon K, Williams R H, Hoehn M, et al: Second International Congress Heterocyclic Chemistry, Montpellier, France, July 10, 1969, abstract C-30
197. Streightoff F, Nelson J A, Cline J C, et al: Ninth Conference on Antimicrobial Agents and Chemotherapy, Washington D C, abstract 18, 1969
198. Gralla R J, Currie V E, Goldberg R B, Young C W: Phase II therapeutic trial of Pyrazofurin (PZF) in patients with advanced lung cancer. Proc Am Assoc Cancer Res (abstr C230), 1977
199. Young C: Personal communication
200. Ishizula M, Sawa T, Hori S, et al: Biological studies on formycin B. J Antibiotics Tokyo Ser A, 21:5 (abstr), 1968
201. Haneishi T, Okazaki T, Hata T, et al: Oxazinomycin, a new carbon-linked nucleoside antibiotic. J Antibiotics Tokyo Ser A, 24:797–799, 1971
202. Matsuura S, Shiratori O, Katagiri K: Antitumor activity of showdomycin. J Antibiotics Tokyo Ser A, 17:234–237, 1964
203. Chu C K, Watanabe K A, Kyoichi A, Fox J J: Nucleoside XXCII: A facile synthesis of 5-(B-D-ribofuranosyl)-isocytosine (pseudoisocytidine) J Heterocyclic Chem 12:817–818, 1975
204. Burchenal J H, Ciovacco K, Kalaher K, et al: Antileukemic effects of pseudoisocytidine, a new synthetic pyrimidine C-nucleoside. Cancer Res 36:1520–1523, 1976
205. Burchenal J H, Kalaher K, O'Toole T, et al: Antileukemic activity of pseudoisocytidine (4-ICR—A new synthetic C-nucleoside. Proc Am Assoc Cancer Res 17:143 (abstr), 1976

205a. Personal communication

206. Zedeck M S, Chou T C, Vidal P, et al: Pharmacology of pseudoisocytidine, a new antileukemic C-nucleoside. Proc Am Assoc Cancer Res (abstr 471), 1977, p 118
207. Kreis W, Hession C: Enzyme, distribution and combination chemotherapy studies with 1-B-D-arabinofuranosylcytosine (ara-C) plus tetrahydrouridine (THU) in 4 animal neoplasms. Proc Am Assoc Cancer Res 17:83, 1976
208. Philips F: Personal communication

Marcel Rozencweig
Daniel D. Von Hoff
Franco M. Muggia

7
New Agents: Selected Problems in Drug Development and Clinical Testing

Introduction

The successful results that have been obtained with cytotoxic drugs, mainly in hematologic malignancies, indicate a reasonable chance for major advances with this treatment modality in more refractory tumor types. Thus far, however, despite all the progress in cancer chemotherapy, the prognosis of the common tumors in adult patients has been minimally affected.

Most of the presently available drugs have been tested in the most common tumor types. Non small-cell lung cancer has been quite resistant to almost all of them.[1] In colorectal carcinoma, the combination of two moderately active compounds, 5-fluorouracil and MeCCNU, has been more effective than either compound alone, but this treatment still yields only transient tumor shrinkage.[2] Breast cancer is responsive to a substantial number of drugs, particularly when given in combination, but the median duration of remission has not exceeded one year in any study.[3] Furthermore, the increasing use of combination chemotherapy as adjuvant treatment in early breast cancer leaves few chemotherapeutic possibilities for use at the time of disease recurrence.

Thus, after 30 years of cancer chemotherapy, the development of new cytotoxic drugs still remains a task of major priority for cancer research. Over the past 14 years, from 1963 to 1976, the Division of Cancer Treatment of the National Cancer Institute has filed IND (investigational new drug) notices on 167 compounds for use as anticancer agents. Thirty-eight per cent of these agents are still in investigational use, 19 per cent have been marketed as commercial agents and studies with the remaining drugs have been discontinued for a variety of reasons.[4]

This review will be confined to some of the most interesting investigational anticancer drugs that illustrate the practical difficulties encountered in drug development and evaluation of relative clinical activity.

Podophyllotoxin Derivatives

VM-26 and VP-16-213 are two semisynthetic derivatives of podophyllotoxin, a crystalline extract of the May apple. VM-26 is 4′-demethyl-1-0 [4,6-0-(2-thenylidene)-β-D-glucopyranosyl] epipodophyllotoxin and VP-16-213 is 4′-demethyl-1-0 [4,6-0-(ethylidene)-β-D-glucopyranosyl] epipodophyllotoxin. Podophyllotoxin is a well known spindle poison[5,6] that binds to microtubular proteins at the site of colchicine binding[7] and arrests cells in metaphase. In cell cultures, VM-26 and VP-16-213 also arrest the cell cycle in metaphase,[6,8,9] but this phenomenon is rapidly followed by a marked reduction of the mitotic index resulting from a nonreversible inhibition of the entry of cells into mitosis.[6,8-12] The precise molecular action involved in this premitotic block is unknown.

VP-16-213 became available for clinical use after VM-26 on the basis of its apparent superiority over VM-26 in the murine L1210 leukemia system. The comparison of the two agents, however, did not take into account the marked schedule dependency which was subsequently found with both compounds in the L1210 system. In this experimental system, in fact, both compounds achieve increases in life span over untreated controls ranging from <100 per cent to >500 per cent, depending on the schedule investigated.[13,14]

Pharmacokinetic differences between VM-26 and VP-16-213 were found by Allen and Creaven using radio labeled compounds in man.[15] VM-26 plasma decay kinetics followed a triexponential function corresponding to a three-compartment model. The half-life of the terminal phase ranged from 11 to 38 hours. After 72 hours, 44 per cent of the administered dose was recovered in the urine, 9 per cent as unchanged drug and 35 per cent as metabolite. VP-16-213 displayed a biphasic plasma disappearance with a mean half-life of about 11.5 hours. After 72 hours, 44 per cent of the administered dose was also recovered in the urine, but with 29 per cent as unchanged drug and 15 per cent as metabolite. Thus, pharmacologic studies indicate that VM-26 is excreted more slowly, but is metabolized faster than VP-16-213. The actual significance of these features is difficult to interpret insofar as these drugs exhibit a great tendency for protein binding, are rather unstable in physiologic solution and their respective solvents might conceivably interfere with their own pharmacokinetics.

No discrepancy in the spectrum of clinical antitumor activity has been demonstrated between VM-26 and VP-16-213 (Table 7-1). Both drugs are effective in Hodgkin's and non-Hodgkin's lymphoma. VM-26 is active in bladder cancer and possibly in brain malignancies, while VP-16-213 has shown activity in small cell lung cancer, acute nonlymphocytic leukemia and possibly in ovarian cancer. The reported response rate in small cell lung cancer has averaged 40 per cent (ranging from 20 to 52 per cent), and it must be pointed out that these very encouraging results were obtained despite heavy prior treatment with combination chemotherapy. VP-16-213 has shown no activity in breast cancer, head and neck cancer, soft tissue sarcomas or in colorectal cancer and melanoma. Results with VM-26 in these tumors were also not encouraging, although the small number of treated patients with colorectal cancer and melanoma precludes a definite conclusion.

Qualitatively, the pattern of toxic effects induced by both drugs is similar and mainly includes myelosuppression (especially with leukopenia), gastrointestinal disturbances with nausea, vomiting and infrequent diarrhea and alopecia.

Anthracycline Derivatives

The anthracyclines provide another example of the problems of analogue development. Adriamycin was introduced into clinical trials because of its increased experimental antitumor activity as compared to daunomycin. This superiority has not yet been documented in clinical practice, however.[35] The cumulative dose-limiting toxicity of congestive heart failure has greatly hampered the clinical interest in the anthracyclines, and other derivatives endowed with less cardiotoxicity have been actively sought.

Rubidazone results from this development and has been very recently introduced into clinical trials. Rubidazone is the benzoylhydrazone derivative of daunorubicine and is thought to have a similar mechanism of action involving intercalation into DNA. Its activity in animal tumor models resembles that of the other anthracyclines.[36] Studies sponsored by the Drug Evaluation Branch of the National Cancer Institute have shown that the optimal dose of rubidazone in P388 tumor-bearing mice is higher than that of adriamycin and daunomycin. When the therapeutic indices were compared using only survival times as end points, no real differences could be de-

TABLE 7-1. *Single Agent Activity of VM 26 and VP 16-213*

Tumor Type	No. of Responders/No. of Evaluable Patients VM 26	VP 16-213
Hodgkin's disease	15/42[16-18]	5/22[19-21]
Reticulum cell sarcoma	13/31[16-18]	14/64[19-22]
Lymphosarcoma	6/20[16,17]	3/16[19,21,22]
Bladder	10/54[16,23]	1/5 [19]
Brain	4/12[24]	0/2 [19]
Small cell lung	1/1 [24]	33/78[20,25-27]
Acute nonlymphocytic leukemia	1/7 [28]	11/30[20,27,29,30]
Ovary	0/1 [16]	4/26[19,20,27]
Breast	2/22[16]	3/90[19-21,31]
Head and neck	0/16[16]	0/35[19]
Soft tissue sarcoma	0/14[16,32]	0/17[19]
Melanoma	0/3 [16]	0/33[19-21,33]
Colorectal	0/3 [16]	0/45[19-21,34]

tected among the three anthracyclines. Since survival of tumor-bearing mice was the only parameter used to compute these indices, the role of various toxic effects, such as cardiotoxicity, could not be evaluated.

Studies carried out in rats showed that the minimal cumulative cardiotoxic dose of rubidazone was approximately twice that of adriamycin or daunomycin, suggesting that rubidazone was less cardiotoxic than the other two compounds.[37] The practical significance of these results, however, is difficult to ascertain. Higher doses of rubidazone must be used to achieve antitumor activity. In addition, the relevance of the rat model as a predictive tool for clinical purpose has not been demonstrated.

Initial clinical trials in Europe[38,39] and at M. D. Anderson Hospital in Houston[40] have revealed that the pattern of toxic effects induced by rubidazone is qualitatively similar to that observed with the other analogues, but a quantitative comparison must await further investigation. Major problems are, in fact, encountered in this type of clinical testing. The true incidence of congestive heart failure as a function of the cumulative dose is not precisely known for adriamycin. In addition, there are currently no reliable predictive tests for this usually irreversible toxicity. Currently, the only way of determining the cardiotoxicity of a new derivative is to escalate dosage until cardiotoxicity develops; only then can any statement be made relative to its therapeutic index.

ICRF-159

ICRF-159 is a bisdiketopiperazine derivative and belongs to a new class of cytotoxic agents. Its mechanism of action has not yet been fully elucidated. Using phytohemagglutinine-stimulated human lymphocytes in synchronized cell culture, the late prophase and early metaphase (G_2-M) were found to be the most sensitive phases of the cell cycle.[41] In mouse fibroblast cell cultures, the drug inhibits DNA metabolism with little effect on RNA and protein metabolism, following a pattern reminiscent of the activity of X-irradiation and radiomimetic agents.[42]

ICRF-159 is active in a wide range of animal tumors,[43] and experimental antitumor synergism has been reported with X-irradiation[44] and other cytotoxic agents including daunomycin, adriamycin and 5-fluorouracil.[45-47] It should also be mentioned that ICRF-159 was found to reduce the cardiotoxic effects induced by daunomycin and adriamycin in the isolated dog heart.[48]

Thus far, the lack of solubility of ICRF-159 has precluded parenteral administration in man. The first report of its clinical use as an oral drug was published in 1969,[49] but the delay in establishing an optimal dose schedule has hampered full evaluation of the drug.

When the drug is administered at single doses up to 10.5mg/M², only mild and inconsistent myelosuppression is noted, reflecting a peculiar intestinal absorption of the drug and underscoring the usefulness of precise pharmacologic data for oral compounds.[50] When the drug is given in divided doses, leukopenia is clearly dose-related and becomes dose-limiting.[50,51] On subsequent courses, leukopenia is reproducible and remains dose-related. In divided doses, ICRF-159 is generally well tolerated and, besides leukopenia, the toxic effects mainly include mild and transient thrombocytopenia, gastrointestinal intolerance and alopecia.

Data regarding clinical antitumor activity are surprisingly scanty. ICRF-159 is effective in non-Hodgkin's lymphoma[52] and has shown promising activity in colorectal carcinoma, apparently without cross-resistance to either 5-fluorouracil or MeCCNU.[53,54] ICRF-159 appears to have no value in the treatment of non-small cell lung cancer[55] and melanoma.[56] Clearly, additional studies are needed to accurately assess the activity spectrum of this compound as a single agent. In addition, its combination with 5-fluorouracil might be worth investigating in colorectal carcinoma in view of the reported synergism of this combination in the L1210 system.

Other combinations warrant further investigation. Experimental potentiation by ICRF-159 of the antitumor activity of the anthracyclines, as well as the possible decrease of their cardiotoxicity, is an attractive area for clinical studies. Moreover, the promising results with ICRF-159 and radiotherapy in human sarcoma[57] point to the possible radiosensitizing ability of ICRF-159. These findings need confirmation insofar as the many attempts to improve the effectiveness of radiation therapy by concomitant chemotherapy have, to date, been generally disappointing.

Cis-diamminedichloroplatinum

Cis-diamminedichloroplatinum (DDP) is an inorganic complex formed by a central atom of platinum surrounded by chlorine and ammonia atoms in the *cis* position in the horizontal plane. Although numerous studies have been devoted to characterizing this drug, no final conclusion can be drawn concerning its mechanism of action which might be related, at least partially, to alkylating properties.[58]

DDP appears to be one of the most active drugs in testicular cancer, with a reported cumulative overall response rate of 66 per cent (Table 7-2). Strikingly, this activity has been demonstrated in patients who often have received prior chemotherapy with multiple agents. Combinations including DDP are now being widely tested in testicular cancer and, in most of these, DDP can be given at full doses. Some of the most encouraging results were reported by Einhorn and Donohue[69] in a series of 29 evaluable patients. Three induction courses of DDP were given in combination with vinblastine and bleomycin. Twenty-six patients (89 per cent) achieved a "disease-free" status, including 23 complete responders to chemotherapy and three partial responders who underwent surgical removal of residual tumor. Twenty-two of these 26 patients remained alive and disease-free from 4+ to 24+ months.

A series of combinations with vinblastine, actinomycin D, and bleomycin have been developed for germinal tumors at the Memorial Sloan-Kettering Cancer Center. Their latest induction regimen included cytoxan and high doses of DDP.[70] Among 25 evaluable patients, 18 were complete responders and six partial responders were still improving at the time of the report. No relapses were reported but the longest follow-up was limited to 6 months.

The antitumor effectiveness of DDP is not limited to testicular tumors. At present, the efficacy of DDP seems quite well established in bladder [64] and ovarian carcinoma,[65] as well as in head and neck malignancies.[66] In contrast, no activity has been detected in lung cancer,[67] colorectal carcinoma[68] or ALL in children.[62] Additional trials with other dosage schedules may be warranted, however.

The major toxic effects of DDP can be classified as gastrointestinal, audiologic, renal and hematologic. Large scale clinical investigation of DDP was initially hampered by a cumulative renal toxicity which practically precluded lengthy treatments and limited the use of DDP to induction regimens. Preliminary reports of the effect of intravenous hydration and mannitol-induced diuresis[59,60] have

TABLE 7-2. *Single Agent Activity of Cis-Diamminedichloroplatinum (II)*

Tumor Type	No. of Evaluable Patients	No. of Responding Patients (%)	Ref.
Testicular	70	46 (66)	59–63*
Bladder	24	8 (33)	64
Ovary	34	8 (24)	65
Head and neck	26	8 (31)	66
Lung	39	2 (5)	67
Colorectal	32	0	68
Acute lymphocytic leukemia	11	0	62

*Hoogstraten B Personal communication

produced renewed interest. This procedure allows use of higher doses of DDP with a reduction in renal function impairment and no loss of antitumor activity. These data are consistent with an improvement of the therapeutic index, although at this time there is no firm evidence that the pattern of toxicity has been substantially altered.

5-AZACYTIDINE

5-Azacytidine is a ring analogue of the pyrimidine nucleoside cytidine and differs from it only by having a nitrogen atom in place of the fifth carbon atom. It was synthesized in 1964[71] and produced microbiologically in 1966.[72]

Although there have been a number of studies on the mode of action of this drug, there has been no final conclusion on the mechanism of its antineoplastic effect. 5-Azacytidine is thought to act as an antimetabolite through an interference with nucleic acid metabolism.[73-77]

5-Azacytidine has exhibited antileukemic activity against lymphoid leukemia in AK mice.[78] The drug has significant activity in the L1210 mouse leukemia system and is active in sublines resistant to 6-mercaptopurine, aminopterin, and cyclophosphamide.[72] The combinations of 5-azacytidine and cytosine arabinoside have been synergistic in the L1210 system when used in the appropriate schedules.[79] It is of note that the drug has been ineffective in animal solid tumor systems, including Walker 256 and the spontaneous mammary tumor in mice.[80]

In vitro studies showing that the drug has limited stability in infusion solutions have led to recommendations of diluting it in lactated Ringer's for injection (USP) and changing infusion solutions every 3 to 4 hours to avoid administering inactive breakdown products.[81,82]

Pharmacokinetic studies have been performed in man using radioactively labeled 5-azacytidine[83,84] After subcutaneous administration, absorption is rapid and plasma levels within 2 hours are equal to those noted in patients treated with the intravenous drug. The plasma half-life of the labeled 5-azacytidine and its radioactive metabolites was 3 to 6.2 hours after intravenous injection.[83,84] Patients excreted 90 per cent of the total administered radioactivity in the urine within 24 hours.[84,85] The concentration of radioactivity in the CSF was minimal 24 hours after administration, and no significant radioactivity was found in the feces, sputum or expired CO_2.[83,85]

5-Azacytidine was introduced into clinical trials in the United States because of encouraging results noted with the drug in childhood acute lymphocytic leukemia in European clinical studies.[86] Unfortunately, the early European studies used 5-azacytidine in combination with prednisone and it was difficult to determine the role of 5-azacytidine in clinical responses.

To date, the phase II clinical trials have shown that 5-azacytidine has a relatively narrow antitumor spectrum (Table 7-3). Its effectiveness has emerged primarily in the treatment of acute myelogenous leukemia. All of the initial studies used the drug in previously treated patients. Most patients were refractory

TABLE 7-3. *Single Agent Activity of 5-Azacytidine*

Tumor Type	No. of Evaluable Patients	CR	PR	Ref.
Acute myelogenous leukemia	98	23	11	87–91
Acute lymphocytic leukemia	43	2	2	87,89–91
Chronic myelogenous leukemia in blastic transformation	17	0	1	87,90–92
Multiple Myeloma	9	0	0	93
Breast	31	0	3	94,95
Lung	1	0	0	95
Melanoma	31	0	0	90,95*
Lymphoma	4	0	0	90
Colorectal	31	0	1	95,96
Ovarian	4	0	1	95
Renal	1	0	0	95
Hepatoma	1	0	0	95
Tonsil	1	0	0	95
Chordoma	1	0	0	95
Pancreatic	1	0	0	96
Gastric	1	0	0	96

*Bellet R Personal Communication

to conventional antileukemic agents, including combinations of cytosine arabinoside and daunomycin and adriamycin, 6 thioguanine, and occasionally, vincristine and prednisone. The overall response rate to 5-azacytidine in these previously treated patients was 35 per cent (Table 7-3). The median duration of remission ranged from 12 to 14 weeks. Several regimens utilizing the drug in combination chemotherapy have been devised for the treatment of acute myelogenous leukemia. Results for most of these studies are preliminary and, at this point in time, the superiority of a combination regimen including 5-azacytidine versus 5-azacytidine alone remains to be demonstrated.

Trials in the United States with 5-azacytidine in ALL have not confirmed the favorable European experience with this drug (Table 7-3). There has been a glimmer of activity in CML in blast crisis,[92] but the activity of 5-azacytidine against solid tumors has not been encouraging. The drug has no significant clinical activity in breast cancer, in melanoma or in colorectal cancer. The drug has not been adequately tested in a large number of tumor types, but additional data resulting from completed phase II trials will soon be published.

The two most troublesome, usually dose-limiting, toxicities of 5-azacytidine have been nausea and vomiting,[89,94,95,97] and leukopenia.[88,89,91,96,97] The gastrointestinal problems have largely been circumvented by using continuous drug infusion.[98-100] The variable stability of the infusion solutions, however, has caused problems because of the need for frequent changes of intravenous infusion solutions of the drug. Other less common toxicities include thrombocytopenia,[88,96] diarrhea,[96] hepatic toxicity,[101] an unusual neuromuscular syndrome,[88] phlebitis,[102] stomatitis,[102] skin rash,[89] fever,[91] hypotension[102] and possibly hypophosphatemia.[103]

The future of 5-azacytidine seems to rest with its activity in acute myelogenous leukemia. The synergistic activity of cytosine arabinoside and 5-azacytidine in the L1210 system warrants clinical investigation of this combination. The use of 5-azacytidine plus a "cytidine rescue" as described by Hanka and Clark[104] would be of particular interest. In addition, clinical trials are needed in acute myelogenous leukemia using 5-azacytidine in firstline therapy, consolidation, late intensification and maintenance regimens. In children or in patients without venous access, subcutaneous use of the drug could be explored. Finally, the analogue problem will appear again with dihydro-5-azacytidine, a new analogue, which is stable in aqueous solutions over a broad pH range.[105] A major question will be whether these stability properties justify introduction of the analogue into clinical trials, since its animal antitumor activity seems similar to the parent compound.

Discussion

This selected overview of investigational drugs points to some of the emerging general problems in drug development. Repeated emphasis has been placed on the need for evolving a stategy for developing and testing analogues with an aim at decreasing their toxicity, improving their efficacy and broadening their antitumor spectra as compared to the parent compound. Imaginative use of preclinical models to develop rationally designed clinical trials may facilitate this task. A retrospective clinical comparison of existing analogues would be of great help in defining these models but, in general, specific information is lacking and no clear difference can be detected between these analogues.

The evaluation of clinical antitumor activity must consider various parameters, such as the mode of administration and selection of the test population. Premature phase II trials of a new compound may result in completely misleading conclusions. The establishment of a safe mode of administration with predictable and manageable toxicity sometimes requires a considerable amount of time. This is particularly true for drugs which are only given orally or have dose-limiting toxicities other than hematologic effects.

It is now well established that cytotoxic agents must be tested in a panel of so-called signal tumors. The lack of activity in refractory tumors, such as non-small cell lung carcinoma, colon cancer or melanoma, obviously does not preclude high activity in other tumor types. Trials of new drugs in less refractory malignancies are usually performed in the late stage of a disease which is resistant to prior treatment. Under these conditions, lack of activity undoubtedly must be interpreted with caution. It may be argued, however, that drugs of minimal activity are not needed in these tumors and that very effective agents will always be detected even under these unfavorable conditions. The results with VP-16-213 in small-cell lung cancer, *cis*-platinum in testicular cancer and 5-azacytidine in AML seem to substantiate this point.

Improvements in further drug development programs will require higher selectivity of preclinical models and better design of clinical trials. A broader understanding of the mechanism of anticancer drug activity might lead to more rational modes of administration. A close collaboration between experimentalists and clinicians will undoubtedly hasten the achievement of these objectives.

References

1. Cohen M H, Perevodchikova N I: Single agent chemotherapy of lung cancer, in Muggia F M, Rosencweig M (eds): Lung Cancer, Progress in Therapeutic Research. (in press)
2. Moertel C G: Gastrointestinal cancer. Treatment with fluorouracil-nitrosoureas combinations. JAMA 235:2135, 1976
3. Carter S K: Chemotherapy of breast cancer: Current status, in Heuson J C, Mattheiem W M, Rozencweig M (eds): Breast Cancer, Trends in Research and Treatment. New York, Raven Press, 1976, p 193
4. Von Hoff D D, Rozencweig M, Soper W, et al: Whatever happened to NSC? An analysis of clinical results of discontinued anticancer agents. Cancer Treat Rep, 61:759, 1977
5. Cornman I, Cornman M E: The action of podophyllin and its fractions on marine eggs. Ann. N.Y. Acad. Sci. 51:1443, 1951
6. Krishan A, Paika K, Frei E, III: Cytofluorometric studies on the action of podophyllotoxin and epipodophyllotoxins (VM 26, VP 16-213) on the cell cycle traverse of human lymphoblasts. J Cell Biol 66:521, 1975
7. Wilson L, Bamburg J R, Mizel S B, et al: Interaction of drugs with microtubule proteins. Fed Proc 33:158, 1974
8. Stahelin H: 4′-Demethyl-epipodophyllotoxin thenylidene glucoside (VM 26), a podophyllum compound with a new mechanism of action. Eur J Cancer 6:303, 1970
9. Stahelin H: Activity of a new glycosidic lig-

nan derivative (VP 16-213) related to podophyllotoxin in experimental tumors. Eur J Cancer 9:215, 1973

10. Grieder A, Maurer R, Stahelin H: Effect of an epipodophyllotoxin derivative (VP 16-213) on macromolecular synthesis and mitosis in mastocytoma cells in vitro. Cancer Res 34:1788, 1974
11. Huang C C, Hou Y, Wang J J: Effects of a new antitumor agent, epipodophyllotoxin, on growth and chromosomes in human haematopoietic cell lines. Cancer Res 33:3123, 1973
12. Misra N C, Roberts D: Inhibition by 4'-demethyl-epipodophyllotoxin 9-(4,6-0-2-thenylidene-β-D-glucopyranoside) of human lymphoblast cultures in G_2 phase of the cell cycle. Cancer Res 35:99, 1975
13. Venditti J M: Treatment schedule dependency of experimentally active antileukemic (L1210) drugs. Cancer Chemother Rep (3)2:35, 1971
14. Dombernowsky P, Nissen N I: Schedule dependency of the antileukemic activity of the podophyllotoxin-derivative VP 16-213 (NSC 141540) in L1210 leukemia. Arch Path Microbiol Scand 81:715, 1973
15. Allen L M, Creaven P J: Comparison of the human pharmacokinetics of VM-26 and VP-16, two antineoplastic epipodophyllotoxin glucopyranoside derivatives. Eur J Cancer 11:697, 1975
16. European Organization for Research on the Treatment of Cancer, Cooperative Group for Leukaemias and Haematosarcomas: Clinical screening of epipodophyllotoxin VM 26 in malignant lymphomas and solid tumors. Br Med J 2:744, 1972
17. Sonntag R W, Senn H J, Nagel G, et al: Experience with 4'-demethyl-epipodophyllotoxin 9-(4,6-0-2-thenylidene-beta-D-glucopyranoside), VM 26; NSC-122819, in the treatment of malignant lymphosis. Eur J Cancer 10:93, 1974
18. Trempe G, Sykes M, Young C, et al: Phase I trial of the podophyllotoxin derivative VM 26. Proc Am Assoc Cancer Res 11:79, 1970
19. European Organization for Research on the Treatment of Cancer, Clinical Screening Group: Epipodophyllotoxin VP 16-213 in treatment of acute leukaemias, haematosarcomas and solid tumours. Br Med J 3:199, 1973
20. Falkson G, van Dyk J J, van Eden E B, et al: A clinical trial of the oral form of 4'-demethyl-epipodophyllotoxin-β-D ethylidene glucoside (NSC-141540) VP 16-213. Cancer 35:1141, 1975
21. Nissen N I, Larsen V, Pedersen H, et al: Phase I clinical trial of a new antitumor agent, 4'-demethylepipodophyllotoxin 9-(4,6-0-ethylidene-β-D-glucopyranoside) (NSC-141540; VP 16-213). Cancer Chemother Rep 56:769, 1972
22. Jacobs P, King H S, Sealy G R H: Epipodophyllotoxin (VP 16-213) in the treatment of diffuse histiocytic lymphoma. S Afr Med J 49:483, 1975
23. Pavone-Macaluso M and the EORTC Genito-urinary Tract Group A: Single-drug chemotherapy of bladder cancer with adriamycin, VM-26 or bleomycin. Eur Urol 2:138, 1976
24. Sklansky B D, Mann-Kaplan R S, Reynolds A F Jr, et al: 4'-Demethyl-epipodophyllotoxin-β-D-thenylidene-glucoside (PTG) in the treatment of malignant intracranial neoplasms. Cancer 33:460, 1974
25. Eagan R T, Carr T R, Frytak S, et al: VP 16-213 versus polychemotherapy in patients with advanced small cell lung cancer. Cancer Treat Rep 60:949, 1976
26. Hansen M, Hirsch F, Dombernowsky P, et al: Treatment of small cell anaplastic carcinoma of the lung with the oral solution of VP 16-213 (NSC 141540, 4'-demethylepipodophyllotoxin 9-(4,6-0-ethylidene-β-D-glucopyranoside). Cancer 40:633,1977
27. Jungi W F, Senn H J: Clinical study of the new podophyllotoxin derivative, 4'-demethylepipodophyllotoxin 9-(4,6-0-ethylidene-β-D-glucopyranoside) (NSC-141540; VP 16-213) in solid tumors in man. Cancer Chemother Rep 59:737, 1975
28. Goldsmith M A, Carter S K: 4'-Demethyl-epipodophyllotoxin-β-D-thenylidene glucoside (VM 26). A brief review. Eur J Cancer 9:477, 1973
29. Cavalli F, Sonntag R, Brunner K W: Epipodophyllotoxin VP 16-213 in acute non-lymphoblastic leukaemia. Br Med J 4:227, 1975
30. Mathé G, Schwarzenberg L, Pouillart P, et al: Two epipodophyllotoxin derivatives, VM 26 and VP 16-213, in the treatment of leukemias, hematosarcomas and lymphomas. Cancer 34:985, 1974
31. Ahmann D L, Bisel H F, Eagan R T, et al: Phase II evaluation of VP 16-213 (NSC-141540) and cytembena (NSC-104801) in patients with advanced breast cancer. Cancer Treat Rep 60:633, 1976
32. Wilson W W, Bull F, Solomon J: Phase II study of VM 26 in advanced non-lymphomatous sarcoma. Proc Am Assoc Cancer Res 17:250, 1976
33. Ahmann D L, Bisel H F, Edmonson J H, et al: Phase II study of VP-16-213 versus dian-

hydrogalactitol in patients with metastatic malignant melanoma. Cancer Treat Rep 60:1681, 1976

34. Perry M C, Moertel C G, Schutt A J, et al: Phase II studies of dianhydrogalactitol and VP-16-213 in colorectal cancer. Cancer Treat Rep 60:1247, 1976
35. Von Hoff D D, Rozencweig M, Slavik M, et al: Activity of daunomycin in solid tumors. JAMA 236:1693, 1976
36. Maral R, Ponsinet G, Jollès G: Etude de l'activité antitumorale expérimentale d'un nouvel antibiotique semi-synthétique : la rubidazone (22050 RP). CR Acad Sci (D) (Paris) 275:301, 1972
37. Zbinden G, Brändle E: Toxicologic screening of daunorubicin (NSC 82151), adriamycin (NSC 123127) and their derivatives in rats. Cancer Chemother Rep 59:707, 1975
38. Jacquillat C I, Weil M, Gemon-Auclerc M F, et al: Clinical study of rubidazone (22030 RP), a new daunorubicin-derived compound in 170 patients with acute leukemias and other malignancies. Cancer 37:653, 1976
39. Chauvergne J, Durand M: Essai de chimiotherapie de tumeurs solides par la rubidazone. Étude préliminaire de 21 observations. Bordeaux Med. 6:1757, 1973
40. Benjamin R S, Keating M J, McCredie K B, et al: Clinical and pharmacologic studies with rubidazone (R) in adults with acute leukemia (AL). Proc Am Assoc Cancer Res 17:72, 1976
41. Sharpe H B A, Field E O, Hellmann K: Mode of action of the cytostatic agent "ICRF 159". Nature (London) 226:524, 1970
42. Creighton A M, Birnie G D: Biochemical studies on growth-inhibitory bisdioxopiperazines. I. Effect on DNA, RNA and protein synthesis in mouse-embryo fibroblasts. Int J Cancer 5:47, 1970
43. Creighton A M, Hellmann K, Whitecross S: Antitumour activity in a series of bisdiketopiperazines. Nature 222:384, 1969
44. Hellmann K, Murkin G E: Synergism of ICRF-159 and radiotherapy in treatment of experimental tumors. Cancer 34:1033, 1974
45. Woodman R J: Enhancement of antitumor effectiveness of ICRF-159 (NSC-129943) against early L1210 leukemia by combination with *cis*-diamminedichloroplatinum (NSC-119875) or daunomycin (NSC-82151). Cancer chemother Rep 4: (Part 2) 45, 1974
46. Kline I: Potentially useful combinations of chemotherapy detected in mouse tumor systems. Cancer Chemother Rep 4: (part 2) 33, 1974
47. Wampler G L, Speckhart V J, Regelson W: Phase I clinical study of adriamycin-ICRF159 combination and other ICRF-159 drug combinations. Proc Soc Clin Oncol 15:189, 1974
48. Herman E H, Mhatre R M, Lee I P, et al: Prevention of the cardiotoxic effects of adriamycin and daunomycin in the isolated dog heart (36432). Proc Soc Exp Biol Med 140:234, 1972
49. Hellmann K, Newton K A, Whitmore D N, et al: Preliminary clinical assessment of ICRF-159 in acute leukaemia and lymphosarcoma. Br Med J 1:822, 1969
50. Creaven P J, Cohen M H, Hansen H H, et al: Phase I clinical trial of a single-dose and two weekly schedules of ICRF-159 (NSC-129943). Cancer Chemother Rep 58:393, 1974
51. Bellet R E, Mastrangelo M J, Dixon L M, et al: Phase I study of ICRF-159 (NSC-129943) in human solid tumors. Cancer Chemother Rep 57:185, 1973
52. Flannery E P, Corder M P, Sheehan W W, et al: Phase II evaluation of ICRF-159 (NSC-129943) in non-Hodgkin's lymphomas. Proc Am Soc Clin Oncol 16:289, 1976
53. Marciniak T A, Moertel C G, Schutt A J, et al: Phase II study of ICRF-159 (NSC-129943) in advanced colorectal carcinoma. Cancer Chemother Rep 59:761, 1975
54. Bellet R E, Engstrom P F, Catalano R B, et al: Phase II study of ICRF-159 in patients with metastatic colorectal carcinoma previously exposed to systemic chemotherapy. Cancer Treat Rep 60:1395, 1976
55. Eagan R T, Carr D T, Coles D T, et al: ICRF-159 versus polychemotherapy in non-small cell lung cancer. Cancer Treat Rep 60:947, 1976
56. Bellet R E, Catalano R B, Danna V G, et al: A study of antitumor (phase II) and immunosuppressive effects of ICRF-159 in patients with metastatic melanoma. J Clin Pharmacol 16:433, 1976
57. Ryall R D H, Hanham I W F, Newton K A, et al: Combined treatment of soft tissue and osteosarcomas by radiation and ICRF-159. Cancer 34:1040, 1974
58. Rosenberg B: Possible mechanisms for the antitumor activity of platinum coordination complexes. Cancer Chemother Rep 59:589, 1975
59. Hayes D, Cvitkovic E, Golbey R, et al: Amelioration of renal toxicity of high dose *cis*-platinum diammine dichloride (CPDD) by mannitol induced diuresis. Proc Am Assoc Cancer Res 17:169, 1976
60. Merrin C: A new method to prevent toxicity with high doses of *cis* diammine platinum (therapeutic efficacy in previously treated

widespread and recurrent testicular tumors). Proc Am Soc Clin Oncol 17:243, 1976

61. Higby D J, Wallace H J, Jr, Albert D, et al: Diamminodichloroplatinum in the chemotherapy of testicular tumors. J Urol 112:100, 1974
62. Nitschke R, Starling K, Land V, et al: *Cis*-platinum (PDD) in childhood malignancies. Proc Am Soc Clin Oncol 17:310, 1976
63. Osieka R, Bruntsch U, Gallmeier W M, et al: *Cis*-diamino-dichloroplatin (II) in der Behandlung therapieresistenter maligner Hodenteratome. Deutsch Med Woch 101:191, 1976
64. Yagoda A, Watson R C, Gonzalez-Vitale J C, et al: *Cis*-dichlorodiammineplatinum (II) in advanced bladder cancer. Cancer Treat Rep 60:917, 1976
65. Wiltshaw E, Kroner T: Phase II study of *cis*-dichlorodiammineplatinum (II) (NSC-119875) in advanced adenocarcinoma of the ovary. Cancer Treat Rep 60:55, 1976
66. Wittes R E, Cvitkovic E, Shah J, et al: *cis*-dichlorodiammineplatinum (II) in the treatment of epidermoid carcinoma of the head and neck. Cancer Treat Rep 61:359, 1977
67. Rossof A H, Bearden J D III, Coltman C A Jr: Phase II evaluation of *cis*-diamminedichloroplatinum (II) in lung cancer. Cancer Treat Rep 60:1679, 1976
68. Kovach J S, Moertel C G, Schutt A J, et al: Phase II study of *cis*-diamminedichloroplatinum (NSC-119875) in advanced carcinoma of the large bowel. Cancer Chemother Rep 57:357, 1973
69. Einhorn L H, Donohue J P: Improved chemotherapy in disseminated testicular cancer. J Urol 117:65, 1977
70. Cvitkovic E, Hayes D, Golbey R: Primary combination chemotherapy (VAB III) for metastatic or unresectable germ cell tumors. Proc Am Soc Clin Oncol 17:296, 1976
71. Piskala A, Sorm F: Nucleic acids components and their analogues. LI. Synthesis of 1-glycosyl derivatives of 5-azauracil and 5-azacytosine. Collect Czech Chem Commun 29:2060, 1964
72. Hanka L J, Evans J S, Mason D J, et al: Microbiological production of 5-azacytidine. I. Production and biological activity. Antimicrob Agents Chemother 619, October 1966
73. Zadrazil S, Fucik V, Bartl P, et al: The structure of DNA from *Escherichia coli* cultured in the presence of 5-azacytidine. Biochim Biophys Acta 108:701, 1965
74. Cihak A, Tykva R, Sorm F: Incorporation of 5-azacytidine-4-[^{14}C] and of cytidine- [^{3}H] into ribonucleic acids of mouse Ehrlich ascites tumor cells. Collect Czech Chem Commun 31:3015, 1966
75. Karon M, Benedict W F: Chromatid breakage: Differential effect of inhibitors of DNA synthesis during G_2 phase. Science 178:62, 1972
76. Paces V, Doskocil J, Sorm F: Incorporation of 5-azacytidine into nucleic acids of *Escherichia coli.* Biochim Biophys Acta 161:352, 1968
77. Li L H, Olin E J, Buskirk H H, et al: Cytotoxicity and mode of action of 5-azacytidine on L1210 leukemia. Cancer Res 30:2760, 1970
78. Sorm F, Vesely J: The activity of a new antimetabolite, 5-azacytidine, against lymphoid leukemia in AK mice. Neoplasma 11:123, 1964
79. Neil G L, Gray L G, Berger A E: Combination chemotherapy of L1210 leukemia with cytarabine and 5-azacytidine—temporal aspects. Pharmacologist 16:209, 1974
80. Sandberg J, Goldin A: Use of first generation transplants of a slow growing solid tumor for the evaluation of new cancer chemotherapeutic agents. Cancer Chemother Rep 55:233, 1971
81. Pithova P, Piskala A, Pitha J, et al: Nucleic acid components and their analogues. LXVI. Hydrolysis of 5-azacytidine and its connection with biological activity. Collect Czech Chem Commun 30:2801, 1965
82. Lim P, Pont L, Cheung A: Data on 5-azacytidine. NIH Contract 1-CM-33723, December 30, 1974
83. Troetel W M, Weiss A J, Stambaugh J E, et al: Absorption, distribution and excretion of 5-azacytidine (NSC-102816) in man. Cancer Chemother Rep 56:405, 1972
84. Israili Z H, Vogler W R, Mingioli E S, et al: The disposition and pharmacokinetics in humans of 5-azacytidine administered intravenously as a bolus or by continuous infusion. Cancer Res 36:1453, 1976
85. Israili Z H, Vogler W R, Mingioli E S, et al: Studies of the disposition of 5-azacytidine—14C in man. Pharmacologist 16:231, 1974
86. Hrodek O, Vesely J: 5-azacytidine in childhood leukemia. Neoplasma 18:493, 1971
87. Vogler W R, Miller D S, Keller J W: 5-azacytidine (NSC-102816): A new drug for the treatment of myeloblastic leukemia. Blood 48:331, 1976
88. Levi J A, Wiernik P H: A comparative clinical trial of 5-azacytidine and guanazole in previously treated adults with acute nonlymphocytic leukemia. Cancer 38:36, 1976

89. Karon M, Sieger L, Leimbrock S, et al: 5-azacytidine: a new active agent for the treatment of acute leukemia. Blood 42:359, 1973
90. Tan C, Burchenal J H, Clarkson B, et al: Clinical trial of 5-azacytidine. Proc Am Assoc Cancer Res 14:97, 1973
91. McCredie K B, Bodey G P, Burgess M A, et al: Treatment of acute leukemia with 5-azacytidine (NSC-102816). Cancer Chemother Rep 57:319, 1973
92. Canellos G P, DeVita V T, Whang-Peng J, et al: Chemotherapy of the blastic phase of chronic granulocytic leukemia: Hypodiploidy and response to therapy. Blood 47:1003, 1976
93. Quagliana J M, Alexanian R: Personal communication, December 1975
94. Cunningham T J, Nemoto T, Rosner D, et al: Comparison of 5-azacytidine (NSC-102816) with CCNU (NSC-79037) in the treatment of patients with breast cancer and evaluation of the subsequent use of cyclophosphamide (NSC-26271). Cancer Chemother Rep 58:677, 1974
95. Bellet R E, Mastrangelo M J, Engstrom P F, et al: Clinical trial with subcutaneously administered 5-azacytidine (NSC-102816). Cancer Chemother Rep 58:217, 1974
96. Moertel C G, Schutt A J, Reitemeier R J, et al: Phase II study of 5-azacytidine (NSC-102816) in the treatment of advanced gastrointestinal cancer. Cancer Chemother Rep 56:649, 1972
97. Vogler W R, Arkun S, Velez-Garcia E: Writing Committee for the Southeastern Cancer Study Group: Phase I study of twice weekly 5-azacytidine (NSC-102816). Cancer Chemother Rep 58:895, 1974
98. Vogler W R, Miller D, Keller J W: Remission induction in refractory myeloblastic leukemia with continuous infusion of 5-azacytidine. Proc Am Assoc Cancer Res 16:155, 1975
99. Lomen P L, Vaitkevicius V K, Samson M K: Phase I study of 5-azacytidine using 24 hrs continuous infusion for 5 days. Proc Am Assoc Cancer Res 16:52, 1975
100. Lomen P L, Baker L H, Neil G L, et al: Phase I study of 5-azacytidine (NSC-102816) using 24-hour continuous infusion for 5 days. Cancer Chemother Rep 59:1123, 1975
101. Bellet R E, Mastrangelo M J, Engstrom P F, et al: Hepatotoxicity of 5-azacytidine (NSC-102816) (a clinical and pathologic study). Neoplasma 20:303, 1973
102. Von Hoff D D, Slavik M, Muggia F M: 5-azacytidine—A new anticancer drug with effectiveness in acute myelogenous leukemia. Ann Int Med 85:237, 1976
103. Ho M, Bear R A, Garvey M B: Symptomatic hypophosphatemia secondary to 5-azacytidine therapy of acute nonlymphocytic leukemia. Cancer Treat Rep 60:1400, 1976
104. Hanka L J, Clark J J: Use of 5-azacytidine in combination with cytidine in local perfusion. Proc Am Assoc Cancer Res 16:113, 1975
105. Beisler J A, Abbasi M M, Driscoll J S: Dihydro-5-azacytidine hydrochloride, a biologically active and chemically stable analog of 5-azacytidine. Cancer Treat Rep 60:1671, 1976

Acknowledgements

The authors wish to thank William Soper, Sanda Rife, and Audrey Alston for their help in the preparation of this manuscript.

Joseph E. Sokal

8 Immunotherapy of Cancer: Current Status

It is now recognized that there is active host resistance against malignant neoplasms and that the fate of patients with cancer depends not only on the characteristics of the tumor and the action of antitumor agents but also on host defense mechanisms. These have been studied in detail in experimental animal systems and several different types of antitumor activity have been defined (Table 8-1). Tumors carry distinctive antigens not present in the normal adult tissues in which they arise and some defense mechanisms are based on recognition of such "foreign" antigens. Although cytotoxic antibodies and complement may be sufficient to destroy tumor cells in a few experimental systems, cellular defense mechanisms are usually required. These may be brought into play by antitumor antibodies (antibody-directed, cell-mediated cytotoxicity) or may involve cell-to-cell interactions only, with recognition of tumor by specifically sensitized lymphocytes. In addition to defense mechanisms based on recognition of specific antigens on tumor cells, a very potent tumoricidal system is based on antigen-nonspecific recognition of tumor cells by activated macrophages. These host cells recognize an as yet unidentified abnormality of neoplastic cells and can destroy a variety of antigenically different tumors while sparing neighboring normal cells.[1,2]

Studies in experimental systems have demonstrated that: (1) animals can be specifically immunized against individual tumors, (2) "chemotherapeutic cure" of neoplastic disease usually requires an intact immune system,[3] and (3) a variety of immunologic stimulants can increase antitumor resistance. Immunotherapy can lead to the destruction of established neoplasms if administered when tumors are below a critical size.[4,5] In some experimental models, cure of established tumors may be obtained with a combination of chemotherapy and immunotherapy when either modality alone is ineffective.[6]

TABLE 8-1. *Anti-tumor Defense Mechanisms*

Antigen-specific
Cytotoxic antibody + complement
Antibody-directed cell-mediated cytotoxicity
Direct lymphocyte cytotoxicity ("killer" lymphocytes)
Lymphocyte-directed macrophage cytotoxicity
Tumor-specific, Antigen-nonspecific
Tumor cell destruction by activated macrophages

The relative importance of the various antitumor defense mechanisms in human neoplastic disease has not yet been defined. The cellular immune system appears to be much more important, however, than antibody mechanisms. Antitumor antibodies may, in fact, play a role in protection of tumor cells against destruction by specifically sensitized host cells via "blocking" activity.[7] Such activity has been described for antibody, soluble tumor antigen and antigen-antibody complexes. Several types of cancer are associated with impairment of cellular (but not antibody) immune mechanisms, and the fate of patients with cancer often correlates with the status of their cellular immune mechanisms. Such correlations are quite striking for some neoplasms,[8,9,10] (e.g., Hodgkin's disease, head and neck cancer, lung cancer) but are not seen in all types of cancer. The ability to develop hypersensitivity to a new antigen correlates better with antitumor resistance than exhibition of a "memory" response reflecting sensitization earlier in life.[8,9]

The recognition that most, if not all, human tumors have distinctive tumor-associated antigens, as well as the correlations between immune responses and fate in several types of human cancer and the demonstration of effectiveness of immunologic manipulation in a variety of animal models, have led to great interest in clinical immunotherapy. During the past few years there has been very rapid expansion of effort in this field. Enough data are now available to permit some conclusions to be reached and to justify a review of the current status of this new modality of cancer treatment. It must be emphasized, however, that assessment of the potential contributions of immunotherapy to cancer management will not be possible for a number of years. Most current studies cannot yet be evaluated. Very few clinical trials have been in progress as long as 5 years and thus, long-term results can only be guessed at. Particularly troublesome is the fact that we do not know how to determine optimal schedules of administration for most of the immunotherapeutic agents we are using.

A variety of approaches to immunotherapy have had some degree of clinical exploration (Table 8-2). The simplest and best documented of these is local immunotherapy. This depends on induction of a strong delayed hypersensitivity response within the tumor or in its immediate vicinity. Tumor cells within the area of such a response are destroyed, while normal cells are largely spared. Activated macrophages are probably the principal

TABLE 8-2. *Types of Immunotherapy Explored in Man*

1. Local immunotherapy: topical application of sensitizing agents, intralesional injection of BCG or other agents, etc.
2. Administration of agents which stimulate cellular immune mechanisms and/or the reticuloendothelial system: BCG or BCG fractions, *Corynebacterium* parvum, levamisole, synthetic polynucleotides, thymosin, etc.
3. Active tumor-specific immunotherapy
   (a) Possibly specific: vaccination with allogenic cells, cell fractions or purified extracts believed to carry appropriate tumor antigens, to stimulate patients' immunity to their own neoplasms
   (b) Specific: vaccination with autologous tumor cells or cell fractions
4. Passive tumor-specific immunotherapy
   (a) Administration of cells and/or plasma from donors immunized against patients' tumors
   (b) Possibly specific: administration of cells and/or serum from donors presumably cured of similar neoplasms
5. Instructional immunotherapy: administration of dialyzable transfer factor or "immune" RNA prepared from lymphocytes of
   (a) donors presumably cured of similar neoplasms
   (b) animals immunized with patients' tumors
6. "Unblocking" therapy: administration of agents to reduce "blocking activity", which interferes with a patient's immune response against his tumor

mediators of such tumor cell destruction. Obviously, a prerequisite for success with this type of immunotherapy is that the patient be sufficiently immunocompetent to exhibit good delayed hypersensitivity reactions.

Local immunotherapy has been used principally in two situations: (1) Multiple superficial skin cancers or premalignant lesions and (2) superficial metastases of malignant melanoma, breast cancer, etc., accessible to intralesional injection. In the former, the patient is sensitized to an agent which can conveniently be applied to involved areas of skin.[11] A concentration of the agent is used which evokes a moderate reaction in normal skin, and topical applications are repeated periodically. (As a patient's sensitivity increases, the concentration of sensitizer is decreased to avoid excessively severe reactions.) Nitrogen mustard was one of the first agents used topically, and it was thought that a chemotherapeutic effect was being observed. It soon became evident, however, that it was acting via its sensitizing properties. Dinitrochlorobenzene (DNCB) and 5-fluorouracil are more commonly used today. Immunotherapy is now the treatment of choice for patients with recurrent multiple skin neoplasms or premalignant lesions, as in late radiation dermatitis with malignant degeneration and arsenical dermatitis. Patients with many lesions initially require fairly frequent therapy. After good control is achieved, however, an essentially tumor-free state may be maintained with two or three treatments per year.

Morton et al[12] demonstrated that intralesional injection of bacillus Calmette-Guerin (BCG) could result in regression of superficial nodules of malignant melanoma. These observations were confirmed by many other investigators,[13] and intralesional injection of BCG has become a standard form of therapy for disseminated skin involvement with malignant melanoma. An immunologic response to BCG (e.g., tuberculin conversion) is a prerequisite for tumor regression. Intralesional therapy can induce regression of the majority of injected lesions[13] and disappearance of all superficial lesions can be achieved in about half of the treated patients.[14] Infrequently, systemic effects of such therapy are seen, and tumor nodules at sites distant to BCG injection also regress.

Intralesional therapy is equally effective in inducing regression of superficial deposits of other types of tumor, such as skin metastases of breast cancer and malignant lymphoma. It is not necessary to use BCG; regression of superficial neoplasms has also been achieved by intralesional injection of vaccinia virus and of antigens to which the patient is hypersensitive, such as dinitrochlorobenzine (DNCB), purified protein derivative (tuberculin-PPD), and Varidase (streptokinase-streptodornase). In our very limited experience with intralesional therapy, bacterial antigens proved preferable to BCG because they were able to induce regression of lymphomatous deposits without ulceration whereas injection of BCG resulted in ulceration and scarring.

A quite different application of local immunotherapy was developed by McKnealley[15] as an adjunct to surgical therapy for lung cancer. This involves intrapleural administration of BCG, 3 to 6 days after tumor resection. A single instillation is used, and patients are given a course of isoniazid starting 14 days later in order to prevent persistent infection. Presumably, this results in destruction of occult deposits of tumor cells within the chest cavity and thus protects the patient against local or regional recurrence. This treatment appears to be successful in Stage I disease (see Table 8-4 below). To date, no significant benefit has been seen among patients with more advanced disease, however.

Non-specific Immunologic Stimulation

After the demonstration that a variety of immunologic and reticuloendothelial stimulants could increase antitumor resistance in experimental animals, many trials were initiated in man. The agent most commonly used to date has been living BCG. More recently, two fractions of BCG have been tested: MER (methanol extraction residue of killed BCG organisms) and a cell-wall fraction of BCG attached to oil droplets. These materials are quite different, but both appear to be potent immunologic stimulants and both are effective in experimental animal systems. BCG has been given by a variety of routes, in greatly different doses and according to widely varying schedules. This adds to the difficulty of comparing results reported by different investigators. It is generally agreed, however, that BCG is an effective stimulant of delayed hypersensitivity responses in man.[16]

Although BCG is quite well tolerated by most patients with only mild local or systemic side effects, a number of serious complications of its administration have been described. Among immunologically compromised patients, persistent and disseminated infection may result including widespread miliary disease.[17] We have seen two instances of activation of presumably dormant infection with pathogenic acid-fast organisms.[18] A variety of hypersensitivity complications have been described,[17,18,19] including two very severe acute reactions which terminated fatally.[20] Aggravation or induction of allergic or autoimmune phenomena (e.g., bronchospasm) may occur.[18] Use of nonliving fractions of BCG avoids the hazard of persistent infection but not the more common complications associated with hypersensitivity phenomena.

Killed *Corynebacterium parvum* or *granulosum* vaccines have also been used for nonspecific systemic immunotherapy. The immunologic effects of *Corynebacteria* differ from those of BCG, and an increase of delayed hypersensitivity responses has not been recorded by most investigators. There has not been as much experience with these agents as with BCG, but favorable results have been reported by several investigators. These vaccines are usually given subcutaneously or intravenously. The former route frequently causes troublesome pain at the injection site, while the latter can result in chills, fever, cyanosis, hypertension and hypotensive episodes.[21] These complications are acute, usually occurring soon after injection and subsiding within 24 hours.

In contrast to BCG and *C. parvum*, the newest immunologic stimulant to enter clinical trials, levamisole, is taken by mouth and appears to be tolerated quite well. The reported side effects involve the gastrointestinal and central nervous sytems.[21] Levamisole is said to restore cellular immune responses among immunodepressed patients, but not to stimulate normal responses.[22]

Many of the clinical trials of immunotherapy reported to date have utilized nonspecific immunologic stimulation following surgery or in conjunction with chemotherapy or radiation therapy. The early hopes that such adjunctive treatment might substantially prolong remissions and increase cure rates have not been realized, and enthusiasm for immunotherapy has declined measurably during the past year or two. Although the results of most trials are rather disappointing, this type of immunotherapy does appear to have some effectiveness. Most studies in lung cancer, for example, report statistically significant survival benefit for patients receiving immunotherapy (Table 8-3). It is quite evident from these data that: (1) there has been no major breakthrough in the management of advanced lung cancer, and (2) even the most carefully organized clinical studies are subject to considerable variability. The report by Amery illustrates the latter point.[22] All patients in this study were given the same dose of levamisole. The lack of effect among heavier patients is attributed to the lower dose/kg received by these patients which implies a rather unusual dose-response curve for this agent with a very narrow threshold between response and no response. But how does one explain the significant difference in relapse rate between lighter and heavier patients receiving placebo? Despite some inconsistencies in these data, however, it seems reasonable to conclude that nonspecific immunotherapy may modify the course of lung cancer and to predict that, as techniques of immunotherapy are improved, more meaningful differences between treated and control groups will be recorded.

Conflicting data have been reported regarding the effectiveness of nonspecific immunotherapy for other neoplasms. Although there is general agreement regarding the value of intralesional BCG therapy in malignant melanoma, BCG vaccination as an adjunct to surgical therapy for the disease is controversial. One group reported significant benefit,[28] while another reported identical remission and survival curves for immunized and control patients.[29] Two studies of *C. parvum* as an adjunct to combination chemotherapy for advanced breast cancer reported favorable results,[23,30] but both positive and negative results have been reported with BCG. In AML,

TABLE 8-3. *Systemic, Nonspecific Immunotherapy in Lung Cancer*

Author	Patients	Parameter	Stimulant	Result	Controls	Result
Israel[23]	Disseminated epidermoid, Receiving chemotherapy	median survival	*C. parvum*	9.8 mo.*	concurrent, random	5.6 mo*
Yamamura[24]	Stage III	median	BCG cell walls	18 mo.*	historical,	7 mo*
	Stage IV	survival	on oil droplets	12 mo.*	recent	4 mo*
Amery[22]	Resectable tumor,		Levamisole		concurrent,	
	Pt. weight < 70 kg	proven	150 mg/day	2/25*	random,	18/36*
	Pt. weight > 70 kg	relapse	3 da q2wk	15/40	double-blind	7/37
Perlin et al[25]	Stage III, radiation, Chemotherapy	median survival	BCG	10.5 mo	concurrent, random	11 mo
Kerman[26] and Stefani	Locally advanced Inoperable, radiation	median survival	BCG	12 mo*	concurrent, random	8 mo*
Warren et al[27]	Stage II,III,IV	6 mo survival	BCG	59%	concurrent,	59%
	Surgery,	1 yr survival		31%	random	21%
	radiation, Chemotherapy	2 yr survival		24%		14%

*A statistically significant difference between stimulated and control groups.

most investigators report that addition of BCG to combination chemotherapy results in some increase in survival, but without significant numbers of long-term survivors.[31,32,33] There have been several reports on nonspecific immunotherapy in colorectal cancer, but no consensus has yet been reached regarding its value. Evaluation is not yet possible of current studies in malignant lymphoma and a number of other neoplasms.

Specific Immunotherapy

Active immunization of patients against their own tumors has been attempted from time to time through the years. In the past, it was usually tried in patients with advanced, uncontrolled disease as a last-ditch effort to achieve a remission. It became evident some years ago that such efforts are doomed to failure, and more recent trials have focused on patients who are free of grossly evident tumor after surgery, radiation or chemotherapy, but who are at high risk of relapse. Autologous tumor has been used in a few studies, but logistical problems make this a difficult approach. Most investigators have compromised on the use of allogeneic tumor of the same type and carrying similar tumor-associated antigens as that of the patient to be immunized. Vaccines have utilized undamaged tumor cells, irradiated cells, neuraminidase-treated cells, chemically modified cells, cultured cells of established lines and crude or purified antigenic fractions of neoplastic cells. These have been administered alone, in Freund's adjuvant, in conjunction with BCG or other stimulants administered separately, or mixed with BCG. Vaccination schedules have varied considerably.

Patients in remission of ALL or AML have been given frequent injections of irradiated allogeneic blast cells, as well as BCG administered by scarification or multiple puncture. Early reports claimed substantial benefit[34,35] but subsequent experience failed to confirm this. A trial in chronic myelocytic leukemia used cultured lymphoid cells carrying antigens of myeloid leukemia mixed with BCG and injected intradermally. Vaccination schedules were considerably less intensive than in the above trials. Initial evaluation suggested substantial prolongation of survival,[36] but a more recent review reported much less striking data and raised questions regarding efficacy of different vaccination schedules.[18] Preliminary data from a current trial in AML, utilizing intradermal injection of neuraminidase-treated allogeneic myeloblasts, show significant prolongation of remission and survival.[37]

Immunization with native or cultured tumor cells has been tested in malignant melanoma, osteogenic sarcoma and most recently in breast cancer, after primary therapy with surgery or chemotherapy. No important benefit has been reported so far. The most successful application of specific immunotherapy to date appears to be in lung cancer. Takita et al.[38] undertook radical lung resection among patients with locally advanced carcinoma, followed by immunization with autologous neuraminidase-treated tumor cells in Freund's adjuvant. Median survival of 15 patients so vaccinated was about 2 years, significantly better than that of controls managed conventionally. Young[39] has immunized 16 patients with resectable lung cancer with autologous tumor cells mixed with BCG after preliminary stimulation with BCG alone. To date (median followup, 2 years), there has been no tumor recurrence in this group. Stewart et al.[40] have immunized patients postoperatively with a soluble antigen extracted from cancers of the same histologic subtype and administered in Freund's adjuvant. The actuarial 3-year survival rate of immunized patients is 94 per cent—significantly better than the 52 per cent among randomly selected controls not receiving immunotherapy. No benefit was seen among patients with Stage II or III disease, however.

Other Approaches

Passive immunotherapy has been tried among patients with advanced disease. Volunteers were immunized by subcutaneous implants of patients' tumors, after which the patients received circulating cells from the immunized donors. The most thorough study of this approach is probably that reported by

TABLE 8-4. *Effects of Immunotherapy in Stage I Lung Cancer*

Author, technique	Recurrence/Patients Control	Immunotherapy
McKneally et al:[15] intrapleural BCG post-operatively (1 dose)	9/32	1/26
Stewart et al:[41] soluble tumor antigen in Freund's adjuvant (3 doses)	9/24	5/28
Young[40]: frequent BCG ± autologous tumor cells	6/23	3/26
Total	24/79 (30%)	9/80 (11%)
	$p < .01$	

Nadler and Moore,[41] which utilized pairs of patients matched for blood type and tumor histology. Each patient received several tumor transplants from his partner, after which they were repeatedly cross-transfused. These investigators recorded a few dramatic responses, but in the great majority of patients no benefit was evident. Similarly, administration of large numbers of lymphocytes from healthy contacts of patients, who might be immune to tumors of presumed infectious origin, has not resulted in clear-cut benefit.

"Instructional" immunotherapy utilizes a transfer factor prepared from lymphocytes of presumably immune donors or "immune" RNA from lymphocytes of human donors or of animals immunized with the recipient's tumor. The former has been tested in patients with osteogenic sarcoma after potentially curative surgery; to date, no significant reduction in recurrence rate has been reported.[42,43] Pilch et al[44] have tested immune RNA extracted from lymphoid tissues of sheep immunized with the recipients' tumors; apparent benefit was seen in a few patients but it is much too early to attempt evaluation of the clinical utility of such therapy.

Thymosin, a material prepared from animal thymus which may affect cellular immune responses in man, is currently in Phase I trial; no definite antitumor effect is yet evident.[45]

"Unblocking" plasma was tested in a randomized, double-blind trial among patients with Stage II and Stage III malignant melanoma.[46] No benefit was seen, but a few patients developed hepatitis.

CONCLUSIONS

To date, immunotherapy has not had a major impact on the therapy of cancer. Its effectiveness, however, has been demonstrated in a few situations. It is the treatment of choice (and has become conventional therapy) for multiple superficial skin cancers and premalignant lesions, and for multiple superficial metastases of malignant melanoma. Current studies in Stage I lung cancer suggest strongly that postoperative immunotherapy will increase cure rates to 80 to 90 per cent (Table 8-4).

The preponderance of evidence currently available suggests that immunotherapy may be of some value as adjunctive therapy in AML, in advanced lung cancer and in disseminated breast cancer. The effects so far recorded are far from dramatic, but they appear to be significant.

In ALL, immunotherapy seems to have been ineffective to date. In a variety of other areas of clinical oncology, either the available data are conflicting, confirmation of positive reports is not available or studies cannot yet be evaluated.

Immunotherapy cannot be expected to produce improvement in advanced cancer refractory to surgery, irradiation or chemotherapy. At best, its use will achieve nothing; at worst, it may induce serious clinical complications. Among responsive tumors, addition of immunotherapy usually does not increase the remission rate, but may increase duration of remission and survival.

TABLE 8-5. *Parameters of Administration of BCG in Clinical Trials*

Route
Scarification, multiple puncture, intradermal injection, intralesional injection, intracavitary injection, intravenous injection, oral
Dose
Scarification: 10^6 to 5×10^8 colony-forming units
Injection: 2×10^4 to 5×10^8 colony-forming units
Frequency
Once, several times, ... weekly for 3 to 5 years

We do not know the best way to use the immunotherapeutic agents already shown to have some clinical effectiveness. Parameters of the use of one agent are summarized in Table 8-5. It would be most surprising if all of these schedules were effective. I would guess that some of the negative data recorded with BCG are attributable to grossly improper schedules of administration rather than its lack of activity. In particular, there has been a trend to use immunotherapy as aggressively as feasible, which may be a mistake.[18] It seems reasonable to predict that as we improve our techniques of using this new modality of treatment, immunotherapy will make more important contributions to the management of cancer.

REFERENCES

1. Holterman C A, Casale G P, Klein E: Tumor cell destruction by macrophages. J Med 3:305, 1972
2. Mansell P W A, DiLuzio N R, McNamee R, et al: Recognition factors and nonspecific macrophage activation in the treatment of neoplastic disease. Ann N Y Acad Sci 277:20, 1976
3. Mihich E: Modification of tumor regression by immunologic means. Cancer Res 29:2345, 1969
4. Zbar B, Tanaka T: Immunotherapy of cancer: Regression of tumors after intralesional injection of living mycobacterium bovis. Science 172:271, 1971
5. Simmons, R L, Rios A: Immunotherapy of cancer: Immunospecific rejection of tumors in recipients of neuraminidase-treated tumor cells plus BCG. Science 174:591, 1971
6. Glynn J P, Halpern B L, Fefer A: An immunochemotherapeutic system for the treatment of a transplanted Moloney virus-induced lymphoma in mice. Cancer Res 29:515, 1969
7. Rios A, Simmons R L: Comparative effect of mycobacterium bovis- and neuraminidase-treated tumor cells on the growth of established methylcholanthrene fibrosarcomas in syngeneic mice. Cancer Res 32:16, 1972
8. Sokal J E, Aungst C W: Cellular immune responses and prognosis in the malignant lymphomas, in Hall T C (ed): National Cancer Institute Monograph 34, Prediction of Responses to Cancer Therapies, 1971, p 109
9. Eilber F R, Morton D L: Impaired immunologic reactivity and recurrence following cancer surgery. Cancer 25:362, 1970
10. Kerman R, Stefani S: Immunological evaluation of patients with solid tumors before and after radiotherapy, in Crispen R G (ed): Neoplasm Immunity: Mechanisms. Chicago, ITR, 1976, p 109
11. Klein E: Tumors of the skin X. Immunotherapy of cutaneous and mucosal neoplasms. N Y S J Med 68:900, 1968
12. Morton D L, Eilber F R, Malmgren R A, et al: Immunological factors which influence response to immunotherapy in malignant melanoma. Surgery 68:158, 1970
13. Mastrangelo M J, Berd D, Bellet R E: Critical review of previously reported clinical trials of cancer immunotherapy with non-specific immunostimulants. Ann N Y Acad Sci 277:94, 1976
14. Pinsky C M: Presented at a Symposium on Immunotherapy of Solid Tumors, Chicago, 1977
15. McKneally M F, Maver C M, Kausel H W: Regional immunotherapy of lung cancer using postoperative intrapleural BCG, in Terry W D, Windhorst D (eds): Immunotherapy of Cancer. Present Status of Trials in Man. New York, Raven Press, 1978, p 161
16. Sokal J E, Aungst C W, Han T: Effect of BCG on delayed hypersensitivity responses of patients with neoplastic disease. Int J Cancer 12:242, 1973
17. Aungst C W, Sokal J E, Jager B V: Complications of BCG vaccination in neoplastic disease. Ann Int Med 82:666, 1975
18. Sokal J E, Aungst C W, Snyderman M, et al: Immunotherapy of chronic myelocytic leuke-

mia: Effects of different vaccination schedules. Ann N Y Acad Sci 277:367, 1976

19. Sparks F C: Hazards and complications of BCG immunotherapy. Med Clin North Am, 60:499, 1976
20. McKhann C F, Hendrickson C G, Spitler L E, et al: Immunotherapy of melanoma with BCG: Two fatalities following intralesional injection. Cancer 35:514, 1975
21. Hirshaut Y, Pinsky C M, Wanebo J H, et al: Design of phase-1 trials of immunopotentiators for cancer therapy: Levamisole and Corynebacterium parvum. Ann N Y Acad Sci 277:252, 1976
22. Amery W K: Double-blind levamisole trial in resectable lung cancer. Ann N Y Acad Sci 277:260, 1976
23. Israel L: Immunochemotherapy with corynebacterium parvum in disseminated cancer. Ann N Y Acad Sci 277:241, 1976
24. Yamamura Y: Immunotherapy of lung cancer with oil-attached cell wall skeleton of BCG, in Terry W D, Windhorst D (eds): Immunotherapy of Cancer: Present Status of Trials in Man. New York, Raven Press, 1978, p 173
25. Perlin E, Weese J L, Heim W, et al: Immunotherapy of carcinoma of the lung with BCG and allogeneic tumor cells, in Crispen R G (ed): Neoplasm Immunity: Solid Tumor Therapy. Philadelphia, Franklin Institute Press, 1977, p 9
26. Kerman R, Stefani S: Radio and immunotherapy of lung cancer: A preliminary report, in Crispen R G (ed): Neoplasm Immunity: Solid Tumor Therapy. Philadelphia, Franklin Institute Press, 1977, p 29
27. Warren S, Crispen R, Nika B: BCG adjuvant immunotherapy of stage II, III and IV bronchogenic carcinoma, in Crispen R G (ed): Neoplasm Immunity: Solid Tumor Therapy. Philadelphia, Franklin Institute Press, 1977, p 49
28. Gutterman J U, Mavligit G M, Blumenshein G, et al: Immunotherapy of human solid tumors with bacillus Calmette-Guérin: Prolongation of disease-free interval and survival in malignant melanoma, breast, and colorectal cancer. Ann N Y Acad Sci 277:135, 1976
29. Pinsky C M, Hirshaut Y, Wanebo H J, et al: Randomized trial of bacillus Calmette-Guérin (percutaneous administration) as surgical adjuvant immunotherapy for patients with stage-II melanoma. Ann N Y Acad Sci 277:187, 1976
30. Pinsky C, DeJager R, Wittes, R, et al: Corynebacterium parvum as adjuvant to combination chemotherapy in patients with advanced breast cancer, in Crispen R G (ed): Neoplasm Immunity: Solid Tumor Therapy. Philadelphia, Franklin Institute Press, 1977, p 145
31. Vogler W R, Bartolucci A A, Omura G A, et al: A randomized clinical trial of BCG in myeloblastic leukemia, in Terry W D, Windhorst D (eds): Immunotherapy of Cancer: Present Status of Trials in Man. New York, Raven Press, 1978, p 365
32. Gutterman J U, Rodriguez Z, McCredie K B, et al: Chemoimmunotherapy of acute myeloblastic leukemia: 4-year follow-up with BCG, in Terry W D, Windhorst D (eds): Immunotherapy of Cancer: Present Status of Trials in Man. New York, Raven Press, 1978, p 375
33. Whittaker J, Slatter A J: Immunotherapy of acute myelogenous leukemia using intravenous BCG, in Terry W D, Windhorst D (eds): Immunotherapy of Cancer: Present Status of Trials in Man. New York, Raven Press, 1978, p 393
34. Mathé G. Amiel J L. Schwarzenberg L, et al: Active immunotherapy for acute lymphoblastic leukemia. Lancet 1:697, 1969
35. Powles R L, Crowther D, Bateman C J T, et al: Immunotherapy for acute myelogenous leukaemia. Br J Cancer 28:365, 1976
36. Sokal J E, Aungst C W, Grace J T Jr: Immunotherapy in well-controlled chronic myelocytic leukemia. N Y J Med 73:1180, 1973
37. Bekesi J G, Holland J F, Cuttner J, et al: Immunotherapy in acute myelocytic leukemia (AML) with neuraminidase (N'ASE) treated allogeneic myeloblasts with or without MER. Proc Am A Cancer Res 17:184, 1976
38. Takita H, Takada M, Minowada J, et al: Adjuvant immunotherapy of stage III lung carcinoma, in Terry W D, Windhorst D (eds): Immunotherapy of Cancer: Present Status of Trials in Man. New York, Raven Press, 1978, p 217
39. Young W: Immunotherapy of resectable bronchogenic carcinoma. A progress report, in Crispen R G (ed): Neoplasm Immunity: Solid Tumor Therapy. Philadelphia, Franklin Institute Press, 1977, p 55
40. Stewart T H M, Hollinshead A, Harris J, et al: A survival study of specific active immunochemotherapy in lung cancer, in Crispen R G (ed): Neoplasm Immunity: Solid Tumor Therapy. Philadelphia, Franklin Institute Press, 1977, p 37
41. Nadler S A, Moore G E: Clinical immunologic study of malignant disease: Response to tumor transplants and transfer of leukocytes. Ann Surg 164:482, 1966
42. Fudenberg H H: Dialyzable transfer factor in the treatment of human osteosarcoma: An analytic review. Ann N Y Acad Sci 277:545, 1976

43. Ivins J C, Ritts R E Jr, Pritchard D J, et al: Transfer factor versus combination chemotherapy: A preliminary report of a randomized postsurgical adjuvant treatment study in osteogenic sarcoma. Ann N Y Acad Sci 277:558, 1976
44. Pilch Y H, Fritze D, deKernion J B, et al: Immunotherapy of cancer with immune RNA in animal models and cancer patients. Ann N Y Acad Sci 277:592, 1976
45. Schafer L A, Goldstein A L, Gutterman J U, et al: In vitro and in vivo studies with thymosin in cancer patients. Ann N Y Acad Sci 277:609, 1976
46. Wright P W, Hellström K E, Hellström I, et al: Serotherapy of malignant melanoma, in Terry W D and Windhorst D (eds): Immunotherapy of Cancer: Present Status of Trials in Man. New York, Raven Press, 1978, p 135

Julian L. Ambrus
Clara M. Ambrus

9

Anticoagulants, Fibrinolytic Enzymes and Platelet Aggregation Inhibitors in Cancer Chemotherapy

Neoplastic disease and its chemotherapy involves the blood coagulation, fibrinolysin and platelet systems at several levels, and it is likely that patients can benefit from appropriate manipulations of these systems.

Thromboembolic and Hemorrhagic Complications of Neoplastic Disease

In an earlier study[1] we investigated the causes of death of cancer patients in our hospital, the results of which are summarized in Table 9-1. It appears that the category "hemorrhagic and/or thromboembolic complications" was the second most important cause of death (after infections), representing 18 per cent of the "major causes" and 43 per cent of the "contributory causes". Leavey, Kahn and Brodsky,[2] Brodsky et al,[3-6] Bettigole et al[7] and others pointed out the role of disseminated intravascular coagulation (DIC), hemorrhage and thromboembolism in cancer patients, particularly those undergoing certain types of chemotherapy.

In a prospective study we investigated the incidence of thromboembolic episodes in cancer patients over a 5-year period.[8] The incidence was expressed per thousand months of observation (ITE/1000). The data were compared to those obtained from patients who were admitted to the hospital with diagnostic

Table 9-1. *Causes of Death of Patients with Neoplastic Disease (Total No. 486) at RPMI in 1970.*

	Major cause %	Contributory cause %
Infection	36	68
Hemorrhagic and/or thromboembolic episodes	18	43
Organ invasion (including hepatic failure)	16	5
Cachexia	1	0.4
Respiratory failure (including aspiration)	19	3
Cardiovascular failure (including myocardial infarction)	7	3
Other and unknown	5	—

TABLE 9-2. *Control Patients*

Age	Total No. Cases	Clinical TE* No.	%	No. autopsies	TE by autopsy No.*	ITE/1000†
< 40	114	1	0.9	1	1	3.75
40–50	132	4	3	2	1	2.5
50–60	190	5	4	0	0	0.83
60–70	205	10	4.9	3	0	9.41
> 70	159	10	6.3	3	3	16.66
Total or mean	800	30	3.8	9	5	6.625

*TE = thrombo-embolic episodes.
†ITE/1000 = incidence of TE per 1000 months of observation.
From Ambrus J L: J Med 6(5):443, 1975 (with permission).

problems and were found to have nonneoplastic disease of the same organs for which neoplastic disease was studied. Statistical analysis revealed correlation with age. Table 9-2 summarizes age-related incidence of thromboembolism in all nonneoplastic patients. The ITE/1000 was 6.6. Table 9-3 shows that the ITE/1000 in patients with pancreatic carcinoma was 342. Table 9-4 shows that the ITE/1000 for pancreatitis was 8.3, and Table 9-5 indicates an ITE/1000 for gastrointestinal cancer of 119.7; Table 9-6, for lung cancer, 41.5; Table 9-7, for prostatic cancer, 3.0. Table 9-8 summarizes all data and shows that all cancer groups differ significantly from their controls, except for prostatic cancer.

In order to investigate possible causes of this phenomenon we studied the number of morphologically demonstrable cancer cells in the circulation. We succeeded in performing adequate studies in 253 patients. Table 9-9 shows a significant correlation between demonstration of circulating tumor cells and thromboembolic episodes.[8]

On the basis of these data, we have speculated that the majority of circulating tumor cells die off in the circulation (particularly since in many of these patients there was no sign of clinically appreciable metastasis in spite of the fact that circulating tumor cells were observed). These tumor cells then release thromboplastic factors and may initiate intravascular coagulation. The more circulating tumor cells there are and the more rapidly they disintegrate, the higher is the likelihood of the development of thromboembolic complications. We are currently studying the relationship between thromboemolic episodes, disseminated intravascular coagulation and various therapeutic modalities.

In order to elucidate the possible biochemical basis of thromboembolism and/or

TABLE 9-3. *Cancer of the Pancreas.*

Age	Total No. of cases	Clinical TE* No.	No. autopsies	TE by autopsy*	ITE/1000†
< 40	2	2	2	2	1500
40–50	3	0	2	0	0
50–60	7	0	4	0	0
60–70	9	2	7	5	100
> 70	7	3	4	2	110
Total or mean	28	7	19	9	342

*TE = thrombo-embolic episodes.
†ITE/1000 = incidence of TE per 1000 months of observation.
From Ambrus J L: J Med 6(5):443, 1975 (with permission).

TABLE 9-4. *Pancreatitis.*

Age	Total No. of cases	Clinical TE* No.	No. autopsies	ITE/1000†
< 40	2	0	0	0
40–50	3	0	0	0
50–60	1	0	0	0
60–70	2	1	0	41.5
> 70	0	0	0	0
Mean or total	8	1	0	8.3

*TE = thrombo-embolic episodes.
†ITE/1000 = incidence of TE per 1000 months of observation.
From Ambrus J L: J Med 6(5):443, 1975 (with permission).

TABLE 9-5. *Gastrointestinal Cancer*

Age	Total No. cases	Clinical TE No.*	%	No. autopsies	TE by autopsy* No.	%	ITE/100†
< 40	21	5	24	7	2	29	420.9
40–50	69	4	5.8	20	4	20	16.1
50–60	121	6	4.9	29	4	14	3.5
60–70	209	17	8.2	48	20	42	94.25
> 70	245	18	7.4	80	30	38	51.12
Total or mean	665	50	7.5	184	60	33	119.17

*TE = thrombo-embolic episodes.
†ITE/1000 = incidence of TE per 1000 months of observation.
From Ambrus J L: J Med 6(5):443, 1975 (with permission).

TABLE 9-6. *Lung Cancer*

Age	Total No. cases	Clinical TE* No.	%	No. autopsies	TE by autopsy* No.	%	ITE/1000†
< 40	9	0	0	5	2	4	55.5
40–50	33	6	18	18	8	44	68
50–60	113	10	8.9	40	8	20	36
60–70	145	9	6.2	47	8	17	12.5
> 70	62	3	4.8	26	10	38	35
Total or mean	362	28	4.2	136	36	24.6	41.4

*TE = thrombo-embolic episodes.
†ITE/1000 = incidence of TE per 1000 months of observation.
From Ambrus J L: J Med 6(5):443, 1975 (with permission).

TABLE 9-7. *Prostatic Cancer.*

Age	Total No. cases	Clinical TE* No.	%	No. autopsies	TE by autopsy* No.	ITE/1000†
< 40	0	0	0	0	0	0
40–50	6	0	0	2	2	0
50–60	25	2	8	6	3	9
60–70	62	7	11.3	6	1	4.5
> 70	78	3	3.8	6	1	1.5
Total or mean	171	12	4.6	20	7	3

*TE = thrombo-embolic episodes.
†ITE/1000 = incidence of TE per 1000 months of observation.
From Ambrus J L: J Med 6(5):443, 1975 (with permission).

TABLE 9-8. *Occurance of Thrombo-embolic Episodes by Site of Cancer: Expectations Calculated From Rates for RPMI Noncancer Series.*

Diagnosis	No. of patients	No. of thrombo-embolic episodes observed	expected	P
Ca. of stomach	155	38	12.0	< 0.01
Ca. of intestinal tract	399	51	31.1	< 0.01
Ca. of pancreas	28	16	2.9	< 0.01
Ca. of biliary system	29	7	2.4	< 0.01
Other and unclassified g-.i. Ca.	82	14	8.0	< 0.01
Ca. of lung	362	64	26.4	< 0.01
Ca. of prostate	171	19	13.0	N.S.
All sites	1226	209	95.8	< 0.01

From Ambrus J L: J Med 6(5):443, 1975 (with permission).

TABLE 9-9. *Relationship Between Presence of Tumor Cells in the Blood and Thrombo-embolic Episodes.*

	Tumor cells in blood Absent	Present	Total
Without thrombosis	146	107	253
With thrombosis	19	31	50
Total	165	138	303

$\chi^2 = 5.77$ $P < 0.05$

From Ambrus J L: J Med 6(5):443, 1975 (with permission).

TABLE 9-10. *Distribution of 100 Patients with Bronchogenic Carcinoma.*

Males	76
Females	24
	100
Resectable, limited disease	9
Non-resectable, limited disease	20
Metastatic non-resectable disease	71
	100
Squamous cell carcinoma	31
Glandular carcinoma	25
Oat cell carcinoma	19
Anaplastic carcinoma	18
Giant cell carcinoma	5
Bronchiolo-alveolar carcinoma	2
	100

Age range 39–78, mean 57.5 years.

From Brugarolas: J Med 4:96, 1973.

hemorrhage in cancer patients, we have studied 100 patients suffering from bronchogenic carcinoma. Table 9-10 shows distribution of the group according to history and histopathology. Only hematologic changes which differed significantly from the normal control patients will be discussed here.

TABLE 9-11. *Fibrinogen Levels in 100 Patients with Bronchogenic Carcinoma.*

Fibrinogen, mg%	Number of patients
> 500	69
400–500	24
200–400 (normal range)	7

Mean fibrinogen level 598 mg%. Median fibrinogen level 560 mg%.

From Brugarolas: J Med 4:96, 1973.

The most striking difference was an elevation of fibrinogen levels. All but 7 patients in the group had fibrinogen levels above the normal range. Table 9-11 summarizes the distribution of fibrinogen levels. It appears that the majority of patients (93 per cent) had fibrinogen in excess of 400 mg%.

Figure 9-1 shows the antiplasmin levels plotted against the fibrinogen levels. Also included in these data are a small group of patients who suffered from benign pulmonary lesions in addition to the lung cancer patients. Total antiplasmin levels are given which include both the alpha-1-antitrypsin-antiplasmin and the alpha-2-macroglobulin-antiplasmin levels. The graph actually shows a quotient of the total antiplasmin level divided

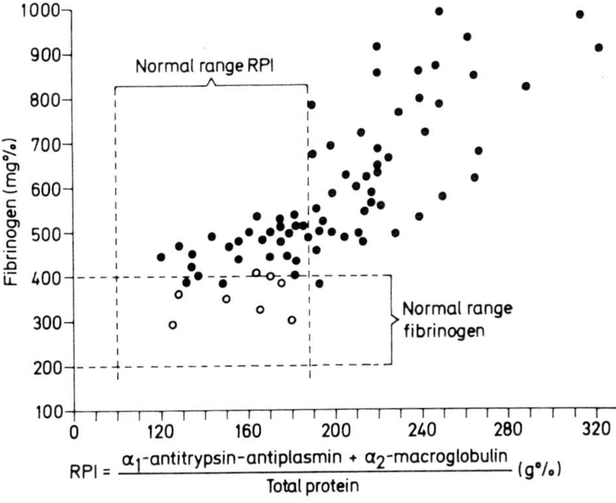

FIG. 9-1. Relationship between plasma fibrinogen levels and relative plasmin inhibitor levels (RPI) in patients with benign and malignant pulmonary lesions. ○ = Patients with benign pulmonary lesions; ● = patients with carcinoma of the lung. From Brugarolas, et al: Blood coagulation and fibrinolysis in patients with carcinoma of the lung. J Med 4:96–105, 1973 (with permission).

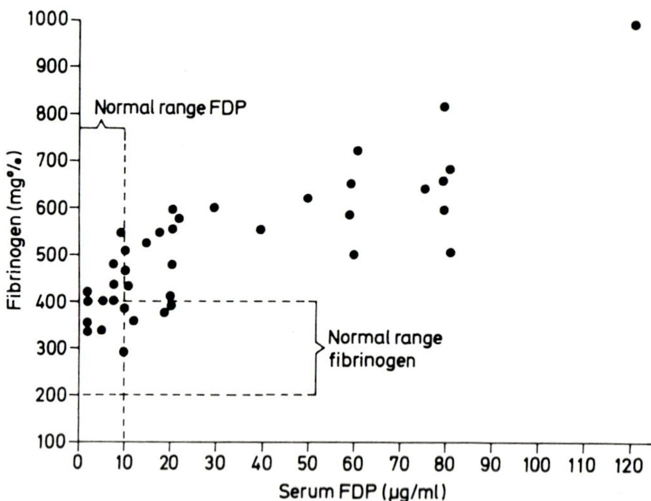

FIG. 9-2. Relationship between plasma fibrinogen and serum fibrinogenfibrin split product (FDP) levels in patients with bronchogenic carcinoma. From Brugarolas, et al: Blood coagulation and fibrinolysis in patients with carcinoma of the lung. J Med 4:96–105, 1973 (with permission).

by total protein level. This quotient was termed "relative plasmin inhibitor level" (RPI). It appears that almost all lung cancer patients had higher than normal antiplasmin levels, while almost all patients with benign pulmonary lesions fell into the normal range. There appears to be a linear relationship between fibrinogen level and antiplasmin level. Figure 9-2 plots the level of fibrinogen-fibrin split products (FDP) against fibrinogen levels. With few exceptions, FDP levels are high in lung cancer patients and these levels appear to be related to the increased fibrinogen levels.

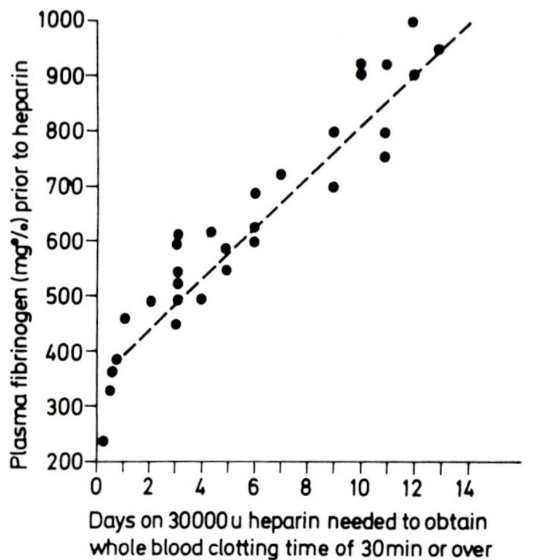

FIG. 9-3. Relationship between fibrinogen levels and time of continuous heparin infusion required for therapeutic heparinization in patients with bronchogenic carcinoma. From Brugarolas, et al: Blood coagulation and fibrinolysis in patients with carcinoma of the lung. J Med 4:96–105, 1973 (with permission).

In the same group of patients, relative clinical susceptibility to heparin was studied in a clinical test. Because of the apparent hypercoagulable state of these patients, heparin therapy appeared to be indicated. The patients were given a standard infusion of 30,000 IU of heparin every 24 hours intravenously. Lee-White coagulation time was taken periodically and the end point of the test was the time period when the clotting time reached 30 minutes or longer. The majority of these patients showed a certain clinical resistance to heparinization. A linear relationship was found between the relative resistance to heparin and the fibrinogen level as shown in Figure 9-3.

On the basis of these findings, the following hypothesis was established: In the tortuous, A-V anastomosis-rich, vasculature of

TABLE 9-12. *Platelet Aggregation Inhibitors in Stumptailed Monkeys.*

Agent	ED_{50}mg/kg	Duration
Prostaglandin E_1	0.005/min	7 min
5-oxo-1-cyclopentene-1 hepatonic acid	40	10 min
Dipyridamole (Persantin®, Ra 8)	20	4 hr
Ra 233	8	6 hr
VK 744	5	6 hr
Cyproheptadine (Periactin®)	1	6 hr
Bencyclan (Fludilat®)	15	5 hr
Pentoxifylline (Trental®)	24	4 hr
Promethazine (Phenergan®)	—	—

(Anesthesia: Sernylan® 2mg/kg i.m., Atropine 0.01mg/kg s.c., Nembutal® 10mg/kg i.v., Heparin 10mg/kg i.v.)

the tumors there is a certain degree of stasis and consequently hypoxia. This may result in relative resistance to radiation therapy. Increased permeability of the vasculature in the tumors and possibly rapid cell turnover rate results in release of thromboplastic enzymes into the circulation of the tumor. Thromboplastins, together with stasis, produce a local defibrination in the vascular bed. There is, also, however, an increased release of tissue activators of the fibrinolysin system. Ossowski et al,[9] Reich,[10] and Unkeless et al[11] have pointed out that neoplastic cells have higher plasminogen activator activity than normal cells. Fibrinolysis is probably responsible for keeping the microvasculature of these tumors open. Fibrinolysis results in increased FDP levels as measured in our studies. It is possible that FDP acts as a feedback control system in the liver increasing the synthesis of fibrinogen and also increasing the synthesis of antiplasmins which will result in a containment of the fibrinolytic process to the vasculature of the tumor.

If this hypothesis is correct, one would expect to find an increased fibrinogen turnover rate in this group of patients. In studies with ^{125}I-labeled fibrinogen we found[12] that in patients with neoplastic disease, fibrinogen turnover is accelerated in comparison with normal individuals. Experiments are also underway to study in isolated perfused liver preparations, whether various FDP fractions indeed influence the production and release of fibrinogen and antiplasmins by the liver.

Hypercoagulability and increased incidence of thromboembolism in cancer patients suggests that prevention by anticoagulants and platelet aggregation inhibitors should be considered, possibly together with therapy by fibrinolytic agents. We have developed a method to study in vivo platelet aggregation inhibitors in primates.[13] Comparative studies are summarized in Table 9-12. Chemical structures of some of the new compounds employed are shown in Figure 9-4. We have also established methods for the in vivo testing of fibrinolytic enzymes in experimental animals with the operative insertion of ^{125}I-labeled human fibrin clots into various blood vessels.[14-16] Figure 9-5 shows an experiment in which four clots were inserted into the femoral and jugular veins of a dog at various time intervals. At the time when treatment with a human urokinase-activated plasmin preparation was initiated, some of the clots were 3 days old, 2 days old, 1 day old and one-half hour old. During a 5-day infusion with a fibrinolytic enzyme preparation, all clots dissolved as shown by disappearance of radioactivity, except for the 3-day-old clot. This was sufficiently organized and endothelialized to prevent effective fibrinolysis. At the same time, radioactive peptides could be recovered from the urine, suggesting that some of the fibrin fragments from fibrinolysis are excreted via the kidneys.

Anticoagulants, platelet aggregation inhibitors and fibrinolytic enzymes may find a

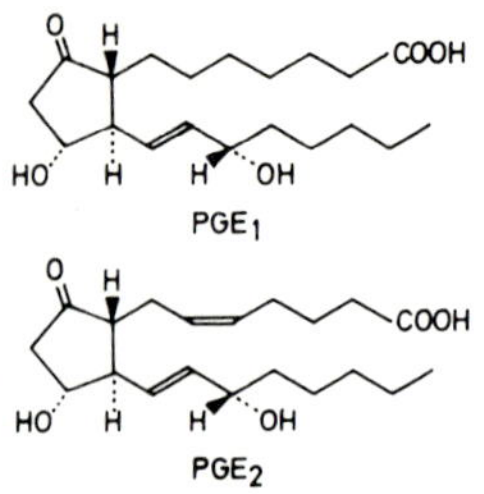

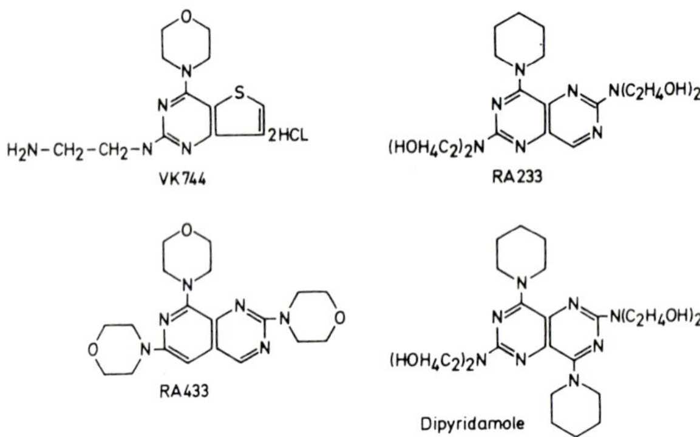

FIG. 9-4. Structural Formula of Prostaglandins E_1 (PGE_1), E_2 (PGE_2) and pyrimido = pyrimidine derivates VK 744, RA 233, RA 433 and dipyridamole (Ra, Persantin). From Ambrus JL, Ambrus CM: Blood coagulation in neoplastic disease, in Gastpar H (ed): Onkohamostaseologie. Stuttgart, FK Schattaver Verlag, 1976, pp 167–193, 1976 (with permission).

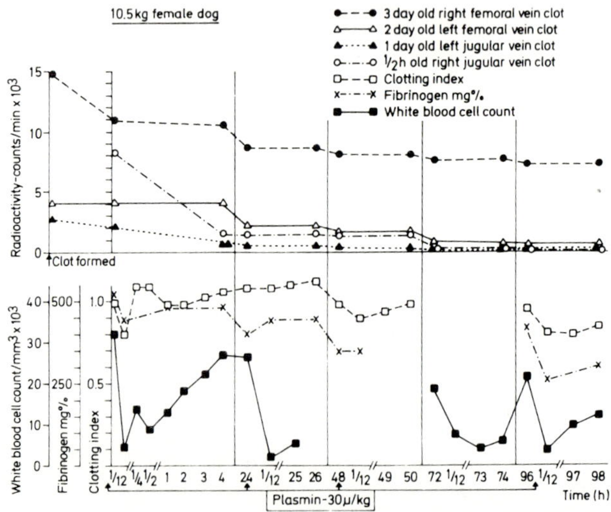

FIG. 9-5. Dissolution of radioactive clots of various ages in a dog treated with 30 RPMI u/Kg of plasmin. Changes in clotting index, fibrinogen and white blood cell count are also shown. From Ambrus JL, Ambrus CM: Blood coagulation in neoplastic disease, in Gastpar H (ed): Onkohamostaseologie. Stuttgart, F K Schattauer Vergal, pp 167–193, 1976 (with permission).

place in the prevention and treatment of thromboembolic complications of neoplastic disease. Some clinical experience is available from this institute.[17-20] The possible use of these agents in other aspects of this problem complex will be discussed later.

Metastasis

Table 9-13 summarizes the role of the blood coagulation, fibrinolysin and platelet systems in metastasis. Cohesive failure may result in the release of cancer cells into the blood stream and lymph. The role of proteolytic enzymes, fibrinolytic enzyme activators, and other related factors are not yet fully clarified. In preliminary studies we have found that cancer cells had generally greater thromboplastic activity than corresponding normal cells. This thromboplastic activity may contribute to the engulfment of metastatic cancer cells into fibrin networks. Platelets aggregate on the rough surface presented and clusters of several tumor cells, surrounded by aggregated platelets and fibrin, may develop. These masses are then arrested in the microcirculation. Tumor cells grow along fibrin fibers breaking through the capillary membranes and penetrating tissues. The newly developed tumors are rapidly vascularized with the aid of the tumor angiogenesis factors and in the resulting tortuous vascularity, defibrination and fibrinolysis develop as described above. High levels of FDP generated in the circulation of the tumor may contribute to the nutrition of tumor cells. In preliminary tissue culture experiments we have obtained some indication that certain fractions of FDP may act as nutrients and/or growth stimulants.

The role of blood coagulation in the settling of metastatic cells was studied in our laboratory with the aid of ^{32}P-labeled Ehrlich ascites cells. Figure 9-6 shows an experiment in which labeled ascites cells were injected into the jugular vein of mice and the circulating radioactivity was continuously recorded over the tail. Labeled, metastatic tumor cells disappeared within 15 minutes from the circulation. When the animals were autopsied immediately after the experiment and the various organs were assayed for radioactivity, most of the activity was found in the lung. In similar experiments in which the animals were fully heparinized prior to the injection of the tumor cells, circulating tumor cells were recorded for up to 7 hours after the original injection. If animals injected with tumor cells were sacrificed 3 weeks after the experiment, metastases were found almost exclusively in the lungs. On the other hand, metastases were found in most organs of heparinized animals. This suggests that anticoagulation helped the tumor cells to pass the capillary filter of the lungs.

TABLE 9-13. *Role of the Blood Coagulation, Fibrinolysin and Platelet Systems in Metastasis.*

1. *Release.* Proteolytic and fibrinolytic
↓ enzymes, "sub-lethal autolysis", cohesive failure (Ca, immune phenomena).
2. *Transport.* Microcirculatory factors,
↓ surface charge.
3. *Lodgement.* Surface charge, TTF,
↓ Tumor cell aggregates (minimum: 3-10 cells) formed with the aid of platelet aggregation and fibrin formation.
4. *Growth and Invasion.* Fibrin network effect TTF, TAF, fibrinolysis, FDP, nutritional factors.

TAF = Tumor angiogenesis factors
TTF = Tumor thromboplastic factors

Accordingly, one could justify the hypothesis that if tumor cells could be kept in the circulation for long periods of time, the majority would probably die off without establishing metastases. Preventing engulfment into a protective layer consisting of platelets undergoing viscous metamorphosis and eventually a fibrin clot, may well increase the ability of chemotherapeutic agents to penetrate the tumor cells. Thus, intravenous chemotherapy, together with "antimetastatic agents," may represent a new approach to the prevention of metastasis formation.

In an earlier report, Gastpar, Ambrus and Thurber[21] have shown that platelet aggregation inhibitors can prolong the circulation lifespan of labeled tumor cells. Gastpar[22] showed that these agents can prevent pulmonary em-

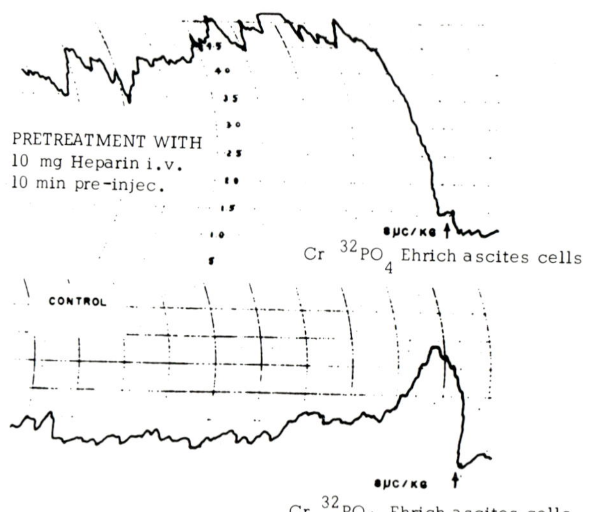

FIG. 9-6 Disappearence of labelled Ehrlich ascites tumor cells from the circulation of mice after i.v. injection. Comparison of a control and a heparinized animal.

bolism and death produced by intravenous injection of certain cancer cells to experimental animals. In current clinical experiments,[23] platelet aggregation inhibitors are used in connection with potentially curative cancer surgery in order to prevent recurrence related to the mobilization of cancer cells into the circulation during surgery.

Agostino et al[24-32] and others[33-62] reported that anticoagulants (both heparin and vitamin K antagonists) and fibrinolytic enzymes can alter metastatic patterns in experimental and clinical situations.

Neoplastic Transformation, Growth and Chemotherapy of Neoplasms

Reich and associates[9-11] reported that neoplastic transformation results in sharp increase of plasminogen activator activity in cell cultures. O'Meara[63-66] indicated increased thromboplastin-like activity in cancer cells. Our studies mentioned above confirm these findings and suggest that consecutive FDP formation may act as nutrient and/or growth stimulator to cancer cells. Inhibition of the blood coagulation-fibrinolysis process in neoplasms may interfere with their invasive capacity.

Laki et al[67,68] pointed out that the fibrin network provides the matrix into which new capillaries grow and along which settled metastatic cancer cells prefer to grow. Agents which inhibit fibrin stabilization interfere with the growth of experimental neoplasms.

Wilkins[69] and others suggested that heparin may act on metastases in part through its ability to impart negative surface charge to circulating tumor cells. Regelson[70] pointed out that heparin and heparinoids may act on tumors in part through their antimitotic activity. Several investigators uncovered suggestions for a direct anti-tumor effect of coumarin derivatives, independent from their anti coagulant activity.[59,71-73]

In this institute, Elias et al[74-76] found that heparinization is synergistic with chemotherapy in cancer patients. Beneficial effects were also reported by Ludwig.[77] Similar results were reported with coumarin derivatives by Kirsch et al[73] and Hilgard et al[78] who found significant potentiation of Bleomycin under experimental conditions. In a clinical trial with 128 patients[53,54] warfarin, as an adjuvant to cancer therapy, significantly increased 2-year survival.

Fibrinolytic therapy probably also involves as yet unclarified mechanisms of action. Plasmin was found to labilize lysosomal hydrolases in animal tumors and to enhance the effect of cytotoxic agents.[79] Human plasmin was found to be cytotoxic to cancer cells in vitro.[80] Several small-scale clinical studies reported encouraging results.[32,60,81]

Streptokinase, a plasminogen activator, and brinase, a proteolytic enzyme of fungal origin, produced complement dependent cytotoxicity[51] and enhanced delayed hypersensitivity.[82] It also interacted with the activation of the complement system.[83]

Preventing the development of fibrin coat on circulating tumor cells, around early clumps of tumor cells growing in tissue and in the vasculature of the tumor or dissolving existing fibrin networks may increase penetration of chemotherapeutic agents into cancer cells. Similarly, prevention of platelet aggregation and development of viscous metamorphosis may eliminate a further barrier to the prevention of certain chemotherapeutic agents.

Further basic and clinical research is required to develop these concepts and bring them to the stage of practical application.

References

1. Ambrus J L, Ambrus C M, Mink I B, Pickren J W: Causes of death in cancer patients. J Med 6:61–64, 1975
2. Leavey R A, Kahn S B, Brodsky I: Disseminated intravascular coagulation—A complication of chemotherapy in acute myelomonocytic leukemia. Cancer 26:142–145, 1970
3. Brodsky I, Conroy T F: Effects of chemotherapy on hemostasis, in Brodsky I, Kahn S B (eds): Cancer Chemotherapy, vol. II. New York, Grune & Stratton, 1972, pp 85–92
4. Brodsky I, Kahn S B, Ross E M, Petkov G: Platelet and fibrinogen kinetics in the chronic myeloproliferative disorders. Cancer 30:1444–1450, 1972
5. Brodsky I, Kahn S B, Vash B, et al: Fibrinogen survival with (^{75}Se) selenomethionone during L-asparaginase therapy. Br J Haem 20:477, 1971
6. Brodsky I, Siegel N H, Kahn S B, et al: Simultaneous fibrinogen and platelet survival with (^{75}Se) selenomethionine in man. Br J Haem 18:347, 1970
7. Bettigole R E, Himelstein E S, Oettgen H F, Clifford G O: Hypofibrinogenemia due to L-asparaginase: Studies of fibrinogen survival using autologous ^{131}-I fibrinogen. Blood 35:195, 1970
8. Ambrus J L, Ambrus C M, Pickren J W, et al: Hematologic changes and thromboembolic complications in neoplastic disease and their relationship to metastasis. J Med 6:433–458, 1975
9. Ossowski L, Unkeless J C, Tobia A, et al: An enzymatic function associated with transformation of fibroblast cultures transformed by DNA and RNA tumor viruses. J Exp Med 137:112–126, 1973
10. Reich E: Tumor associated fibrinolysis. Fed Proc 32:2174–2175, 1973
11. Unkeless J C, Tobia A, Ossowski J P, et al: An enzymatic function associated with transformation of fibroblasts by oncogenic viruses I. Chick embryo fibroblast cultures transformed by avian RNA tumor viruses. J Med 137:85–111, 1973
12. Lyman G H, Bettigole R E, Robson E, et al: Fibrinogen kinetics in patients with neoplastic disease. Cancer 41(3):113–122, 1978
13. Ambrus J L, Ambrus C M, Gastpar H, et al: Study of platelet aggregation in vivo I. Effect of bencyclan. J Med 7(6):439-447, 1976
14. Ambrus J L, Back N, Mihalyi E, Ambrus C M: Quantitative method for the in vivo testing of fibrinolytic agents: Effect of intravenous trypsin on radioactive thrombi and emboli. Circulation Res 4(4):430–443, 1956
15. Back N, Ambrus J L, Goldstein S, Harrisson J W E: In vivo fibrinolytic activity and pharmacology of various plasmin (fibrinolysin) preparations. Circulation Res 4(4):440–443, 1956
16. Back N, Ambrus J L, Simpson C L, Shulman S: Study on the effect of streptokinase-activated plasmin (fibrinolysin) on clots in various stages of organization. J Clin Invest 37(6):864–871, 1958
17. Ambrus J L, Ambrus C M, Back N, et al: Clinical and experimental studies on fibrinolytic enzymes. Ann N Y Acad Sci 68(1):97–136, 1957
18. Sokal J E, Ambrus J L, Ambrus C M: Treatment of thrombosis with fibrinolysis (plasmin). JAMA 168(10):1314-1323, 1958
19. Ambrus J L, Ambrus C M, Sokal J E, et al: Clinical pharmacology of various types of fi-

brinolytic enzyme preparations. Am J Cardiol 6(2):462–475, 1960

20. Lippschutz E J, Ambrus J L, Ambrus C M, et al: Controlled study of the treatment of coronary occlusion with urokinase-activated human plasmin. Am J Cardiol 16(1):93–98, 1965
21. Gastpar H, Ambrus J L, Thurber L E: Study of platelet aggregation in vivo II: Effect of bencyclan on circulating metastatic tumor cells. J Med 8(1):53056, 1977
22. Gastpar H: Die hemmung der "cancer cell stickiness" durch Bencyclanhydrogen fumarat. Fortschr Med 33:1232, 1973
23. Gastpar H: Unpublished report of current studies, 1977
24. Cliffton E E, Grossi C E: Effect of human plasmin on tonic effect and growth of blood-borne metastasis of Brown-Pearce carcinoma and VX_2 carcinoma of the rabbit. Cancer 9:1147, 1956
25. Grossi C E, Agostino D, Cliffton E E: The effect of human fibrinolysin on pulmonary metastases of Walker 256 carcinosarcoma. Cancer Res 20:605, 1960
26. Grossi C E, Agostino D, Melamed E, Cliffton E E: Survival of Walker 256 carcinosarcoma cells in the blood: Effect of human fibrinolysin. Cancer 14:957–969, 1969
27. Agostino D, Grossi C E, Cliffton E E: Effect of heparin on the circulating Walker 256 carcinoma cells. J Med Cancer Inst 27:17–24, 1961
28. Agostino D, Cliffton E E: Anticoagulants and the development of pulmonary metastasis. Arch Surg 84:87–91, 1962
29. Agostino D, Cliffton E E: Trauma as a cause of localization of blood-borne metastases. Ann Surg 161:970102, 1965
30. Agostino D, Cliffton E E, Girolami A: Effects of prolonged coumadin treatment on production of pulmonary metastases in the rat. Cancer 19:284, 1966
31. Agostino D, Cliffton E E: Fibrinogen levels and pulmonary metastases in rats. (effect of tissue damage). Arch Path 87:141–145, 1969
32. Cliffton E E, Grossi C E: The rationale by anticoagulants on the treatment of cancer. J Med 5(1-3):107, 1974
33. Ryan J J, Ketchman A S, Wexler H: Warfarin treatment of mice bearing autochthonous tumors: Effect on spontaneous metastases. Science 162:1493, 1968
34. Ryan J J, Ketcham A S, Wexler H: Reduced incidence of spontaneous metastases with long-term coumadin therapy. Ann Surg 168:163–168, 1968
35. Ryan J J, Ketcham A S, Wexler H: Warfarin therapy as an adjunct to the surgical treatment of malignant tumors in mice. Cancer Res 29:2191–2194, 1969
36. Miller R C, Ketcham A S: The effect of heparin and warfarin on primary and metastatic tumors. J Med 5(1-3):23, 1974
37. Michaels L: Cancer incidence and mortality in patients having anticoagulant therapy. Lancet 2:832–835, 1964
38. Michaels L: The incidence and course of cancer in patients receiving anticoagulant therapy. Retrospective and prospective studies. J Med 5:98, 1974
39. Kudrjashor B A, Kalishevskaya T M, Kolomina S M: Blood and coagulating system and malignant tumors. Nature 222:548–550, 1969
40. Boeryd B: Action of heparin and plasminogen inhibitor (EACA) on metastatic spread in an siologous system. Acta Pathol et Microbiol Scand 65:395–404, 1965
41. Boeryd B: Effect of heparin and plasminogen inhibitor (EACA) in brief and prolonged treatment on intravenously injected tumour cells. Acta Pathol et Microbiol Scand 68:347–354, 1966
42. Hagmar B: Effect of heparin, E-aminocaproic acid and coumarin on tumor growth and spontaneous metastasis formation. Path Europ 3:622–630, 1968
43. Hagmar B: Effect of heparin, coumarin and E-aminocaproic acid (EACA) on spontaneous metastasis formation. Path Europ 4:283–292, 1969
44. Hagmar B, Boeryd B: Distribution of intravenously induced metastases in heparin and coumarin-treated mice. Path Europ 4:103–111, 1969
45. Hagmar B, Norrby K: Evidence for effects of heparin on cell surfaces influencing experimental metastases. Int J Cancer 5:72–84, 1970
46. Hagmar B: Tumour growth and spontaneous metastasis spread in two syngeneic systems. Acta Pathol et Microbiol Scand 78:131–142, 1970
47. Hagmar B: Experimental tumour metastases and blood coagulability (review). Acta Pathol et Microbiol Scand 78:1–38 (suppl 211), 1970
48. Hagmar B: Defibrination and metastasis formation: Effects of arvin on experimental metastases in mice. Europ J Cancer 8:17–28, 1972
49. Boeryd B, Hagmar B: Disappearance of circulation tumour cells in mice treated with heparin, coumarin and EACA. Acta Pathol et Microbiol Scand 80:303–307, 1972
50. Thornes R D, Edlow D W, Wood S: Inhibition of locomotion of cancer cells in vitro by anticoagulation therapy. John Hopkins Med J 123:305–316, 1968
51. Thornes R D, Deasy P F, Carrall R, et al: The

use of the proteolytic enzyme brinase to produce autocytotoxicity in patients with acute leukemia and its possible role in immunotherapy. Cancer Res 32:280–284, 1972
52. Thornes R D: Anticoagulant therapy in patients with cancer. J Ir Med Assoc 62:426, 1969
53. Thornes R D: Warfarin as maintenance therapy for cancer. J Ir Coll Physicians Surg 2:41, 1972
54. Thornes R D: Fibrin and cancer. Br Med J 1:110, 1972
55. Wood S: Experimental studies on the spread of cancer, with special reference to fibrinolytic agents and anticoagulants. J Med 5:7, 1974
56. Retik A B, Arons M S, Ketcham A S, Mantel N: The effect of heparin on primary tumors and metastases. J Surg Res 2:49, 1962
57. Suemasu K, Ishikawa S: Inhibitive effect of heparin and dextran sulfate on experimental pulmonary metastases. Gann 61:125, 1970
58. Kiricuta I, Todorutiu C, Muresian T, Risca R: Prophylaxis of metastases formation by unspecific immunologic stimulation associated with heparin therapy. Cancer 31:1392, 1973
59. Brown J M: A study of the mechanism by which anticoagulation with warfarin inhibits blood-borne metastases. Cancer Res 33:1217, 1973
60. Larsen V B, Mogensen B, Amris C J, Storm O: Fibrinolytic enzyme in the treatment of patients with cancer. Dan Med Bull 11:137, 1964
61. Clery A P, Hogan B L, Holland P D J, et al: Early experience in a controlled clinical trial using streptokinase induced fibrinolysis during resections for colon and rectal carcinomas in an attempt to prevent haematogenous metastasis. J Ir Coll Physicians Surg 1:91, 1972
62. Gasic G, Gasic T, Galanti N, et al: Platelet tumor-cell interactions in mice. The role of platelets in the spread of malignant disease. Int J Cancer 11:704, 1973
63. O'Meara R A Q: Coagulative properties of cancers. Ir J Med Sci 394:474–479, 1958
64. O'Meara R A Q: The growth pattern in carcinomas. Arch de Vecchi 31:365–384, 1960
65. O'Meara R A Q, Jackson R D: Cytological observations on carcinoma. Ir J Med Sci 391:327–328, 1958
66. O'Meara R A Q, Thornes R D: Some properties of the cancer coagulative factor. Ir J Med Sci 423:106–112, 1961
67. Laki K: Fibrinogen and metastases. J Med 5:32–37, 1974
68. Yancey S T, Laki K: Transglutaminase and tumor growth. Ann NY Acad Sci 202:344–348, 1972
69. Wilkins D J: Interaction of charged colloids with the RES. Advanc Exp Med Biol 1:25, 1967
70. Regelson W: The antimitotic activity of polyanions: heparin and heparinoids. J Med 5:50, 1974
71. Ryan J J, Ketcham A S, Wexler H: Warfarin treatment of mice bearing autochthonous tumors: Effect on spontaneous metastases. Science 162:1493, 1968
72. Lisnell A, Mellgren J: Effect of heparin, protanune dicoumarol, streptokinase and epsilon-amino-M-caproic acid on the growth of human cells in vitro. Acta Pathol Microbiol Scand 57:145, 1963
73. Kirsch W M, Schulz D, van Buskirk J J, Young H E: Effects of sodium warfarin and other carcinostatic agents on malignant cells: A study of drug synergy. J Med 5:69, 1974
74. Elias, Elias G, Sepulveda F, Mink I B: Increasing the efficiency of cancer chemotherapy with heparin: Clinical study. J Surg Oncol 5:189–193, 1973
76. Brugarolas A, Elias E G: Incidence of hyperfibrinogenemia in 1961 patients with cancer. J Surg Oncol 5:359–463, 1973
77. Ludwig H: Antikoagulation beim fortgeschrittenen carcinom. Gynakologe 7:1, 1974
78. Hilgard P, Schulte H, Wetzig G, et al: Oral anticoagulation in the treatment of a spontaneously metastasising murine tumor (3LL). Br J Cancer 35(1):78–86, 1977
79. Shimoyama H, Niitani H, Taniguchi T, et al: The role of lysosomes in cancer chemotherapy. III. Influence of plasmin on the cytocidal effect of mitomycin-C. Gann 60:33, 1969
80. Thornes R D, Martin W T: The cytopathic effect of fibrinolytic agents and human placental fractions on Hela cells. Ir J Med Sci 431:487, 1961
81. Cliffton E E: Fibrinolytic therapy for thromboembolic disease. Principles and practice. J La State Med Soc 118:309, 1966
82. Thornes R D, Smith H, Browne D, Holland P D J: B C G plus protease in malignant melanoma. Lancet 1:1386, 1973
83. Brown D L: Complement and coagulation. Br J Haem 30:377, 1975

LUTHER W. BRADY

10
Multi-Modality Therapy

The original approach to cancer diagnosis and treatment is undergoing a quiet revolution based on a combination of quantitative laboratory measurements, computer technology, mathematical analysis, the advent of new chemotherapeutic combinations and the application of these data in combined modality treatment programs. The results will be a new level of precision in accomplishment of diagnosis, tumor localization and specific patient treatment. In part, these results have already begun to appear, although followup times are still short.

Various research groups have been concerned with each of the aspects of this revolution. The development of mathematical models describing the distribution of chemotherapeutic drugs has evolved so that the concentration of the drug can be predicted at the site of action, allowing for manipulation of the concentration to improve results and diminish toxicity. The inclusion of physiologic information in the overall patient evaluation allows for individual physiologic differences to be taken into account in the treatment. The linkage of such models to laboratory and patient data allows for a more rapid integration of these concepts into active ongoing clinical trials. The organization of decision procedures based on this quantitative base and the statistical evaluation of the results, combined with long-term followup, allows for adequate evaluation of the efficacy of each of the combinations of treatment.

These approaches are of practical and significant importance in deriving the best results from what we have learned through research, so that they may be applied to the treatment of the individual patient.

Four major approaches have been developed, and are aimed at increased quantification and precision in diagnosis and treatment programs in cancer:

1. Mathematical models can describe the proliferation of cancer cells and normal cells. These models are designed to identify biological differences in cell behavior which can be used to predict how certain chemotherapeutic agents act and to improve the strategies for their administration in conjunction with other treatment programs. Wrba presents a schematic representation of the relationship between tumor size and cell number on the one hand, and the stage of development of the illness on the other. (Fig. 10-1)[1] Based on this presentation, improvement in local therapy is a significant and important concept in reduction of the tumor cell bur-

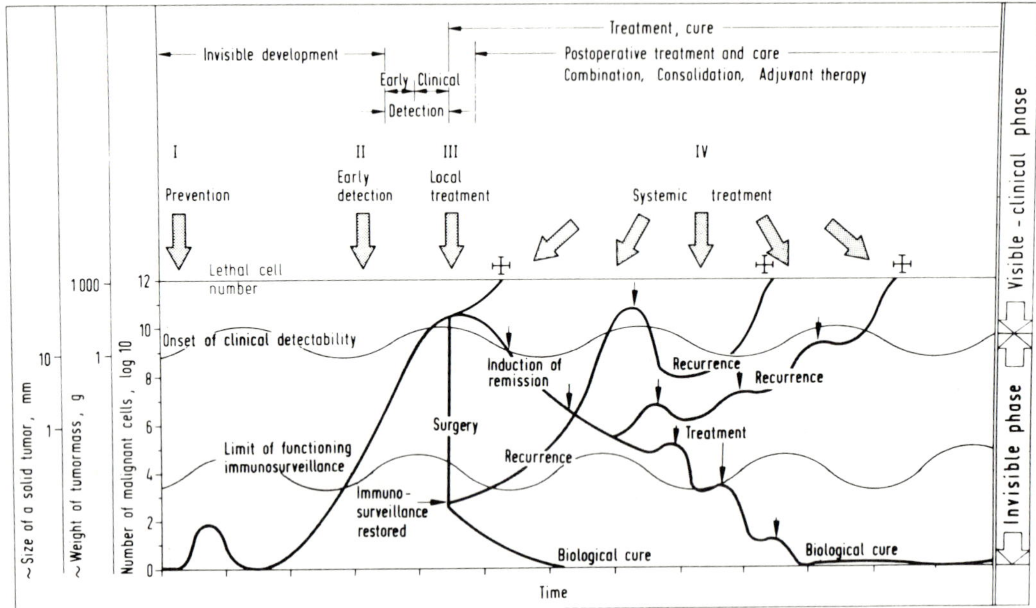

FIG. 10-1. Schematic representation of the relationship between tumor size and cell number on the one hand and the stage of development of the illness on the other. From Wrba H: Main issues in oncology (editorial). Oncology 33(3):103, 1976 (with permission). Editorial, Vol. 33, No. 3, 1976.

den. Involved within this is an attempt to determine the proliferation kinetics of the primary tumor under consideration. It is obvious from Wrba's presentation that local treatment, whether by surgery or by radiation therapy, has a major and dramatic impact upon the reduction of tumor cell burden. The introduction of subsequent treatment regimens in the patient's treatment program has a greater potential for effect when the tumor cell burden is at its lowest level. The data from Whitmore et al[2] as well as Shabal et al[3] suggests that radiation and chemotherapy have their effect by reduction of tumor cell burden by several logs. Therefore, the sequential implementation of each of these treatment programs is critically important to achieve the maximum potential for cure. It has been suggested by Pilch that immunotherapy is most effective when applied at a point where the tumor cell burden consists of 10^6 cells or less. The sensitivity of the treatment program, therefore, indicates that sequential application of treatment mechanisms is of critical importance in maximizing the potential for control of the tumor. The objectives of the treatment programs relate to the biological fate of most patients and the fact that the critical period follows the first specific treatment, after the attempted curative surgical operation, radiotherapy or after the first induction of a remission using the chemotherapeutic compounds. It becomes imperative to gain valid data in order to decide the fateful question of quality and intensity of necessary post-treatment programs and rehabilitation specifically suited to each patient. The analysis suggested by Wrba indicates that the tumor quantitatively is specifically related to its particular response to each therapeutic regimen. Therefore, the appropriate sequential introduction to treatment programs may prove to be the most effective means of treatment when these factors are considered in the overall management of the patient.

2. Mathematical models of drug distribution have evolved that accurately reflect the exposure of cells and tissues to particular

chemotherapeutic agents, thereby allowing for maximum utilization of all treatment techniques.

3. The statistical analysis of patients' specific risk factors, to improve our ability to choose among alternatives to treatment, now plays a major part of the decision-making process relative to cancer management.
4. The analysis of data related to the functions and activities of cells of the immune system allows for more accurate characterization of the biological behavior of tumors.

The implementation of combined programs of management using chemotherapy and radiation therapy, radiation and surgery or chemotherapy, radiation therapy and surgery requires a broad basic understanding of the biologic effects of each of the treatment programs being carried out. Into this understanding must be interjected the influence of the factors relative to the radiation therapy, such as fractionation, protraction, dose rate and total dose in the biologic effects as well as problems of hypoxia. Also to be evaluated is surgery under the influence of the surgical management and its impact upon the dramatic reduction in tumor cell burden. The basic understanding of the chemotherapeutic response and its timing when the tumor cell burden is at its lowest level must be evaluated, as well as factors of administration of the chemotherapeutic agents including the manner and mechanism of delivery. Upon this background of basic information can be developed the evaluation of interaction of these various treatment programs.

The chemotherapeutic agents currently being employed in the treatment of cancer need further study relative to their effect on the repair of radiation damage, the reoxygenation of tumor cell systems, the redistribution of cells about the cell cycle and the repopulation of normal tissues. As the planning and implementation of cancer chemotherapy in combination with radiation is strewn with complexities and limitations as well as strong potential, this rapidly developing field requires the urgent attention of all oncologists in both clinical and laboratory investigations. This would result in optimal advantage for the cancer patient for the use of these combined modalities.

TABLE 10-1. *Causes of Treatment Failure in Cancer Management*

1. Disease status—stage, histology, etc.
2. Tumor cell burden at the time of initiation of treatment
3. Sanctuary sites
   a. anatomical
   b. physiologic
   c. iatrogenic
   d. traumatic
4. Ineffectively administered treatment program
   a. surgery
   b. radiation therapy
   c. chemotherapy
   d. immunotherapy
5. Inappropriate combination of treatment modalities
6. Non-responsiveness to treatment
   a. radiosensitivity
   b. chemosensitivity

The disappointing results occur because of failure to control the tumor in the primary site, the regional lymph nodes, the distant visceral sites or a combination of these various compartments. Table 10-1 illustrates the potential causes of treatment failure in cancer management. These include the disease status, the tumor cell burden at the time of the initiation of each treatment program, the potential relative to sanctuary sites as well as factors related to the manner in which the treatment programs are carried out. Chemotherapeutic manipulation may be used so as to sensitize tumor cells in the primary region to radiation, or in the hope of controlling subclinical metastases in those tumors where such dissemination carries a high probability. Table 10-2 presents the area of greatest response for the various treatment techniques.

Radiation Therapy and Surgery

The application of the two most important modalities of cancer therapy, surgery and radiotherapy, has not produced a substantial im-

TABLE 10-2. *Influence of Treatment on Tumor Control*

	Local (T)	Regional (N)	Distant (M)
Surgery	+	+	—
Radiation therapy	+	+	—
Chemotherapy			
Alone	±(variable)	±(variable)	+
Postsurgery	−	±(variable)	+
Postradiation	−	±(variable)	+
Immunotherapy	±	±	±

provement in the results of cancer treatment in the last decade. Part of this has resulted from the failure to analyze the reasons for local and regional failure, as well as the potential for disseminated failure. Theoretical speculations, as well as experimental studies in some clinical trials, have yielded sufficient information suggesting that combined therapy could improve not only the results obtained by a single modality of therapy, but also would result in preservation of function and cosmesis. The failure to demonstrate the real value of the combination of surgery and radiation therapy is probably related to the indescriminate application to every patient, including possibly inappropriate groups of patients in the treatment program. Patients in whom the disease was too advanced locally and regionally are not appropriate in all cases for combined surgery and radiation therapy. Inadequate application of the techniques and treatment also would contribute to inappropriate utilization.

Surgery will fail in the control of a malignant tumor because of the following factors:

1. There is tumor at the resected margins.
2. There is subclinical spread of tumor beyond the operative field in lymphatic, vascular or perineural structures.
3. There are lymph node metastases beyond the operative field where an end-block dissection is not possible.
4. There is seeding locally or into the blood stream, produced at the time of the surgical program.

The failure of radiation therapy when used alone is related to the following factors:

1. Tumors with too large a tumor cell burden may make tumor eradication impossible.
2. Inadequate volume being irradiated for the true extent of the tumor may give rise to failure.
3. There are hypoxic subpopulations of tumor cells unresponsive to the radiation injury.
4. There may be inhomogeneity in the dose distribution within the tumor volume, preventing maximization of the potential for control.
5. Specific cell types may not respond to the radiation event.
6. The dose needed to sterilize the tumor may be limited by the tolerance of the surrounding normal tissues.

In order that improvement in tumor control may be achieved, attention should be given to the integrated therapeutic action of surgery to control the massive central tumor, and radiation therapy to eradicate the residual disease at the periphery of the tumor and in the regional node distribution.

The rationale for preoperative radiation therapy relates to: (1) the potential for eradication of subclinical disease beyond the margins of surgical resection, thus diminishing tumor implantation by decreasing the number of viable cells within the operative field, (2) sterilization of lymph node metastases outside the operative field to increase the possibility of resectability and (3) to decrease the potential for dissemination of tumor cells that might lead to distant metastatic disease.

Experimental data suggests that preoperative irradiation may be more effective than postoperative irradiation. This is related to the potential to displace the tumor cells outside of the operative field that were not irradiated postoperatively, and the fact that surgical trauma may interfere with the vascular supply of the tissues, thereby rendering the residual tumor cells hypoxic.

The main disadvantages for preoperative irradiation is that it interferes with normal healing of the tissues. Such interference, however, is negligible when the radiation dosages are 5000 rads in 5 weeks or less.

The rationale for postoperative irradiation relates to the fact that it is possible to treat the known residual, unresected tumor by destroying subclinical foci of tumor cells following the surgical procedure, by eradication of new disease in adjacent areas by sterilization of the subclinical foci of cancer (including lymph node metastases), and the deliverance at higher dosages than can be achieved by preoperative irradiation with the higher dose being directed to the area of high risk or known residual disease.

The potential disadvantages for postoperative irradiation are related to the delay imposed on the initiation of radiation therapy until healing of the wound is completed. In addition, theoretical and experimental evidence suggests that the radiation effect may be impaired by changes produced in the tumor bed by the surgical act.

The combination of surgery and radiation therapy has demonstrated significant and important advances in the local and regional control in breast cancer, soft tissue sarcomas, in various anatomical cancers in the head and neck, urinary bladder cancer, rectal cancer, lung cancer, testicular tumors, kidney tumors and carcinomas of the endometrium and uterine cervix.

The main combination of surgery and radiation therapy are related to (1) preoperative, postoperative or intraoperative radiation therapy, (2) surgery or irradiation alone for the primary, (3) irradiation or surgery for the lymph node metastases or (4) less than conventional surgery followed by irradiation for residual subclinical disease.

The indications for combined surgery and radiation therapy for the primary are: (1) those tumors where low cure rates by either surgery or irradiation alone are achieved, (2) anaplastic tumors or tumors with a high tendency toward vascular invasion, (3) where there is a high percentage of local-regional failure by either modality, (4) where residual tumor after either surgery or irradiation alone is of great probability, (5) where high morbidity or poor functional results occur after surgery or radiation or (6) where the degree of radiation therapy or surgery can be diminished to preserve cosmesis or function.

Combined surgery and radiation therapy are indicated in the treatment of lymph node metastasis where more than one node is present, where the node involving the tumor is greater than 2 cm in size, where there is a high risk of subclinical disease within the lymph nodes or where the lymph nodes are inaccessible to the combined treatment programs.

The area of the addition of chemotherapy to combined surgery and radiation therapy needs to be investigated in depth. By the combination of all treatment techniques, it may be possible to diminish the radiation dose or the extent of surgery, and thereby preserve function and cosmesis. Chemotherapy has a high probability for treating the distant subclinical disease uninfluenced by surgery or radiation therapy. The addition of chemotherapy to the treatment regimens is a reasonable area for investigation that could be immediately developed. A variety of tumors might benefit from this integrated, sequential, multimodal treatment program. These include cancers of the head and neck, carcinoma of the rectosigmoid, carcinoma of the urinary bladder and kidney and soft tissue sarcomas where the distant metastatic component is a significant and important part of the disease process.

Combined Radiation Therapy and Chemotherapy

The success of cancer chemotherapy in palliation, remission and potential cure of certain hematologic and other malignancies has led to the rapid introduction of anticancer chemotherapeutic agents into the treatment of a wide spectrum of malignancies, including

TABLE 10-3. *Techniques to Modify Radiosensitivity*

A. Increased yield of irreversible radiochemical lesions
   1. Oxygen
   2. Nitrous oxide, organic nitroxides
   3. Metranidazole (Flagyl), nitrofurans, RO-51-0582
   4. High LET particulate radiations
B. Increased intrinsic sensitivity of target DNA
   1. Halogenated pyrimidine analogues (BUdR, BCdR, IUdR)
   2. Possible potentiation of BCdR by tetrahydrouridine
   3. Purine starvation
C. Inhibition of repair
   1. Hyperthermia
   2. Chemical inhibition of single-strand break repair (Actinomycin-D)
   3. High LET particulate radiations
D. Partial synchronization in cycle-dependent sensitive states
   1. Fractionated radiotherapy timed to mitotic delay
   2. Colchinine, *Vinca* alkaloids, mitotic spindle poisons
E. Differential radioprotection of normal tissues

those primarily treated by radiotherapy. This practice has developed because of disappointing results with the use of a single modality in terms of local and regional control, as well as a large number of failures which occurred because of distant metastases.

Those chemotherapeutic agents currently being employed in the treatment of neoplastic disease need further study relative to their effect on the various mechanisms of radiation injury. Much research needs to be pursued in the planning and implementation of combined chemotherapy and radiation treatment programs because of the complexities and limitations of such combinations.

Chemotherapeutic manipulation may be used so as to sensitize tumor cells in the primary region to radiation, or in the hope of controlling subclinical metastases in those tumors where such dissemination is of high probability. Table 10-3 defines the techniques to modify radiation sensitivity.

The inability to control the tumor in the primary site remains a significant factor in treatment failure. Depending upon the primary site and histology, local failure of control by surgery and/or radiation therapy is a significant problem in many tumor sites. There appears to be three major approaches to combination chemotherapy and radiation therapy: (1) augmentation of local and regional radiation effects, (2) control of subclinical metastases by chemotherapy and (3) the use of radiation to sterilize sanctuary sites or bulky disease in primarily chemotherapeutically treated patients. The success of combined treatment using radiation and chemotherapy in the past has fallen primarily into the second and third groups. Radiation therapy and chemotherapy can augment each other for the control of advanced disease in the local (T) or regional (N) compartment and in a supplementary or complementary manner for subclinical metastases (metastatic (M) compartment).

A number of chemotherapeutic agents have been identified which are active in each of the various tumor sites. Essentially all prior or ongoing clinical trials that have combined radiation therapy and chemotherapy began with agents which were known to be active against the tumor being studied. Only a few of the roughly 25 active drugs, however, have been tested for their potential for interaction with radiation effects. A large number of combined radiotherapeutic-chemotherapeutic trials are underway in a wide range of solid tumors. At the moment, however, the number of such trials is significantly less than those involving other combined treatment modalities, such as multiple drug combinations. Certain significant advances have been recorded with adjuvant chemotherapy and this makes it urgent that these kinds of studies be rapidly expanded.

The effects of combined radiation therapy-chemotherapy can be described as separate, additive, or interactive (Table 10-4). The interaction of radiation and chemotherapy may occur at the cellular level, where the two major effects of either strict additivity or of interaction with enhanced killing or, perhaps, decreased killing could occur. Thus, various agents may cause additive or enhanced radiation damage, while others may actually cause decreased damage. Great skill, therefore, is needed in predicting whether a combined treatment will indeed lead to an enhanced therapeutic ratio. This requires extensive clinical data and properly designed clinical trials.

The potential impact of a program of combined radiation therapy-chemotherapy on the morbidity and mortality of cancer is immense. Metastatic disease currently accounts for the majority of deaths from cancer. Control of metastatic disease remains, therefore, our greatest challenge. Combination chemotherapy and radiation therapy offers a potential solution to at least a part of this challenge. An added benefit may be the enhanced control of local and regional disease in some cancer types so that the treatment may be more effective in all combinations of the T, N and M compartments.

At the level of the organism there are significant effects that take place during combined modalities outside of the hope for enhancement in the therapeutic ratio for local and regional control, as well as the control of subclinical distant metastases. Decreases in the immune response, suppression of the bone marrow and general debilitation resulting from combination treatments may adversely affect the outcome of treatment if not properly controlled and accounted for. These are some of the limitations in planning and implementing combined modality treatment.

Sequencing of radiation therapy and chemotherapy has varied from site to site with the use of chemotherapy before, during and after irradiation. There has been little consistency to, or rationale for, this approach in the past. In general, these have been selected in terms of limiting toxicity, with particular emphasis on bone marrow tolerance. Wrba's data[1] suggests that sequencing of treatment at the appropriate time has a significant relationship on the residual tumor cell burden at the point of introduction of each new treatment program (Fig. 10-1).

Chemotherapy, applied before radiation therapy, has been used in order to cause maximum tumor regression prior to irradiation in the attempt to reduce the tumor cell burden and hopefully increase local control. It also affects subclinical disease outside of the irradiated volume. Applications of this method, and, in particular, the application of MTX to head and neck cancer treatment programs before radiotherapy, has not enhanced local control. It is highly possible that the drug acts on the cells which are most radiosensitive with no overall gain. It is also possible that the drug is introduced at an inappropriate time since the tumor cell burden is at its maximum point at the onset of treatment.

TABLE 10-4. *Modes of Action of Combination Chemotherapy and Radiation Therapy*

1. Adjunctive Action
2. Synergistic Action
   - A. Alkylating agents
   - B. Purine and pyrimidine antagonists
   - C. Antibiotics
   - D. *Vinca* alkaloids
   - E. Cell Synchronizers
3. Radiation Sensitizers
   - A. Oxygen
   - B. Electron-affinitive compounds (Flagyl, RO-07-0582)
4. Anticoagulants
5. Secondary Irradiators

The use of chemotherapy during radiotherapy has a strong rational basis in that it would interact with local treatment in terms of additivity and even interaction, as well as affecting subclinical disease at an early time in the treatment. Approaches in this manner have been limited, although the initial results of the brain tumor group and of some of the preliminary trials with bleomycin in head and neck cancer are encouraging. Here, however, one must remember that the combination of the treatments may cause excessive normal tissue toxicity. Therefore, investigations of these combinations need to be carefully carried out.

Chemotherapy, added after irradiation, has been primarily used for control of subclinical disease. This approach, in conjunction with its administration during treatment, however, has been used in Wilm's tumor, in embryonal rhabdomyosarcoma, Ewing's sarcoma, osteogenic sarcomas and in some breast cancers. At the moment, based on clinical trials, this has been the most successful use of combined radiotherapy and chemotherapy.

Based on the data suggested by Wrba,[1] this sequential application of treatment programs results from their introduction at a point when the tumor cell burden has been reduced significantly by the previously used treatment program. A number of studies combining radiation and several alkylating agents seem to indicate the combination to be a good model of pure additive effects.

Because the interaction of chemotherapy and radiation involves additivity and interaction with tumor and normal tissues, it is necessary to develop a number of systems which look at both the cellular level and the tissue level for evidences of completely separate effects. Additive effects and interactive effects, are both augmented and inhibited. This requires the concomitant measurement of the radiation damage in normal tissues and in the tumor. If dose-modifying factors or dose-effect factors are then determined experimentally, they can be compared and the gain factor of the therapeutic ratio can then be calculated from the modifying factors for tumor and normal tissue. Although these represent artificial models in animals, they may help to predict changes in the therapeutic ratio in human tumors. All of these actions indicate the complexity of using radiation in combination with chemotherapy. The immense gains to be achieved by aggressive chemotherapy added to the high local cell-kills achievable by radiotherapy outweigh these risks, however.

Many agents have been used in combination with radiation therapy. Radiation sensitizers are chemical compounds which have the capacity to increase the lethal properties of ionizing radiation when administered in conjunction with the radiation event. In the ideal case they increase radiosensitivity without being toxic and they significantly increase the radiosensitivity of the cancer over that of normal tissues.

Several classes of radiosensitizing compounds have been identified:

1. Electron-affinitive compounds share the property of setting the stage for increased free radical production much as oxygen does. They hold the promise of minimizing the oxygen effect as a cause for failure in the irradiation of hypoxic tumors. Examples of these compounds are Metronidazol (RO-07-0582 Roche).
2. Certain pyrimidine analogues, when incorporated into DNA, have the property of increasing its fragility to ionizing radiation, whereas others interfere with the repair of radiation-induced damage to DNA.
3. Other derivatives, such as actinomycin-D, bleomycin and adriamycin act with diverse mechanisms, adding to the radiation effect rather than acting as true radiation sensitizers.

Table 10-4 offers a classification of compounds by their mode of action when used in combination with radiation therapy. A major program has been initiated in the development of radiation sensitizers in terms of new compounds and the evaluation of existing compounds. These programs have been given high priority in terms of the development of subsequent programs. Major emphasis is being placed on the implementation of the evaluation of radiation sensitizers in combination with radiation therapy during 1978, with the Phase I studies already underway and the progression to Phase II and Phase III studies planned as soon as the data from the Phase I studies are available.

The development of new hypoxic cell-sensitizers for radiation therapy is being actively stimulated, and programs, such as the one at the Gray Laboratories at the Mount Vernon Hospital, illustrate the value of the center-directed efforts toward development and evaluation of new compounds having potential as hypoxic cell-sensitizers. Programs, such as this, allow for: (1) the synthesis of new or analogue compounds having predicted electron affinity, (2) the measurement of electron affinity by pulse radiolysis, (3) the measurement of lipid solubility, (4) screening for activity, in vitro, with mammalian cells as a function of drug concentration, (5) measurement for toxicity in vitro and (6) measurements for toxicity and sensitization of a mouse tumor with significant hypoxic cell fractions in vivo in at least one or more systems. The valuation of these data would then allow for widespread mouse tumor testing, subsequent review of that data, large animal toxicity evaluation and subsequent initiation of clinical trials.

Because of the potential for combined

treatment techniques in the management of the patient with cancer, it is important to develop rapid and in-depth biological studies. These data must soon be integrated into the design of clinical trials, combining the modalities of radiation, chemotherapy and surgery.

The goals for combined radiation therapy and radiation sensitizer clinical studies are directed toward: (1) improvement in the methods of measurement, recording, reviewing and reporting the response of tumors and normal tissues to combination radiation and chemotherapy trials, (2) the rapid application of basic concepts from laboratory research programs into clinical study design and (3) a widespread multidisciplinary approach to the failure pattern in all tumor sizes and the enhancement of tumor cure rates in all cancer sites and histologies, in which T, N or M failure is a major problem.

These goals can be achieved by expansion of protocol studies to include individuals actively pursuing basic studies, as well as clinicians in the design of basic studies relevant to clinical programs. With the elucidation of basic mechanisms and X-ray drug interaction, clinical studies can be pursued more effectively and with a better scientific base.

The utilization of radiation sensitizers offers the possibility of improving the radiation damage in the tumor by increasing radiosensitivity.

Various problems need to be studied and include:

1. The toxicology and pharmacology of the existing radiation sensitizing compounds
2. The development of new compounds
3. The perturbation of cell kinetics as a function of dose-modifying agents
4. The development of methodologies for monitoring drug localization with respect to site and time, as well as methodology for monitoring the parameters of cell kinetics in the clinic.
5. The performance of clinical trials using the electron-affinitive compounds to study the biology of hypoxic cells and the mechanisms of reoxygenation in tumor.

The potential impact of a program of combined radiation therapy and chemotherapy on the morbidity and mortality of cancer is immense. Data now suggest that one can utilize each treatment program in a combined fashion at a point when the response potential is at the highest degree of probability. Such integrated sequential applications of treatment modalities have the greatest potential for ultimate cure of the cancer patient.

Strategies relative to cancer should be aimed at optimization of local and regional treatment. Delineation of subsets of patients with high risk for recurrence would have a significant impact upon which such adjunctive systems of therapeutic management should be evaluated. The initiation of adjuvant therapy studies has great potential for improving the control rate in cancer.

In disseminated disease, or where the probability of dissemination is high, evaluation of any realistic potential combination of treatment for tumor control should be pursued. It is not only necessary to delineate optimal palliative therapy where tumor control is not possible, but also to test new drugs, immunotherapeutic tools and combination regimens in all such situations where the disseminated compartment of the disease is of high probability.

Only under such circumstances will the most practical and important optimization of treatment programs be achieved. The development of the above basic attributes for each tumor type need to be studied so that the protocols can be developed with a clear understanding of the nature of disease, conditions to be studied and the general therapeutic strategies to be followed. This type of disease orientation and study includes the essentials necessary to make appropriate decisions. These data include adequate diagnostic evaluation, adequate clinical and pathologic staging, pathologic review, delineation of relapse and recurrence patterns, criteria of response delineation, standarized followup routine and adequate data retrieval and analysis techniques to maximize the acquisition of appropriate information necessary to change treatment programs in the appropriate manner. Through such mechanisms, new therapeutic regimens can be demonstrated, tried and implemented for the benefit of the cancer patient.

REFERENCES

1. Wrba H: Main issues in oncology (editorial). Oncology 33(3):102–104, 1976
2. Whitmore G F: Some radiation effects on mammalian cells in tissue culture, in Kallman R F, (ed): Research in Radiotherapy. National Academy of Sciences–National Research Council, (no. 888) Washington D C, 1961
3. Schabel F M: Experimental basis for adjuvant chemotherapy, in Salmon S E, Jones S E (eds): Adjuvant Therapy in Cancer. Amsterdam, Elsevier/North Holland Biomedical Press, 1977 pp 3–14
4. Mathe G, Halle-Pannenko O, Florentin I, et al: Experimental and rational bases for immunology as cancer adjuvant therapy, in Salmon S E, Jones S E (eds): Adjuvant Therapy in Cancer. Amsterdam, Elsevier/North Holland Biomedical Press, 1977 pp 29–48

Part I I

The Solid Tumors

Ezra M. Greenspan

11 The Chemotherapy of Breast Cancer

A major change in the clinical management of breast cancer has been underway since the recent recognition that 250,000 women in the United States could be potential beneficiaries of combination chemotherapy given either postoperatively or as treatment for metastatic recurrent cancer. The average American woman, after operation, now realizes that several cancerous lymph nodes in the axilla indicate a continuous future threat to her life. Her numerous questions, stimulated by the constant intrusion of diverse management concepts from the laiety and the news media, have added a mounting burden to the medical oncologist. The evaluation of chemotherapy vis-a-vis the other modalities of cancer management has thus become a most pressing psychological and therapeutic problem for all concerned.

Control of breast cancer seems currently to be approaching a horizon close to that attainable with Hodgkin's disease and the lymphomas as a result of progressive developments in polychemotherapy. We published detailed data as early as 1963 indicating the striking regressions and clinical advantages of combination chemotherapy in the majority of patients with metastatic breast.[1] Now, major objective regressions can be induced in 75 to 85 per cent of "fresh" previously untreated metastases with complex four-to-six drug combination regimens at tolerable toxic doses.[2] Since this high proportion of patients with diverse clinical strata of metastatic disease show objective regressions, it can be assumed that nondetectable micrometastases in postoperative patients would also be suppressed in an equal proportion and with probably even more efficiency due to the smaller tumor load. Because of these high objective regression rates and the widespread favorable publicity for prophylactic chemotherapy, thousands of patients now at risk are expecting, and even demanding, early combinations of chemotherapy. These usually consist of three major categories of agents: (1) alkylating agents, (2) cell cycle-specific antimetabolites and (3) cell "synchronizers" or mitotic inhibitors (at times accompanied by hormones and anabolic agents).

Critical analysis of the results of combination chemotherapy in recurrent or advanced metastatic breast cancer requires a more detailed clinical stratification, based on predominant presenting metastatic patterns

Supported in part by a grant from The Chemotherapy Foundation to the Division of Medical Oncology, Department of Medicine, Mount Sinai School of Medicine.

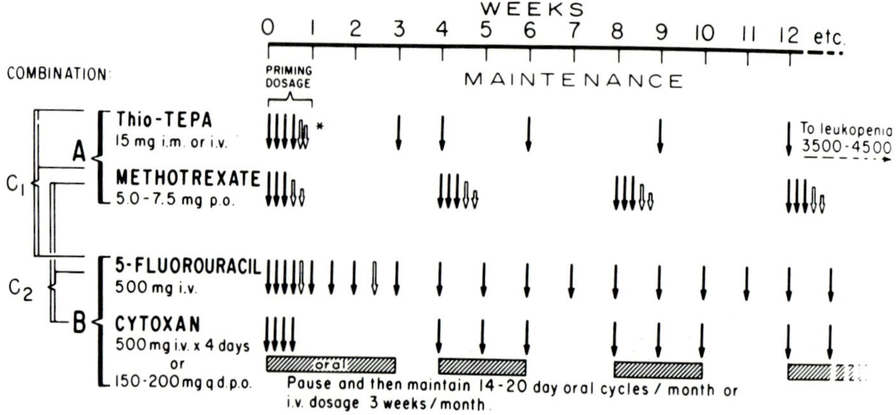

FIG. 11-1 Scheme of combination chemotherapy employed in early (1959-1963) studies with couplets of (a) Thio-TEPA and MTX (since 1959) and (b) Cytoxan and FU (since 1961). Triple therapy combination C_1 and C_2 adopted in 1963. From Greenspan E M: Clinical Cancer Chemotherapy. New York, Raven Press, 1975 (with permission).

(M_1-M_9) in accordance with progressive threat to life, Table 11-1) rather than the classical 3-part classification of soft tissue, osseous or visceral metastases. The old classification accounts for much of the ambiguity inherent in the analysis of results of single drug therapy of advanced cancer, well summarized by Carter.[3] As most new agents have appeared, some degree of antitumor activity has been demonstrated but, even after adriamycin, the rate of good partial or complete regression does not exceed the 25 to 40 per cent range. The duration of induced regressions from single drugs has also been short—usually 3 to 7 months. No clear distinctions have been recognized to establish a preference for any one of the seven or eight major different agents over another, even though there are some biologic and clinical data indicating selective penetration and action of certain agents on different organ metastases. Although the addition of a corticosteroid to a single agent, such as chlorambucil[4] or FU,[5] does increase the initial regression rate, no valid therapeutic reason exists any longer for patients to be treated with only a single one of the drugs, which are relatively ineffective when used alone.

Our early retrospective studies[1,6,7] showed that couplets (Fig. 11-1) of an alkylating agent (i.e., thio-TEPA) and a cell cycle-specific antimetabolite (i.e., MTX) raised regressions up to a 60 per cent rate without corticosteroids or androgen support. Secondary regressions induced after crossing over to a "non-cross-resistant" secondary combination of cytoxan plus FU were also observed in 30 to 40 per cent of diverse metastatic patients for 3 to 5 months after resistance had developed to thio-TEPA and MTX.[7] The potential value of triple therapy was clearly demonstrated in 1964[6] by combining 5-FU, at that time known alone to inhibit some liver metastases,[8] into a regimen which markedly improved the control of the strata (M-8) presenting with predominant metastatic hepatomegaly. Triple therapy raised the response rate of all strata of fresh cases to a 75 per cent level from the previous 60 per cent response rate with the two-drug combinations. Cytoxan was also noted by us[7] and others[9] to be a better alkylating agent for osseous metastases (M-3) than standard alkyl-

TABLE 11.1. *Mammary Carcinoma: A Nine Level Clinical Stratification (Staging) According to Predominant Presenting Metastatic Patterns*

Course	Strata	Predominant metastatic sites	Est. patients (%)	Est. med.* survival (months)
Chronic indolent	M1A	Skin and chest wall subcutaneous nodular ulcerative	35	24+
	B	Lymph node regional (cervical, axillary)		24+
Subacute intermediate	M2A	Lung, pleural effusion		?
	B	Nodular parenchymal	15	12-24
	M3A	Bone:focal <four sites		12-24
	B	diffuse >four sites	20	6-12
	M4	Inflammatory	5	6-12
	M4	Inflammatory	5	6-12
	M5	Intraabdominal	7	3-12
Acute, life-threatening	M6	CNS	3	2-6
	M7	Lymphangitic pulmonary	3	2-6
	M8	Massive hepatomegaly	6	2-6
	M9	Generalized, three or more dire sites	6	2-6

*Prior to era of combination chemotherapy.
From Greenspan E M: Clinical Cancer Chemotherapy. New York, Raven Press, 1975 (with permission).

ating agents (thio-TEPA or chlorambucil). Inflammatory cancer (M-4) was reported to be exquisitively responsive to thio-TEPA and MTX, since 15 of the first 16 patients in this stratum rapidly regressed, and 12 of 16 were controlled for more than a year. Thio-TEPA was given repeatedly with multiple small daily oral dose-cycles of MTX to produce mild acute predictable toxicity (mucositis).[7] Wright previously had noted that less than one-third of patients with skin metastases responded to MTX alone.[10] The clinical strata presenting with cerebral metastases (M-6) showed relatively short-term responses to the thio-TEPA and oral MTX (at the height of MTX toxicity), but the use of whole-brain radiation after initial induction chemotherapy prolonged survival for 1 to 2 years in this group. Subsequent clinical recurrence was most often manifested terminally outside the brain. Thus, the critical evaluation of therapy in advanced mammary cancer can be distinctly enhanced by employing the nine-level (Table 11-1) clinical stratification based on predominant organ metastatic patterns presenting at onset of chemotherapy. The worst strata (M3B-M9) represent life-threatening categories analogous to those designated as "dire" by Cutler[11] and associated prior to the era of chemotherapy with a median life expectancy of about 5 months.[2]

In a brief abstract reported in 1969 Cooper described the induction of 80 to 85 per cent regressions by using vincristine and prednisone with cytoxan, MTX and FU (CMFVP) in fresh cases of X-radiation and/or hormonal failures.[12] Although this "Cooper regimen" accelerated the acceptance of polychemotherapy it was never precisely imitated in either the national or international studies of various combinations of the so-called CMF or CMFVP (A) regimens. The detailed flow sheet of the dosage scheme (Fig. 11-2) of the Cooper regimen was not published until 1975.[2] The differences in the Cooper regimen and in our regimen as compared to the CMF regimens are several, and are especially notable by comparison of the specific scheduling of the "schedule dependent" FU and MTX (Fig. 11-3). Only fluorouracil was primed initially by Cooper with four daily doses (Fig. 11-3), whereas we primed both MTX and FU daily at onset of chemotherapy. Cooper gives MTX and FU steadily once weekly after priming

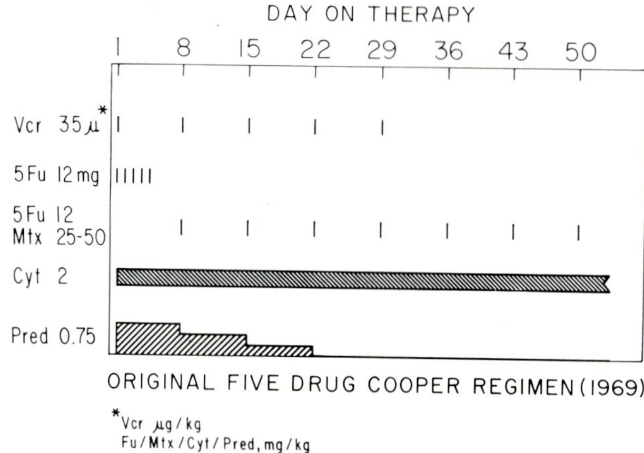

FIG. 11-2. Flow diagram of Cooper regimen. Drug dosage expressed in mg/kg, except for Vincristine, in units/kg.

with weekly vincristine until a leukopenic nadir becomes discernible. Thereafter, drug dosages are cut back or omitted and later resumed. Our regimen has included not only initial daily dosages of both FU and MTX for induction[2] but short pulses of oral MTX every 1 to 2 months. Prednisone dosages in the Cooper regimen are high only for the first week and then are rapidly reduced during the initial induction phase of chemotherapy and suspended after three weeks. Cytoxan is given steadily by Cooper until interruption or until signs of bone marrow intolerance developed. Vincristine is given weekly until reflexes are diminished. The regimens thus employed by Cooper and by us are more intense during the first 4 to 8 weeks of treatment and are individually custom-tailored to develop early tolerable toxicity. FU and MTX are employed more intensively than in the usual CMF regimens.

A recent randomized comparative ECOG

DIFFERENCES IN FU AND MTX INDUCTION SCHEDULES

	1	2	3	4	5	6	7	8
EMG FU	↓↓↓↓	↓↓	↓	↓	↓	↓	↓	↓
EMG MTX	IIII		IIII			IIII		
"COOPER" FU	↓↓↓↓	↓	↓	↓	↓	↓	↓	↓
"COOPER" MTX		I	I	I	I	I	I	I
"CMF" Carbone Bonadonna FU	↓	↓			↓	↓		
"CMF" Carbone Bonadonna MTX	I	I			I	I		
"CMF" Leone FU	↓	↓	↓	↓	↓	↓	↓	↓
"CMF" Leone MTX	I	I	I	I	I	I	I	I
WEEKS	1	2	3	4	5	6	7	8

FU ↓
MTX I

FIG. 11-3. Differences in aggregate dosage and scheduling of FU & MTX in Cooper regimen and our (EMG) regimen compared to CMF-Bonadonna, ECOG and CALGB protocols.

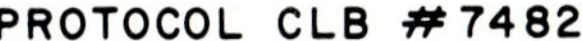

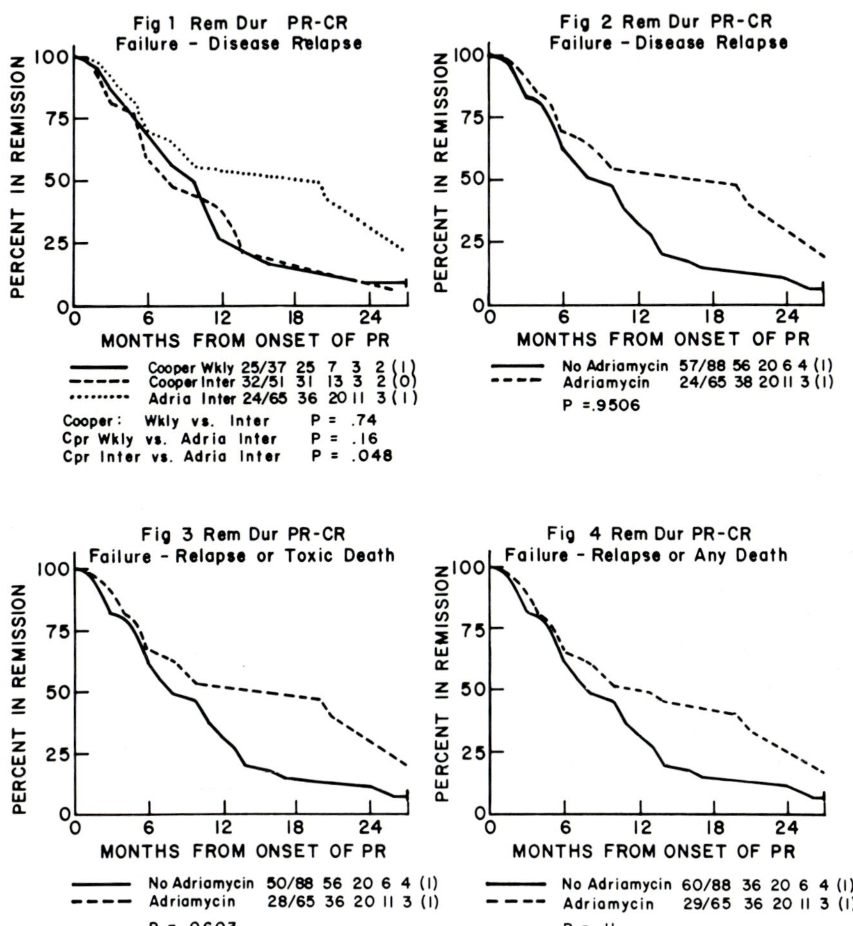

FIG. 11-4. More sustained response in remission between 12-18 months in patients receiving adriamycin plus CMFVP shown in dotted line curves.

study indicates that prednisone does indeed add to overall effectiveness of CMF therapy. No comparable data is available to delineate the additional contribution of vincristine to polychemotherapy. Our policy has been to employ corticosteroids only for the life-threatening clinical metastatic patterns (M_{3b}-M_9). The lack of daily induction of the schedule-dependent FU and the several other differences in the randomized protocol regimens of ECOG, CALGB and the Milan groups could account for the fact that at best, a 55 to 60 per cent regression induction rate was observed. This lower-than-expected rate is not necessarily due to differences of criteria for response.

Despite the various differences in protocol versus individualized dosage schemes and differences in regression rates, the 2-year survival rate in all large heterogenous series using 3 to 5 drug regimens has been disappointing. Randomized studies of Carbone, Tormey and others[13,14,15] and Cooper's data show that not more than 20 per cent of patients treated for recurrent metastatic cancer remained alive (Fig. 11-4) after 2 years, less than 10 per cent after 3 years and probably less than 5 per cent after 5 years. The individualized dosage-tai-

TABLE 11-2. *Guide Lines for Selection of Drugs for Combination Chemotherapy*

Strata	Predominant metastatic site(s)	"Standard" alkylating agent*	CTX	FU	MTX	ADR	VCR	BCNU/ CCNU
M1	Skin and subcutaneous	+	+	+	++	+	??	+
M2	Pulmonary nodular, or pleural effusion, or both	+	++	+	+	++	+ ??	+ +
M3	Osseous (diffuse)	+	++	+	+	??	+	+
M4	Inflammatory	+	+	+	++	+	??	+
M5	Intraabdominal	+	+	++	+	++	??	+
M6	CNS	??	??	??	++	??	+	+
M7	Lymphangitic	+	++	+	+	++	+	+
M8	Liver	+	++	++	+	++	+	+
M9	Generalized (three or more dire sites)	+	++	++	++	++		

* Thio-TEPA, chlorambucil, phenylalanine mustard, mustargen.
+=Clinically useful inhibition.
++=Significant, more frequent inhibition.
??=Probable antitumor action not clinically demonstrable on a regular basis.
From Greenspan E M: Clinical Cancer Chemotherapy. New York, Raven Press, 1975 (with permission).

loring in our patients did not yield more than 30 per cent survivors after 2 years, prior to the advent of adriamycin. Thus, it became more and more obvious that earlier treatment in the early postop period with combined agents and newer different agents lacking cross-resistance in a program of longer (up to 2 years) maintainance therapy until relapse, would be required to make a major impact on survival in metastatic breast cancer. Although a more relevant selection of drugs vis-a-vis metastatic patterns (Table 11-2) might improve survival of selected clinical strata, it seemed unlikely that major increases in long-term 3 to 5 year survival could be expected once recurrences appear.

Since 1973, the chemotherapists' armamentarium has been visibly strengthened by adriamycin, not so much when used as a single agent, but when combined with 3 to 4 other agents. The attainment of secondary or tertiary regressions in at least 25 to 40 per cent of patients after primary or secondary drug failures with adriamycin combinations can be regularly achieved, but only 3 to 5 months of survival has been added when reliance is placed on this agent in the late phase of recurrent metastases. Adriamycin and vincristine as an initial induction couplet has also been disappointing (Table 11-3), yielding only 6 to 9 months of median survival compared to 12 to 18 months for CMF and 18 to 22 months for CMFP and CMFVP. More frequent, sustained and better quality remissions, however, have been reported since 1976 over the 12 to 18 month interval from onset of therapy in a complex CALGB regimen involving adriamycin plus CFVP in induction, followed in 6 months by CMFVP, as compared to those not receiving any adriamycin in the induction regimen (Fig. 11-4). Unfortunately after 24 months on C(M)FVP(A) the survival differences with or without adriamycin disappear although, for the first time, metastatic patients (Fig. 11-4) are apparently showing a 2-year survival above 40 per cent by this use of CMFVP (with or without adriamycin). Steadier polychemotherapy by more skilled groups of physicians may account for this improving outlook in "advanced" cancer, but a slightly earlier use of combination chemotherapy (Fig. 11-5) in better patients with a lower tumor load cannot be excluded as the significant factor. According to Tormey and Weiss (unpublished to date) the better quality of the survival in remission at 12 to 18 months associated with adriamycin in the induction period seems to reflect the contribution of a cross-over in the six-drug regimen. In our private clinical practice well over 50 per cent of metastatic recurrent patients are currently surviving over 2 years from onset of therapy but it is still too early to guess what the survival at 4 to 5 years will be with the six drugs. Most observers doubt that it can be maintained at a 30 to 40 per cent level despite partial plateauing of the survival curve after 2 years. Thus, the average patients treated for recurrent metastases might now be expected to survive about 2½ years rather than the 2 years, on six-drug combinations and sequences. Before 1960 the median survival without any chemotherapy had been 10 to 12 months.

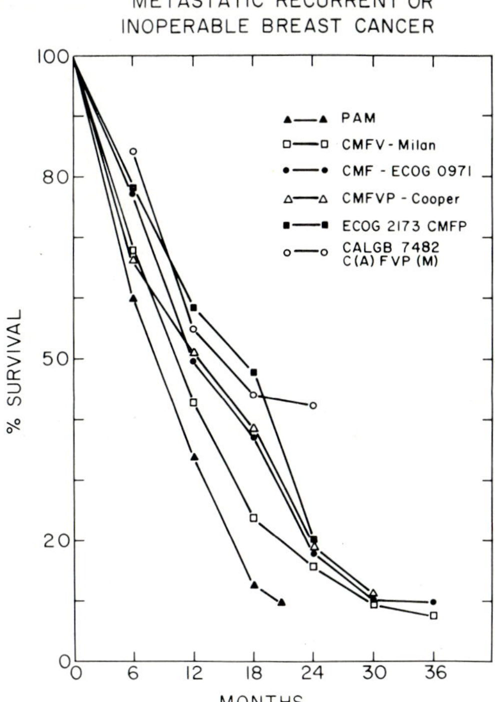

FIG. 11-5. Results of "Cooper" regimen and five different randomized trials varying from 1 drug (PAM) to the five- and six-drug regimens CALGB #7482 shows best survival (courtesy Tormey-see text).

SURGICAL ADJUVANT THERAPY

The concept of early postoperative chemotherapy was explored by certain surgical cooperative groups under Moore's direction prior to 1970.[16] Thio-TEPA, FU and other single agents were used but dosages and schedules were grossly inadequate and ignored the modern concepts of cellular kinetics, the cell-kill hypothesis and combination chemotherapy. The superiority of three different drugs (CMF) compared to one agent (phenylalanine mustard) was confirmed in the early 1970's in a randomized advanced cancer study of ECOG, but this did not prevent a large adjuvant study of a single alkylating agent (phenylalanine mustard) from being launched.[17]

TABLE 11-3. *Metastatic Breast Cancer-ECOG Protocols Median in Months*

	TTF*	Resp. Duration	Survival
F			
F+Prem	1.5-3.2	3.5-5.7	10-14
Pa			16-25
A			7-11
CMF			12-18
CMFP	5.0-7.0	5.2-7.7	18-22
AV			6-9

*TTF=time to failure.

From Tormey D, et al: Breast cancer survival in single and combination chemotherapy trials since 1968. For the Eastern Cooperative Oncology Group (ECOG). Cancer Abstr Proc ASCO, Denver, Col, 1977 (with permission).

TABLE 11-4. *Milan-Bonadonna: "CMF" at Three Years*

		Recurrences		
	Deaths	ALL	4+	1-3 nodes
Control	21%	45%	65%	40%
CMF	10%	25%	42%	19%

Recurrence and survival after surgical adjuvant CMF regimen by Bonadonna in Milan.

In the postmenopausal group CMF suppressed recurrences for only 1 year in the 4+ node group and had no effect on 1-3+ node group. From Greenspan E M: Clinical Cancer Chemotherapy. New York, Raven Press, 1975 (with permission).

The outcome of this postoperative adjuvant trial was disappointing despite much premature favorable publicity in the media. Currently the cooperative surgical groups are again involved in what appears to be a somewhat outdated comparison of two drugs, PAM + FU versus CMF. In the well known large randomized study of CMF conducted postoperatively in Milan, Italy, by Bonadonna et al[18] the CMF schedule seems to us unpredictable in quickly reaching the toxic therapeutic potential of the cell cycle-specific agents (MTX and FU), but it is obviously more convenient than the Cooper regimen. Only the aggregate dosage of the alkylating agent, cytoxan, appears adequate in this CMF regimen. Survival and recurrence data 2 years after the 1 year of CMF chemotherapy were acclaimed as "monumental" by Holland, i.e., at long last proving the effectiveness of surgical adjuvant combination chemotherapy for a common major adult cancer.[19] The now available recurrence and survival data after 3 years are disappointing, however, since the disquieting fact was revealed that the suppression of micrometastases was very transient in postmenopausal women (average age 58 years), although it remains relatively of much more significance in premenopausal women.[18] The overall death rate in both pre- and postmenopausal was 21 per cent in the controls at 3 years compared to 10 per cent after CMF therapy, given only during the first postoperative year (Table 11-4).

The major clinical and statistical impact of CMF in Bonadonna's study appears in premenopausal women with either 4+ or 1 to 3 positive nodes at operation. After 3 years without any chemotherapy, 65 per cent of all the women in the control series with 4+ nodes showed recurrence, whereas only 42 per cent of the CMF-treated patients recurred. The difference among all with 1 to 3 positive nodes was 19 per cent compared to 40 per cent for the controls. In the postmenopausal patients after 12 to 18 months, the delay to recurrence was unfortunately of no statistical significance whatsoever.

Analysis of the premenopausal patients in the CMF study at Milan did not reveal any recurrence differences between those developing drug-induced amenorrhea compared with those who continued to menstruate. Thus the factor of age and the clinical features of breast cancer in the older woman could be playing a more significant role than menopausal status per se in response to chemotherapy. Obviously, a better and more sustained program of chemotherapy continuing into the second year, perhaps with a fixed crossover at 6 to 12 months employing other agents including adriamycin and vincristine, might provide better control among the older women. The therapeutic index for cytotoxic agents and thus the response to chemotherapy in older women is usually inferior to that in younger women.

The previously ignored differences in drug stoichiometrics of the original Cooper regimen compared to CMF-Milan or various American CMFVP regimens may account for the striking results of a 4 to 7 year followup of 100 patients with 4+ nodes first reported by Cooper at a Chemotherapy Foundation Symposium in October of 1976.[20] Survival free of clinical (Fig. 11-6) metastases was reported in more than 70 per cent of these patients after 4 years. In this study 27 of 100 patients received conventional chest wall deep-radiotherapy after operation and were then sent for chemotherapy. The onset of polychemotherapy was delayed from a median of 23 days postoperatively in 73 patients receiving only chemotherapy to 57 days postoperatively in the 27 patients first receiving radiotherapy before chemotherapy. Recurrences in the radiotherapy group were much higher and appeared earlier than in the chemotherapy-only patients (Fig. 11-7). The delay of onset of the chemotherapy appears more likely to account for the unfavorable affects of postop radiotherapy rather than the modest required reduction of chemotherapy dosages, although delayed but protracted effects on immunity could also play a major role.

Cooper's data has been retrospectively analyzed by Holland and Glidewell.[21] No differences were found in the comparison of input variables in both groups. It appears that initial postop radiation therapy with delay in chemotherapy markedly diminishes a patient's chance for apparent clinical cure. This study provides additional support to Sternsward's recent review of the negative effects of postop radiotherapy on survival in five different European centers.[22] Most important is the startling possibility that only several weeks delay and perhaps a better use of schedule-dependent antimetabolites, as we and Cooper advocate, could make a vital difference in the survival of thousands of women.

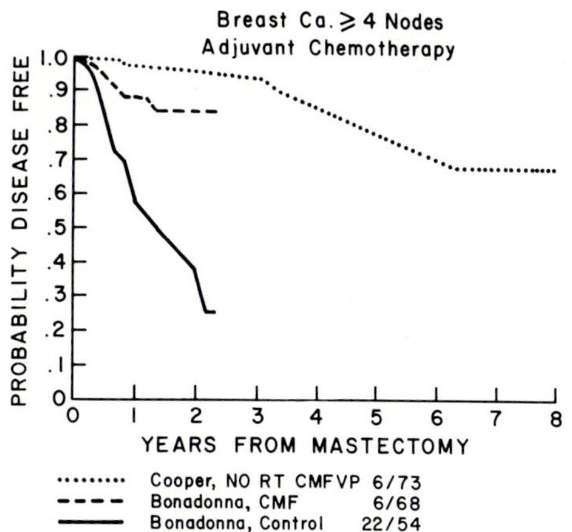

FIG. 11-6. Survival curves of Cooper regimen (top curve) on patients with four or more nodes compared to results of CMF in Milan (middle curve) versus several historical control series with one or more nodes positive.

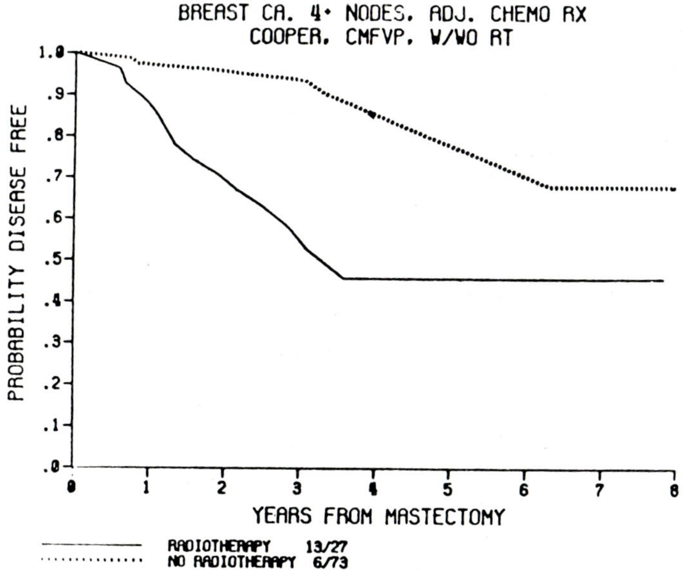

FIG. 11-7. Actuarial analysis of survival in 27 patients receiving radiotherapy (bottom) prior to chemotherapy compared to 73 patients (top) receiving only chemotherapy by Cooper.

It is becoming obvious that surgeons must now candidly and promptly advise patients of their nodal status and of the inadequacy of surgery to control breast cancer (regardless of the type of surgical procedure employed!). Although surgical cure is achieved in 45 to 50 per cent by whatever surgical procedure, less than 5 per cent of all patients have a life expectancy which could be influenced by the type of surgical procedure chosen by either patient or physician.

Radiotherapists must also soon acknowledge that an essentially local modality could have deleterious systemic and survival effects. Postoperative radiotherapy has not cured any statistically (>5%) recognizable or predictable cohort of patients. Although electron-beam therapy and superficial radiation may avoid immunosuppression and potential compromise of the bone marrow, it cannot significantly alter survival. It must be reiterated that chest wall recurrence[18] is well-suppressed by combination chemotherapy. After 75 years of debate, argument and interminable studies on the various types of radiation therapy and surgery, no data has convincingly made an impact on the 5 per cent zone of borderline statistical significance.

The time is at hand to face the fact that the management of breast cancer, like Hodgkin's disease and lymphomas, appears to be becoming a predominantly chemotherapy-oriented process from the moment of diagnosis in almost all patients, and certainly in those with three or more nodes positive at mastectomy. The most important contribution derived from Fischer's surgical adjuvant group studies establishes that those with three or more involved nodes are likely to die in 5 years.[17] Even with current conventional CMF therapy, patients with four or more nodes may still be likely to die of breast cancer within 4 years. The urgent need today is to improve, modify and extend our combinations of chemotherapeutic agents, our sequences of chemotherapy and especially to confirm Cooper's results. The era of a chemo-prophylaxis for breast cancer may well be on the horizon, encouraged by the inconsequential incidence of late chemotherapy-induced second neoplasms 4 to 7 years after, thus far reported following surgical adjuvant programs.

Nonspecific immunotherapy as an effective adjuvant to chemotherapy is still not established, although striking examples of unexpected clinical regression in breast cancer cannot be ignored in this regard. Documented regression of recurrent metastases have been seen shortly after bacterial infections, nonspecific immunization, allergic skin reactions and hepatitis. In a small group of patients previously recovered from pulmonary tuberculosis, chemotherapy has been noted to be associated with an unusually long responsive and indolent course of metastatic breast cancer.[23] None of these impressions nor any of the detailed studies of comparative chemo-immunotherapy, have as yet put immunotherapy on a scientific or reproducible basis. Immunotherapy thus still appears as a "will of the wisp," without an established therapeutic rhythm or dosage and with varying therapeutic components.

The future enhancement of chemotherapy in breast cancer requires emphasis on early treatment. Studies on clinical metastatic disease will continue to be frustrating in the long run despite randomization unless a more pertinent clinical stratification is incorporated at onset of protocols. Prospective randomized protocol chemotherapy trials by large committees and diverse physicians and institutions should certainly tell us which of two effective regimens appears better, but it certainly will not tell us what regimen is the best one for the individual patient. Inevitably the best regimen should be one that is custom-tailored to the individual patient's tolerance to cyclically-induced tolerable toxicity with treatment given at the earliest possible time, intensive at the outset, consistent with the doubling time of the tumor and with combinations of 3 to 6 drugs acting by different mechanisms according to modern concepts of cellular kinetics. The clinical concepts of acute, subacute and chronic breast cancer, and the relationship of age and recurrence-free interval may be as important for the optimal management of the recurrent inoperable or metastatic patient as the nodal status is for the postoperative patient. The best combination and sequential chemotherapy in the future may ultimately be based on proof that certain of the drugs on our chemotherapists' shelf are to be preferred in accordance with the location of the major metastatic disease.

References

1. Greenspan E M, Fieber M, Lesnick G, Edelman S: Response of advance breast carcinoma to the combination of the antimetabolite methotrexate and the alkylating agent thio-TEPA. J Mt Sinai Hosp 30:246–267, 1963
2. Greenspan E M: Clinical Cancer Chemotherapy. New York, Raven Press 1975
3. Carter S K: Single and combination non-hormonal chemotherapy in breast cancer. Cancer 30: 1543–1555, 1972
4. Freckman H A, Fry H R, Mendez F L, Maurer E R: Chlorambucil-prednisone therapy for disseminated breast cancer. JAMA 189:23–26, 1964
5. Moore F D, Woodrow S I, Aliapoulios M A, Wilson R E: Carcinoma of the breast. N Eng J Med 227:343–350, 411–416, 460–468, 1967
6. Greenspan E M: Regression of metastatic hepatomegaly from mammary carcinoma. Cytotoxic combination chemotherapy with 5-fluorouracil. NYSJ Med 64:2442–2449, 1964
7. Greenspan E M: Combination cytotoxic chemotherapy in advanced disseminated breast carcinoma. J Mt Sinai Hosp 33:1–27, 1966
8. Dao T L, Grinberg R: Fluorinated pyrimidines in treatment of breast cancer patients with liver metastases. Cancer Chemother Rep 27:71–77, 1963
9. Nemoto T, Dao T: Fluorouracil and cyclophosphamide in disseminated breast cancer. NYSJ Med 554–558, 1971
10. Wright J C, Cobb J P, Golomb F M, et al: Chemotherapy of disseminated carcinoma of the breast. Ann Surg 150:2, 221–229, 1959
11. Cutler S J, Asire A J, Taylor S G: Classification of patients with disseminated breast cancer. Cancer 24:864–869, 1969
12. Cooper R G: Combination chemotherapy in hormone resistant breast cancer. Cancer Res (abstr 57 AACR), 1969
13. Tormey D, Carbone P, Bauer M, Band P: Breast cancer survival in single and combination chemotherapy trials since 1968 for the Eastern Cooperative Oncology Group (ECOG). Cancer Abstract Proceedings ASCO, Denver, Col, 1977
14. DeLena M, DePalo G M, Bonadonna G, Bjetta G B: Terapia del carcinoma mammario metostatizzato conciclofosfamide, methotrexate, vincristine E fluorouracilia. Tumori 59:11–24, 1973
15. Tormey D C, Neifeld V P: Chemotherapeutic approach to disseminated breast cancer, in Stoll B A (ed): Breast Cancer Management—Early and Late. London, Heinemann Medical Books, 1977
16. Moore G E, Pickran J W: Response of breast cancer to triethylene thio-phosphoramide. JAMA Arch Path 65:98, 1958
17. Fisher B, Carbone P, Economou S G, et al: L-phenylalanine mustard (L-Pam) in the management of primary breast cancer. A report of early findings. N Eng J Med 292:117–122, 1975
18. Bonadonna G, Ross A, Valagussa P et al: The CMF program for operable breast cancer with positive axillary nodes. N Eng J Med (in press), 1977
19. Holland J H: Guest editorial. N Eng J Med 194:1346, 1976
20. Cooper R: Abstract, Symposium Chemotherapy Foundation, New York, October, 1976
21. Cooper R G, Holland J F, Glidewell O: Breast cancer: Surgery and chemotherapy as primary treatment. (in press), 1978
22. Stjernsward J: Decreased survival related tc irradiation postoperatively in early operabl(breast cancer. Lancet 2:1284–1286, 1974
23. Greenspan E M: Personal observations

Allan J. Schutt

12
Chemotherapy of Gastrointestinal Neoplasms

About 170,000 Americans will be found to have digestive tract cancer this year and over 100,000 will ultimately die of their cancer.[1] The causes and measures needed to prevent most cases of cancer of the GI and hepatobiliary tracts are as yet only vague theory. Surgical cure rates have shown little change over the past 25 years despite efforts at earlier diagnosis and improvement in surgical techniques. Only chemotherapy has established value as systemic treatment of their malignant disease. While immunotherapy has shown activity in experimental animal tumor systems and theoretically should have its greatest potential in the surgical adjuvant setting, this modality as yet has not been shown to have a role in the management of GI cancer.

In the two decades since 5-FU was introduced as the first agent with significant activity against GI carcinoma, progress has been painfully slow. Most remissions after chemotherapy have proven to be transient and incomplete in nature without significant improvement in survival. A few agents have now been identified which can produce temporary shrinkage and symptomatic improvement in digestive tract carcinoma. Combination chemotherapy regimens have more recently been developed that, in early trials, have suggested increased activity compared to single-agent treatment. Only through the development of treatment programs that can eliminate the low tumor cell burdens present in the surgical adjuvant setting, can significant improvement be made in the cure rate of gastrointestinal cancer. The chemotherapy of digestive tract cancer should not be considered routine treatment but should be best directed at developing more effective regimens through controlled studies.

Agents Active in Treating GI Cancer

Only a few of the many agents studied have shown evidence of significant activity in GI cancer. Objective regression has been defined as at least 50 per cent decrease in the product of the two longest perpendicular diameters of the most clearly measurable tumor mass for at least 2 months without enlargement of other areas of disease or new lesions appearing. For liver metastases, the sum of liver measurements extending below the costal margin or xiphoid at quiet respiration must decrease at least 30 per cent. Since introduction of 5-FU, no other drug has been identified as capable of achieving objective regression rates in the common GI cancers that are clearly superior to the 17 per cent response rate of 5-FU alone.

The wide variety of dosage schedules and routes of administration of 5-FU that have been tried have not exceeded the therapeutic index of standard intensive course treatment when the dosage was adjusted to mild, tolerable toxicity. Oral 5-FU treatment has been markedly inferior (13 to 18 per cent response rate) to intravenous therapy (24 to 38 per cent response rate) in multiple controlled comparisons.[2,3] Even more striking was the shorter duration of response with oral 5-FU in colorectal carcinoma metastatic to the liver in our study (8.5 weeks oral versus 28 weeks IV).[4] Weekly 5-FU, without an initial intensive "loading" course, has been demonstrated in controlled comparison to be inferior to intermittent intensive course treatment (12 versus 38 per cent response).[3] In addition to leukopenia, less common 5-FU toxicity induces alopecia, esophagitis, reversible cerebellar ataxia,[5] peripheral neuritis and perhaps transient cardiotoxicity.[6] 5-FU does have the advantage of lacking cumulative marrow toxicity and very reproducible toxicity once a dosage has been established.

The nucleoside 5-fluoro-2′-deoxyuridine (5-FUDR) has activity in GI cancer of a similar magnitude to 5-FU, but is far more expensive. While FUDR is marketed for use in hepatic artery infusion, there is no evidence that it has any therapeutic advantage to justify its much higher cost.

The close structural analogue of 5-FUDR, ftorafur, was developed in the Soviet Union and is now undergoing clinical testing in the United States. Ftorafur has only very mild myelotoxic potential but produces dose-limiting CNS toxicity.[7]

Nitrosourea Agents

The nitrosourea drugs have shown broad, but modest activity against GI cancer as primary therapy but are useless as secondary treatment.[8]

BCNU, administered intravenously, is active against gastric adenocarcinoma. MeCCNU given as a single oral dose every 7 to 8 weeks yields response rates in colorectal carcinoma comparable to 5-FU, but of significantly shorter duration. CCNU is also given orally, but has shown disappointing response rates in GI cancer. In addition to troublesome acute nausea and vomiting, these nitrosoureas produce unique delayed bone marrow suppression with a double nadir of leukopenia and thrombocytopenia and potentially cumulative marrow toxicity.

Streptozotocin is an antibiotic containing a nitrosourea moiety which is active against islet cell carcinoma and perhaps against carcinoid tumors.[9] This agent is given intravenously either in intensive courses every 6 weeks, or weekly. Streptozotocin can produce intolerable vomiting. It has little tendency for bone marrow toxicity and can be combined with marrow toxic drugs such as 5-FU at near full doses. Streptozotocin can produce dosage-limiting renal tubular toxicity. This nephrotoxic potential can be minimized by adequate hydration, close monitoring of renal function and appropriate reduction of dosage and frequency of administration. Streptozotocin is toxic to normal islet cells, particularly in some animal species. Fortunately, in humans, clinical diabetes is rarely seen though mild transient hypoglycemia is common.

Mitomycin C

Mitomycin C, an alkylating antibiotic of Japanese origin has shown activity in gastric cancer, but is only marginally active in other GI cancers. Mitomycin C should not be used as a single agent in GI cancer in view of the short (2 month average) regressions produced and marked tendency for cumulative bone marrow toxicity. This agent should be most useful in combination regimens where lower dosage and less frequent administration may minimize its toxic potential.

Adriamycin

Adriamycin has little activity in colorectal cancer, but it is active in hepatoma[10] and gastric carcinoma.[11] Adriamycin is usually administered in a single intravenous dose every 3 or 4 weeks. As the primary excretion pathway of adriamycin is hepatic, toxicity is markedly increased in jaundiced patients and the dosage must be reduced. Adriamycin toxicity includes leukopenia, thrombocytopenia, a striking degree of alopecia, occasional stomatitis and the potential for myocardial damage. The total dosage of adriamycin should not exceed 550 mg/m^2 to reduce the incidence of myocardiopathy.

ICRF-159

ICRF-159 is a unique synthetic compound that is administered orally every 8 hours for 3 days every 3 weeks. Toxicity pattern is similar to that of an alkylating agent with early onset of leukopenia and thrombocytopenia and rapid recovery. Activity has been seen in colorectal cancer in initial studies at American Oncologic Hospital[12] and at Mayo Clinic.[13] ICRF is currently being evaluated in ongoing trials as a single agent in gastric and pancreatic cancer and as a component of combination programs in GI cancer.

Triazinate

Triazinate (Baker's antifol, BAF, or TZT) like MTX, is a potent dihydrofolate reductase inhibitor that may have the advantage of entering the CSF in higher concentration. In initial Phase II trials at Mayo Clinic[14] and M. D. Anderson Institute[15] this agent produced objective regressions in 9 of 53 patients (17 per cent) with colorectal carcinoma on a 3-day schedule every 3 weeks. Moderately severe myelosuppression is seen with a nadir at 12 days. Triazinate is currently being evaluated for single-agent activity in gastric carcinoma and in combination with other agents active in colorectal carcinoma.

Chemotherapy of Advanced Gastrointestinal Carcinoma

Colorectal Carcinoma

The experience of our group with single-agent chemotherapy of measurable advanced colorectal carcinoma is detailed in Table 12-1. Other investigators have also reported that single-agent treatment of colorectal carcinoma tends to produce discouragingly low response rates of limited duration for most patients. Our earlier drug combinations were failures (Table 12-2) with only the combination of 5-FU and mitomycin C equaling the response rate of 5-FU alone. In 1974, Falkson's group in South Africa reported a 43 per cent response rate in metastatic colon cancer to the combination of 5-FU, DTIC, vincristine, and BCNU.[16] DTIC was eliminated as it has limited activity in colon cancer and produces severe nausea and vomiting. As me-CCNU is more active in colorectal cancer, it was substituted for BCNU. In our initial controlled study of 80 patients in 1975, the combination of 5-FU, me-CCNU, and vincristine produced a 43.5 per cent objective response rate compared to 19 per cent with an intensive course of 5-FU alone.[17] The following year Falkson and Falkson reported a 37 per cent response rate to a combination of these three drugs as compared to 22 per cent with 5-FU alone,[18] while the Georgetown group reported a 40 percent response rate in 25 patients with advanced colorectal cancer treated with a combination of these three drugs including 5-FU given weekly.[19] With experience now in 101 colorectal patients treated with the 5-FU, me-CCNU and vincristine combination, our objective response rate at 2 months has fallen to 32 per cent compared to 16 per cent in 62 patients treated with 5-FU plus me-CCNU without the addition of vincristine. The controlled study of the Southwest Oncology Group, using 5-FU on a weekly IV schedule, found a 30 per cent response rate in 128 patients treated with 5-FU plus me-CCNU, compared to a 14 per cent response rate in the 36 who received 5-FU alone.[20] While the combination of 5-FU, me-CCNU and vincristine may offer some improvement in response rates compared to either 5-FU alone or in combination with me-CCNU, this advantage may not be apparent with greater experience and in no study does this translate into increased survival for patients with advanced metastatic colorectal cancer.

Gastric Carcinoma

Gastric carcinoma appears to be more responsive to chemotherapy than the other common digestive tract carcinomas. In our studies of single-agent treatment of gastric carcinoma, the drugs with the most significant activity include: 5-FU, with an objective response rate at 2 months of 26 per cent in 72 patients, BCNU, with 18 per cent of 33 patients responding, and adriamycin to which 44 per cent of 16 patients treated responded. Median duration of these responses varied from 4 to 5 months. Activity of mitomycin C against gastric carcinoma was suggested by the three objective responses seen in 11 patients though the median duration was only 2.7 months. These four drugs also stand out in the recent

TABLE 12-1. *Colorectal Carcinoma—Single Drug Treatment*

Agent	Number Treated	Percent Objective Response (2 mo.)
Inactive Drugs		
Adriamycin	56	5
5-Azacytidine	27	0
Benzcarbimine	20	0
Bleomycin	15	0
Camptothecin	49	4
Chromomycin A_3	27	0
Cyclophosphamide	25	8
Cytembena	25	0
Emetine	18	6
Fluorometholone	18	6
FUDR; 24 hr.	64	6
Galactitol	30	0
Hydroxyurea	22	0
Ifosphamide	21	0
Imidazole Carboxamide	17	0
Methotrexate, p.o.	38	5
Platinum (CACP)	33	3
Pyrazofurin	35	0
Streptonigrin	27	0
Streptozotocin	18	6
TIC mustard	22	0
Vincristine	9	0
VP-16	28	0
Active Drugs		
FUDR, Rapid IV	147	22
Methyl CCNU	38	18
Triazinate	28	18
5-FU	359	17
Mitomycin C	69	12
ICRF-159	25	12
BCNU	69	10
CCNU	75	9

TABLE 12-2. *Colorectal Carcinoma—Ineffective Drug Combinations*

Combination	Number Treated	Percent Objective Response (2 mo.)
5-FU + Mitomycin C	23	17
BCNU + Mitomycin C	25	8
CCNU followed by 5-FU	28	7
5-FU + BCNU + Mitomycin C	22	5
5-FU + BCNU	25	4
Actinomycin D + Cyclophosphamide	11	0

From Schutt A J, et al: Combination chemotherapy of colorectal cancer. Proceedings of the XI International Cancer Congress, No. 354, vol. 6. Florence, Excerpta Medica Amsterdam, 1974 (with permission).

review by Carter and Comis[21] of the chemotherapy of gastric carcinoma as the most active single agents studied (Table 12-3). Me-CCNU with a 7 per cent objective response rate in 55 patients, and CCNU with only a single response in 35 patients, showed no significant activity as single agents in gastric carcinoma.

Combination drug treatment of gastric cancer offers the most exciting prospect for the oncologist treating the common gastrointestinal neoplasms. In an earlier study we noted a high response rate in a small group of gastric cancer patients who received 5-FU plus BCNU. In a controlled study involving 85 patients with advanced gastric cancer, we found 5-FU plus BCNU to produce an increase in long-term survival for the first time in patients with advanced gastrointestinal cancer.[22] Eighteen months after initiation of chemotherapy 27 per cent of patients treated with 5-FU plus BCNU combination were alive compared to just 7 per cent of those who received 5-FU or BCNU alone. The Eastern Cooperative Oncology Group (ECOG) has also reported an increase in survival of patients treated with 5-FU and me-CCNU compared to those who received me-CCNU alone.[23] Table 12-4 summarizes reports of studies from five different centers which suggest that combination chemotherapy may be a significant breakthrough in the treatment of unresectable gastric carcinoma.[24,25,26]

TABLE 12-3. *Gastric Carcinoma—Active Single Drugs*

Drugs	Number Treated	Percent Objective Response
5-FU	448	22
Mitomycin C	221	30
BCNU	33	18
Adriamycin	27	26

Pancreatic Carcinoma

Unfortunately, pancreatic carcinoma is now both a more common neoplasm than gastric cancer and has proven to be far more resistent to our chemotherapy approaches. 5-FU is the most active agent against pancreatic cancer with a 15 per cent objective response rate in the 39 patients we treated. Median duration of response was only 2.5 months. We noted responses to mitomycin C in 2 of 9 patients treated. Carter and Comis found a 27 per cent response rate in 44 patients collected from the literature.[27] Three responses were noted in 27 patients treated with streptozotocin.

In a controlled study of 82 patients we found a 33 per cent objective response rate in the 30 patients with pancreatic carcinoma treated with 5-FU plus BCNU, compared to 16 per cent of the 31 who received 5-FU alone.[22] No responses were noted in 21 patients receiving only BCNU. Survival was not increased in any group. Two of 4 patients treated with a combination of 5-FU plus streptozotocin responded. This combination is now being studied by the ECOG. The only glimmer of light in this discouraging disease would appear to be the preliminary report from the Georgetown group of a 47 per cent partial response rate in 17 patients with measurable advanced pancreatic carcinoma treated with an 8-week-cycle of combined streptozotocin, mitomycin C and 5-FU (SMF).[28]

TABLE 12-4. *Gastric Carcinoma—Active Drug Combinations*

Drug Combination	Group	Number Treated	Percent Objective Response
5-FU + BCNU	Mayo	34	41
5-FU + MMC* + Ara C	Memorial	32	38
5-FU + Methyl CCNU	ECOG	30	40
5-FU + MMC + Ara C	Aichi, Nagoya	27	55
5-FU + MMC + ADR**	Georgetown	18	50

*Mitomycin C
**Adriamycin

Hepatocellular Carcinoma

Hepatoma is an extremely aggressive cancer, particularly in Orientals, black Africans and patients with cirrhosis. Median survivals are measured in a few weeks. We have observed objective responses in 33 per cent of 18 patients with hepatocellular carcinoma treated with 5-FU plus BCNU including two responses exceeding 3 years. Livingston and Carter collected 60 patients from the literature with hepatoma and found that 30 per cent responded to treatment with an intensive course of 5-FU.[29] African hepatoma proved totally resistant to chemotherapy until the reports from Uganda of objective responses in 11 of 14 patients with hepatoma treated with adriamycin.[30] Adriamycin appears also to have definite activity in American hepatoma. Combination of adriamycin with 5-FU and a nitrosourea seems to offer an attractive possibility of increasing response of hepatoma to chemotherapy.

Biliary Carcinoma

As carcinoma of the bile ducts and gallbladder is both rare and rarely measurable, experience with chemotherapy of these cancers is scattered and limited. Utilizing a variety of agents, we have observed an overall objective response rate of 23 per cent in 56 patients with biliary tract cancer. Included are responses to 5-FU in 24 per cent of 17 patients, 2 of 5 to mitomycin C and 2 of 4 to BCNU alone. The ECOG is evaluating intensive courses of 5-FU given orally or by T-tube, either alone or in combination with streptozotocin or me-CCNU in this class of neoplasms.

Endocrine Gastrointestinal Carcinomas

These unusual and fascinating neoplasms have widely varied manifestations and provide the frosting on the gastrointestinal oncologist's cake.

The malignant carcinoid syndrome includes flushing, diarrhea, elevation of urinary 5-hydroxy-indole acetic acid, and right heart disease. We have observed objective responses in 40 per cent of 15 patients with malignant carcinoid treated with an intensive course of 5-FU alone and 3 of 6 with streptozotocin alone. These two drugs combined in near full dosage produced responses in 6 of the first 9 patients we treated. It is particularly important to reduce the dosage of the initial course of chemotherapy in patients with florid carcinoma syndrome (urinary 5-HIAA excretion in excess of 150 mg/24 hrs) to avoid precipitating a fulminant, possibly lethal carcinoid crisis.

The hormones produced by islet cell carcinoma may lead to severe hypoglycemia, the Zollinger-Ellison syndrome, watery diarrhea hypokalemia (WDHA) syndrome or the even rarer hyperglycemia and dermatitis of glucogonoma.[31] In the series of patients with islet cell carcinoma treated with streptozotocin reported from the National Cancer Institute, objective responses were seen in 50 per cent of 30 functioning and 5 of 8 nonfunctioning tumors.[9] Of the 39 patients evaluable for functional response, 64 per cent improved. We have observed objective responses in 3 of 6 patients treated with streptozotocin alone and in 6 of 8 with the combination of 5-FU plus streptozotocin. In early studies adriamycin has shown activity against both malignant carcinoid syndrome and islet cell carcinoma.

Squamous Cell Carcinoma of the Gastrointestinal Tract

We have not observed responses of squamous cell carcinoma of the esophagus to bleomycin as reported from Japan. Of 19 patients with squamous carcinoma of the esophagus that we treated with CCNU, 16 per cent had objective response of measurable metastases. Responses have also been seen with MTX and 5-FU. A rare squamous cell carcinoma of pancreatic origin responded to adriamycin. We have also observed dramatic regression in a few patients with metastatic squamous cell and basaloid (transitional) carcinoma of the anus treated with CCNU following a prior course of bleomycin.

Regional Chemotherapy

Interest in regional chemotherapy of GI carcinoma has been largely confined to hepatic artery infusion with either 5-FU or 5-FUDR for hepatocellular carcinoma or metastatic liver disease. While attractive in theory and enthusiastically endorsed by some practitioners, this modality has not gained widespread acceptance. The significant morbidity and mortality reported, practical problems and expense compared to systemic treatment and, particularly, the failure to demonstrate increased survival in either hepatocellular[32] or metastatic[33] carcinoma patients treated by this method likely accounts for the poor acceptance by most oncologists.

Locally Unresectable Gastrointestinal Carcinoma

We conducted a prospective, randomized, double-blind study of 177 patients with locally unresectable gastric, pancreatic or colorectal carcinoma. Addition of 15 mg/kg body weight IV of 5-FU on each of the first 3 days of cobalt-60 or linear accelerator treatment (3500-4000 rads) significantly increased survival over that of radiotherapy alone.[34] This concept has been confirmed by other groups.

Adjuvant Chemotherapy

In five large randomized clinical trials of either 5-FU or 5-FUDR given for from 6 weeks to 1½ years to a total of 1723 patients after "curative" resection of colorectal cancer, no significant increase in survival was noted in those groups receiving chemotherapy as compared to concurrent untreated control groups.[35] Similarly disappointing results have been experienced in six large surgical adjuvant studies conducted by the Stomach Cancer Study Group of the National Hospitals in Japan.[36] Therapeutic benefit was suggested only in a few subgroups of patients treated with mitomycin C.

Summary

Chemotherapy of advanced gastrointestinal carcinoma is of very limited effectiveness and has the potential for such severe toxicity that its use should be restricted to research efforts directed toward developing more effective treatment. Combination chemotherapy is more effective than single-drug therapy of GI cancer. Chemotherapy added to radiation therapy of locally unresectable GI cancer increases survival over that with radiation therapy alone. No chemotherapy has yet been demonstrated to increase survival in patients undergoing potentially curative resection of GI cancer. It seems likely that chemotherapy can be developed that is capable of eradicating the low tumor cell burden of patients with micrometases. Controlled studies of surgical adjuvant treatment should identify this curative potential of surgical adjuvant chemotherapy if programs active enough to kill all residual cancer cells are developed.

References

1. National Cancer Institute: Third national cancer survey; cancer statistics, 1975. Cancer 25:8, 1975
2. Bateman J R, Irwin L E, Pugh R P, et al: Comparison of intravenous (IV) and oral (PO) administration of 5-fluorouracil (5-FU) for colorectal carcinoma. Proc Am Assoc Cancer Res 16:242, 1975
3. Ansfield F, Klotz J, Nealon T, et al: A phase III study comparing the clinical utility of four regimes of 5-fluorouracil. Cancer 39:23, 1977
4. Hahn R G, Moertel C G, Schutt A J, et al: A double-blind comparison of intensive course 5-fluorouracil by oral vs. intravenous route in the treatment of colorectal carcinoma. Cancer 35:1031, 1975
5. Moertel C G, Reitemeier R J, Bolton C F, et al: Cerebellar ataxia associated with fluorinated pyrimidine therapy. Cancer Chemother Rep 41:15, 1964
6. Roth A, Koloric K, Popovic S: Cardiotoxicity of 5-fluorouracil (NSC-19893). Cancer Chemother Rep 59:1051, 1975
7. Valdivieso M, Bodey G P, Gottlieb J A, et al:

Clinical evaluation of ftorafur (pyrimidine-deoxyribose N,−2′-furanidyl-5-fluorouracil). Cancer Res 36:1821, 1976
8. Moertel C G: Therapy of advanced gastrointestinal cancer with the nitrosoureas. Cancer Chemother Rep 4:27, 1975
9. Broder L E, Carter S K: Pancreatic islet cell carcinoma. Results of therapy with streptozotocin in 52 patients. Ann Int Med 79:108, 1973
10. Vogel C L, Bayley A C, Brooker R J, et al: A phase II study of adriamycin (NSC 123127) in patients with hepatocellular carcinoma from Zambia and the United States. Cancer 39:1923, 1977
11. Frytak S, Moertel C G, Schutt A J, et al: Adriamycin (NSC-123127) therapy for advanced gastrointestinal cancer. Cancer Chemother Rep 59:405, 1975
12. Bellet R E, Engstrom P I, Catalano R B, et al: Phase II study of ICRF-159 in patients with metastatic colorectal carcinoma previously exposed to systemic chemotherapy. Cancer Treat Rep 60:1395, 1976
13. Marciniak T A, Moertel C G, Schutt A J, et al: Phase II study of ICRF-159 (NSC-129943) in advanced colorectal carcinoma. Cancer Chemother Rep 59:761, 1975
14. McCreary R H, Moertel C G, Schutt A J, et al: A phase II study of triazinate (NSC-139105) in advanced colorectal carcinoma. Cancer 40:9-13, 1977
15. Rodriguez V, Richman S P, Benjamin R S, et al: Phase II study with Baker's antifol in solid tumors. Cancer Res 37:980, 1977
16. Falkson G, van Eden E B, Falkson H C: Fluorouracil, imidazole carboxamide dimethyl triazeno, vincristine, and bis-chloroethyl nitrosourea in colon cancer. Cancer 33:1207, 1974
17. Moertel C G, Schutt A J, Hahn R G, et al: Therapy of advanced colorectal cancer with a combination of 5-fluorouracil, methyl-1, 3-cis (2-chlorethyl)-1-nitrosourea, and vincristine. J Nat Cancer Inst 54:69, 1975
18. Falkson G, Falkson H C: Fluorouracil, methyl CCNU and vincristine in cancer of the colon. Cancer 38:1468, 1976
19. Macdonald J S, Kisner D F, Smythe T, et al: 5-fluorouracil (5-FU), methyl CCNU, and vincristine in the treatment of advanced colorectal cancer: Phase II study utilizing weekly 5-FU. Cancer Treat Rep 60:1597, 1976
20. Baker L H, Matter R, Talley R, et al: 5-FU vs. 5-FU and MeCCNU in gastrointestinal cancer. Proc Am Assoc Cancer Res 16:229, 1975
21. Carter S K, Comis R L: Gastric cancer: Current status of treatment. J Nat Cancer Inst 58:567, 1977
22. Kovach J S, Moertel C G, Schutt A J, et al: A controlled study of combined 1, 3-bis (3-chloroethyl)-1-nitrosourea and 5-fluorouracil therapy in advanced gastric and pancreatic cancer. Cancer 57:563, 1974
23. Moertel C G, Hanley J A: Phase II-III studies in chemotherapy of advanced gastric cancer. Proc Am Assoc Cancer Res 16:260, 1975
24. DeJager R L, Magill G B, Golbey R B, et al: Combination chemotherapy with mitomycin C, 5-fluorouracil, and cytosine arabinoside in gastrointestinal cancer. Cancer Treat Rep 60:1373, 1976
25. Ota K, Kurita S, Nishimura M: Combination therapy with mitomycin C (NSC-26980), 5-fluorouracil (NSC-19893), and cytosine arabinoside (NSC-63878) for advanced cancer in man. Cancer Chemother Rep 56:373, 1972
26. Macdonald J, Schein P, Ueno W, et al: 5-fluorouracil (5-FU), mitomycin C (MMC) and adriamcyin (ADR)-FAM: A new combination chemotherapy program for advanced gastric carcinoma. Proc Am Assoc Cancer Res 17:264, 1976
27. Carter S K, Comis R L: The integration of chemotherapy into a combined modality approach for cancer treatment. Pancreatic adenocarcinoma. Cancer Treat Rev 2:193, 1975
28. Wiggans G, Smythe T, Ueno W, et al: Streptozotocin (strep), mitomycin C (MMC) and 5-fluorouracil (5-FU), SMF, chemotherapy for advanced pancreatic carcinoma: Phase II trial. Proc Am Assoc Cancer Res 18:304, 1977
29. Livingston R B, Carter S K: Single Agents in Cancer Chemotherapy. New York, Plenum, 1970
30. Olweny C L M, Toya T, Katongole-Mbidde E, et al: Treatment of hepatocellular carcinoma with adriamcyin. Cancer 36:1250, 1975
31. Broder L E, Carter, S K: Pancreatic islet cell carcinoma. Clinical features of 52 patients. Ann Int Med 79:101, 1973
32. Davis H L, Ramirez G, Ansfield F J: Adenocarcinomas of stomach, pancreas, liver and biliary tracts. Cancer 33:193, 1974
33. Ansfield F J, Ramirez G, Skibba J L, et al: Intrahepatic arterial infusion with 5-fluorouracil. Cancer 28:1147, 1971
34. Moertel C G, Childs D S, Reitemeier R J, et al: Combined 5-fluorouracil and supervoltage radiation therapy of locally unresectable gastrointestinal cancer. Lancet 2:865, 1969
35. Moertel C G: Fluorouracil as an adjuvant to colorectal cancer surgery; the breakthrough that never was. J Am Med Assoc 236:1935, 1976
36. Koyama Y, Kimura T: Controlled clinical trials of chemotherapy as an adjuvant to surgery in gastric carcinoma. Report from Cancer Chemother Coop Res Unit Nat Hosp, Japan 1, 1976

Martin H. Cohen
202-389-7275

13
Chemotherapy of Bronchogenic Carcinoma

Chemotherapy shows great promise in small-cell bronchogenic carcinoma. For this histologic cell type, response rates to chemotherapy alone or with radiation therapy approach 80 to 90 per cent. Approximately 30 to 40 per cent of responses are complete. Survival of complete responders generally exceeds 1 year and prolonged disease-free survivals after completion of induction or maintenance therapy are beginning to be reported.[1,2]

Chemotherapy in patients with epidermoid carcinoma, adenocarcinoma and large-cell anaplastic carcinoma is generally employed when systemic metastases are documented or when there is disease recurrence after radiation therapy. Development of effective chemotherapy regimens for these histologies is proceeding slowly. Recent pilot studies do, however, demonstrate improved response rates with survival prolongation for responding patients. These studies require confirmation.

Because of disappointing results of surgical adjuvant trials using single-agent chemotherapy, there is little activity at present in this area. As new effective drug combinations are discovered, however, one can expect renewed interest in adjuvant trials. Autopsy study[3] of individuals dying within 1 month of curative surgery and a staging laparotomy series[4] both indicate that systemic metastases are commonly present at the time of initial presentation. Chemotherapy will presumably be necessary to control this disease.

In this review of lung cancer chemotherapy, prognostic factors that influence patient response and survival will be emphasized since patient selection can greatly influence therapeutic results. Variations in the way in which data is reported will also be considered since criteria for patient evaluability and response to treatment may vary from one trial to another.

Surgical Adjuvant Trials

Surgical adjuvant trials in non small-cell lung cancer have been limited by defects in study design and by a lack of highly effective single drugs and drug combinations. To determine whether adjuvant treatment is beneficial, one needs comparable patients in the treatment and control groups. This is best accomplished by a suitably stratified, prospectively randomized study design. Use of retrospective controls is suboptimal since there have been recent improvements in staging techniques, changes in staging nomenclature and improvements in supportive care techniques for the lung cancer patient.

Randomized surgical adjuvant trials are listed in Table 13-1. Cyclophosphamide is the

TABLE 13-1. *Randomized Surgical Adjuvant Studies*

Study Plan	Drug Dose and Schedule	Stratification	# of Patients Studied	Results	Reference
Cytoxan vs Placebo	CTX 6mg/kg/d × 5 Repeat 5 weeks later at 8mg/kg/d × 5	"Curative" vs. "Paliative" Resection	1,008	Benefit in small cell patients. No benefit for other histologies	VA Surgical Adjuvant Lung Group[9]
Cytoxan vs. Placebo	CTX 12mg/kg/w for 8 or 9 doses every 4 months for 2 years	None. But results reported by histology, type of surgery and by patient age.	189	Rate of recurrence higher in cytoxan groups	Swiss Group[11]
Cytoxan vs. Placebo	CTX 50-200 mg PO qd for 21 months	Only reports on Epidermoid cancer. No stratification	106	Possible benefit for Cytoxan. Follow up about 1 year	Poulson[8]
Cytoxan vs Busulfan vs. Placebo	CTX 75-200mg PO qd Busulfan 1.5-4mg PO qd for 24 months	None. But results reported by histology, age, sex, type of surgery and by whether mediastinal nodes were involved	492	No benefit for either chemotherapy	British Medical Research Council[7]
Cytoxan vs Alternating Cytoxan-Methotrexate vs Placebo	CTX 8mg/kg/d × 5, q5w alone or alternating with methotrexate 10mg qd × 5, q5w for 18 months	None. But patients had a poor prognosis based on histology or local or regional tumor extension	377	No benefit for either treatment	VA Surgical Adjuvant Lung Group[6]

Cytoxan vs Thiotepa vs Placebo	CTX 1 gm IV q5d to dose of 8-12 gm or thio tepa 20 mg qod to 280-380mg. 50% of drug dose pre-op, 50% post-op	None	301	Benefit for all cell types except adenocarcinoma	Pavlov[10]
Vinblastine vs Placebo	0.1 mg/kg/w or more based on hematologic toxicity for 3 months	None	63	Possible benefit for patients with regional mode involvement and for small cell cancer at 1 year.	Crosbie[12]
Nitrogen Mustard vs Placebo	HN2 0.3-0.4mg/kg divided dose over 3-4 days starting on day of surgery	Stage (Univ. Group) "Curative" vs "Palliative" resection(VA)	2,334	No benefit	University group[13] VA Surgical Adjuvant Group[14]
Combination Chemotherapy vs Placebo	CTX 12mg/kg, 5FU 12mg/kg MTX 0.5 mg/kg. V1b 0.1 mg/kg qwx3 every months	Stage, Histology	83	Benefit for Stage I patients at 1 year Follow up	Austrian Group[128]
CCNU vs Placebo	CCNU 130mg/m² q6w for 2 years	Stage, Histology	Ongoing		Working Party for Lung Cancer
CCNU + Hydroxyurea vs Placebo	CCNU 70mq/m² + HU 1 gm/m² biw for 1 year		Ongoing		VA Surgical Adjuvant Group

most often studied drug. Unfortunately, even this drug has not had an adequate trial. Current concepts for adjuvant treatment indicate that treatment should be given intermittently to avoid a prolonged immunosuppressive effect and that therapy should be continued for a sufficiently long duration to ensure eradication of residual tumor (12-24 months).[5] Using these criteria, only one cytoxan study was therapeutically adequate.[6] Two studies used daily oral drug administration[7,8] while in another two trials patients were treated for only a short period of time.[9,10] One study used weekly parenteral cytoxan administration for 8 or 9 doses every 4 months.[11] Similar criticisms of drug treatment schedules could be made for other single-agent trials utilizing busulfan,[7] vinblastine[12] and nitrogen mustard.[13,14]

Analysis of the above studies is also hampered by a lack of breakdown of treatment and control groups by important prognostic variables. Thus, it is difficult to tell if the various treatment groups in any study are comparable. The primary prognostic variable for surgical adjuvant studies is stage of disease. This is best recorded in the TNM system.[15] Besides the recorded stage, one must also consider the precision with which the stage of disease is established. Patients who are staged after a vigorous preoperative work-up should have a better prognosis than individuals staged less intensively. A second prognostic variable is whether or not a "curative" tumor resection is possible. This is influenced by the location of the tumor, by the age of the patient and by the presence and extent of preexisting lung disease.[16,18] A third prognostic variable relates to the pathologic features of the resected lung specimen, including whether or not there was vascular or lymphatic invasion and whether, if any lymph nodes were involved, was involvement intranodal or did the disease extend into perinodal tissues.[17,19] For surgical adjuvant studies tumor histology, possibly excluding small-cell carcinoma,[20] is of lesser prognostic importance. Several studies indicate that 5-year survival after an apparently curative resection is similar for all histologies.[21-23] Performance status is also of lesser importance since nearly all patients are ambulatory.

During the next several years treatment priorities for operable lung cancer patients can probably be assigned as follows. In Stage I disease,[15] interest will probably lie in immunotherapy trials because of the positive results of the trial of McKneally and co-workers with intrapleural BCG.[24] In Stage II well and moderately well differentiated epidermoid cancer, it would appear reasonable to restudy postoperative radiation therapy because of the low metastatic potential of this histologic cell type[3] and because of promising results of nonrandomized trials.[25,26] It should be pointed out that while randomized trials have not demonstrated benefit for postoperative radiation,[27,28] there are deficiencies in study design in these trials similar to those pointed out for surgical adjuvant chemotherapy studies. For Stage II adenocarcinoma and large-cell anaplastic carcinoma, and for Stage III patients (based on positive ipsilateral mediastinal lymph nodes), chemotherapy is an appropriate surgical adjuvant because of the high probability that the tumor has already spread systemically at the time of surgery.[3,25]

Chemotherapy Plus Radiation Therapy

Radiation therapy is used with curative intent in patients who are nonresectable because of regional tumor extension. While local control of disease within the radiation field may be achieved in 30 to 40 per cent of treated patients[29-33] survival gain has been less impressive.[34,35] The primary reason for the slight survival increase is the presence of subclinical metastatic disease. Consequently, trials of combined chemotherapy plus radiation therapy were undertaken. Table 13-2 lists those trials showing benefit for the combined approach in patients with non-small-cell cancer. Four trials demonstrate benefit when single chemotherapeutic agents are added to radiation therapy.[36-39] As opposed to these results, however, there are four trials comparing radiation therapy alone or with cyclophosphamide in which there was no advantage to the added chemotherapy[40-43] and there are five trials in which no survival benefit accrued to the addition of 5-FU to radiation therapy.[40,44-

TABLE 13-2. *Radiation Therapy Plus Chemotherapy in Non-small Cell Lung Cancer Trials with Positive Results*

Study Design	Radiation Dose/ Duration	Chemotherapy Dose and Schedule	# of Patients	Characteristics of Patients	Results	Reference
RT ± Cytoxan	4000R/4 Weeks	CTX 1 gm/m^2 q3w for 4 or 8 courses	74	Previously untreated Limited disease Adenocarcinomas excluded	Median survival of CTX+RT 327d vs 223d for RT alone. Delay in appearance of systemic metastases with cytoxan treatment	Bergsagel[36]
RT ± 5 FU	4500-5000/4-5 weeks continuous or split	5FU 10 mg/kg/d ×5. Only 1 course with continuous RT, 2 courses with split	30	Previously untreated Limited disease	Benefit in Adenocarcinoma 2yr survival 27% vs 5%	Carr[38]
RT ± Methotrexate	3000R/12 days	MTX 5 mg/IV daily during RT	20	Previously untreated Limited disease Epidermoid cancer only	Improved survival with Methotrexate treatment P = 0.1	Tucker[37]

TABLE 13-2. (continued)

Study Design	Radiation Dose/ Duration	Chemotherapy Dose and Schedule	# of Patients	Characteristics of Patients	Results	Reference
RT ± Bleomycin	2000R/5 days, 3 weeks rest, 2000R/5 days	Bleo 10mg/m^2 biw × 12 doses	30	Previously untreated Limited disease Epidermoid only	Improved response rate and median survival with Bleomycin	Chan[39]
RT + Bleomycin, Vincristine, Methotrexate	3000R/2 weeks, 4 week rest, 3000R/2 weeks RT started after first course of chemo	Bleo 15u biw × 6 doses VCR 2 mg qw × 3 MTX 25-30 mg biw × 6	27	21-Epidermoid 6-Adeno-limited disease, Ambulatory	Response rate 56% median survival responders 70+ weeks vs 26 weeks for nonresponders	Samuels[57]
RT + Cytoxan, Adriamycin, Methotrexate, Procarbazine	3000-4500R/2-3 weeks in 19 of 23 pts	CTX 300 mg/m^2, ADR 20mg/m^2 MTX 15mg/m^2, PROC 100mg/m^2 CAM given day 1 & 8 q 28d PROC given day 1-10 q28d	26	Previously untreated Extensive disease Ambulatory	Response rate of 23 evaluable patients was 48% median survival 12.5 months for responders & stable disease	Bitran[58]

TABLE 13.3. *Bronchogenic Carcinoma—Response to Commonly Used Drugs*

Drug	No. of Patients	Response %	Response Range
Cyclophosphamide	1,513	20	0–63
Mechlorethamine	1,442	31	0–68
Hexamethylmelamine	485	18	10–30
Methotrexate	416	22	3–43

[47] Other studies showed no survival benefit when nitrogen mustard,[48,49] chlorambucil,[50] hydroxyurea,[51-54] vinblastine[55] or procarbazine[54,56] was added to radiation therapy.

Recent pilot studies suggest that radiation therapy plus combination chemotherapy might be beneficial for patients with both limited and extensive disease. As indicated in Table 13-2. Samuels and co-workers obtained a response rate of 50 per cent with significant prolongation of survival in responding patients.[57] Bitran and co-workers obtained corresponding response rates and patient survival in patients with disseminated disease.[58] Both of these studies employed prognostically favorable patients. All of the study patients were ambulatory and none had received prior therapy. Other trials of combination chemotherapy with radiation therapy have been less successful with a suggestive survival disadvantage for the addition to radiotherapy of cyclophosphamide plus MTX for adenocarcinoma patients and nitrogen mustard plus MTX for epidermoid cancer and large-cell anaplastic carcinoma patients.[59]

CHEMOTHERAPY OF NON-SMALL-CELL BRONCHOGENIC CARCINOMA

A major difficulty in the evaluation of chemotherapy results in non-small-cell lung cancer is illustrated in Table 13.3. This table, modified from reports of Selawry [60-62] indicates the range of response rates reported for each of four commonly used single agents in lung cancer patients. Response rates with these agents varied from 0 to 70 per cent. An important cause for the observed variation in response is the type of patient studied in these various trials. Inclusion of good prognosis patients will increase response rates and survival, while study of poor prognosis patients will have the opposite effect. Important prognostic factors are stage of disease,[63] performance status,[64] prior treatment[65] and immune status.[66,67] Histology is of lesser importance although there are slight differences in responsiveness to radiation therapy[68] and to chemotherapy[61,62] in the non-small-cell lung cancers. Good prognosis patients have tumors confirmed to chest, are asymptomatic and completely ambulatory, have received no prior therapy and have intact delayed hypersensitivity measured both in vivo and in vitro. Poor prognosis patients have metastatic disease, are bedridden because of tumor symptoms, have received prior radiotherapy and/or chemotherapy and have impaired reactivity to delayed hypersensitivity tests.

Table 13-4 lists several promising pilot studies in non-small-cell lung cancer. All of these trials require confirmation by other investigators. Characteristics of study patients are recorded in Table 13-4. Generally patients with no prior therapy were studied. The majority of patients were ambulatory and most had metastatic disease. Since response rates in these trials were generally less than 50 per cent, one would expect little change in median survival for the total study population. The results are, therefore, reported as median survival of responding patients compared to survival of nonresponding patients. While this type of reporting may be criticized as selecting out a favorable group of patients who would do well irrespective of therapy, it does provide an indication of drug activity. Furthermore, it provides an indication of the toxicity of treatment since regimens yielding a high response rate with little difference in

TABLE 13-4. *Chemotherapy of Non-Small Cell Lung Cancer*

Regimen	No. of Patients	Characteristics of Study Patients	Response Rate %	Median Survival (Months) Overall	Responders	Non-Responders	Reference
Methotrexate plus citrovorum factor	11	Half had limited disease. Most had no prior therapy	90% (not all had 50% tumor shrinkage).	7	7	4.5	Djerassi[69]
Cytoxan, Fluorouracil, methotrexate vinblastine, rufochromomycin	188	Extensive disease Ambulatory and non-ambulatory	—	7.2 epid 5.2 adeno	—	—	Israel[78]
Cytoxan, 5FU, 6TG Methotrexate, Vincristine ± Heparin	28	Limited and extensive All had prior therapy	Heparin 50 Chemo alone 0	—			Elias[71]
Cytoxan, Vincristine, Methyl-CCNU and Bleomycin (Comb)	58	No prior therapy limited and extensive disease Epidermoid and adeno	epid. 37 adeno 11	2 epid 5.5 adeno	3 epid 10 adeno	2 5	Livingston[79]
Bleomycin, Adriamycin CCNU, Vincristine, Nitrogen Mustard (Bacon)	50	76% Extensive 24% Limited All performance levels	Extensive 45 Limited 33	4 Ext 7.5 Ltd	6 —	2 —	Livingston[80]
Methotrexate, Cytoxan Procarbazine, Vincristine,	118	32 pts had prior therapy Majority of patients were	Epidermoid; simultaneous 33 sequential 13 small cell		11 small 11 epid Responders and stable	4	Alberto[81]

simultaneous or sequential		ambulatory. About 50% had limited disease	simultaneous 65 sequential 36		disease		
Cytoxan, Methotrexate	28	26 with extensive disease 9 with prior radiation 22 ambulatory	Large cell 5/7=70 Adeno 5/8=62 Small 10/11=90	12 7 12	—	—	Straus[74]
Adriamycin, 5FU, Methotrexate	11	Extensive disease. Approx. half had prior therapy. Only adenocarcinoma	5/11=45	—	2+ - 7+	0.5	Lowitz[82]
Adriamycin, CCNU Hydroxyurea	28	Extensive disease. 4 patients had prior therapy.	Epid 1/11 = 10 Large Cell 3/7 = 43 Small 3/5 = 60 Adeno 0/3 = 0	—	4-32	1-5	Alberto[83]
CCNU, Adriamycin Hexamethylme lamine	8	Extensive disease 3 had prior radiation	Epid 3/3 Anaplastic 3/3	—	4-15	—	Wilson[84]
Cytoxan or Nitrogen Mustard, Methotrexate vs. CCNU, Cytoxan or Nitrogen Mustard Methotrexate	206	Extensive disease No prior therapy	Epid and Large Cell 10% on 2 or 3 drugs. Small cell 3 drugs 56 2 drugs 38 Adeno, 3 drugs 38 2 drugs 6	—	8.5 small 8 Adeno	3 6	Hansen[75]
Methotrexate, Adriamycin, Cytoxan, CCNU	31	Not stated	Epid 4/9 Adeno 4/13 Small 2/3 Large 2/3	—	3-15	—	Chahinian[85]

TABLE 13-5. *Non Small-Cell Bronchogenic Carcinoma Ineffective Drug Regimens As Tested*

Regimen	Reference
Bleomycin, Cytoxan, Vincristine, Methotrexate 5-Fluorouracil	Lanzotti[86]
Hexamethylmelamine, CCNU, Methotrexate	DiBella[87]
Meccnu, Cytoxan, Vinctistine, Methotrexate Bleomycin	McMahon[88]
Meccnu, Vincristine or Meccnu, Vincristine Methotrexate	Richards[89]
Vincristine, Bleomycin, Adriamycin	Eagan[90]
Nitrogen Mustard, CCNU	Edmonson[91]
Heparin, Cytoxan	Edlis[72]

survival of responders versus nonresponders are likely to be highly toxic.

Four of the reports in Table 13-4 include new treatment approaches. Djerassi indicates that high-dosage MTX with citrovorum factor rescue was beneficial in a small number of patients.[67] Unfortunately, a recent attempt to confirm this data has been unsuccessful.[70] Elias has shown that combination chemotherapy plus heparin yields tumor shrinkage, while the same drugs without heparin does not.[71] Two attempts to confirm the efficacy of heparin administration in prolonging response and survival of cyclophosphamide-treated patients have been unsuccessful.[72,73] The report by Straus is interesting in that dosage modifications for hematologic toxicity were different than those usually employed.[74] As a result, considerably more drug could be administered for comparable degrees of hematologic toxicity. Perhaps this explains the 62 per cent response rate in adenocarcinoma in this study as compared to a 6 per cent response rate in adenocarcinoma in Hansen's trial,[75] in which doses of cytoxan and methotrexate were conventionally modified for hematologic toxicity.

The Eastern Cooperative Oncology Group is attempting to confirm Straus' results. Finally, Dimitrov has utilized a combined chemotherapy-immunotherapy approach. He found that concomitant administration of *Corynebacterium parvum* with adriamycin was associated with decreased hematologic toxicity and with prolonged survival when compared to a randomized control group receiving adriamycin alone.[76]

If one looks at the drug combinations listed in Table 13-4, it is evident that adriamycin is present in a number of active combinations. This is in contrast to its relatively limited activity as a single agent in lung cancer.[77] Other pilot studies yielding favorable results are included in the table.[78-85]

In contrast to the above reports, several newly tested drug combinations have not demonstrated any beneficial effect. These are listed in Table 13-5.[86-91] Several of these combinations include vincristine and bleomycin, suggesting that these two drugs may have only limited utility in non small-cell lung cancer.

SMALL-CELL CARCINOMA

Small-cell (including oat-cell) bronchogenic carcinoma is highly responsive to many chemotherapeutic agents and to radiation therapy. Active drugs include cyclophosphamide, nitrogen mustard, procarbazine, nitrosoureas, adriamycin,[92] vincristine,[93] hexamethylmelamine[94] and VP-16-316 (epipodophyllotoxin ethylidene glucopyranoside).[95,96] When these drugs are combined together in any of several two-to-four-drug combinations, response rates of up to 90 per cent have been reported. Unfortunately, survival gain has been less impressive and for patients with metastatic disease, median survival is generally less than 1 year.

In evaluating clinical trials in small-cell cancer, one must be aware of the prognostic factors that influence therapeutic response and survival. As in other lung cancer studies, stage of disease at presentation and patient performance status are the two principal prognostic variables. Prior therapy and immune reactivity are also important.

Because small-cell cancer generally presents as disseminated disease, neither surgery nor radiation therapy alone is optimal therapy.[97] Chemotherapy is the principal therapeutic modality for this disease. An important question being asked in many of the current small-cell cancer therapy trials is whether addition of radiation therapy to chemotherapy will prolong survival. In present trials radiation therapy is usually directed to sites of bulk disease (the presenting lung lesion and mediastinum) and to chemotherapy sanctuaries (the brain). It is clear that one generally obtains higher response rates in protocols using combined chemotherapy-radiation therapy than with chemotherapy alone. There is also the suggestion that recurrence of disease within the thorax may be delayed. Unfortunately, there is little to no information from postmortem studies on the frequency of tumor sterilization within the irradiated field. This information is critical for planning future therapeutic trials. The price paid for the use of radiation therapy in these studies includes decreased tolerance to chemotherapy (proportional to radiation dose, fractionation and field size),[98] an increased incidence of chemotherapy side effects, especially in regimens using adriamycin[99] and a decreased ability, because of the frequent occurrence of radiation pneumonitis and fibrosis, to use the chest roentgenogram for following changes in tumor size.[100]

Table 13-6 lists chemotherapy and combined chemotherapy radiation therapy trials in small-cell cancer.[101-121] A problem with developing drug combinations for small-cell cancer is that all of the active single agents enumerated earlier, except vincristine and to a lesser extent hexamethylmelamine, have myelosuppression as their principal toxicity. Thus, as the number of drugs in a combination increases, one must decrease the optimal single dose of each drug proportionately. If the combination does not include vincristine, a three-drug combination may be optimal, and if vincristine is included, then four drugs may be used together. Table 13-6 indicates the popularity of three-drug combinations compared to trials utilizing two or four drugs. Since current median survival with chemotherapy alone or with radiation therapy is 6 to 8 months for patients with extensive disease and 10 to 14 months for patients with limited disease, new treatment approaches are necessary. From the chemotherapy standpoint, one approach is to use non-cross-resistant drug combinations in fixed alternating sequences so as to delay development of drug resistance.[122] Intensive induction therapy to considerable leukopenia appears to be of greater utility than more standard induction therapy, both in terms of initial response rates and patient survival.[104] With regard to radiation therapy, further study of optimal dosage and fractionation of therapy are necessary. The timing of radiation therapy administration relative to chemotherapy also has to be studied.

The aim of small-cell cancer treatment is to obtain a complete response (defined as complete disappearance of all evident tumor). Lesser degrees of response are unlikely to be associated with prolonged survival. In this regard, one must be concerned with the type of evaluation employed to determine completeness of response. For intrathoracic disease, bronchoscopy provides independent information from the chest roentgenogram.[123] For systemic disease, routine evaluation usually includes bone, brain and liver scans and bone marrow aspiration and biopsy. Any of these tests that are initially abnormal should be repeated before considering the patient as a complete responder. An important aspect of future therapeutic trials will be the evaluation of newer diagnostic procedures to determine the presence of abdominal disease including peritoneoscopy for liver evaluation,[124] computerized axial tomography[125] and abdominal sonography.[126,127]

A final aspect of lung cancer chemotherapy trials relates to variations in the way in which data is reported. It is necessary that uniform criteria of response be adopted. In addition, if patients with stable disease are included as responders, this should be clearly specified. It is necessary in survival calculations to indicate the starting point for these calculations. Is it day one of treatment—the date of diagnosis or the date of first symptoms? Criteria for patient evaluability must also be indicated. Are all eligible patients evaluable or does the study exclude patients who die before a specified time? Exclusion of these patients will serve to increase response rates and survival.

Perhaps, in the future, guidelines for the reporting of lung cancer trials will be adopted.

TABLE 13-6. *Combination Chemotherapy for Small Cell Lung Cancer*

Regimen	Prognostic Factors	No. of Patients	Response Rate %	Median Survival (Months)	Reference
2 Drug Combinations					
Cytoxan, CCNU	17% Limited disease 81% Ambulatory 51% No prior therapy	110	43	5	Edmonson [101]
Cytoxan, Methotrexate, + Radiation Therapy for Limited disease	50% Limited disease No prior therapy	8	100	12 Limited 7.5 Extensive	Hansen[102]
Cytoxan, Methotrexate	100% Extensive disease No prior therapy	24	38	8 mo. for Responders 3 mo. for Non-responders	Hansen[75]
Cytoxan, Methotrexate	100% Extensive disease 2 had prior radiation 9 Ambulatory	11	90	10	Straus[74]
Cytoxan, Vincristine + radiation therapy for limited disease	41% Limited disease 97% Ambulatory 94% No prior therapy	39	94 Limited 64 Extensive	12 Limited 6 Extensive	Holoye[103]
3 Drug Combinations					
Cytoxan, Methotrexate CCNU (Standard Dose)	100% Extensive disease No prior therapy	30	56	9	Hansen[75]
Cytoxan, Methotrexate CCNU (High Dose)	88% Extensive disease No Prior therapy 90% Ambulatory	32	96	11	Cohen[104]
Cytoxan, Vincristine Methotrexate, Radiation	84% Extensive	30	85	9.5	Eagan[105]
Cytoxan, Vincristine, Methotrexate, Radiation	94% Extensive	18	72	11 (Responders) 2 (Non-responders)	Bitran[106]

Adriamycin, Cytoxan Vincristine, Radiation BCG	72% Extensive dis. No prior therapy	29	100	6+	Hornback[107]
Cytoxan, Adriamycin DTIC	Not given	13	75	Not Given	Lowenbraun[108]
Cytoxan, Adriamycin Vincristine, Radiation for 12 weeks	52% Limited disease No Prior therapy	21	95 Complete	10 + Limited 6 + Extensive	Johnson[109]
Cytoxan, Procarbazine Vincristine ± Radiation	33% Limited disease	18	78	12 Responders	Davis[110]
MeCCNU, Cytoxan Vincristine ± Radiation	31% Prior therapy	26	54	10	Taylor[111]
Vincristine, Bleomycin, Adriamycin	No prior therapy	13	38	8	Eagan[95]
Cytoxan, Adriamycin VP-16, MER	No information	11	73	Too soon	Aisner [112]
CCNU, Cytoxan Vincristine, Radiation	No prior therapy	19	94	10+ CR 7+ PR	Comis[113]
Cytoxan, Adriamycin Vincristine, Radiation	32% Limited disease	100	67	6 Extensive 5+ Limited	Livingston[114]
		4 or More Drugs			
BCNU, Cytoxan, Vincristine, Procarbazine ± Radiation	14% Prior therapy 26% Limited disease	43	53	7+	Abeloff[15]

TABLE 13-6. *Combination Chemotherapy for Small Cell Lung Cancer (continued)*

Regimen	Prognostic Factors	No. of Patients	Response Rate %	Median Survival (Months)	Reference
Cytoxan, Vincristine, Procarbazine, Prednisone ± Radiation	7% Prior Therapy 54% Limited disease	28	93	10	Nixon[116]
Bleomycin, Adriamycin Cytoxan, Vincristine	No prior therapy 14% Limited disease	29	72	8	Einhorn[117]
Methotrexate, Cytoxan Procarbazine, Vincristine	Ambulatory About 30% had prior therapy 50% limited disease	53	80 Limited 50 Extensive	10	Alberto[81]
Cytoxan, CCNU, Methotrexate, Vincristine	No information	49	83	9	Hansen[118]
Cytoxan, Adriamycin Methotrexate, CCNU Alternate with Bleomycin Vincristine, Dehydroemetine	No information	24	83	8 partial 17+ complete	Israel[119]
Procarbazine, Vincristine Cytoxan, CCNU, Radiation	No information	39	not given	11	Glatstein[120]
Cytoxan, CCNU, Procarb, Adriamycin, Vincristine Methotrexate, Radiation	29% Limited disease	17	90	5.5 extensive	Levitt[121]

REFERENCES

1. Cohen M H, Fossieck B E, Creaven P J, Minna J D: Intensive chemotherapy of small cell bronchogenic carcinoma. Proc Am Soc Clin Oncol 16:273, 1976
2. Johnson R E, Brereton H D, Kent H C: Small cell carcinoma of the lung. Attempt to remedy causes of past therapeutic failure. Lancet 2:289–291, 1976
3. Matthews M J, Kanhouwa S, Pickren J, Robinette D: Frequency of residual and metastatic tumor in patients undergoing curative resection for lung cancer. Cancer Chemother Rep 4:63–67, 1973
4. Bell J W: Abdominal exploration in 100 lung carcinoma suspects prior to thoracotomy. Ann Surg 167:199–203, 1968
5. Carter S K: Some thoughts on surgical adjuvant studies in lung cancer. Cancer Chemother Rep 4:109–117, 1973
6. Shields T W, Robinette D, Keehn R J: Bronchial carcinoma treated by adjuvant cancer chemotherapy. Arch Surg 109:329–333, 1974
7. Stott H, Stephens R J, Fox W, Roy D C: 5 year follow-up of cytotoxic chemotherapy as an adjuvant to surgery in carcinoma of the bronchus. Br J Cancer 34:167–173, 1976
8. Poulson O: Cyclophosphamide. An evaluation of its cytostatic effects on surgically treated carcinoma of the lung. J Int Coll Surg 37:177–187, 1962
9. Higgin G A Jr: Use of chemotherapy as an adjunct to surgery for bronchogenic carcinoma. Cancer 30:1383–1387, 1972
10. Pavlov A, Pirigov A, Trachtenberg A, et al: Results of combination treatment of lung cancer patients. Surgery plus radiotherapy and surgery plus chemotherapy. Cancer Chemother Rep 4:133–135, 1973
11. Brunner K W, Marthaler T, Muller W: Effects of long term adjuvant chemotherapy with cyclophosphamide (NSC 26271) for radically resected bronchogenic carcinoma. Cancer Chemother Rep 4:125–132, 1973
12. Crosbie W A, Kamdar H H, Belcher J R: A controlled trial of vinblastine sulphate in the treatment of cancer of the lung. Br J Dis Chest 60:28–35, 1966
13. Slack N H: Bronchogenic carcinoma: Nitrogen mustard as a surgical adjuvant and factors influencing survival. University surgical adjuvant lung project. Cancer 25:987–1002, 1970
14. Shields T W: Status report on adjuvant cancer chemotherapy trials in the treatment of bronchial carcinoma. Cancer Chemother Rep 4:119–124, 1973
15. Mountain C F, Carr D T, Anderson W A: A system for the clinical staging of lung cancer. Am J Roentogenol 120:130–138, 1974
16. Watson W L: Extended surgical procedures at Memorial Hospital, in Watson W L (ed): Lung Cancer. A study of 5000 Memorial Hospital Cases. St. Louis, C V Mosby, 1968 p 299–307
17. Bergh N P, Schersten T: Bronchogenic carcinoma. A follow-up study of a surgically treated series with special reference to the prognostic significance of lymph node metastases. Acta Chir Scand Suppl 347:1–42, 1965
18. Shields T W, Higgins G A, Keehn R J: Factors influencing survival after resection of bronchogenic carcinoma. J Thorac Cardiovasc Surg 64:391–399, 1972
19. Spjut H J, Roper C L, Butcher H R: Pulmonary cancer and its prognosis. A study of the relationship of certain factors to survival of patients treated by pulmonary resection. Cancer 14:1251–1258, 1961
20. Mountain C F: Keynote address on surgery in the therapy of lung cancer: Surgical prospects and priorities for clinical research. Cancer Chemother Rep 4:19–24, 1973
21. Ashor G L, Kern W H, Meyer B W, et al: Long term survival in bronchogenic carcinoma. J Thorac Cardiovasc Surg 70:581–589, 1975
22. Higgins R A, Shields T W, Keehn R J: The solitary pulmonary nodule. 10 year follow-up of Veterans Administration-Armed Forces cooperative study. Arch Surg 110:570–575, 1975
23. Vincent R G, Takita H, Lane W W, et al: Surgical therapy of lung cancer. J Thorac Cardiovasc Surg 71:581–591, 1976
24. McKneally M F, Maver C, Kausel H W: Regional immunotherapy of lung cancer with intrapleural BCG. Lancet 1:377–379, 1976
25. Kirsh M M, Kahn D R, Gago O, et al: Treatment of bronchogenic carcinoma with mediastinal metastases. Ann Thorac Surg 12:11–18, 1971
26. Green N, Kurohara S A, George F W III, Crews Q E Jr: Postresection irradiation for primary lung cancer. Radiology 116:405–407, 1975
27. Bangma P J: Postoperative radiotherapy, in Deeley T H(ed): Modern Radiotherapy. Carcinoma of the Bronchus. New York, Appleton-Century-Crofts, 1971, p 163–170
28. Patterson R, Russell M H: Clinical trials in malignant disease. IV. Lung cancer. Value of postoperative radiotherapy. Clin Radiol 13:141–144, 1962

29. Bloedorn F G, Cowley C A, Cuccia R, et al: Preoperative irradiation in bronchogenic carcinoma. Am J Roentgenol 92:77–87, 1964
30. Shields T W, Higgins G A Jr, Lawton R, et al: Preoperative x-ray therapy as an adjuvant in the treatment of bronchogenic carcinoma. J Thorac Cardiovasc Surg 59:49–61, 1970
31. Abadir R, Muggia F M: Irradiated lung cancer. An autopsy analysis of spread pattern. Radiology 114:427–430, 1975
32. Rissanen P M, Tikka U, Holsti L R: Autopsy findings in lung cancer treated with megavoltage ratiotherapy. Acta Radiol (Ther) (Stockholm) 7:433–441, 1968
33. Guttman R: Radical supervoltage therapy in inoperable carcinoma of the lung, in Deeley T J (ed): Modern Radiotherapy Carcinoma of the Bronchus. New York, Appleton-Century-Crofts, 1971, p 181–195
34. Roswit B, Patno M E, Rapp R, et al: The survival of patients with inoperable lung cancer. A large scale randomized trial of radiation therapy versus placebo. Radiology 90:688–697, 1968
35. Wolf J, Patno M E, Roswit B, D'Esopo N: Controlled study of survival of patients with clinically inoperable lung cancer treated with radiation therapy. Am J Med 40:360–367, 1966
36. Bergsagel J E, Jenkin R D T, Pringle J F, et al: Lung cancer: Clinical trial of radiotherapy alone vs. radiotherapy plus cyclophosphamide. Cancer 30:621–627, 1972
37. Tucker R D, Sealy R, Van Wyk C, et al: A clinical trial of methotrexate (NSC 740) and radiation therapy for squamous cell carcinoma of the lung. Cancer Chemother Rep 4:157–158, 1973
38. Carr D T, Childs D S Jr, Lee R E: Radiotherapy plus 5FU compared to radiotherapy alone for inoperable and unresectable bronchogenic carcinoma. Cancer 29:375–380, 1972
39. Chan P Y M, Byfield J E, Kagan A R, Aronstam E M: Unresectable squamous cell carcinoma of the lung and its management by combined bleomycin and radiotherapy. A clinical study of the enhanced results. Cancer 37:2671–2676, 1976
40. Gollin F F, Ansfield F J, Vermund H: Continued studies of combined chemotherapy and irradiation in inoperable bronchogenic carcinoma. Cancer Chemother Rep 51:189–192, 1967
41. Brouet D: Results of a trial using radiotherapy and chemotherapy in bronchial cancer. Eur J Cancer 4:437–445, 1968
42. Host H: Cyclophosphamide (NSC 26271) as an adjuvant to radiotherapy in the treatment of unresectable bronchogenic carcinoma. Cancer Chemother Rep 4:161–164, 1973
43. Kaung D T, Wolf J, Hyde L, Zelen M: Preliminary report on the treatment of nonresectable cancer of the lung. Cancer Chemother Rep 58:359–364, 1974
44. Hosley H F, Marangoudakis S, Ross C A, et al: Combined radiation–chemotherapy for bronchogenic carcinoma—Pilot study. Cancer Chemother Rep 16:467–471, 1962
45. Hall T C, Dederick M M, Chalmers T C, et al: A clinical pharmacologic study of chemotherapy and x-ray therapy in lung cancer. Am J Med 43:186–193, 1967
46. Cohen J L, Krant M J, Shnider B I, et al: Radiation plus 5-fluorouracil (NSC 19893): Clinical demonstration of an additive effect in bronchogenic carcinoma. Cancer Chemother Rep 4:253–258, 1971
47. Holsti L R: Alternative approaches to radiotherapy alone and radiotherapy as part of a combined therapeutic approach for lung cancer. Cancer Chemother Rep 4:165–169, 1973
48. Krant M J, Chalmers T C, Dederick M M, et al: Comparative trial of chemotherapy and radiotherapy in patients with non resectable cancer of the lung. Am J Med 35:363–373, 1963
49. Durrant K R, Ellis F, Black J M, et al: Comparison of treatment policies in inoperable bronchial carcinoma. Lancet 1:715–719, 1971
50. Horwitz H, Wright T L, Perry H, Barrett C M: Suppressive chemotherapy in bronchogenic carcinoma. A randomized prospective clinical trial. Am J Roentgenol 93:615–638, 1965
51. LePar E, Faust D S, Brady L W, Beckloff G L: Clinical evaluation of the adjunctive use of hydroxyurea (NSC 32065) in radiation therapy of carcinoma of the lung. Radiol Clin Biol 36:32–40, 1967
52. Landgren R C, Hussey D H, Barkley H T Jr, Samuels M L: Split-course irradiation compared to split course irradiation plus hydroxyurea in inoperable bronchogenic carcinoma. Cancer 34:1598–1601, 1974
53. Scheer A C, Wilson R F, Kalisher L: Combined radiotherapy and hydroxyurea in the management of lung cancer. Clin Radiol 25:415–418, 1974
54. Hall T C, Pocock S, Horton J: Procarbazine and hydroxyurea as radiosensitizers in lung cancer. Medical Pediat Oncol 1977, (in press)
55. Coy P: A randomized study of irradiation and vinblastine in lung cancer. Cancer 26:803–807, 1970
56. Landgren R C, Hussey D H, Samuels M L, Leary W V: A randomized study comparing

irradiation alone to irradiation plus procarbazine in inoperable bronchogenic carcinoma. Radiology 108:403–406, 1973

57. Samuels M L, Barkley H T, Holoye P Y, et al: Combination chemotherapy with bleomycin (NSC 125066), vincristine (NSC 67574), and methotrexate (NSC 740) plus split-course radiotherapy in the treatment of non-oat cell bronchogenic carcinoma. Cancer Chemother Rep 59:377–383, 1975
58. Bitran J D, Desser R K, DeMeester T R, et al: Cyclophosphamide adriamycin, methotrexate and procarbazine (CAMP): Effective 4 drug combination chemotherapy for metastatic non-oat cell bronchogenic carcinoma. Cancer Treat Rep 60:1225–1230, 1976
59. Hansen H H, Selawry O S: Personal communication
60. Selawry O S: On chemotherapy of lung cancer, in Israel L, Chahinian A P (eds): Lung Cancer Natural History, Prognosis and Therapy. New York, Academic Press, 1976, 205–239
61. Selawry O S: The role of chemotherapy in the treatment of lung cancer. Semin Oncol 1:259–272, 1974
62. Selawry O S: Monochemotherapy of bronchogenic carcinoma with special reference to cell type. Cancer Chemother Rep 4:177–188, 1973
63. Lanzotti V J, Thomas D R, Boyle L E, et al: Survival with inoperable lung cancer. An integration of prognostic variables based on simple clinical criteria. Cancer 39:303–313, 1977
64. Zelen M: Keynote address on biostatistics and data retrieval. Cancer Chemother Rep 4:31–42, 1973
65. Zelen M: Importance of prognostic factors in planning therapeutic trials, in Staquet M J (ed): Cancer Therapy: Prognostic Factors and Criteria of Response. New York, Raven Press, 1975, p 1–6
66. Israel L, Muggica J, Chahinian P H: Prognoses of early bronchogenic carcinoma. Survival curves of 451 patients after resection of lung cancer in relation to the results of preoperative tuberculin skin test. Biomedicine 19:68–72, 1973
67. Oldham R K, Weese J L, Herberman R B, et al: Immunological monitoring and immunotherapy in carcinoma of the lung. Int J Cancer 18:739–749, 1976
68. Salazar O M, Rubin P, Brownn J C, et al: Predictors of radiation response in lung cancer. A clinico-pathobiological analysis. Cancer 37:2636–2650, 1976
69. Djerassi I, Rominger C J, Kim J S, et al: Phase I study of methotrexate with citrovorum factor in patients with lung cancer. Cancer 30:22–30, 1972
70. Minna J, Pelsor F, Ihde D, Cohen M: High dose methotrexate—Citrovorum factor rescue treatment of adeno and large cell carcinoma of the lung. Proc Am Assoc Cancer Res and ASCO 18:289, 1977
71. Elias E G, Shukla S K, Mink I B: Heparin and chemotherapy in the management of inoperable lung cancer. Cancer 36:129–136, 1975
72. Edlis H E, Goudsmit A, Brindley C, Niemetz J: Trial of heparin and cyclophosphamide (NSC 26271) in the treatment of lung cancer. Cancer Treat Rep 60:575–578, 1976
73. Conroy J, Brodsky I, Kahn S B, Elias E: Anticoagulation in the treatment of inoperable lung cancer. Proc Am Soc Clin Oncol 17:277, 1976
74. Straus M J: Combination chemotherapy in advanced lung cancer with increased survival. Cancer 38:2232–2241, 1976
75. Hansen H H, Selawry O S, Simon R, et al: Combination chemotherapy of advanced lung cancer. A randomized trial. Cancer 38: 2201–2207, 1976
76. Dimitrov N V, Singh T, Conroy J, Suhrland G L: Combination therapy with *C. parvum* and adriamycin in patients with lung cancer. Proc Am Assoc Cancer Res and ASCO 17:292, 1976
77. Selawry O S: Response of bronchogenic carcinoma to adriamycin (NSC 123127). Cancer Chemother Rep 6:349–351, 1976
78. Israel L, Depierre A, Chahinian P: Combination chemotherapy in 418 cases of advanced cancer. Cancer 27:1089–1093, 1971
79. Livingston R B, Einhorn L H, Bodey G P, et al: COMB (cyclophosphamide, oncovin, methyl CCNU and bleomycin): A four-drug combination in solid tumors. Cancer 36:327–332, 1975
80. Livingston R B, Einhorn L H, Burgess M A, et al: Combination chemotherapy with bleomycin (NSC 125066), adriamycin (NSC 123127) CCNU (NSC 79037), vincristine (NSC 67574) and mechlorethamine (NSC 762) (BACON) in squamous cell lung cancer. Experience with 50 patients. Cancer Chemother Rep 6:361–367, 1975
81. Alberto P, Brunner K W, Martz G, et al: Treatment of bronchogenic carcinoma with simultaneous or sequential combination chemotherapy, including methotrexate, cyclophosphamide, procarbazine and vincristine. Cancer 38:2208–2216, 1976
82. Lowitz B B: Phase II trial of 5-fluorouracil

(NSC 19893), adriamycin (NSC 123127) and methotrexate (NSC 740) in lung adenocarcinoma. Cancer Treat Rep 60:623–624, 1976

83. Alberto P, Barreler L, Chapuis B, Garcia B: A combination of adriamycin, CCNU and hydroyurea in the treatment of disseminated bronchogenic carcinoma. Eur J Cancer 11:795–799, 1975
84. Wilson W L, Andrews N C, Frelick R W, et al: Preliminary report on the use of CCNU (NSC 79037), adriamycin (NSC 123127), and hexamethylmelamine (NSC 13875) in carcinoma of the lung. Cancer Treat Rep 60:269–271, 1976
85. Chahinian P, Cohen J, Purpora O, Jaffrey I S: Chemotherapy of bronchogenic carcinoma with methotrexate, adriamycin, cyclophosphamide and CCNU. Proc Am Assoc Cancer Res and ASCO 17:287, 1976
86. Lanzotti V J, Thomas D R, Holoye P Y, et al: Bleomycin (NSC 125066) followed by cyclophosphamide (NSC 26271), vincristine (NSC 67574), methotrexate (NSC 740) and 5-fluorouracil (NSC 19893) for non-oat cell bronchogenic carcinoma. Cancer Treat Rep 60:61–68, 1976
87. DiBella N J, Nelson R A, Norgard M J: Combination chemotherapy with CCNU (NSC 79037), hexamethylmelamine (NSC 13875) and methotrexate in advanced bronchogenic carcinoma. Oncology 32:82–85, 1975
88. McMahon L J, Jones S E, Durie B G M, Salmon S E: Combination chemotherapy with methyl-CCNU (NSC 95441) cyclophosphamide (NSC 26271), vincristine (NSC 67574) methotrexate (NSC 740) and bleomycin (NSC 125066) in advanced bronchogenic carcinoma. Cancer Letters 1:97–102, 1975
89. Richards F II, Cooper M R, Muss H B, et al: Methyl-CCNU alone and in combination with vincristine, or vincristine and methotrexate, in advanced bronchogenic carcinoma. Cancer 38:1077–1082, 1976
90. Eagan R T, Carr D T, Coles D T, et al: ICRF-159 versus polychemotherapy in non-small cell lung cancer. Cancer Treat Rep 60: 947–948, 1976
91. Edmonson J H, Lagakos S, Stolbach L, et al: Mechlorethamine (NSC 762) plus CCNU (NSC 79037) in the treatment of inoperable squamous and large cell carcinoma of the lung. Cancer Treat Rep 60:625–627, 1976
92. Wasserman T H, Comis R L, Goldsmith M, et al: Tabular analysis of the clinical chemotherapy of solid tumors. Cancer Chemother Rep 6:399–419, 1976
93. Dombernowsky P, Hansen H H, Sorenson P G, Hainau B: Vincristine (NSC 67574) in the treatment of small cell anaplastic carcinoma of the lung. Cancer Treat Rep 60:239–242, 1976
94. Takita H, Didolkar M S: Effect of hexamethylmelamine (NSC 13875) on small cell carcinoma of the lung. Cancer Chemother Rep 58:371–374, 1974
95. Eagan R T, Carr D T, Frytak S, et al: VP-16-213 versus polychemotherapy in patients with advanced small cell lung cancer. Cancer Treat Rep 60:949–951, 1976
96. Cohen M H, Broder L E, Fossieck B E, et al: Phase II trial of weekly administration of 4-demethylepipodophyllotoxin 9-(4,6-0-ethylidene-3-D-glucopyranoside) (NSC 141540, EPEG, VP-16-213) in small cell bronchogenic carcinoma. Cancer Treat Rep 61: 489–490, 1977
97. Miller A B, Fox W, Tall R: Five year follow-up of the Medical Research Council trial of surgery and radiotherapy for the primary treatment of small celled or oat-celled carcinoma of the bronchus. Lancet 2:501–505, 1969
98. Lewis C L, Paterson E: Leukopenia after postmastectomy irradiation. JAMA 235: 747–748, 1976
99. Greco F A, Brereton H D, Kent H, et al: Adriamycin and enhanced radiation reaction in normal esophagus and skin. Ann Int Med 85:294–296, 1976
100. Lamoureux K B: Diagnostic problems after radiotherapy involving the lung. South Med J 66:1388–1392, 1973
101. Edmonson J H, Lagakos S W, Selawry O S, et al: Cyclophosphamide and CCNU in the treatment of inoperable small cell carcinoma and adenocarcinoma of the lung. Cancer Treat Rep 60:925–932, 1976
102. Hansen H H, Muggia F M, Andrews R, Selawry O S: Intensive combined chemotherapy and radiotherapy in patients with non-resectable bronchogenic carcinoma. Cancer 30:315–324, 1972
103. Holoye P Y, Samuels M L: Cyclophosphamide, vincristine and sequential split-course radiotherapy in the treatment of small cell lung cancer. Chest 67:675–679, 1975
104. Cohen M H, Fossieck B E, Creaven P J, Minna J D: Intensive chemotherapy of small cell bronchogenic carcinoma. Proc Am Assoc Cancer Res and ASCO 17:273, 1976
105. Eagan R T, Maurer L H, Forcier R J, Tulloh M: Small cell carcinoma of the lung: Staging, paraneoplastic syndromes, treatment and survival. Cancer 33:527–532, 1974
106. Bitran J, Golomb H H, Desser R K, Colman M: Prolonged survival of patients with exten-

sive oat-cell carcinoma treated with radiotherapy and cyclophosphamide (NSC 26271), vincristine (NSC 67574), and methotrexate (NSC 740). Cancer Treat Rep 60:221–223, 1976

107. Hornback N B, Einhorn L, Shidnia H, et al: Oat-cell carcinoma of the lung. Early treatment results of combination radiation therapy and chemotherapy. Cancer 37:2658–2664, 1976

108. Lowenbraun S, Krauss S, Smalley S, Huguley C: Randomized study of cyclophosphamide (CTX) alone versus CTX, adriamycin (ADR) and dimethyl triazeno imidazole carboxamide (DTIC) in small cell lung carcinoma. Proc Am Soc Clin Oncol 15:246, 1975

109. Johnson R E, Brereton H D, Kent H C: Small cell carcinoma of the lung: Attempt to remedy causes of past therapeutic failure. Lancet 2:289–291, 1976

110. Davis H L Jr, Prout M M: Combination chemotherapy for oat-cell carcinoma of the lung. Proc Am Soc Clin Oncol 16:243, 1976

111. Taylor S G IV, Donavan M A, Sponzo R W, et al: Treatment of small cell carcinoma of the lung using methyl-CCNU (NSC-95441) combined with cyclophosphamide (NSC-26271) and vincristine (NSC-67574) in a 3 week schedule. Cancer Chemother Rep 59:1127–1130, 1975

112. Aisner J, Esterhay R J Jr, Wiernik P H: Treatment of oat-cell carcinoma of the lung with cyclophosphamide, adriamycin, epipodophyllotoxin VP-16-213 and methanol extracted residue (MER) of BCG Proc Am Soc Clin Oncol 16:261, 1976

113. Comis R, Ginsberg S, Goldberg J, et al: CCNU/cytoxan/vincristine (CCV) plus radiotherapy (XRT) in small cell carcinoma of the lung. Proc Am Soc Clin Oncol 17:280, 1976

114. Livingston R B, Moore T N: Combined modality treatment of oat-cell carcinoma of the lung. Proc Am Assoc Cancer Res 16:152, 1976

115. Abeloff M D, Ettinger D S, Baylin S B, Hazra T: Management of small cell carcinoma of the lung. Therapy, staging, and biochemical markers. Cancer 38:1394–1401, 1976

116. Nixon D W, Carey R W, Suit H D, Aisenberg A C: Combination chemotherapy in oat-cell carcinoma of the lung. Cancer 36:867–872, 1975

117. Einhorn L H, Fee W H, Farber M O, et al: Improved chemotherapy for small cell undifferentiated lung cancer. JAMA 235: 1225–1229, 1976

118. Hansen H H, Hansen M: A comparison of 3 and 4 drug combination chemotherapy for advanced small cell anaplastic carcinoma of the lung. Proc Am Assoc Cancer Res and ASCO 17:129, 1976

119. Israel L, Depierre A: Long duration of complete response to immunochemotherapy in oat-cell carcinomas of the lung. Proc Am Soc Clin Oncol 16:239, 1976

120. Glatstein E: Combined chemotherapy-radiotherapy of oat-cell cancer of the lung. Proc Am Soc Clin Oncol 17:262, 1976

121. Levitt M, Meikle A, Weinerman B: Intensive combined modality therapy in oat-cell carcinoma of lung (OCCL). Proc Am Soc Clin Oncol 17:308, 1976

122. Cohen M H, Ihde D C, Fossieck B E, et al: Intensive chemotherapy of small cell bronchogenic carcinoma (SCBC). Proc Am Assoc Cancer Res and ASCO 18:286, 1977

123. Ihde D C, Bernath A B, Cohen M H, et al: Utility of fiberoptic bronchoscopy in assessing response to combination chemotherapy in small cell carcinoma of the lung. Proc Am Assoc Cancer Res and ASCO 18:290, 1977

124. Hansen H H, Muggia F M: Staging of inoperable patients with bronchogenic carcinoma with special reference to bone marrow examination and peritoneoscopy. Cancer 30:1395–1401, 1972

125. Ledley R S, DiChiro G, Luessenhop A J, Twigg H L: Computerized transaxial tomography of the human body. Science 186:207–212, 1974

126. Freimanis A K: Ultrasonic imaging of neoplasms. Cancer 37:496–502, 1976

127. Carson P L, Wenzel W W, Avery P, Hendee W R: Ultrasonic imaging as an aid to cancer therapy. Int J Radiat Oncol 1:119–132, 1975

128. Karrer K, Pridun N, Zwintz E: Chemotherapeutic studies in bronchogenic carcinoma by the Austrian Study Group. Cancer Chemother Rep 4:207–213, 1973

Elaine M. Bunick, and Leslie I. Rose (I,II)
Linda A. Haegele (III)

14 Endocrine Neoplasia

I. Detection and Management of Irradiation-Induced Thyroid Neoplasms

Carcinoma of the Thyroid Following Low-Dose Irradiation to the Head and Neck

Lack of knowledge about the oncogenic potential of low-dose irradiation to the head, neck and chest led many therapists to believe that this mode of therapy was safe and effective for treatment of tinea capitis, tonsil and adenoid hypertrophy, acne and thymic enlargement. With the advent of the atomic bomb came concern for long-term biologic effects due to radiation exposure. In 1950, Duffy and Fitzgerald postulated a relation between irradiation of the thymus and thyroid carcinoma in children.[1] Subsequently, more patients with carcinoma of the thyroid were noted to have a history of neck irradiation in childhood. Studies were undertaken to establish the relation between age, dose, and time of occurrence of thyroid abnormalities.

Silverman and Hoffman,[2] in their review of seven major epidemiologic studies, found the estimated risk of radiation-induced thyroid neoplasms to be 2.2 to 5.5 cases per million children/rad/year for those who had thymic irradiation; 0 to 6.1 cases per million children/rad/year for those who received irradiation for tinea capitis; 2.9 cases per million children/rad/year for survivors in Hiroshima and Nagasaki; and 2.1 cases per million children/rad/year for those on Rongelap Atoll (Marshall Islands) exposed to radioactive fallout.

An unusually high number of patients with benign adenomas were found in one of the Japanese groups irradiated for tinea capitis and in the Rongelap group. The estimated minimum dose to the thyroid gland associated with increased risk of thyroid malignancy was 6.5 rad.

Refetoff et al[3] examined 100 patients approximately 20 years after they were irradiated before age 10 with 300 to 1600 rad to thyroid carcinomas. According to a Framingham study,[4] the prevalence of one thyroid nodule is 1.6 per cent, and new nodules in normal glands occurred in 1.3 per cent over a 15-year period. Of the thyroid nodules removed, carcinoma was found in 10 to 15 per cent.

Certain diagnostic procedures were also evaluated with respect to the amount of irradiation delivered to the thyroid gland in adults. An ^{131}I thyroid uptake is estimated to deliver about 10.5 rad to the thyroid, and an

^{131}I thyroid scan, 100 to 200 rad.[2] Since the number of rad absorbed by the thyroid varies widely with age and the effect is much greater in children than in adults, indiscriminate use of these procedures in children may also increase their risk of thyroid neoplasms.

A cooperative thyrotoxicosis therapy follow-up study reported in 1974 that patients treated with ^{131}I before the age of 20 had an increased risk of both benign and malignant tumors of the thyroid.[5]

Experiments with rats confirmed the theory that proliferating thyroid glands are more susceptible to neoplastic changes after irradiation. Doniach showed that no tumors developed in unirradiated young rats.[6] A few follicular adenomas were noted in those rats whose thyroids were irradiated with 100 to 250 rad. If 500 rad was delivered to the thyroid, follicular carcinomas were noted. There was a decrease in tumor production rate following irradiation of rats given thyroxin in doses sufficient to suppress thyroid-stimulating hormone (TSH) production. Conversely, when rats were given 0.1 per cent aminotriazole to decrease thyroxine production but increase TSH production, the tumor production rate increased even in those rats that were not irradiated. Thus, TSH may also play a role in tumorigenesis; when patients have elevated TSH levels during low-dose irradiation, the incidence of neoplastic change is markedly increased.

It has been well documented that irradiation to the proliferating thyroid gland in young people is associated with neoplastic changes. Since irradiation for tinea capitis, acne, and hypertrophy of tonsils, adenoids or thymus was performed from the late 1920s to the early 1960s, any person with a history of this mode of therapy should have a periodic evaluation of the thyroid gland and prompt attention should be paid to any nodule found.

In light of these facts, the following guidelines are suggested: when the history is taken, the clinician should obtain as much information as possible about the clinical reason for radiation therapy, the age when therapy was begun and the dose administered. After a complete physical examination is performed, with careful palpation of the thyroid gland, those with palpable nodules should be referred immediately for subtotal thyroidectomy and subsequently placed on a replacement dose of thyroxine. Patients with no palpable abnormality of the thyroid gland should have measurements of serum thyroxine (T4) and resin T3 uptake, radioactive ^{123}I uptake, and a technetium pertechnetate (Tc^{99}) thyroid scan. If there is any suspicious area on the thyroid scan, a subtotal thyroidectomy should be performed and the patient maintained on a replacement dose of thyroxine. If all results of the thyroid studies are normal, it is advisable to have the patient take a replacement dose of thyroxine daily to suppress thyroid function, thus markedly reducing the risk of thyroid carcinoma. This therapy should be continued for life, and a complete reevaluation should be made every year.

References

1. Duffy B J, Fitzgerald P J: Cancer of the thyroid in children: A report of twenty-eight cases. J Clin Endocrinol Metab 10:1296-1308, 1950
2. Silverman C, Hoffman D A: Thyroid tumor risk from radiation during childhood. Prev Med 4:100-105, 1975
3. Refetoff S, Harrison J, Karanfilski B T, et al: Continuing occurrence of thyroid carcinoma after irradiation to the neck in infancy and childhood. N Engl J Med 292:171-175, 1975
4. Vander J B, Gaston E A, Dawber T R: Significance of solitary nontoxic thyroid nodules: Preliminary report. N Engl J Med 251:970-973, 1954
5. Dobyns B M, Sheline G E, Workman J B, et al: Malignant and benign neoplasms of the thyroid in patients treated for hyperthyroidism: A report of the cooperative thyrotoxicosis therapy follow-up study. J Clin Endocrinol Metabol 38:976-998, 1974
6. Doniach I: Carcinogenic effect of 100, 250, and 500 rad x-rays on the rat thyroid gland. Br J Cancer 30:487-495, 1974

II. The Management of Adrenal Cortical Carcinoma

Carcinoma of the adrenal cortex is a rare and lethal neoplasm. It is estimated to develop in two out of every million persons.[1] In one study of all patients with malignant tumors approximately 0.2 per cent were found to have adrenal cortical carcinoma.[2] The left and right adrenals appear to be involved with equal frequency. Although there is no sex predominance, the average age at time of diagnosis was 28 to 40 years for women but 45 to 50 years for men.[3,4] This malignancy may also develop in children. The youngest patient reported in the literature was 8 months of age.[5] Survival rates depend on the extent of disease and the mode of therapy, but females in general survive longer than males.

The most frequent complaints encountered on initial presentation are abdominal pain, weakness, weight loss, anorexia and nausea.[4] Upon physical examination, the most common signs are abdominal mass, lymphadenopathy, hepatomegaly and edema of the lower extremities.

On endocrinologic examination, the patient may have Cushing's syndrome, with centripetal obesity, red-purple striae, rosy, "moon" facies, thin skin that bruises easily, muscle-wasting, carbohydrate intolerance, hypertension, acne, hirsutism, edema and psychosis. Some females may show virilization, for example, clitoral hypertrophy, severe hirsutism, including development of sternal hair and male escutcheon, development of skeletal muscles, bitemporal balding, deepening voice, breast atrophy and menstrual irregularity. Others may have both virilization and Cushing's syndrome.

To establish the diagnosis, the following studies are performed; the patient should be on NO medication:

1. Plasma cortisol level, at 7 a.m. and 7 p.m.
2. 24-hour urinary 17-ketosteroid (17-KS) and 17 hydroxycorticosteroid (17-OH) levels, total urine volume and creatinine collected as two consecutive 12-hour samples from 7 a.m. to 7 p.m. and 7 p.m. to 7 a.m. to determine diurnal variation.
3. Plasma testosterone, estradiol, follicle-stimulating hormone (FSH) and luteinizing hormone (LH) if the patient shows virilization.
4. Daily morning plasma cortisol levels, testosterone and estradiol if patient shows virilization, and daily 24-hour urine collections for levels of 17-KS, 17-OH, total urine volume and creatinine during the 2-mg dexamethasone suppression test (0.5 mg by mouth every 6 hours for 8 doses) and the 8-mg dexamethasone suppression test (2.0 mg by mouth every 6 hours for 8 doses).
5. Scout x-ray of abdomen to determine whether there are any masses.
6. Intravenous pyelogram after dexamethasone tests are completed.
7. Biochemical profile, electrolytes, creatinine and hemogram.

A carcinoma of the adrenal cortex is considered to be present if any of the following conditions prevail:

1. Excess cortisol is produced with loss of normal diurnal variation and cannot be suppressed with the 8-mg dexamethasone test.
2. The 17-KS or 17-OH levels (or both) are markedly elevated and cannot be suppressed with the 8-mg dexamethasone test.
3. The testosterone or estradiol levels are markedly elevated and cannot be suppressed with the 8-mg dexamethasone test.

Once the diagnosis of carcinoma of the adrenal has been made, appropriate studies are performed in search of metastases. The areas most commonly involved are lungs, liver, lymph nodes, bone, local extension into kidneys, pancreas, peritoneum, retroperitoneum and spleen. Three patients were reported to have had spontaneous rupture of a carcinoma of the adrenal gland.[2]

On gross examination, adrenal carcinomas vary in size and shape and may contain areas of hemorrhage and necrosis.[4] Histologically, these tumors can be designated as either differentiated (that is, polygonal cells arranged in sheets, trabeculae, nests or ribbons) or undifferentiated (that is, pleomorphic cells forming bizarre patterns). On occasion, both differentiated and undifferentiated histologic types have been found in the same adrenal tumor.

The response to the various modes of therapy, surgery radiation and chemotherapy, whether used alone or in combination, is poor in most cases. The reported 5-year survival rate ranges from 9 to 33 per cent.[2,4] There is no standard method for staging carcinoma of the adrenal. No protocol studies of the therapeutic modalities have been reported. Thus, it is difficult to determine the best mode or combination of modes to use in treating all patients with carcinoma of the adrenal.

Surgical removal of the tumor appears to be the treatment of choice because it is the only modality consistently associated with prolonged survival. The benefits of radiation therapy remain controversial. Early studies of this mode of therapy did not show a demonstrable effect on this tumor. More recently, Percarpio and Knowlton reported that metastases of adrenal cortical carcinoma can respond to palliative doses (3000 to 4000 rad given for 2 to 3 weeks) of irradiation and therefore should be considered part of the therapeutic regimen.[6]

Numerous chemotherapeutic agents have been evaluated, including vinblastine, L-arcolysine, MTX, 5-FU, medroxyprogesterone acetate, hydroxyurea, daunomycin, cyclophosphamide, me-CCNU, adriamycin, aminoglutethimide and mitotane (o,p'-DDD). Only the last two compounds have been found effective in alleviating symptoms, and none has consistently been shown to prolong life.[2,4] Aminoglutethimide interferes with the conversion of cholesterol to pregnenolone. As a result, the amount of steroid synthesized by the adrenal carcinoma is decreased. Since it does not cause destruction of the tumor, aminoglutethimide can provide only symptomatic relief.

Mitotane, whose chemical formula is 1,1-dichloro-2-(ortho-chlorophenyl)-2-(parachlorophenyl)ethane, usually referred to as o,p'-DDD, acts directly on the adrenal glands to suppress steroid production by inhibiting secretion of glucose-6-phosphate dehydrogenase as well as steroid. It also inhibits the enzymes involved in metabolism of steroid hormones in peripheral tissues. Hutter and Kayhoe assessed the results of treatment with o,p'-DDD in 138 patients.[7] They found the maximal daily dose to be between 8 and 10 grams since, at that dose, 88 per cent of the patients manifested one or more signs of toxicity; anorexia, nausea, vomiting, diarrhea, lethargy, somnolence, dizziness, visual disturbances, headache, confusion, weakness and skin rash were the most frequent. No liver or bone marrow toxicity was observed in any of these patients. Seventy-two per cent of the patients were considered to be steroid responders, as evidenced by a 30 per cent or greater reduction in levels of 17-OH or 17-KS, or both. The onset of steroid reduction occurred within 30 days after o,p'-DDD was started. Only 34 per cent of the patients had a measurable disease response. The mean dose for inducing a steroid response was 8.5 gm, with a mean duration of 7 months. No patient with a measurable disease response was without an associated steroid response, but every patient with a steroid response did not have an associated measurable disease response. At autopsy, varying degrees of necrosis, hemorrhage and fibrosis were found in the adrenal cortex.

Ostuni and Roginsky reported a case in which a young female had been given o,p'-DDD and fluorouracil for 5 months because of metastases to her right adrenal, liver and lung within 1 year of removal of a 1520-gram adrenal carcinoma from the left adrenal; no evidence of tumor was found at autopsy, 9 years after chemotherapy.[8]

Because adrenal carcinoma is such a lethal neoplasm, aggressive therapy combining all the available therapeutic modalities—surgery, radiation and o,p'-DDD—should be undertaken in an attempt not only to alleviate symptoms but also to prolong the patient's life.

REFERENCES

1. Hutter A M, Kayhoe D E: Adrenal cortical carcinoma. Am J Med 41:572-580, 1966
2. Bradley E L: Primary and adjunctive therapy in carcinoma of the adrenal cortex. Surg Gynecol Obstet 141:507-511, 1975
3. Huvos A G, Hajdu S I, Brasfield R D, et al: Adrenal cortical carcinoma: Clinicopathologic study of 34 cases. Cancer 25:354-361, 1970
4. Hajjar R A, Hickey R C, Samann N A: Adrenal cortical carcinoma. Cancer 35:549-554, 1975
5. Stewart D R, Jones P H M, Jolleys A: Carcinoma of the adrenal gland in children. J Pediatr Surg 9:59-67, 1974
6. Percarpio B, Knowlton A H: Radiation therapy of adrenal cortical carcinoma. Acta Radiol 15:288-292, 1976
7. Hutter A M, Kayhoe D E: Adrenal cortical carcinoma: Results of treatment with o,p'-DDD in 138 patients. Am J Med 41:581-592, 1966
8. Ostuni J A, Roginsky M S: Metastatic adrenal cortical carcinoma. Arch Intern Med 135:1257-1258, 1975

III. Classification and Chemotherapeutic Management of Apudomas and Other Endocrine Neoplasms*

The APUD Concept

Since embryologic studies with tissue culture techniques showed that autonomic neurons and adrenal chromaffin cells are derived from the neural crest,[1] the entire field of endocrine neoplasia has undergone critical review.

Pearse and other investigators performed cytochemical studies to delineate a group of cells of possible endodermal and oral ectodermal origin with characteristic enzymatic and amine-uptake properties, namely, amine precursor uptake and decarboxylation (APUD) (Table 14-1).[2] Similar cytochemical capabilities in both neuroectodermal cells and APUD cells support the concept of the common origin of neuroendocrine cells.[3]

Thus, the concept of a unified cellular origin evolved, with emphasis on the homogeneity of a group of tumors, both adenomas and carcinomas, "apudomas," which arise from cells of the APUD type. Orthoendocrine syndromes develop when an apudoma secretes excessive amounts of the normal polypeptide or amine products of the cells of origin, whereas paraendocrine syndromes denote production of APUD cellular material foreign to the cells of origin. Other apudomas may secrete substances that are characteristic of non-APUD cells, such as prostaglandins, histamine, and erythropoietin (Table 14-2).[3,4]

Multiple Endocrine Adenomatoses

Many derivatives of neural crest tissue are involved in the neurocutaneous syndromes and multiple endocrine adenomatoses (MEA), which represent hyperplastic or neo-

TABLE 14-1. *Characteristics of APUD Cells*

Cytochemistry
Fluorogenic amine content and/or
Amine precursor uptake
Amine acid decarboxylase
Side-chain carboxyl groups
Nonspecific esterases and/or cholinesterases
Alpha-glycerophosphate dehydrogenase
Specific immunofluorescence
Ultrastructure
Low levels of rough (granular) endoplasmic reticulum (ER)
High levels of smooth ER in the form of vesicles
High content of free ribosomes
Electron dense mitochondria
Fixation labile mitochondria
Membrane-bound secretion vesicles

*Supported by Grants Nos. CA17963-03 and CA13611-03 from the National Cancer Institute, National Institutes of Health, Bethesda, Maryland.

TABLE 14-2. *APUD Tumors and Complex Neuroectodermal Disorders*

Organ	Tumor	Secretory Product	Endocrine Syndrome	
			Ortho	Para
Hypothalamus	None identified			
Pineal	Pinealoma	Unknown		
Adenohypophysis	Pituitary adenoma	Unknown	Cushing's disease Acromegaly Galactorrhea-amenorrhea	
Autonomic nervous system	Neurocytoma Neuroblastoma Ganglioneuroma	ACTH Vasoactive intestinal peptide (VIP)		Cushing's syndrome Verner-Morrison syndrome
Adrenal medulla	Pheochromocytoma	Catecholamines	MEA Type II	
		ACTH		Cushing's syndrome
		Calcitonin		
		Insulin		Hypogylcemia
Carotid body	Paraganglioma	Catecholamines	Hypertension	
		ACTH		Cushing's syndrome
		Calcitonin		
Thyroid	Medullary carcinoma	Calcitonin	MEA Type II	
		ACTH		Cushing's syndrome
		Insulin		Hypogylcemia
Skin	Melanoma	Melanin		
		ACTH		Cushing's syndrome
		Gastrin		Zollinger-Ellison
Stomach				
EC Cell	Carcinoid	5-HT	Malignant carcinoid	Atypical carcinoid
		Kallikrein		
		Histamine		
		ACTH		Cushing's syndrome
G Cell	Hyperplasia	Gastrin	Zollinger-Ellison I	
	Carcinoma			
Pancreas				
Cell types	Hyperplasia	Insulin	Hypoglycemia	
B	Adenoma	Glucagon	Diabetes	
A	Adenomatous hyperplasia	Gastrin	Zollinger-Ellison II	
D		ACTH		Cushing's syndrome

TABLE 14-2. (continued)

Organ	Tumor	Secretory Product	Endocrine Syndrome	
			Ortho	Para
Pancreas	Carcinoma	VIP		Verner-Morrison
		Parathormone		Hyperparathyroidism
		Antidiuretic hormone		Schwartz-Bartter syndrome
Small intestine				
EC Cell	Carcinoid	5-HT	Malignant carcinoid	
		Kallikrein		
		VIP		Verner-Morrison

Abbreviations: MEA, multiple endocrine adenomatases; VIP, vasoactive intestinal peptide; 5-HT, 5-hydroxytryptamine (serotonin).

plastic proliferations that are sometimes familial.[3] Wermer's syndrome (MEA type I) comprises tumors of the pituitary, pancreatic islet cells, and parathyroid; MEA type II includes Sipple's syndrome (medullary thyroid carcinoma, pheochromocytoma, and hyperparathyroidism) as well as the mucosa-neuroma syndrome in which the same tumors are associated with neural proliferation in the oral mucosa, gastrointestinal tract, and bronchi (Table 14-3).[5]

Although the theory of a common ancestral cell is supported by the existence of multiple tumors of various endocrine structures, it does not separate the multiple endocrine adenomatoses into two discrete entities, especially since hyperparathyroidism is common to both syndromes. Phenotypic expression may be modified by hormonal or metabolic interaction and therefore the clinical course of the genetically determined disease may be influenced; other aspects, such as hyperparathyroidism, may represent reactive phenomena elicited by the peripheral effects of the primary tumor.[6]

The extensive cytochemical and genetic investigations of these endocrine neoplasms have not only provided a fascinating etiologic

TABLE 14-3. *Multiple Endocrine Adenomatoses Syndromes*

	MEA I (Wermer's Syndrome)	MEA II (Sipple's Syndrome)
Organ involvement	Pituitary	Thyroid
	Pancreas	Adrenal medulla
	Parathyroid	
Principal neoplasms	Pituitary adenoma	Medullary thyroid carcinoma
	Islet cell adenoma or carcinoma	Pheochromocytoma
	Parathyroid adenoma or hyperplasia	Parathyroid adenoma or hyperplasia
Associated neoplasm	Adrenal cortical adenoma	Mucosal neuroma
	Renal cortical adenoma	
	Thyroid adenoma or hyperplasia	
	Carcinoid	
	Lipoma	
	Gastric polyp	
	Mediastinal endocrine neoplasm	

model for many disorders—the diagnostic approach to these entities has been refined considerably. In addition, there is the attractive suggestion that multiple functionally discrete neoplasms may respond to similar chemotherapeutic agents. Unfortunately, until recently, the response of these tumors to pharmacologic therapy has been extremely disappointing.

Improvements in chemical assay procedures have improved the clinician's ability to monitor the response of these diseases to various modes of therapy, and several promising drugs are being developed for clinical trial.

Chemotherapy of endocrine neoplasms

Apudomas of the Alimentary Tract. Carcinoid. Variations in the clinical expression of carcinoid tumors may reflect the embryologic derivation of the lesion. Carcinoids of the bronchus, stomach and pancreas arise in the foregut and typically are argyrophil-positive and argentaffin-negative. They are frequently associated with signs of the carcinoid syndrome. Midgut lesions involving the small intestine through the midtransverse colon are both argyrophil- and argentaffin-positive, and are manifested by clinical symptoms. Often they are multicentric, whereas hindgut carcinoids of the descending colon and rectum are rarely argyrophil- or argentaffin-positive, are not multicentric, and are rarely manifested by symptoms. Colbert has reported the simultaneous occurrence of primary carcinoids of the ileum and rectum, and has emphasized the heterogeneity of these embryologically distinct lesions. Multicentricity of carcinoid tumors is therefore usually restricted to a specifically defined subdivision of the gastrointestinal tract.[7]

Review of a group of relatives who had more malignant disease than unrelated groups has demonstrated several cases of metastasizing carcinoid, thus supporting the possibility of genetic predisposition.[8]

Analysis of a large population before chemotherapeutic intervention produced a wide range of 5-year survival rates, from 99 per cent for appendiceal primaries to 33 per cent for sigmoid colon lesions.[9] As early as 1965, Mengel and coworkers reported measurable antitumor effects with cyclophosphamide and subsequently improved response rates with cyclophosphamide and methotrexate or melphalan alone. Significant side effects included a transitory exacerbation of symptoms and increased 5-hydroxyindoleacetic acid (5-HIAA).[10,11]

The early success of streptozotocin therapy in insulinomas, as well as acceptance of the apudoma concept, prompted trials of this agent in patients with metastatic carcinoid. Alleviation of symptoms frequently preceded reduction of 24-hour urinary excretion of 5-HIAA and diminution of hepatic size, without evidence of the transitory exacerbations noted with other agents.[12] Protocols are now being used for evaluating the possible potentiation of streptozotocin effectiveness by other agents, including 5-fluorouracil.

Pancreatic Islet Cell Apudomas. Insulinoma. In one series of carefully executed autopsies, as many as 1.5 per cent of cases had pancreatic islet cell adenomas, although most of these were not clinically manifest. Excessive insulin secretion by an insulinoma elicits the most commonly observed clinical symptom complex. Approximately 3 per cent of these tumors are extrapancreatic, within the splenic hilum, duodenum or surrounding pancreatic structures. At the time of initial diagnosis, 10 per cent of these lesions are obviously malignant, with distant metastases, whereas another 10 per cent are multiple benign adenomas or hyperplasia.[13]

Little correlation has been shown between the severity of symptoms, caused by the amount of insulin production, and the size of the tumor; diagnosis depends on several factors, including recurrent symptomatic hypoglycemia relieved with glucose, concomitant hyperinsulinemia, and the absence of plasma insulin antibodies. Challenge with prolonged fasting or the intravenous tolbutamide test is infrequently indicated and must be closely supervised. Diagnosis should be made in accordance with strict criteria.[14]

Chemical differentiation of adenomas and carcinomas may ultimately be possible, since various researchers have observed higher concentrations of a proinsulin-like component in patients with carcinoma when compared with such levels in patients with adenomas.[13] In patients with clinical evidence of functional islet cell tumor, ectopic production of chorionic gonadotropin and its subunits may result from malignant derepression of the genome. Elevated values of HCG do not distinguish islet cell carcinoma from other carcinomas.[15]

Although metastatic malignant insulinomas may have an indolent clinical course, the median survival without chemotherapy is less than 1 year. Tumor localization makes surgical resection difficult. In an estimated 25 per cent of patients with suspected insulinoma, no neoplasm is demonstrated at operation. Partial pancreatectomy is not indicated in these individuals since the distribution of adenomas is uniform throughout the organ.[13]

Medical palliation was initially attempted with diazoxide, in view of its direct inhibition of insulin release.[16] One report suggests the possible clinical efficacy of diphenylhydantoin, which impedes insulin release from labile and storage beta cell pools.[17] Somatostatin administration also reduces circulating insulin levels, but the hyperglycemic effect is not sustained.[18] Since none of these agents possesses any antitumor property, the primary lesion will continue to proliferate and metastasize despite this therapy.

The depression of protein synthesis elicited by L-asparaginase is well documented, and reduction in plasma insulin levels was observed in one case of refractory malignant insulinoma after this agent was administered. No objective reduction in tumor mass was achieved during this treatment.[13]

At present, the most effective agent for the treatment of pancreatic islet cell carcinoma is streptozotocin, an antibiotic isolated from *Streptomyces achromogenes* and composed of a methylated nitrosourea moiety linked to glucosamine. Its primary effect[19] is inhibition of DNA synthesis by depressing metabolism of nicotinamide-adenine dinucleotide (NAD) and nicotinamide-adenosine dinucleotide phosphate (NADH). Uptake by the pancreatic beta cell may be facilitated by the glucose portion of the molecule.[20]

Since hepatic metabolism, urinary excretion, and spontaneous degradation of streptozotocin combine for a half-life of only 15 minutes, up to 20 per cent of the total dose may be excreted within an hour. Renal toxicity occurs frequently, with early signs of proteinuria, usually reversible once therapy is stopped. Continued streptozotocin administration may induce glycosuria and renal tubular acidosis, with progressive damage to the proximal tubules.[21]

By both biochemical and measurable-disease parameters, the overall response of patients who have islet cell carcinomas when they are treated with streptozotocin approaches 60 per cent; there is an attendant significant improvement in survival, even in patients experiencing partial remissions.

Tests of serial fasting insulin levels document a rapid insulin response to this therapy (median of 17 days) at a total dose of 2 gm per square meter of body surface area, although the maximal effect[19] may not occur prior to the fifth week of therapy or a total dose of 4 gm/m^2. Quantitative reductions of circulating proinsulin-like material have also been described during remissions.[20]

Clinical diabetes has not been demonstrated after streptozotocin therapy for non-insulin-secreting neoplasms; this implies possible drug resistance of normal beta cells or benign adenomas.[13]

Glucagonoma and Somatostatinoma. Malignant glucagonoma is an uncommon functional islet cell neoplasm. Characteristically, patients with these tumors have erythematous skin eruptions, with progressive superficial bullous formation, and mild diabetes. Streptozotocin therapy has been reported to resolve the skin rash, normalize the oral glucose tolerance test, and reduce measurable metastases.[22]

The demonstration of somatostatin production by D cells of the pancreatic islets forecast the existence of the somatostatinoma, with its resultant hyperglycemia, hypoinsulinemia, hypoglucagonemia, and hypersomatostatinemia. Immunofluorescent techniques were positive in one patient, and cultured tumor cells released somatostatin into the culture medium. Although complete resection was successful in this patient, these lesions may require chemotherapeutic intervention.[23]

The Verner-Morrison Syndrome. The syndrome of "pancreatic cholera," initially described by Verner and Morrison, includes the clinical features of profuse watery diarrhea with subsequent hypokalemia and gastric achlorhydria (WDHA syndrome) in as-

TABLE 14-4. *Differential Diagnosis of Gastrin Levels*

Normal	Mildly Elevated	Elevated
Control	Gastric ulcer	Obstructing duodenal ulcer
Duodenal ulcer	Gastric carcinoma	Retained gastric antrum
Postresection	Primary hyperparathyroidism	Secondary hyperparathyroidism
	Postvagotomy	Pheochromocytoma
	Vitiligo	Atrophic gastritis
	Rheumatoid arthritis	Pernicious anemia
		Zollinger-Ellison

sociation with a non-gastrin-secreting, non-beta islet cell tumor of the pancreas. Half of these lesions are benign and are amenable to curative surgical resection. Temporary amelioration of symptoms in patients with unresectable disease may be achieved with glucocorticoids or 5-fluorouracil, but patients eventually die because of fluid and electrolyte imbalance.[24] Malignant lesions invariably metastasize before surgical exploration; the mean survival time is 14 months.[13]

Excessive secretion of vasoactive intestinal peptide (VIP) produces the characteristic symptoms of this syndrome. There is some debate as to the specificity of VIP as a tumor marker.[25,26]

Intravenous or intraarterial streptozotocin therapy has been used for several patients with VIP-secreting malignancies; one case report documents clinical and biochemical response as well as regression of measurable disease.[27,28]

Zollinger-Ellison Syndrome. The initial description of excessive gastrin production secondary to non-beta islet cell tumors associated with gastric hypersecretion and ulceration was fairly explicit, but further experience with large patient populations has supplied nuances in the approach to diagnosis and in observed clinical variations. In less than 25 per cent of patients with Zollinger-Ellison syndrome, the location of the ulceration is atypical; 60 per cent of all such patients have single gastric or duodenal ulcers.[13] Symptoms of diarrhea and abdominal pain related to gastric hypersecretion must be differentiated from similar complaints evoked by excessive VIP secretion in the Verner-Morrison syndrome.

There are significant elevations of serum gastrin levels in several disease entities (Table 14-4).[29] In individuals with renal disease and secondary hyperparathyroidism, hypergastrinemia probably reflects failure of renal inactivation of gastrin rather than abnormalities of renal excretion.[29]

Since 20 per cent to 50 per cent of patients with the Zollinger-Ellison syndrome have concomitant multiple endocrine adenomatoses, including hyperparathyroidism and medullary thyroid carcinoma, the stimulatory effects of hypercalcemia on gastrin secretion may evoke a particularly malignant synergism.[30] The interhormonal relation between calcitonin and gastrin may inhibit gastrin secretion by calcitonin or may cause excessive calcitonin stimulation by gastrin.[31]

Analogous to the elevation of serum proinsulin-like material observed in patients with insulinomas, heterogeneity of circulating gastrin may exist in the Zollinger-Ellison syndrome.[13] Approximately one-third of all patients may have normal serum gastrin levels, and ultimately calcium infusion or secretin challenge may be required to establish the diagnosis. Secretin provocation may differentiate this syndrome from hypergastrinemia of antral origin and thus provide insight into the clinical evolution of the Zollinger-Ellison syndrome.[32]

Recognition of the clinical similarity between antral G-cell hyperplasia and non-beta islet cell gastrinomas has made possible the etiologic subclassification of the Zollinger-Ellison syndrome (Table 14-5).[29]

Sixty percent of gastrin-secreting islet cell tumors are malignant, and half of these have metastasized prior to diagnosis; less than 25 per cent are amenable to simple surgical

TABLE 14-5. *Etiologic Subclassification of the Zollinger-Ellison Syndrome*

Feature	Type 1	Type 2
Tumor	Absent	Gastrinoma (pancreas or duodenum) or islet hyperplasia
Antral G cells	Hyperplastic	Normal
Serum gastrin	Very high	High
Clinical duration	Brief	Extended

resection. Total gastrectomy, which results in longest survival,[13] produces palliation of peripheral tumor effects and does not decrease tumor burden.

Although initial trials with intravenous streptozotocin therapy were extremely disappointing,[33,34] there has been a significant clinical and biochemical response in one patient after 4 gm of intraarterial streptozotocin via the celiac axis. Subsequently, urinary excretion diminished and the renal toxicity of the drug was reduced.[35] Recent evaluation of the effect of streptozotocin on gastrin release in patients with carcinoid tumors and malignant insulinomas, who ostensibly had normal gastrin-producing G cells, has suggested that the drug may actually stimulate gastrin release.[36] Further studies into the pharmacologic capabilities of streptozotocin is certainly warranted.

Chemotherapy with tubercidin (7-deazaadenosine), an antimetabolite adenosine analogue, which may be incorporated into DNA and RNA as a fraudulent purine, has produced an objective remission in one patient with Zollinger-Ellison syndrome. The necessity of incubating the drug in vitro with the patient's own red blood cells prior to administration by transfusion, as well as its renal toxicity, has drastically curtailed clinical experience with this agent.[37]

Protocol studies are under way to assess the efficacy of 5-FU and streptozotocin or adriamycin in particularly resistant lesions.

Thyroid Neoplasms

The implication of prior cervical irradiation in the genesis of thyroid neoplasia is reviewed in another part of this volume, and the standard techniques of thyroid ablation by means of radiation therapy and hormonal manipulation are described in endocrine textbooks.

Medullary Thyroid Carcinoma. Unique among thyroid neoplasms, this lesion may be familial through autosomal dominant inheritance, although most patients do not give such a family history. The clinical course after initial therapeutic resection is variable, and metastatic involvement of regional lymph nodes may denote advanced or fairly aggressive disease, necessitating rigorous therapy.[38]

Since serum calcitonin elevations do not ordinarily produce significant symptoms, the refinement of calcitonin assay procedures has introduced a valuable diagnostic aid and permits early documentation of postoperative metastases.[39,40] Provocative stimulation of calcitonin secretion after calcium infusion detected lesions in 30 per cent of individuals at risk in one study.[41] Glucagon and pentagastrin infusions are also utilized, but none of these maneuvers can distinguish the specific source of hypercalcitoninemia.[42]

Enzymatic studies demonstrated the correlation between increased serum histaminase levels and tumor extension beyond the thyroid gland, although attempts to block histaminase activity by using the inhibitor aminoguanidine were not clinically effective.[43] Dopa-decarboxylase, an enzyme known to be present in pheochromocytomas, has been isolated from medullary thyroid carcinoma in patients with Sipple's syndrome; this fact emphasizes the complex biochemical interrelations of these neoplasms.[43]

Immunologic elucidation of cellular immune response to tumor antigen in patients with medullary thyroid carcinoma, and in individuals who are genetically at risk, may support the existence of some element of clinical protection influencing the expression of the disease.[44]

Medical therapy of these lesions has proved disappointing, with the exception of one case report of regression after administration of triiodothyronine.[45]

Chemotherapy of Advanced Thyroid Carcinoma. Because there are few effective chemotherapeutic agents, radiation therapy and hormonal manipulation have remained the mainstay of the nonsurgical treatment of thyroid carcinoma.[46] Although the most effective dosage of radioiodide to produce thyroid ablation[47] and the use of drugs such as lithium[48] as practical adjuncts in ^{131}I therapy is controversial, the principles remain constant. Most difficulties arise in those patients whose tumors have become resistant to this conventional therapy or who present with clinically aggressive disease.

Anaplastic giant-cell thyroid carcinoma constitutes 11 per cent to 16 per cent of all thyroid cancers, and is one of the most resistant neoplastic lesions. Few patients survive more than a year from the time of diagnosis. Review of one large population reveals that 73 per cent of patients had concomitant thyroid tumors, which supports the hypothesis that these lesions arise from preexisting differentiated thyroid carcinoma.[49]

Regression of primary tumor was achieved in all patients who received both external radiation and intraarterial or intravenous methotrexate, although severe complications of therapy were observed and the lesions recurred when the medication was stopped. Median survival was significantly extended from 2.5 months to 9.4 months.[50]

Local disease was controlled for 2 or more years after treatment with a combination of extensive surgical resection; postoperative irradiation (6000 rad to a single field encompassing the neck, supraclavicular regions, and superior mediastinum); and multiple courses of actinomycin D, 0.5 mg twice weekly until toxicity developed. Extensive primary lesions larger than 5 cm in diameter remained resistant.[49]

Adriamycin has produced significant remissions in patients with advanced refractory metastatic thyroid carcinoma of various histologic cell types, including medullary thyroid carcinoma, which had been notoriously resistant to therapy. Pulmonary metastases were most responsive, with some beneficial effect noted in bone and soft-tissue metastases but none in hepatic disease. The subsequent median duration of response was 7 months.[51]

After administration of a total dose of adriamycin or demonstration of progressive disease, disease control has been attempted with bleomycin or methyl-CCNU, which is 1-(2-chloroethyl)-3-cyclohexyl-1-nitrosourea, with no objective effect.[51] The documented efficacy of cis-diamine-dichloroplatinum in testicular tumors and other neoplasms has encouraged the evaluation of this agent in combination with adriamycin in a controlled protocol study.[52]

Adrenal Neoplasms

The diagnostic criteria and therapy of adrenal cortical carcinoma are discussed in another chapter of this volume.

Pheochromocytoma. Although the voluminous literature on pheochromocytoma describes diagnostic and surgical procedures, as well as mechanisms of palliative adrenergic blockade, the prevailing lack of knowledge regarding chemotherapy results from the dearth of effective agents for this disorder and the low incidence of malignancy (2 to 15 per cent).[53] Despite the frequent association of pheochromocytoma with other endocrine neoplasms, chiefly as a constituent of Sipple's syndrome, reliable assessment of malignancy is still dependent upon the demonstration of distant metastases.

Recent efforts to control malignant metastatic pheochromocytoma with streptozotocin therapy were prompted by the variable success of this agent with the other apudomas. No biochemical improvement or reduction in tumor mass has been documented.[54]

Pituitary Neoplasms

Approximately 10 per cent of all intracranial tumors arise in the pituitary, and the clinical expression of the lesion reflects the specific hormone that may be excessively produced. Suprasellar extension of tumor parallels elevated CSF adenohypophyseal hormone concentration and may be utilized to indicate the efficacy of therapy.[55]

Surgery, irradiation and hormonal manipulation remain the primary modes of treatment for all pituitary neoplasms, since the effects of chemotherapy have not been definitively evaluated.[56]

Parathyroid Neoplasms

In patients with multiple endocrine adenomatoses, especially Sipple's syndrome, parathyroid adenoma and hyperplasia may represent a compensatory reaction to excessive calcitonin production by medullary thyroid carcinoma, although the incidence of hyperparathyroidism is also increased in Wermer's syndrome, in the absence of the thyroid lesion.[38]

Parathyroid carcinoma is encountered in 0.5 to 4 per cent of all cases of primary hyperparathyroidism, and has only recently been described in association with the MEA complex. Simultaneous occurrence of parathyroid carcinoma and hyperplasia is rare.[57]

Medical management of parathyroid carcinoma includes control of hypercalcemia with phosphate, mithramycin or calcitonin after surgical resection of the primary lesion. Glucocorticoids have been used to sustain the calcitonin effect.[58] No other chemotherapy has been attempted, and the 5-year survival[57] approaches 50 per cent, with a 10-year survival of 13 per cent.

References

1. Weston J A: The migration and differentiation of neural crest cells. Adv Morphol 8:41, 1970
2. Pearse A G E: The APUD cell concept and its implications in pathology. Pathol Annu 9:27, 1974
3. Tischler A S, Dichter M A, Bioles B, et al: Neuroendocrine neoplasms and their cells of origin. N Engl J Med 296:919, 1977
4. Welbourn R B, Pearse A G E, Polak J M, et al: The APUD cells of the alimentary tract in health and disease. Med Clin N Am 58:1359, 1974
5. Carney J A, Go V L W, Sizemore G W, et al: Alimentary tract ganglioneuromatosis. N Engl J Med 295:1287, 1976
6. Deftos L J, Parthemore J G: Secretion of parathyroid hormone in patients with medullary thyroid carcinoma. J Clin Invest 54:416, 1974
7. Colbert P M: Primary carcinoids of the ileum and rectum. JAMA 236:2201, 1976
8. Moertel C G, Dockerty M B: Familial occurrence of metastasizing carcinoid tumors. Ann Intern Med 78:389, 1973
9. Godwin J D: Carcinoid tumors. An analysis of 2837 cases. Cancer 36:560, 1975
10. Mengel C E, Kelly M G, Carbone P O: Clinical and biochemical effects of cyclophosphamide in patients with malignant carcinoid. Am J Med 38:396, 1965
11. Lotito C A, Mengel C E: Effects of melphalan in the malignant carcinoid syndrome. Arch Intern Med 124:36, 1969
12. Feldman J M, Quickel K E, Marecek R L, et al: Streptozotocin treatment of metastatic carcinoid tumors. South Med J 65:1325, 1973
13. Schein P S, DeLellis R A, Kahn C R, et al: Islet cell tumors: Current concepts and management. Ann Intern Med 79:239, 1973
14. Service F J, Dale A J D, Elvebach L R, et al: Insulinoma: Clinical and diagnostic features of 60 consecutive cases. Mayo Clin Proc 51: 417, 1976
15. Kahn C R, Rosen S W, Weintraub B D, et al: Ectopic production of chorionic gonadotropin and its subunits by islet cell tumors. N Engl J Med 297:565, 1977
16. Graber A L, Porte E, Williams R H: Clinical use of diazoxide and mechanism for its hyperglycemic effects. Diabetes 15:143, 1966
17. Brodows R G, Campbell R G: Control of refractory fasting hypoglycemia in a patient with suspected insulinoma with diphenylhydantoin. J Clin Endocrinol Metab 38:159, 1974
18. Curnow R T, Carey R M, Taylor A, et al: Somatostatin inhibition of insulin and gastrin hypersecretion in pancreatic islet cell carcinoma. N Engl J Med 292:1385, 1975
19. Broder L E, Carter S K: Pancreatic islet cell carcinoma. II. Results of therapy with streptozotocin in 52 patients. Ann Intern Med 79:108, 1973
20. Schein P, Kahn R, Gorden P, et al: Streptozotocin for malignant insulinomas and carcinoid tumor. Arch Intern Med 132:555, 1973

21. Sadoff L: Nephrotoxicity of streptozotocin. Cancer Chemother Rep 54:457, 1970
22. Mallinson C M, Bloom S R, Warin A P, et al: A glucagonoma syndrome. Lancet 2:1, 1974
23. Ganda O P, Weir G C, Soeldner J S, et al: "Somatostatinoma": A somatostatin-containing tumor of the endocrine pancreas. N Engl J Med 296:963, 1977
24. Verner J V, Morrison A B: Endocrine pancreatic islet cell disease with diarrhea: Report of a case due to diffuse hyperplasia of nonbeta islet tissue with a review of 54 additional cases. Arch Intern Med 133: 492, 1974
25. Bloom S R, Polak J M: The role of VIP in pancreatic cholera, in Thompson J C (ed): Gastrointestinal Hormones. Austin, University of Texas Press, 1975, pp 635-642
26. Said S I, Faloona G R: Elevated plasma and tissue levels of vasoactive intestinal polypeptide in the watery diarrhea syndrome due to pancreatic, bronchogenic, and other tumors. N Engl J Med 293:155, 1975
27. Kahn C R, Levy A G, Gardner J D, et al: Pancreatic cholera: Beneficial effects of treatment with streptozotocin. N Engl J Med 292:941, 1975
28. Gagel R F, Costanza M E, DeLellis R A, et al: Streptozotocin-treated Verner-Morrison syndrome. Arch Intern Med 136:1429, 1976
29. Cryer P E, Kissane J M: Metastatic pancreatic islet cell carcinoma with peptic ulcer disease and hypercalcemia. Am J Med 63:142, 1977
30. Snyder N, Scurry M, Hughes W: Hypergastrinemia in familial multiple endocrine adenomatoses. Ann Intern Med 80:321, 1974
31. Sizemore G W, Go V L W, Kaplan E L, et al: Relations of calcitonin and gastrin in the Zollinger-Ellison syndrome and medullary carcinoma of the thyroid. N Engl J Med 288:642, 1973
32. Lamers C B, Buis J T, vanTongeren J: Secretin-stimulated serum gastrin levels in hyperparathyroid patients from families with multiple endocrine adenomatoses. Ann Intern Med 86:719, 1977
33. Sadoff L, Franklin D: Streptozotocin in the Zollinger-Ellison syndrome. Lancet 2:504, 1975
34. Lamers C B H, vanThongeren J: Streptozotocin in the Zollinger-Ellison syndrome. Lancet 2:1150, 1975
35. Hayes J R, O'Connell N, O'Neill T, et al: Successful treatment of a malignant gastrinoma with streptozotocin. Gut 17:285, 1976
36. Stadil F, Stage J G: Effect of streptozotocin on gastrin release. Scand J Gastroenterol 37:67 (suppl), 1976
37. Bisel H F, Ansfield F J, Mason J H, et al: Clinical studies with tubercidin administered by direct injection. Cancer Res 30:76, 1970
38. Hill C S, Ibanez M L, Samaan N A, et al: Medullary carcinoma of the thyroid gland: An analysis of the M.D. Anderson experience with patients with the tumor, its special features, and its histogenesis. Medicine 52:141, 1973
39. Deftos L J: Radioimmunoassay for calcitonin in medullary thyroid carcinoma. JAMA 227:403, 1974
40. Goltzman D, Potts J T, Ridgway E C, et al: Calcitonin as a tumor marker. N Engl J Med 290:1035, 1974
41. Jackson C E, Tashjian A H, Block M A: Detection of medullary thyroid cancer by calcitonin assay in families. Ann Intern Med 78:845, 1973
42. Hennessey J F, Wells S A, Ontjes D A, et al: A comparison of pentagastrin injection and calcium infusion as provocative agents for the detection of medullary carcinoma of the thyroid. J Clin Endocrinol Metab 39:487, 1974
43. Keiser H R, Beaven M A, Doppman J, et al: Sipple's syndrome: Medullary thyroid carcinoma, pheochromocytoma, and parathyroid disease. Ann Intern Med 78:561, 1973
44. Rocklin R E, Gagel R, Felman Z, et al: Cellular immune responses in familial medullary thyroid carcinoma. N Engl J Med 296:835, 1977
45. Wahner H W, Cuello C, Aljure F: Hormone-induced regression of medullary (solid) thyroid carcinoma. Am J Med 45:789, 1968
46. Halnan K E: The non-surgical treatment of thyroid cancer. Br J Surg 62:769, 1975
47. McCowen K D, Adler R A, Ghaed N, et al: Low-dose radioiodide thyroid ablation in postsurgical patients with thyroid cancer. Am J Med 61:52, 1976
48. Gershengorn M C, Izumi M, Robbins J: Use of lithium as an adjunct to radioiodine therapy of thyroid carcinoma. J Clin Endocrinol Metab 42:105, 1976
49. Rogers J D, Lindberg R D, Hill C S, et al: Spindle and giant cell carcinoma of the thyroid. A different therapeutic approach. Cancer 34:1328, 1974
50. Jereb B, Stjernswärd J, Löwhagen T: Anaplastic giant-cell carcinoma of the thyroid. Cancer 35:1293, 1975
51. Gottlieb J A, Hill C S: Chemotherapy of thyroid cancer with adriamycin. N Engl J Med 290:193, 1974
52. Rozencweig M, vonHoff D D, Slavik M, et al: Cis-diaminedichloroplatinum: A new anticancer drug. Ann Intern Med 86:803, 1977

53. Öhman U, Granberg P O, Hjern B, et al: Pheochromocytoma: Diagnosis, management and follow-up in twenty patients. Acta Chir Scand 140:660, 1974
54. Hamilton B P M, Cheikh I E, Rivera L E: Attempted treatment of inoperable pheochromocytoma with streptozotocin. Arch Intern Med 137:762, 1977
55. Jordan R M, Kendall J W, Seaich J L, et al: Cerebrospinal fluid hormone concentration in the evaluation of pituitary tumors. Ann Intern Med 85:49, 1976
56. Ontjes D A, Ney R L: Pituitary tumors. Ca 26:330, 1976
57. Mallette L E, Bilezikian J P, Ketcham A S, et al: Parathyroid carcinoma in familial hyperparathyroidism. Am J Med 57:642, 1974
58. Au W Y W: Calcitonin treatment of hypercalcemia due to parathyroid carcinoma. Arch Intern Med 135:1594, 1975

Gerald P. Murphy

15

Chemotherapy of Renal, Bladder, and Prostate Cancer

The American Cancer Society recently estimated that neoplasms of the urogenital tract, including the prostate, bladder, and kidney, would be diagnosed in 100,000 instances as new cancer cases.[1]

Chemotherapy has been infrequently used in the urogenital tract, and in some instances, in the opinion of some, has played a minimal role or none at all in producing increased survival rates by various therapeutic means. Carter and former associates of the National Cancer Institute have recently reviewed some of the sparse material available on the effects of chemotherapeutic agents on these very deadly tumors.[1]

There are additional modalities of therapy, as well as chemotherapy, however, that have potential for overall intervention. Additional clinical results in certain urogenital cancers recently obtained with chemotherapy give reasonable basis for updating current clinical information. Moreover, on the basis of some of the recent cooperative study results, the initial pessimistic approach to the role of chemotherapy for urogenital cancer today seems unwarranted.[1] A review of basic principles of therapy as they relate to the urogenital tract would be in order. Basic knowledge of pharmacodynamics can be expected to be minimally available to the clinician urgently in need of a therapeutic regimen effective in the individual clinical situation. Generalizations thus might seem inappropriate. In the rapidly expanding field of chemotherapy today, however, some basic principles remain true regardless of the site of effectiveness of the agent. These must be brought to mind for application, if possible, whether it is on a controlled basis, a cooperative group study between institutions or under intensive and selective investigation at a comprehensive center or even within the National Cancer Institute itself.[1]

Prostatic Cancer

There have been recent reviews of beneficial chemotherapeutic results in prostate cancer.[1,2] For the most part, we are speaking today of the use of such agents as cytoxan or 5-FU under controlled conditions, in patients with Stage D or widely metastatic prostatic cancer who have relapsed after other types of hormonal therapy. The present status of chemotherapy, in terms of nonhormonal treat-

Supported in part by United States Public Health Service Grant #RR-05648-10 from the National Institutes of Health

ment, is not such that one can concern oneself with the possible implementation of nonhormonal agents at earlier stages of the disease. There is much that we do not understand about the development of prostatic cancer,[2,3] that will perhaps be clarified in the next few years as a result of the multiple activities sponsored by the National Cancer Institute and the National Prostatic Cancer Task Force.

Some authorities believe that radiation therapy has a definite role at various stages of prostatic cancer, particularly in those patients who may have been on hormonal therapy and have a local extension of the tumor.[4]

Implantation of radioactive agents including ^{125}I has also recently been reported.[5] There is, however, no final data at present to suggest that any synergism exists between these modalities of treatment and that of chemotherapy.

The hormonal effects of new agents in man, such as antiandrogens, to date remain to be further elucidated.[6] We may not know the mechanism of action of hormonal or noncytotoxic agents, however, but we still may be able to employ them effectively in prostatic cancer patients. The action of exogenous estrogens in the treatment of prostatic cancer patients is still a matter that is relatively unsettled.[7] Analogues of diethylstilbestrol have been manufactured and may have some synergistic effect with chemotherapy,[8] but at present, this is a speculative matter. The action of diethylstilbestrol on DNA in experimental in vitro systems may shed more light on their action.[9] A call for a reconsideration of the biology of carcinoma of the prostate has been made,[10] and a response in terms of new agents and new therapies, especially chemotherapy, seems to be unfolding. It is unfortunate, perhaps, that palliative effects of hormonal therapy still remain a matter of ongoing concern for many physicians treating prostatic cancer. The effects of new agents of a hormonal nature are important. The ultimate answer, however, in terms of cell-kill does not seem to be altered.[11]

Chemotherapy in general is not discussed in most reviews on the management of carcinoma of the prostate.[12] Steroid therapy is, however, important, and one does not wish to diminish its role in the palliative management of carcinoma of the prostate.[13] We must recognize from the outset, because of lack of technical and research data and despite the availability of adrenalectomy or hypophysectomy, that even some clinical aspects of these areas are incomplete.[13,14] Current clinical results do not involve large numbers of patients. Moreover, such advanced hormonal techniques, e.g., adrenalectomy or hypophysectomy, have not resulted in an overall increased survival of the patients despite over 30 years of experience with this approach. Newer agents, such as medroxyprogesterone, appear to have no greater benefit at this time.[15]

Hormones apparently participate, even at an early stage, in the formation of immune responses of the host.[16] This must be taken into consideration in the chemotherapy of prostatic cancer.[17] Whereas such evaluations at present are involved with clinical investigations, they will be a practical matter for routine consideration in the near future. A most promising new compound, an estradiol mustard combination (Estracyt*), appears to offer better results in patients who have relapsed, in comparison to those receiving standard hormonal therapy or even hypophysectomy and adrenalectomy.[18] The experience of a randomized study conducted at Roswell Park Memorial Institute, comparing the effects of Estracyt, has provided sufficient evidence that good long-term responses are obtained with this oral medication and result in better patient performance by objective criteria in operative measures such as bilateral adrenalectomy or hypophysectomy. Most other studies currently using the oral form of this agent report a total response rate close to or exceeding 40 per cent.[1]

The National Prostatic Cancer Task Force Treatment Group has evaluated several protocols. In their earliest studies comparing the effectiveness of standard treatment to 5-FU and cyclophosphamide, the group determined that, in patients in advanced stages with relapse after all forms of available therapy, a significant effectiveness of cyclophosphamide could be demonstrated.[19] Equally important in this particular initial observation on a controlled trial basis was the fact that chemo-

*Estracyt (estradiol-3-N[bis-(2-chlorethyl)]-carbamate-17-dihydrogenphosphate) AB Leo Company, Helsingborg, Sweden.

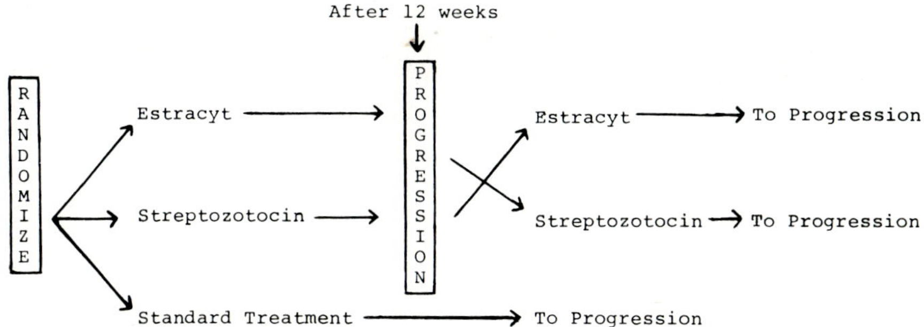

FIG. 15-1. PROTOCOL 200. - Treatment Schema: Estracyt; (600 mg/M^2 p.o. daily in three divided doses), Streptozotocin (500 mg/M^2 I.V. daily for five days every six weeks) or Standard treatment. A cross-over will be done at progression unless death intervenes.

therapeutic agents gave better relief from pain and other palliative benefits than the standard regimens that were being used at the various institutions.[19] Results from other cooperative studies are as yet incomplete and unavailable for critical evaluation. These trials encompass a most encouraging approach in prostatic cancer. The earlier history of chemotherapy in advanced prostatic cancer is limited principally to anecdotal observations, which are of sufficient merit for further review.

Since its inception, however, the National Prostatic Cancer Project has treated over 500 patients following their first protocol. Figure 15-1 illustrates Protocol 200. This protocol was derived to utilize chemotherapeutic agents in patients undergoing radiation therapy who could not tolerate cytotoxic activity. In this case again, estracyt has shown the greatest number of objective and subjective responders. Additional drugs are still underway in their initial evaluation in Protocol 300 (Fig. 15-2). In this protocol, both DTIC and cytoxan have shown activity. Other protocols are shown in Figure 15-3 (Protocol 400), Figure 15-4 (Protocol 500), and Figure 15-5 (Protocol 600). In Protocols 500 and 600, as a result of earlier observations, the National Prostatic Cancer Project is now treating patients who are newly diagnosed as having been in a state of metastatic or Stage D disease; or patients who have been in a stable state. Such chemotherapeutic randomized trials will compare the initial impact of chemotherapy with that of hormonal therapy on an equal and objective basis. The combination treatments also illustrated in these protocols have continued to indicate beneficial impact that will be described upon completion of their review.

Bloom and Hendry observed that a limited response of prostatic cancer to various alkylating agents has been reported.[20] They noted the work of Weyrauch and Nesbet in 1959, of Fox in 1965, and of Flocks in 1969; pain relief and temporary remission occurred in 6 of 12 patients with disseminated disease treated with small dosages of nitrogen mustard by Flocks. Bloom and Hendry have found that a combination of nitrogen mustard and 5-FU on an intermittent basis obtained subjective improvement for up to one year in 11 of 12 patients. The difficulty in discussing response rates in patients with such advanced disease, of course, always relates to the criteria for remission. These have been firmly established on a reasonable basis for the National Prostatic Cancer Task Force.[19] Bloom and Hendry also felt that decreases in serum-acid phosphatase levels in five of their patients who initially had raised levels, were objective signs of response.[20] The majority of workers in this field would agree with this viewpoint. Most, however, feel that multiple agents, e.g., hydroxyurea, remain to be tested.

Kogler, in a review of chemotherapy of prostatic cancer, confirmed several of the earlier observations recounted in this report.[21] In addition, in an unpublished phase I study, he found that the agent carbesterol, used in 18 patients at a dosage of 2.5 to 200 mg/day, resulted in remissions in 2 patients. This compound apparently has estrogenic activity with additional antitumor activity and, in Kogler's opinion, may merit further testing.[21]

We have so far talked mainly about agents

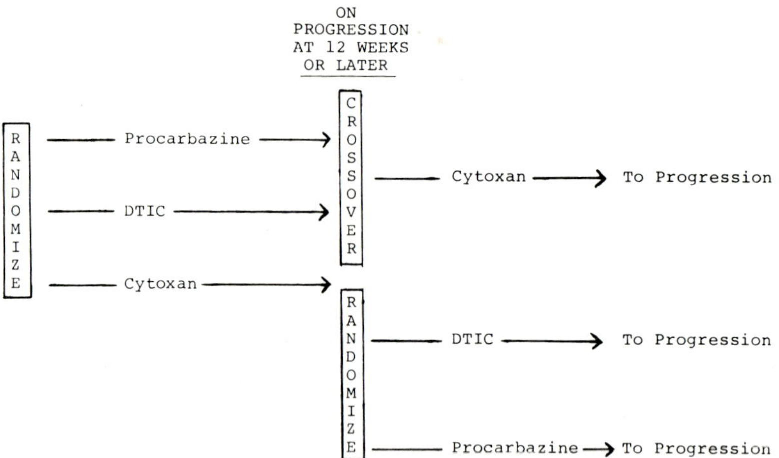

FIG. 15-2. PROTOCOL 300. - Treatment Schema: DTIC (200 mg/M² I.V. Days 1-5, 21 days rest, then repeat cycle), Procarbazine (100 mg/M² p.o. daily days 1-22, 3 weeks rest. Rx days 44-65; 3 weeks rest etc.) or Cytoxan (1 gm/M² I.V. every three weeks). A cross-over will be done at progression unless death intervenes.

that are given orally or intravenously. There is some initial evidence suggesting that arterial infusion of 5-FU may also have a beneficial effect for local extensive Stage C as well as Stage D lesions of prostatic cancer.[22] Intraprostatic injections of various antitumor agents have been attempted on an experimental basis but have not shown any long-lasting effect in man.[23]. One must recall that in all of these patients we are dealing with a relatively older population, already beset with chronic heart and lung disease in many instances and with a limited bone marrow capacity. This is in marked contrast to other genitourinary tumors that may occur in younger age groups.

Prostatic cancer does, however, infrequently occur in young adults, and perhaps chemotherapy may have a more hopeful outlook in some of these rare instances.[24] At Roswell Park Memorial Institute, our own results of a randomized study utilizing 5-FU, cytoxan and adriamycin have shown a decrease in pain, improvement in performance status and stabilization of the disease in a significant number of patients (Table 15-1). These initial results favored cytoxan and adriamycin (Table 15-1). Others have described good results using only one of the agents at a time, e.g., cytoxan or 5-FU.[19] Thus, it appears that chemotherapy may now be indicated for careful use in patients with advanced prostatic cancer with relapse after other conventional forms of therapy. Its future role remains to be determined and can be aggressively pursued under properly conducted controlled trials, as well as in earlier stages of the disease.

Other combination therapeutic studies with prostatic cancer have utilized as many as

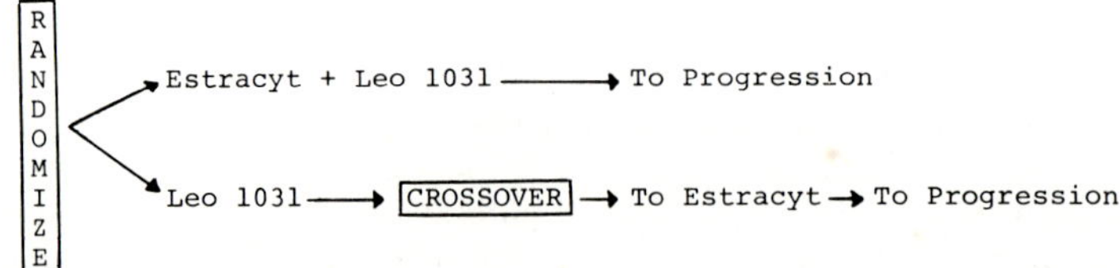

FIG. 15-3. PROTOCOL 400 - Treatment Schema: Estracyt (600 mg/M² p.o. daily in three divided doses plus Leo 1031, 30 mg/day p.o. in three divided doses for six days out of every seven days) or Leo 1031 (30 mg/day p.o. in three divided doses for six days out of every seven days).

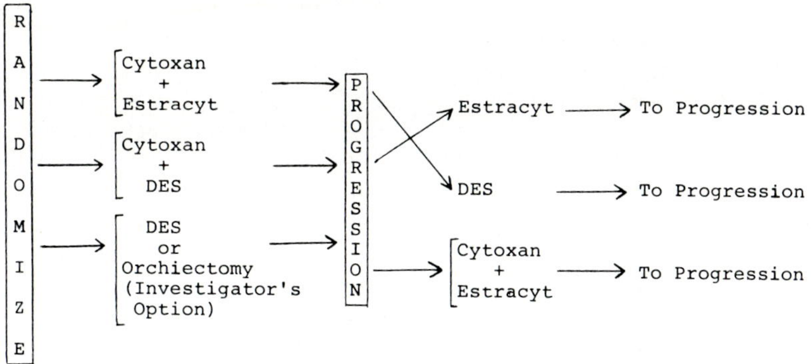

FIG. 15-4. PROTOCOL 500 - Treatment Schema: Cytoxan (1 gm/M² I.V. every three weeks) plus Estracyt (600 mg/M² p.o. daily in three divided doses), Cytoxan (1 gm/M² I.V. every three weeks) plus Diethylstilbestrol (1 mg t.i.d. p.o.) *or* Diethylstilbestrol (1 mg t.i.d. p.o.) *or* Orchiectomy. Patients whose disease progresses after the initial 12 weeks of therapy will be crossed over.
(Protocol 500 is for the treatment of patients with newly diagnosed clinical Stage D carcinoma of the prostate who have not had prior hormonal therapy).

five drugs. The criteria for objective and subjective responses in advanced disease with multiple toxic agents are difficult to evaluate, however, and must be watched with caution. Other combinations have yet to be used to suitably treat an adequate number of patients on a randomized basis in order to permit objective assessment at this time.

BLADDER CANCER

Chemotherapy of bladder cancer in most instances has been limited to the advanced cases, i.e., Stage D, where the tumor has spread beyond the bladder and is present in metastatic sites. Conventional chemotherapeutic agents have been evaluated under such conditions.

Prout et al, in a study with a bladder surgical adjuvant group, did not find benefit with 5-FU used in various stages, either preoperatively or postoperatively.[25] As shown in Table 15-2, from data collected by Carter and Wasserman,[1] 5-FU has been the drug most studied in this disease state. Despite conflicting reports, it appears to have some activity. The difference of opinion relates chiefly to

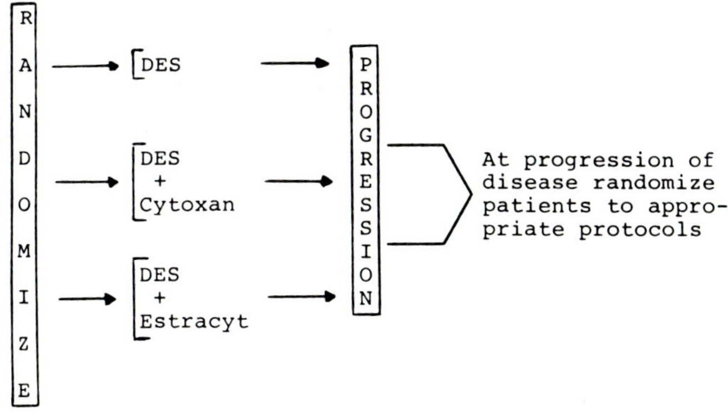

FIG. 15-5. PROTOCOL 600 - Treatment Schema: Diethylstilbestrol (1 mg t.i.d. p.o.), Diethylstilbestrol (1 mg t.i.d. p.o.) plus Cytoxan (1 gm/M² I.V. every three weeks) or Diethylstilbestrol, (1 mg t.i.d. p.o.) plus Estracyt (600 mg/M² p.o. daily in three divided doses). (Protocol 600 is for the treatment of patients with non-progressing metastases).

TABLE 15-1. *Results at Roswell Park Memorial Institute of Chemotherapy of Prostatic Carcinoma Stage D, with 5-FU + Cytoxan and Adriamycin +Cytoxan**

	5-FU + Cytoxan†	Adriamycin + Cytoxan§
Objective response	2	3
Subjective response	5	5
Stable	1	3
Progression	3	0
Total	11	11

*Follow-up of one year.

†5-FU 8 mg/kg/day for 5 days every month; cytoxan 4 mg/kg/day for 5 days every month.

§Adriamycin 40 mg/m² every 3 weeks; cytoxan 200 mg/day for 4 days every 3 weeks.

the timing and the amount to be given. Hopefully, the new National Bladder Task Force will further elucidate this difficult problem. Earlier studies have suggested that adriamycin may have some activity in bladder cancer, but the response rates are relatively variable and not entirely clear.[1] Cyclophosphamide, chlorambucil, hydroxyurea and procarbazine have all been tried but without impressive response rates in patients with advanced disease.[1] It would appear that MTX treatment for advanced bladder cancer has been successful in the hands of several authors.[26] Published reports that have been collected indicate a combined response rate of above 36 per cent. These objectives responses have been seen in advanced cases and these results have been duplicated in the Royal Marsden Hospital se-

TABLE 15-2. *5-Fluorouracil Therapy of Bladder Cancer Data Accumulated by Carter and Wasserman (1975)*[1]

Investigator	Drug Schedule*	No. of Patients Evaluable	Responses
Olson and Greene	S	3	1
Lemon	12-15 mg/kg/day × 3-6 days, 1 g/day × 5	3	1
	days (daily 8 hr IV infusion)	2	0
Wilson	S	12	9†
Young et al	S	4	1
Kennedy and Theologides	S	2	0
Weiss et al	S	6	0
Staley et al	S	3	1
Vaitkevicius et al	S	3	0
Ansfield et al	S	7	1
Hall and Good	S or 15 mg/kg/day × 3 days then 7.5 mg/kg on day 4 and day 5, followed by 7.5 mg/kg biweekly × 4-6 wk	2	0
Choy et al	S	1	0
Field	S except 7.5-10 mg/kg/wk as maintenance	9	1‡
Glenn et al	S	7	4§
Cressy and Schell	S	1	1
Moore et al	S	9	6
Total		74	26

*S = Standard loading dose (15 mg/kg/day IV for 4 to 5 days, then 7.5 mg/kg for 2 to 3 days to toxicity, repeated monthly).

†Responses include only marked objective regression.

‡Response > 1 year duration.

§Patients with superficial lesions had significant improvement; those with invasive tumors failed to respond.

Includes 1 complete and 5 partial responses.

1. Carter S K, Wasserman T H: The chemotherapy of urologic cancer. Cancer 36:729 (Suppl), 1975

ries.[26] This given considerable hope for further employment of 5-FU and MTX combined.

In our own institution, good results have been obtained combining cyclophosphamide and adriamycin. In a randomized study comparing the effects of cyclophosphamide alone and adriamycin alone with a combination of adriamycin and cyclophosphamide, regression of metastases, subjective improvement and stabilization of advanced disease states were frequently observed (Table 15-3). Such regimens, in our opinion, can now be used effectively in advanced disease states and may have a role to play in earlier stages of the disease. We have utilized mitomycin C in 27 patients with advanced Stage D carcinoma at Roswell Park. Of these, 19 were considered evaluable, and an objective response occurred in 21 per cent for a sufficiently long period of time. The major toxicity involving myelosuppression and occasional nephrotoxicity, however, is such that this single-agent regimen is no longer being pursued.[27]

In superficial bladder tumors, multiple papillomas have presented a problem. Since Veenema's earliest observation of thio-TEPA, this agent appears to be the one most useful for topical chemotherapy or instillation into the bladder of patients with recurrent bladder papilloma.[28] Veenema's earlier results have been confirmed in a variety of institutions world-wide and by a variety of individuals.[29] The frequency of administration per urethral catheter directly into the bladder to treat multiple well-differentiated papillary bladder tumors appears to be well established. The urinary bladder naturally lends itself to topical therapy, as a high local concentration of the drug can usually be obtained with minimal toxicity.[28] While some may disagree about the indications for use of thio-TEPA, most would agree that there may be some indication for use in the treatment of small multiple super-

TABLE 15-3. *Results at Roswell Park Memorial Institute of Chemotherapy of Advanced Bladder Carcinoma with Adriamycin and Cytoxan**

Responses	Cytoxan† No., %	Cytoxan† Stage	Adriamycin‡ No., %	Adriamycin‡ Stage	Cytoxan + Adriamycin§ No., %	Cytoxan + Adriamycin§ Stage	No. of Patients
Objective response	8	A 4	2	A 2	8	A 5	18
	38%	B 4	28.5%	B 0	53.3%	B 0	
		C 0		C 0		C 0	
		D 0		D 0		D 3	
Subjective response	7	A 2	2	A 0	4	A 1	13
	33.3%	B 1	28.5%	B 1	26.6%	B 1	
		C 1		C 1		C 0	
		D 3		D 0		D 2	
Stable	4	A 1	0	A 0	0	A 0	4
	19%	B 2		B 0		B 0	
		C 0		C 0		C 0	
		D 1		D 0		D 0	
Progression	2	A 1	3	A 0	3	A 0	8
	9.5%	B 0	43%	B 0	20%	B 0	
		C 0		C 0		C 0	
		D 1		D 3		D 3	
Total	21		7		15		43

*Follow-up of one year.
†1 g/m² every three weeks.
‡75 mg/m² every three weeks.
§ADR 40 mg/m² every three weeks; CYT 800 mg/m² every three weeks.

ficial papillary tumors and perhaps as a prophylaxis to minimize recurrence in patients with a pattern of multiple tumor recurrence. A recent review found thio-TEPA to be effective when properly applied in about 2 of 3 patients, with 1 of 3 patients receiving complete remission.[1] It is felt by some that the recurrence of failures of the thio-TEPA regimen in some circumstances may be related to immunologic aspects locally present in the bladder.[30]

Chemotherapy of bladder cancer is still in an early stage of development, and it would appear that cytoxan, adriamycin, 5-FU and mitomycin C have some evidence of activity. Their proper combination and application in the management of bladder carcinoma remain to be studied under additional controlled situations. As has been stated, the primary need of bladder cancer therapy is an effective modality capable of eradicating tumor cells remaining after surgery or radiotherapy or both, and accomplishing the major cell-kill function.[1] The various chemotherapeutic agents discussed seem to offer this opportunity.

Renal Cell Carcinoma

Unresectable or metastatic renal cell carcinoma is a relentless disease which kills 11,000 Americans annually. This tumor has proven to be one of the least responsive to additional local or systemic therapy. In a series of patients reviewed by Talley et al in 1969, the radioresistance of renal cell carcinoma was reaffirmed.[31] A review of the chemotherapy at that time was not encouraging, however. Talley reviewed the subject again in 1973 and found little change in the status of therapy.[32] Nevertheless, hormonal therapy of hypernephroma was often attempted and responses are occasionally seen.[31] Alberto and Senn found hormonal therapy of no detectable value in a study published in 1974.[33] A recent Eastern Cooperative Oncology Group (ECOG) study also showed an unequivocally negative result with progestational agents.[34] At a number of centers an organized preclinical screening approach to the testing of cytotoxic agents and combinations has been instituted. An important part of this approach has been the development of hormonally independent renal tumor models. Hrushesky and Murphy have characterized a spontaneous murine renal adenocarcinoma model that was transplantable in an inbred mouse strain.[35] The data obtained with this model at Roswell Park Memorial Institute and by Shefner and Marlow at the National Cancer Institute has supported several trials of agents yielding some apparent clinical activity in this tumor (see Table 15-1).[33,34,36,37,38,39]

Before detailed evaluation of the various therapeutic modalities is made, a comment concerning the spontaneous regression of renal carcinomas in man is in order. The true incidence of this occurrence is exceedingly hard to obtain, and the incidence of histologically confirmed complete regression is a figure even harder to determine. H.J.G. Bloom has written extensively on this tumor type and has reported a single, well-documented case in experiences of over 200 patients.[40] The incidence of this phenomenon is believed to be perhaps substantially below 1 per cent.

Hormonal Therapy

A review of the literature of hormonal therapy of renal carcinoma is difficult to interpret because of markedly differing response criteria. Hormonal manipulations have been the mainstay of therapy in advanced disease, both because of their lack of serious toxicity and because of quoted response rates which may be inaccurately high. Early enthusiasm for androgenic and progestational therapies was generated by reviews which seldom clearly separated response data into subjective and objective categories. Furthermore, objective response criteria were often ill-defined. In reviewing hormonal therapy in this disease, it becomes clear that as stricter response criteria have been applied to this study population, response rates have shrunk. Therefore, literature prior to 1971 and since 1971 are reviewed with this in mind.[41]

There are nine studies in the literature prior to 1971 which separate subjective from objective responses.[31,42,43,44,45,46,47,48,49] Some of these studies, however, do not clearly define an objective response. Each of these studies includes a progestational agent, except that of Jenkin which used androgens alone.[43] The studies range in size from 4 patients to 80 patients and a total of 228 patients are included, 40 of which responded. Objective response rates range from 7 per cent (1 of 15 patients treated by Jenkin with androgens alone) to 33 per cent (4 of 12 patients treated by Papac with progestins followed by androgens).[43,46] The response rates of most of the other studies hover very closely around the mean of a 17 per cent objective response. It should be emphasized that objective response in these studies is not a partial remission and does not necessarily represent 50 per cent tumor regression or improved survival. It may be stabilization, i.e., a less than 50 per cent tumor regression, or a mixed response. Table 15-4 summarizes the reported objective response data between 1967 and 1971.[41]

Studies done since 1971 have not demonstrated so great a benefit from progestational or androgenic hormonal therapy.[32,33,34,50,51] Two of these studies are randomized ECOG studies, as is the study of Alberto and Senn.[33,34,50]

The other two studies are more recent unselected series of patients treated with hormonal therapy alone.[32,51] Talley has reported 98 patients treated exclusively with hormonal therapy, 7 of whom showed objective response.[32] A 1973 ECOG study is referenced in Legha's review of hormonal therapies.[50] Twenty-one patients in one arm of this randomized study of advanced renal cell carcinoma received provera (100 mg tid p.o.) alone with a single brief response. In the study by Alberto and Senn in 1974, 58 consecutive patients were treated with hormonal therapy without a single objective response.[33] Lokich and Harrison likewise treated 73 consecutive patients without a response.[51] A 1976 ECOG study treated a large series of patients with chemotherapy alone or chemotherapy plus depo-provera and demonstrated no additional benefit to any of the 166 patients hormonally treated.[34] Table 15-5 shows the data collected between 1971 and 1976 and demonstrates a markedly decreased objective response rate for hormonally treated patients when compared to the years 1967 to 1971. In the latter group, 416 patients are included, 8 of whom showed objective evidence of response or 1.8 per cent.[41]

Single Agent-Chemotherapy

Data available for the evaluation of single agents in this disease come from published reports and reports made directly to the National Cancer Institute Cancer Therapy Evaluation Program. Almost none of the agents have been evaluated sufficiently to allow definitive statements concerning their activity in this tumor. Only vinblastine has been used in more than 100 patients. One hundred thirty-five patients have been treated with vinblas-

TABLE 15-4. *1967-1971—Progestins and/or Androgens Hormonal Treatment of Advanced Renal Carcinoma**

Investigator	Patients Evaluated	Responses
Woodruff et al., 1967 [49]	4	1 (25%)
Melander et al., 1967 [44]	20	4 (20%)
Jenkin, 1967 [43]	15	1 (7%)
Samuels et al., 1968 [47]	23	4 (17%)
Talley et al., 1969 [31]	16	2 (12%)
Papac, 1969 [46]	12	4 (33%)
Paine et al., 1970 [45]	15	3 (20%)
Wagle and Murphy, 1971 [48]	43	8 (17%)
Bloom, 1971 [42]	80	13 (16%)
Total	228	40 (17%)

*Hrushesky W J, Murphy G P: Current status of the therapy of advanced renal carcinoma. J Surg Oncol 9(3):277–288, 1977.

TABLE 15-5. *1971-1976—Progestins and/or Androgens Hormonal Treatment of Advanced Renal Carcinoma**

Investigator	Patients Evaluated	Objective Responses
Alberto and Senn, 1974 [33]	58	0
Eastern Cooperative Oncology Group, 1976 [34]	166	0
Lokich and Harrison, 1975 [51]	73	0
Talley, 1971 [32]	98	7 (7%)
Eastern Cooperative Oncology Group, 1973 [50]	21	1 (4%)
Total	416	8 (<2%)

*Hrushesky W J, Murphy G P: Current status of the therapy of advanced renal carcinoma. J Surg Oncol 9(3):277–288, 1977.

tine as a single agent and 33 (25 per cent) of these have shown evidence of objective response. The next most adequately evaluated drug is meCCNU in which seven responses have been seen in 79 patients treated. If the nitrosoureas are taken as a group, 99 patients have been treated with a response rate of under 10 per cent. Other alkylating agents have also shown poor activity in moderate numbers of patients. Cytoxan has registered no response in 44 patients treated. Nitrogen mustards fared slightly better with 10 per cent activity, or 4 of 35 patients responding. Other drugs which have been used to treat more than 25 patients are the antimetabolites, 5-FU, and 6-mercaptopurine (6-MP). These two agents each register about a 10 per cent activity with five of 51 and two of 26 responses respectively. Hydroxyurea is the only other agent which has been used in any number of patients. Five responses have been seen in 45 patients treated or about 11 per cent. All other agents must be considered as totally inevaluable by virtue of the very small number of patients treated with each agent (Table 15-6).[41]

Vinblastine is the only agent which has received moderately extensively trial in this disease and is the most active single agent.

Combination Chemotherapeutic and Hormonal Therapy

Three studies involving a combination of chemotherapy plus some form of hormonal therapy are described in Table 15-7.[41] Alberto and Senn combined vinblastine, 5-FU, and medroxyprogesterone in 20 patients with advanced renal cell carcinoma and saw no objective remissions.[33] The Eastern Cooperative Oncology Group ran a four-armed study comparing vinblastine alone, with meCCNU alone and with each of these agents plus a progestin. Responses were seen in all four arms, but hormones did not add significantly to the effectiveness of the cytotoxic agent.[34] The most recent combination study was done by Lokich and Harrison at the Sidney Farber Cancer Center.[51] In this study, 4 patients were treated with cytoxan, MTX, 5-FU and vincristine plus prednisone. No responses were seen. The overall objective response rate of 7 per cent for combination chemotherapeutic and hormonal therapy is not encouraging and is somewhat worse than the best single-agent chemotherapy data. This 7 per cent activity is, however, somewhat better than the review of hormonal therapy reported since 1971 (Table 15-5).

Combination Chemotherapy

Multiple-agent chemotherapy of renal cell carcinoma has been understandably slow in development due to the lack of active or even evaluated single agents (Table 15-6).

Five studies appear in Table 15-8.[41] Merrin et al compared meCCNU plus vinblastine with CCNU plus vinblastine.[39] Fifteen patients with advanced disease were given the first combination and a single objective remission was observed.[39] Six patients were treated with CCNU and vinblastine and again

TABLE 15-6. *Single Agent Chemotherapy of Renal Cell Carcinoma**

Drugs	Patients Evaluated	>50% Objective Response
Alkylating Agents		
Cytoxan	44	0
Nitrogen mustards	35	4
BCNU	2	0
CCNU	18	0
MeCCNU	79	7
Hydroxyurea	45	5
Thiotepa	22	2
Azotepa	2	0
Dimethyltriazeno Imidazole Carboxamide	4	0
Sulfonic acid esters	9	0
AB 132	14	0
AB 103	6	1
Hexamethylamine	17	1
Dianhydrogalactitol	11	1
Antimetabolites		
5-FU	51	5
5-FUDR	4	1
6-Mercaptopurine	26	2
Arabinoside-C	2	0
5-Azacytidine	4	0
Hadacin	3	0
Thiocarzolamide	1	0
Pyrazo pyrimidines	1	0
Vitamin Analogues		
Methotrexate	5	0
5-Aminonicotinamide	7	2
Antibiotics		
Adriamycin	3	0
Mithramycin	4	0
Actinomycin D	4	0
Mitomycin C	2	0
Bleomycin	3	0
Plant Alkaloids		
Vinblastine	135	33
Vincristine	6	0
Epidophylotoxin VP16	5	0
Metals		
Cis platinum	20	0

*Hrushesky W J, Murphy G P: Current status of the therapy of advanced renal carcinoma. J Surg Oncol 9(3):277–288, 1977.

a single objective response was observed.[39] No responses have been seen in 4 patients given vincristine, bleomycin and Cis platinum by Samson et al[52] Johnson et al treated 15 patients with hydroxyurea plus vincristine with no response, and Lokich and Harrison treated 3 patients each with adriamycin plus dimethyltriazeno imidazole carboxamide (DTIC) and mitomycin C plus 5-FU and no responses were seen.[51,53]

Altogether, 46 patients have been treated with various combinations of chemotherapeu-

TABLE 15-7. *Advanced Renal Cell Carcinoma Combination Chemotherapy and Hormone Therapy**

Investigator	Chemotherapy	Hormone	Patients Evaluated	Objective Response
Alberto and Senn 1974 [33]	Vinblastine + 5-FU	Medroxyprogesterone	20	0
Eastern Cooperative Oncology Group, 1976 [34]	MeCCNU	Depo-Provera	38	4
Eastern Cooperative Oncology Group, 1976 [34]	Vinblastine	Depo-Provera	38	3
Lokich and Harrison, 1975 [51]	Cytoxan Methotrexate 5-Fluorouracil Vincristine	Prednisone	4	0
		Total	100	7 (7%)

*Hrushesky W J, Murphy G P: Current status of the therapy of advanced renal carcinoma. J Surg Oncol 9(3):277–288, 1977.

tic agents. Two objective responses (5 per cent) were seen. This poor objective response record is significantly worse than the best single agents, e.g., vinblastine. Whether the lack of activity of these combinations reflects accurately the lack of activity of each of the constituent agents is impossible to say, since virtually no single-agent data exists for many of the drugs used in these combinations. A further reason for the lack of activity of the combination regimens is that the toxicity caused by administration of the inactive agents within the combination may have caused decreased dosage of the active agent or agents given.

ANALYSIS OF VINBLASTINE ACTIVITY

Vinblastine, as stated, appears effective. It may be valuable, therefore, to study in greater detail the only agent so far clinically evaluated which has shown significant activity. Table 15-9 details each of the thirteen

TABLE 15-8. *The Combination Chemotherapy of Advanced Renal Cell Carcinoma**

Investigator	Chemotherapy	Patients Evaluated	Objective Response
Merrin et al [39]	MeCCNU + Vinblastine	15	1
Merrin et al [39]	CCNU + Vinblastine	6	1
Samson et al [52]	Vinblastine + Bleomycin + Cis-dichlorodiammine-platinum (II)	4	0
Johnson et al [53]	Vincristine + Hydroxyurea	15	0
Lokich and Harrison [51]	Adriamycin + Dimethyltriazeno imidazole carboxamide	3	0
Lokich and Harrison [51]	Mitomycin C + 5-Fluorouracil	3	0
	Total	46	2 (5%)

*Hrushesky W J, Murphy G P: Current status of the therapy of advanced renal carcinoma. J Surg Oncol 9(3):277–288, 1977.

studies in which vinblastine was used as a single agent weekly.[31,32,34,38,51,54,55,56,57,58,59,60,61] The table is arranged with those studies using the highest dose of vinblastine appearing first. One hundred and thirty-five patients were treated in these thirteen studies. Three complete remissions of up to 4 years duration were seen. Twenty-three partial remissions, i.e., greater than 50 per cent decrease of all disease with appearance of no new lesions, were seen, while seven cases of less than 50 per cent regression or stabilization of rapidly progressive disease were registered. One hundred and two patients progressed while on vinblastine therapy. A total of 25 per cent or 33 of 135 patients treated showed evidence of objective remission. It becomes apparent from Table 15-9 that the patients receiving the highest weekly doses of vinblastine were the most likely to respond.[38,58]

Vinblastine in Combination Therapy

Table 15-10 outlines the details of treatment of four series of patients given combinations containing vinblastine.[41] Drugs used in combination with vinblastine included CCNU, 5-FU plus progestins, bleomycin plus Cis-platinum and finally provera.[33,34,39,55] Sixty-eight patients were treated with combination therapy which included vinblastine. Four of these patients had 50 per cent tumor regressions, 9 had either less than 50 per cent regressions or stabilization of previously progressive disease, and 55 of the patients progressed while on therapy. The overall objective response rate is 18 per cent in 13 of 68 patients. It is of interest that where combination therapy required the dose or frequency of vinblastine to be decreased, no objective regressions were seen.[33,55] This would lead one to suspect that the vinblastine may very well be the most important element within these combination regimens.

Summary

This report describes the current status of chemotherapy of prostate, bladder and renal cancer. As stated, there are few randomized trials, limited Phase I and Phase II reports, and some anecdotal information. There are intimations, nevertheless, despite this paucity of reported information, that indicate effectiveness in prostate cancer. Among these agents are Estracyt, cytoxan, 5-FU, and per-

TABLE 15-9. *Tabular Analysis of Results of Trials Using Vinblastine as a Single Agent Weekly for Advanced Renal Cell Carcinoma*

Weekly Dose	Patients Evaluated	Complete Remission	Partial Remission (>50%)	Stable or Regression of <50%	Progression	Reference
0.3 mg/kg	35	1	10	0	24	38
0.2 mg/kg	4	0	1	1	2	58
0.15 mg/kg	1	0	1	0	0	54
0.15 mg/kg	4	0	1	2	1	56
0.15 mg/kg	1	0	0	0	1	59
0.15 mg/kg	1	0	0	0	1	51
5 mg/m^2	44	2	3	0	39	34
0.1 mg/kg	15	0	2	0	13	32
0.1 mg/kg	13	0	3	0	10	31
0.1 mg/kg	7	0	0	4	3	61
0.1 mg/kg	2	0	1	0	1	60
N.A.	4	0	1	0	3	57
N.A.	4	0	0	0	4	55
Total	135	3	23	7	102	

Objective responses in 33 of 135 or 25%

TABLE 15-10. *Tabular Analysis of Results of Trials Using Vinblastine Containing Combinations for Advanced Renal Cell Carcinoma**

Regimen	Patients Evaluated	Complete Remission	Partial Remission (>50%)	Stable or >50%	Progressive	Reference
Vinblastine 0.2 mg/kg qwk + CCNU 130 mg/m² qbwk	6	0	1	3	2	39
Vinblastine 0.15 mg/kg biw + 5-FU 0.15 mg/kg biw + Progestin	20	0	0	6	14	35
Vinblastine 6 mg/m² biw + Bleomycin 15 mg biw + Cis-dichlorodiammine-platinum (II) 15 mg/m² biw	4	0	0	0	4	55
Vinblastine 5 mg/m² qwk + Provera	38	0	3	0	35	34
Total	68	0	4	9	55	
	Objective responses in 13 of 68 or 18%					

*Hrushesky W J, Murphy G P: Current status of the therapy of advanced renal carcinoma. J Surg Oncol 9(3):277–288, 1977.

haps DTIC. Further clinical trials will doubtless support this observation. In terms of bladder cancer, limited information indicates that 5-FU, cytoxan, adriamycin, mitomycin C and perhaps MTX may have some activity. The agents are listed in their order of preference at the current time according to our understanding. Other agents have been described, but reports at this time are limited. In terms of renal cell carcinoma, the nitrosoureas have less activity than vinblastine and its analogues. Vinblastine appears to be the drug of choice as compared with hormonal agents. Some of these trials could be improved if the agents were used as adjunctive forms of therapy at an earlier stage of the disease.

REFERENCES

1. Carter S K, Wasserman T H: The chemotherapy of urologic cancer. Cancer 36:729 (suppl), 1975
2. Murphy G P: Prostatic cancer, in Murphy G P, Mittelman A (eds): Chemotherapy of Urogenital Tumors. Springfield, IL, Thomas, 1975, p 26
3. Akazaki K: Comparative histological studies on the latent carcinoma of the prostate under different environmental circumstances. International Agency for Research on Cancer Scientific Publications 18:89, 1973
4. Ray G R, Bagshaw M A: The role of radiation therapy in the definitive treatment of adeno-

carcinoma of the prostate. Annual Review of Medicine, vol. 26. Palo Alto, CA, Annual Reviews, 1975, p 567
5. Whitmore W F Jr, Hilaris B, Grabstald H, et al: Implantation of ^{125}I in prostatic cancer. Surg Clin North Am 54:887, 1974
6. Schoonees R, Schalch D S, Murphy G P: The hormonal effects of antiandrogen (SH-714) treatment in man. Invest Urol 8:635, 1971
7. Szendröi Z, Kocsár L, Karika Z, et al: Recent data on the mechanism of action of oestrogens in the treatment of prostatic tumour patients. Int Urol Nephrol 5:311, 1973
8. Lawson J E, Dennis R D, Majewski R F, et al: Diarylcyclobutane analogs of diethylstilbestrol. J Med Chem 17:383, 1974
9. Blackburn G M, Flavell A J, Thompson M H: Oxidative and photochemical linkage of diethylstilbestrol to DNA in vitro. Cancer Res 34:2015, 1974
10. Williams G, Wallace D M, Bloom H J G: A reconsideration of the biology of carcinoma of the prostate. Br J Urol 46:61, 1974
11. Zimel H, Bocancea D: Treatment of prostatic carcinoma with stilbostat. Neoplasma 21:101, 1974
12. Abercrombie G F: Carcinoma of the prostate. Ann R Coll Surg Engl 54:16, 1974
13. Williams D C: Steroid therapy of carcinoma of the prostate, in Raven R W (ed): Modern Trends in Oncology-1, Part I: Research Progress, vol. 1. Toronto, Butterworth, 1973, p 209
14. Thompson J B, Greenberg E, Pazianos A, et al: Hypophysectomy in metastatic prostate cancer. NY State J Med 74:1006, 1974
15. Rafla S, Johnson R: The treatment of advanced prostatic carcinoma with medroxyprogesterone. Curr Ther Res 16:261, 1974
16. Maor D, Englander T, Eylan E, et al: Participation of hormone in the early stages of the immune response. Acta Endocrinol 75:205, 1974
17. Catalona W J: Host-tumor interactions during 5-fluorouracil therapy for prostatic carcinoma. Urology 4:287, 1974
18. Welvaart K, Merrin C E, Mittelman A, et al: Stage D prostatic carcinoma. Survival rate in relapsed patients following new forms of palliation. Urology 4:283, 1974
19. Scott W W, Gibbons R P, Johnson D E, et al: The continued evaluation of the effects of chemotherapy in patients with advanced carcinoma of the prostate. J Urol 116:211, 1976
20. Bloom H J G, Hendry W F: Treatment of prostatic carcinoma, in Raven R W (ed): Modern Trends in Oncology-1, Part 2: Clinical Progress, vol. 2. Toronto, Butterworth, 1973, p 143
21. Kogler J: Chemotherapy of prostatic cancer. A review of the literature. Wadley Med Bull 4:32, 1974
22. Nevin J E III, Melnick I, Baggerly J T, et al: Arterial infusion of 5-fluorouracil as a treatment for carcinoma of the prostate. J Urol 112:114, 1974
23. Firstater M, Meshorer A: Intraprostatic injections of various antitumoral compounds into rats. Urol Res 2:49, 1974
24. Chiu C L, Weber D L: Prostatic carcinoma in young adults. JAMA 230:724, 1974
25. Prout G R Jr, Slack N H, Bross I D J: Irradiation and 5-fluorouracil as adjuvants in the management of invasive bladder carcinoma. A cooperative group report after 4 years. J Urol 104:116, 1970
26. Hall R R, Bloom H J G, Freeman J E, et al: Methotrexate treatment for advanced bladder cancer. Br J Urol 46:431, 1974
27. Early K, Elias E G, Mittelman A, et al: Mitomycin C in the treatment of metastatic transitional cell carcinoma of the urinary bladder. Cancer 31:1150, 1973
28. Veenema R J, Dean A L Jr, Roberts M, et al: Bladder carcinoma treated by direct instillation of thio-TEPA. J Urol 88:60, 1962
29. Currò S, Foti E: Local antiblastic chemotherapy in tumours of the bladder. Panminerva Med 15:298, 1973
30. Corrado F, Lalanne G, Pizza G C: Chemoprophylaxis of bladder cancer recurrence: Immunological aspects. Panminerva Med 16:85, 1974
31. Talley R W, Moorhead E L, Tucker W G, et al: Treatment of metastatic hypernephroma. J Am Med Assoc 207:322, 1969
32. Talley R W, Chemotherapy of adenocarcinoma of the kidney. Cancer 32:1062, 1973
33. Alberto P, Senn H J: Hormonal therapy of renal carcinoma alone and in association with cytostatic drugs. Cancer 33:1226, 1974
34. Hahn R G, Brodovsky H: Methyl CCNU, Velban and Depo-Provera treatment trials in advanced renal cancer. Proc Am Assoc Cancer Res and Am Soc Clin Oncol 17:246 (abstr #C-38), 1976
35. Hrushesky W J, Murphy G P: Investigation of a new renal tumor model. J Surg Res 15:327, 1973
36. Hrushesky W J, Murphy G P: Evaluation of chemotherapeutic agents in a new murine renal carcinoma model. J Natl Cancer Inst 52:1117, 1974
37. Shefner A M, Marlow M: Preliminary drug trials in a renal cell carcinoma animal model. Cancer Chemother Reports 5:145, 1975
38. Hagan K, Trapp J D, Rhamy R K, et al: Treatment of metastatic renal cell carcinoma.

Southern Med J 67:1175, 1974
39. Merrin C, Mittelman A, Fanous N, et al: Chemotherapy of advanced renal cell carcinoma with vinblastine and CCNU. J Urol 113:21, 1975
40. Bloom H J G: Adjuvant therapy for adenocarcinoma of the kidney: Present position and prospects. Br J Urol 45:237, 1973
41. Hrushesky W J, Murphy G P: Current status of the therapy of advanced renal carcinoma. J Surg Oncol, 9(3):277–288, 1977
42. Bloom H J G: Medroxyprogesterone acetate (Provera) in the treatment of metastatic renal cancer. Br J Cancer 25:250, 1971
43. Jenkin R D T: Androgens in metastatic renal adenocarcinoma. Br Med J 1:361, 1967
44. Melander O, Notter G, T von Schreeb: Hormonbehandling av metastaserande renal kancer. Nordisk Med 78:1309, 1967
45. Paine C H, Wright F W, Ellis F: The use of progestogen in the treatment of metastatic carcinoma of the kidney and uterine body. Br J Cancer 24:277, 1970
46. Papac R J: Hormonal therapy of renal carcinoma. Proc Am Assoc Cancer Res 10:67, 1969
47. Samuels M L, Sullivan P, Howe C D: Medroxyprogesterone acetate in the treatment of renal cell carcinoma (hypernephroma). Cancer 22:525, 1968
48. Wagle D G, Murphy G P: Hormonal therapy in advanced renal cell carcinoma. Cancer 28:318, 1971
49. Woodruff M W, Wagle D, Gailani S D, et al: The current status of chemotherapy for advanced renal carcinoma. J Urol 97:611, 1967
50. Legha S: Nafoxidine in antiestrogen for the treatment of breast cancer. Cancer 38:1535, 1976
51. Lokich J J, Harrison J H: Renal cell carcinoma: Natural history and chemotherapeutic experience. J Urol 114:371, 1975
52. Samson M K, Baker L H, Devos J M, et al: Phase I clinical trial of combined therapy with vinblastine (NSC-49842), bleomycin (NSC-125066) and cisdichlorodiammineplatinum (II) (NSC-119875). Cancer Treat Rep 60:91, 1976
53. Johnson D E, Rodriguez L, Holoye P Y, et al: Combination vincristine (NSC-67574) and hydroxyurea (NSC-32065) for metastatic renal carcinoma. Cancer Chemother Rep 59:1159, 1975
54. Dorn W III, Gladden M P, Rankin E A: Regression of a renal-cell metastatic osseous lesion following treatment. J Bone and Joint Surg 57-A:869, 1975
55. Frei E III, Franzino A, Shnider B I, et al: Clinical studies of vinblastine. Cancer Chemother Rep 12:125, 1961
56. Hahn D, Schimpff S, Wiernik P, et al: Single agent therapy for hypernephroma: CCNU, vinblastine, thiotepa and bleomycin. Proc Am Assoc Cancer Res and Am Soc Clin Oncol 17:82 (abstr #327), 1976
57. Hill J, Loeb E: Treatment of leukemia lymphoma and other malignant neoplasms with vinblastine. Cancer Chemother Rep 15:41, 1961
58. Horn Y, Hochman A: The alkaloids of *vinca rosea linn* in malignant tumors. Oncology 21:214, 1967
59. Schellhammer P F, Smith M J V: Renal cell carcinoma in children. Southern Med J 66:1345, 1973
60. Smart C R, Rochlin D B, Nahum A M, et al: Clinical experience with vinblastine sulfate (NSC-49842) in squamous cell carcinoma and other malignancies. Cancer Chemother Rep 34:31, 1964
61. Wright T L, Hurley J, Korst D R, et al: Vinblastine in neoplastic disease. (Midwest Cooperative Chemotherapy Group). Cancer Res 23:169, 1963

M. L. Samuels, V. J. Lanzotti,
L. E. Boyle, P. Y. Holoye,
D. E. Johnson

16

An Update of the Velban-Bleomycin Program in Testicular Neoplasia with a Note on Cis-Dichlorodiammineplatinum

This report will be limited to 92 Stage III nonseminoma germinal cancer patients who were treated with the most recent modification of the Velban-bleomycin program.[1,2,3] The method of administration of bleomycin was changed in July 1973 to a continuous infusion technique. This program, termed the VB-3 program, initially consisted of pulse doses of Velban totaling 0.4 mg. given on days 1 and 2 with continuous infusion bleomycin starting on day 2 at a dosage rate of 30 mg/24 hours times 5 days; the program thus takes 6 days to complete. With the use of concomitant intravenous hyperalimentation, it is possible to give a second course in 14 to 21 days and, indeed, even a third. In practice, however, a 3-week rest period follows the first two cycles, and then the entire program is repeated for two to four additional cycles. If complete remission is to be obtained, it usually will be seen at this time. Documentation of complete response must be thorough and include all biochemical markers of disease (β-HCG, α-fetoprotein, isoenzymes of lactic dehydrogenase and alkaline phosphatase). In addition to normal routine x-ray studies, tomograms of the lung may be necessary for questionable residuals and must be negative. Special serial X-ray studies, such as inferior vena cavogram for right-sided testicular lesions, are very important. Serial lymphangiograms are done but even if negative, documentation of a tumor-free retroperitoneum requires surgery. Thus, the restaging program is rigorous and expensive, but necessary.

Remarks On Stage III Presentations

It has become quite clear that patients with Stage III metastatic disease may present in strikingly different ways and these presentations have prognostic implications.[3] Thus, we have proposed a pragmatic stratification of Stage III disease as follows:

III-A Disease limited to lymph nodes in the left supraclavicular area. There is no mediastinal adenopathy. There may be disease in the right supraclavicular area as well, but this finding is unusual.

IIIB-1 Gynecomastia, unilateral or bilateral, manifested as a measurable "button". There may be galactorrhea, but this is unusual. Human chorionic gonadotropin titers are frequently elevated, but may be normal. There is no grossly detectable tumor.

TABLE 16-1. *Stage and Histology—92 Patients Treated with VB-3*

	A	B1	B2	B3	B4	B5	Total
Embryonal	2	2	10	12	12	6	44
Teratoma	—	—	—	—	—	1	1
Teratoma, Mixed	1	—	7	16	10	4	38
Choriocarcinoma*	—	—	3	3	1	2	9
Total	3	2	20	31	23	13	92

*1 pure choriocarcinoma; remainder choriocarcinoma plus embryonal carcinoma.

IIIB-2 Minimal pulmonary disease. There may be up to five metastatic masses in each lung, with the largest diameter of any single mass not exceeding 2 cm.

IIIB-3 Advanced pulmonary disease. Any mediastinal or hilar mass ± left supraclavicular mass, neoplastic pleural effusion or intrapulmonary mass greater than 2.0 cm.

IIIB-4 Advanced abdominal disease. Any palpable mass, ureteral displacement by enlarged para-aortic nodes or obstructive uropathy.

IIIB-5 Visceral disease (excluding lung), for example, liver, G.I. tract and brain. Liver usually has positive retroperitoneal nodal disease and constitutes over 75 per cent of this group.

In addition, there is a group of Stage III patients who will have received prior radiotherapy to the para-aortic retroperitoneal lymph nodes. The dose will have varied from 3000 to 4500 rads and node dissection may have been done prior to the radiotherapy or within a frame of two separate courses (split or sandwich technique[4]). These patients now constitute 43 per cent of our study group and are more difficult to treat with aggressive chemotherapy. In addition, there were 4 patients presenting with incomplete retroperitoneal node dissections but without prior radiotherapy. They were started on dactinomycin as primary chemotherapy by their local physicians. They presented to us with uncontrolled abdominal disease and represent the second type of failed Stage II patients, constituting 48 per cent of the study population.

RESULTS

Table 16-1 summarizes the distribution of patients by histology and substage. Note that the minimal disease presentations (IIIA, IIIB-1, IIIB-2) constitute only 25 patients or 27 per cent of the study population. Embryonal carcinoma is the most frequent histological type (47 per cent) while teratocarcinoma "mixed," usually with added embryonal carcinoma, is not significantly different at a 41 per cent incidence.

Table 16-2 gives the complete response rate by histological group. As has been previously documented,[1,2,3] embryonal carcinoma is the most responsive with a 70 per cent complete response rate, while there is an appreciable difference with teratocarcinoma and choriocarcinoma. Table 16-3 separates complete response by individual substage presentation. The minimal pulmonary presentation (IIIB-2) shows a 90 per cent complete response rate, while advanced lung and abdomen presentations (IIIB-3, IIIB-4) show a 50 per cent complete response rate. Presently, abdominal exploration is routinely done to confirm complete response. The abdominal visceral presentations (IIIB-5) constituting liver and/or gastrointestinal tract metastases are responsive but documentation of complete response is difficult. Figure 16-1 shows such a response in a patient who received high-dose Velban therapy (0.6 mg/kg) with continuous infusion bleomycin and intravenous hyperalimentation. Four courses of chemotherapy resulted in a normalization of baseline abnormalities and multiple liver biopsies at laparatomy disclosed only regenerating liver tissue. Table 16-4 shows the effect of Velban dosage on the complete response rate. With high-dose Velban, the complete response rate rises to 80 per cent irrespective of presentation. Those patients receiving low-dose Velban (<0.4 mg/kg) initially had diminished bone marrow reserve from prior chemotherapy or major radiotherapy.

TABLE 16-2. *Histology and Complete Response—VB-3 to 1/77*

Histology	Total No.	C.R.
Embryonal Carcinoma	44	30 (68%)
Teratocarcinoma	39	18 (46%)
Choriocarcinoma	9	4 (44%)
TOTAL	92	52 (57%)

TOXICITY

Significant side reactions are summarized in Table 16-5. Fourteen patients developed 17 episodes of bacteriologically proven septicemia. Six of these infections were caused by *Staphylococcus aureus*, one *Candida albicans* and 10 were caused by gram negative organisms with *Pseudomonas aeruginosa* predominating. There was one death caused by *Serratia marcescens* that occurred in a 53-year-old patient during the fifth course of chemotherapy who was a non-responder to VB-3 and DDP. Induction chemotherapy was being pursued in this patient with high-dose Velban and continuous infusion bleomycin. All of the remaining patients with septicemia promptly responded to appropriate antibiotic therapy with no sequelae.

Classical bleomycin interstitial pneumonitis was observed in only 2 patients, both of whom showed minimal findings with normal arterial PO_2 at rest,[5] and both recovered. In addition, 2 patients developed a peculiar hypersensitivity pneumonitis as proven by open-lung biopsy. Both of these patients responded dramatically to corticosteroid therapy and have received additional Velban-bleomycin with added predinisone coverage. The lung biopsy of these 2 patients showed intense infiltration with eosinophils.

Radiation enteritis with small bowel obstruction supervened in 5 of 40 patients who had received prior irradiation to the para-aortic lymph nodes. Laparotomy with bypass procedures was done in 4 patients, but only one survived. The 12.5 per cent incidence of this complication is unacceptably high and chemotherapy could possibly be contributory.

Malignant hypertension resulting in death from congestive failure and uremia was observed in only 1 patient and resulted from obstruction of the left renal artery by tumor. Peripheral renin blood levels were very high

TABLE 16-3. *Presentation and Response—VB-3 to 1/77*

	Total No.	No. C.R.	(%)	C. R. Failures Relapse	C. R. Failures Dead	Mean Survival (wks)
Minimal Lung (3B-2)	20	18	(90)	1	3	82
Advanced Lung (3B-3)	31	16	(51)	2	6	60
Advanced Abdomen (3B-4)	23	12	(52)	0	2	65
Visceral (exclude lung) (3B-5)	13	1*		—	—	43
	2					
Gynecomastia Only (3B-1)	2		0	0		
						80
Supraclavicular Nodes Only (3A)	3	3		0	0	
TOTAL	92	52	(57)			

*Partial responses 6; 8 presented with liver metastasis.

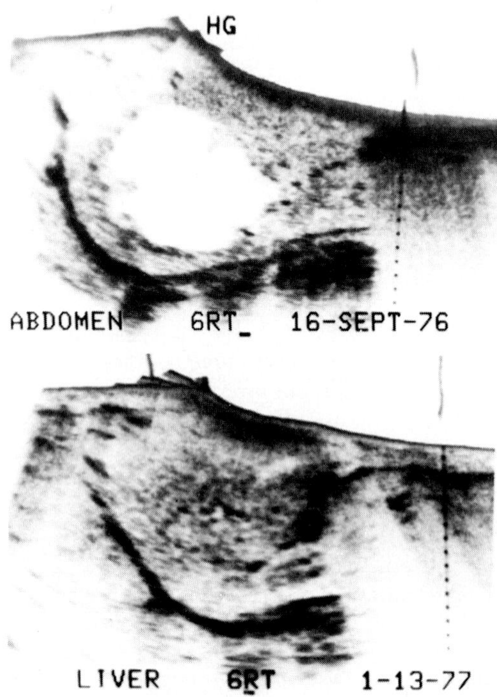

FIG. 16-1. Sonogram of liver before and after four courses of VB-3 (Velban high dose, 0.6 mg/kg per course). Note disappearance of massive liver metastases. Verified by multiple liver biopsies and laparotomy.

and temporary control of the hypertension was finally achieved with the combination of Minoxidil, Lasix, and Propanol. The histology and presentation of the tumor was teratocarcinoma plus embryonal carcinoma, IIIB-4, and there was no response to chemotherapy. All of the deaths listed under the heading Other Major Complications in Table 16-5, are considered chemotherapy failure deaths.

MAINTENANCE THERAPY AND REMISSION DURATION

Immunotherapy with BCG was given to 28 patients. The technique of administration and dose of BCG was by skin scarification with 2×10^6 organisms applied each week between courses and then every 2 weeks after complete remission was obtained. Twenty patients completed a minimum of 10 BCG applications with therapy still continuing in those achieving complete remission without recurrence. A comparison of the survival curves of the BCG group with the remaining 72 patients showed no significant difference in the complete response rates or in the survival ($P = 0.82$, Wilcoxson two-tailed test). The value of BCG remains very doubtful.

Maintenance chemotherapy has not been utilized in the present study. Our aim is to achieve a documented complete response by maximum dosage with first-line drugs and then to discontinue chemotherapy, provided a minimum of four courses have been given. If complete response comes slowly, if further surgery is necessary to remove a mass that proves not to be teratoma, or if the initial presentation was IIIB-3 or worse, an additional two to three courses of therapy will follow beyond the point of established complete response. Further therapy with polypharmacy drug programs using suboptimal dosages of primary drugs or second-line drugs, such as dactinomycin and Leukeran, is unproven at this time and could interfere with reinduction therapy should it become necessary.

Figure 16-2 gives the survival curves by presentation for the 92 patients. There is a significant difference between advanced lung or IIIB-3 versus the minimal lung or IIIB-2 presentation ($P = 0.02$). There is no significant difference between the advanced lung

TABLE 16-4. *Effect of Velban Dose on Response and Survival*

Velban mg/kg	C. R./Total	Failed C. R.	Alive/Total
<0.4	10/23 (43%)	5 Dead (50%)	7/23 (30%)
0.4-0.5	34/59 (57%)	6 Dead (18%)	31/59 (53%)
>0.5-0.65	8/10 (80%)	0	10/10 (100%)

TABLE 16-5. *Complications by Age Group (to 1/77)*

Age Group	No. Patients with Septicemia Total		No. Bleomycin Lung	Other Major Complications
15-20	4/22*	(18%)	2-hypersensitivity pneumonitis recovered	Malignant hypertension, Dead
21-30	6/56**	(10%)	1-recovered	1. Ruptured aorta, Dead 2. Bleeding peptic ulcer, Dead 3. Radiation enteritis, 4 Dead
31-40	0/7			1. Bleeding peptic ulcer, Dead 2. Radiation enteritis, Alive
>40	4/7 1 dead	(57%)	1-recovered	Myocardial infarction, Dead

* staphylococcus aureus—3.
**staphylococcus—3.

and advanced abdomen presentations, but there is a significant difference between these two groups and the IIIB-5 group (P = 0.04). Therefore, three groups are clearly separable by survival with advanced lung and advanced abdomen merging together into one group. Figure 16-3 compares the survival of complete response versus partial and non-responders. There is a highly significant difference (P = <0.01) between the two curves.

CIS-DICHLORODIAMMINE-PLATINUM (DDP)

Credit must be given to Highby, Wallace and Albert et al who clearly demonstrated the activity of this drug in testicular germinal neoplasia.[6] While DDP is unquestionably a first-line drug, the correct strategy for its optimum use has yet to be demonstrated. Using the recommended dosage of 100 mg/M² for three or four courses, minimal high-frequency hearing loss (10-20 decibels) is not unusual. Serious permanent hearing loss is rare, however. Tinnitus is an infrequent finding and, peculiarly, while it is not necessarily associated with any degree of hearing loss, it may be severe

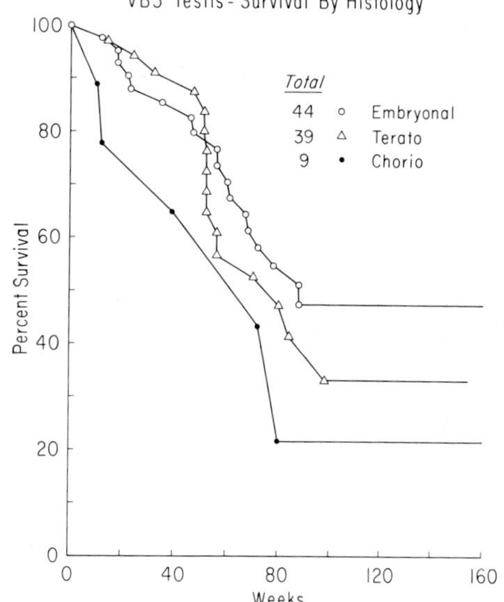

FIG. 16-2. Survival curves by substage presentation. There is a significant difference between minimal lung and advanced lung presentations. There is also a significant difference between advanced lung and advanced abdomen presentations versus the visceral presentation (predominantly liver). As can be readily appreciated, advanced lung and advanced abdomen have similar survival. (See text.)

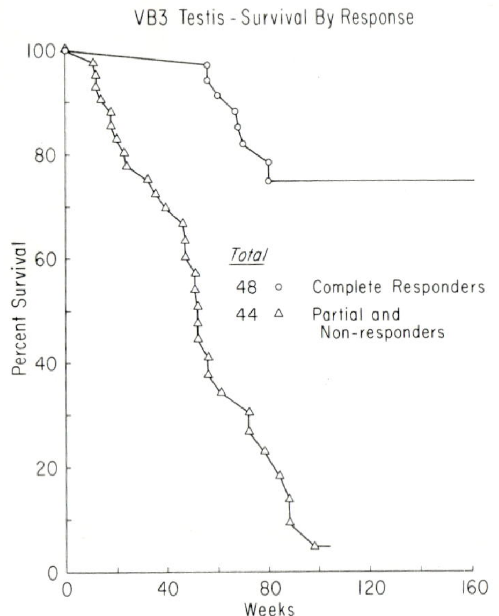

FIG. 16-3. Survival curves by response. The complete responder is significantly better than the partial and nonresponder (P<0.01).

enough to cause delay in treatment. Chronic uremia with serum creatinine at or near 2 mg per cent is seen in at least 15 to 20 per cent of patients receiving the full three to four courses. Dentino[7] has noted subclinical renal damage in all patients at 1 year with a mean fall of creatinine clearance to 50 per cent of baseline values. We have had one death from uremia and a near death in another patient. All patients develop intense vomiting which can be protracted for as long as 3 days. We have observed severe diarrhea in 1 patient who developed a cholera-like syndrome and shock, but recovered. Myelosuppression is an infrequent major side effect, as is peripheral neuritis.

Highby, Wallace and Albert reported a 36 per cent complete remission rate with DDP alone but the responses were brief, except for seminoma.[6] Cvitkovic, Hayes and Golbey have used DDP in combination protocols with improvement in their response rates.[8] Einhorn has added DDP to our two-drug program, but gives a much lower dose of bleomycin.[9] His overall complete response rate appears to be no better than our own and, indeed, may be inferior for advanced presentations since it leaves no room for acceleration of Velban dosage.

In our view, there are presently two emerging indications for cis-platinum. The first is Stage III seminoma, postradiotherapy status. Table 16-6 summarizes our recent experience with 5 patients, all failures to radiotherapy or prior chemotherapy, and poor candidates for further aggressive chemotherapy. The first 3 patients received DDP at a dosage of 100 mg/M^2 at 7- to 10-day intervals for three doses. The responses were striking and unquestionably, patients 1 and 2 had been salvaged. Patients 4 and 5 received a lower dosage of cis-platinum (40 mg/M^2) with full dose Adriamycin and showed no response. Clearly then, further seminoma trials must include full dose DDP. The second major indication is in the extragonadal group of tumors that are primary in either the retroperitoneum, anterior mediastinum or occasionally in the presacral area. We have recently treated 5 patients, 2 of whom were VB-3 failures (Table 16-7). One achieved a complete response of 1-year duration and the second achieved pain

TABLE 16-6. *Seminoma and Cis-Platinum (PDD)*

Patients/Age	Prior Therapy	No. Courses PPD + Mannitol	Response	Survival (weeks)
1. E. P./40	XRT-abdomen	4	C. R.*	34 Alive
2. T. J./37	XRT B-COMF	3	C. R.	40 Alive
3. W. H./50	XRT	3	Pain Control (bone disease)	37 Alive
4. J. R./41	B-COMF	Adriamycin + PPD	N. R.	104 Dead
5. J. T./43	B-COMF	Adriamycin + PPD	N. R.	78 Dead

*C. R. is complete response; N. R. is no response.

TABLE 16-7. *Cis-Platinum and Extragonadal Primary Tumors*

Patient/Age	Histology	Prior Therapy and Response	No. Courses Cis-Platinum	Response	Toxicity	Survival
1. T. R./23	Embryonal Retroperitoneal	VB-3 Partial Response	Adria-Platinum × 2 Cis-Platinum + Mannitol	P. R. Pain Control	1) Severe nausea + Vomiting 2) Uremia, severe 3) Leukopenia	42 weeks Dead
2. T. B./33	Embryonal Retroperitoneal	VB-3 Apparent complete response	Adria-Platinum × 1 Cis-Platinum + Mannitol × 3	C. R.	1) Nausea + Vomiting 2) Uremia	56 weeks Alive
3. P. Q./26	Embryonal Anterior Mediastinum	Surgery	VB-3 + Platinum × 3	C. R. (relapse)	1) Nausea + Vomiting	26 weeks Alive
4. R. W./25	Embryonal Anterior Mediastinum	XRT	VB-3 + Platinum × 3	<P. R.	1) Nausea + Vomiting	26 weeks Dead
5. B. W./23	Embryonal	VB-3 × 5 Apparent complete response	Cis-Platinum + Mannitol × 3 VB-3 + Platinum × 3	C. R.	1) Nausea + Vomiting 2) Uremia	44 weeks Alive

control for a brief period. The remaining 3 patients received VB-1 plus 100 mg/M^2 DDP on day 14 to 18 and two achieved a complete response. One has failed after 26 weeks, and one has sustained a complete response with negative abdominal exploration. These results are clearly encouraging and further trials will proceed, although a major improvement in salvage is not expected.

Discussion

There are currently three programs in active use in metastatic testicular cancer. Our present two-drug program plus intravenous hyperalimentation represents the first major change since the original and first combination chemotherapy program of Li reported in 1960.[10] Dactinomycin was considered the primary active drug of this program and there followed a decade of its intensive use with a 5 per cent ultimate salvage rate.[3] Thus, by modern standards, we do not consider Dactinomycin a first-line drug. The Memorial Hospital group has now altered their program to include a very complicated six-drug polypharmacy,[8] in which first-line drugs (bleomycin and DDP) are mixed with second-line drugs (Leukeran, Dactinomycin, Cytoxan and very low dose Velban) in a time sequence that is arbitrary and therefore predicated by patient tolerance. A 66 per cent complete response rate has been reported. Comparison of this study with our results is difficult because of failure to comparably substratify Stage III presentations. We would emphasize that any program using two first-line drugs in full dosage can be expected to give a high complete response rate in minimal disease presentations. The major problem is the advanced presentations.

Einhorn[9] has recently promulgated a program using the three major first-line drugs but has had to alter the dosage and timing of one drug, bleomycin, to a once per week schedule. DDP is at full dosage and Velban is at our initial recommendation of 0.4 mg/kg (which we now consider inadequate for advanced presentations). With this program, there is a 65 per cent complete response rate (28 of 43 patients) but 7 patients have failed from 4 to 20 months. Unfortunately, there is a 15 per cent death rate from therapy and there were four chemotherapy deaths in complete responders. We have never had a chemotherapy death in a complete responder and would regard this as a very serious contraindication for minimal disease presentation or as adjuvant therapy in Stage II disease. Furthermore, only seven of Einhorn's patients (16 per cent) had prior radiotherapy (as opposed to 43 per cent in our present series) and most of his patients were of the favorable embryonal carcinoma cell type with pulmonary presentations. Also, he is using BCG and Velban for maintenance. With all this, we fail to really see an improvement in complete response rate and there is no significant survival data at this time.

We would hasten to add that we consider our program unsatisfactory for advanced presentations. The current initial dosage of Velban has been significantly increased to 0.6 mg/kg and we try to accelerate this dosage in those with acceptable tolerance from 0.7 to 0.8 mg/kg. Intravenous hyperalimentation becomes mandatory and the program can only be given in oncology centers, which is a major disadvantage. DDP will find use in close sequential application so that all three drugs (DDP, Velban and bleomycin) can be used in maximal dosage. We are currently engaged in a randomized study of the Velban-bleomycin program versus Velban-bleomycin sequential DDP. Hopefully, the three-drug program at full dosage will prove superior.

References

1. Samuels M L, Holoye P Y, Johnson D E: Bleomycin combination chemotherapy in the management of testicular neoplasia. Cancer 36:318–326, 1975
2. Samuels M L, Johnson D E, Holoye P Y: Continuous intravenous bleomycin (NSC-125066) therapy with vinblastine (NSC-49842) in stage III testicular neoplasia. Cancer Chemother Rep 59:563–570, 1975
3. Samuels M L, Lanzotti V J, Holoye P Y, et al:

Combination chemotherapy in germinal tumors. Cancer Treat Rev 3:185–204, 1976

4. Johnson D E, Bracken R B, Wallace S, et al: Urologic cancer, in Clark R L, Howe C D (eds): Cancer Patient Care. Chicago, Year Book Medical Publishers, 1976, p 390–396
5. Samuels M L, Johnson D E, Holoye P Y, Lanzotti V J: Large dose bleomycin therapy and pulmonary toxicity: A possible role of prior radiotherapy. JAMA 235:1117–1120, 1976
6. Highby D J, Wallace J W Jr, Albert D J, Holland J F: Diamminochloroplatinum: A phase 1 study showing response in testicular and other tumors. Cancer 33:1219–1225, 1974
7. Dentino M E, Yum M N, Rohn R J, et al: The long-term effect of cis-platinum diamminedichloride (CPDD) on renal function in man. Proc Am Assoc Cancer Res 18:116, 1977
8. Cvitkovic E, Hayes D, Golbey R: Primary combination chemotherapy for metastatic or unresectable germ cell tumors. Proc Am Assoc Cancer Res 17:296, 1976
9. Einhorn L H, Furnas B: Improved chemotherapy in disseminated testicular cancer: Part 2. J Clin Hematol Oncol 7:662–671, 1977
10. Li M C: Effects of combined drug therapy in metastatic cancer of the testis. JAMA 174:1271–1299, 1960

Thomas V. Sedlacek

17
Chemotherapy of Gynecologic Malignancies

As recently as 10 years ago, chemotherapy for gynecologic cancer was considered a novelty and, by some, a passing fad. During the past decade, an interest in the application of cytotoxic agents in gynecologic malignancies has been awakened. Medical and gynecologic oncologists are developing and participating in controlled studies of a multitude of single-agent and multiple drug regimens. It is now clear that chemotherapy is a very important component of our therapeutic armamentarium in gynecologic oncology. Great strides have been made recently and we now cannot practice quality gynecologic oncology without a thorough understanding and practical knowledge of chemotherapy and its uses.

A detailed comprehensive discussion of chemotherapy in gynecologic cancer is not the ultimate goal for this communication. Such a treatise would be bulky and quickly outdated. The purpose of this section will be to explore the important concepts of the natural history of the major gynecologic malignancies as they relate to chemotherapy, the methods of chemotherapy available today and their successes and failures, some guidelines for the application of chemotherapy, and a brief glimpse of potential methods for the future.

Gestational Trophoblastic Disease

It is appropriate that the discussion should begin with gestational trophoblastic disease, the first human cancer successfully treated by chemotherapy. We now understand a great deal more about gestational trophoblastic disease than we have in the past. Gestational trophoblastic disease is a manifestation of a spectrum of histologic changes ranging from the benign hydatidiform mole through the chorioradenoma destruens and concluding with the frankly invasive choriocarcinoma. The common denominator in this disease entity appears to be chromosomal aneuploidy and proliferation of abnormal trophoblasts.[1] It is felt that these abnormal trophoblasts may be a product of endoreduplication of the second polar body during mitosis. As a result of this process, abnormal trophoblasts develop. They are defective in cellular regulation capacity, stimulation of vascular endothelium, and the normal control mechanisms of nonmalignant trophoblasts. As a result of the failure to stimulate vascularization, the metabolic by-products of the cell accumulate causing a so-called hydropic or edematous degeneration of villi.

The hydatidiform mole is characterized

by hydropic villi with trophoblastic proliferation and absence of the typical stromal vascular pattern within the villi as seen in normal placental villi. This is essentially a benign process, but if not treated properly may result, over a period of time in progressive dedifferentiation to more malignant components of gestational trophoblastic disease.

The chorioadenoma destruens or malignant mole is also characterized by hydropic villi. Trophoblastic proliferation, however, is somewhat increased and there is, as a rule, increased cellular atypia manifested by bizarre-shaped nuclei, increased chromatin clumping, and decreased cytoplasm. One may also see abnormal penetration of uterine musculature with local tissue destruction and necrosis. This condition may occasionally metastasize, but it is generally characterized by local spread. There may be a lethal outcome caused by local tissue destruction and erosion into the large vessels of the uterus.

The frankly invasive choriocarcinoma, the most malignant portion of the spectrum, is characterized by absence of placental villi, sheets of extremely atypical trophoblasts, hemorrhage and tissue necrosis. This disease entity is lethal if untreated and is commonly associated with metastatic disease. Common sites of metastasis are the lung and vagina.

The clinical management of a patient with gestational trophoblastic disease should be based on tissue histology, the clinical behavior of the patient and the serum HCG titres.[2]

It is important to understand that it is extremely difficult to differentiate invasive potential or degree of malignant neoplasia of a specific lesion on histologic grounds alone. Trophoblasts are normally invasive cells and exhibit the cellular morphologic characteristics of malignant cells in a normal state. The degree of cellular atypia, especially nuclear atypia, however, can be used as a guideline in that such atypia roughly correlates with the malignant potential.

Clinical signs such as persistence of bleeding, continued malaise or persistent metastatic masses in spite of adequate therapy are important elements in shaping decisions related to management of gestational trophoblastic disease. Such signs should serve to keep us alert and to maintain a high degree of suspicion of invasive persistent neoplasm.

The single, most consistent, parameter to be followed in patients with gestational trophoblastic disease is the serum HCG titres, especially the B-Sub-Unit assay. It is wise to assume that persistent elevated HCG titres mean persistent trophoblastic disease.

We may categorize gestational trophoblastic disease into two general categories. The nonmetastatic trophoblastic disease, which is represented by the more benign hydatidiform mole and chorioadenoma destruens, will respond to conservative surgical therapy, i.e., evacuation or hysterectomy, and result in remission following such therapy in approximately 85 per cent of the cases.[6]

The second category includes those patients with metastatic gestational trophoblastic disease. This group can be subdivided into the patients at low risk and the patients at high risk. The significance of this subcategorization is that patients with low risk of metastatic disease can be treated with single-agent chemotherapy and a remission rate of 95 to 100 per cent can be expected. Patients in the high-risk category will respond to single-agent therapy only approximately 40 to 50 per cent of the time.[4]

The factors with which we associate an increased risk are age over 40 years, duration of disease greater than 4 months, metastases to liver and/or brain and an initial HCG titre greater than 100,000 mIU/mm.

As a general guideline, then, we can establish our criteria for treatment. Patients with the histologic diagnosis of chorioadenoma destruens or choriocarcinoma should be treated with chemotherapy. If metastatic disease is documented, it should then be classified into high-risk or low-risk groups and treated accordingly. All patients with evidence of metastatic disease should be treated with chemotherapy regardless of the histologic diagnosis. Patients with rising HCG titres, stable HCG titres or titres not within the normal range within one month after initial therapy should be treated with chemotherapy. In the absence of high-risk factors, single-agent chemotherapy is a method of choice.

Available therapy can cure metastatic trophoblastic disease in three fourths of patients in the United States.[23] The agents of choice are actinomycin-D and MTX. Undoubtedly other agents are equally effective; however,

TABLE 17-1. *Triple Agent Chemotherapy for High-Risk or Poor Prognosis Patients with Metastatic Trophoblastic Disease*

Smith JP (B1)	
Actinomycin D	0.5 mgm IV daily × 5
Methotrexate	10–15 mgm IV daily × 5
Cyclophosphamide	150–250 mgm IV daily × 5
Repeated as soon as toxicity has resolved	
Hammond CB (J)	
Methotrexate	15 mgm IM daily × 5
Actinomycin D	0.5 mgm IV daily × 5
Chlorambucil	10 mgm PO daily × 5
Repeated with a minimum of 10 days between courses	

in close to 90 per cent of cases MTX or actinomycin-D are curative. Actinomycin-D is given in a dose of 10 to 15 mgm/kg/day for 5 days. MTX is given in a dose of 0.4 mgm/kg/day for 5 days. Unless toxicity intervenes, the drug is repeated every 2 weeks until the HCG titres are normal. Other schedules include MTX 1.5 mg/kg I.M. on alternate days for 4 doses, with Citrovorum rescue (6 mg/m^2 I.M. on alternate days) for 4 doses. Smith has reported a sequential regimen utilizing actinomycin-D and MTX.[24] MTX is given at a dosage of 15 to 30 mgm/day I.V. for 5 days, alternating with actinomycin-D at a dosage of 0.5 mgm/day I.V. for 5 days. The agents are given sequentially and alternately as soon as toxicity from the preceding course has resolved.

Patients assigned to the high-risk category should be treated with triple-agent chemotherapy. These regimens usually include MTX, actinomycin-D and an alkylater. Typical regimens are presented in Table 17-1. These programs are complicated by greatly increased toxicity and treatment-related deaths. In addition, when either the brain or liver is involved, whole organ irradiation to 2,000 rads should be repeated every 10 to 14 days with dosage modification because of marrow toxicity.

When a patient with malignant trophoblastic disease is treated successfully HCG titres must be returned to normal levels. It should be recalled that a tumor burden of less than 10^9 cells cannot be detected by physical examination, conventional radiographs or nuclear scans. HCG titres, however, correlate well with tumor burdens approaching very low levels. Experience indicates that when the HCG titre is normal and remains normal for six months, the patient is cured.

OVARIAN CARCINOMA

The ovarian carcinomas can be classified into three broad categories. The first is comprised of the germ cell cancers which arise from the totipotent germ cells of the ovary. These are tumors primarily of young women in adolescence or early adulthood. They constitute 0 to 5 per cent of all ovarian cancers and are, as a rule, extremely lethal. Entodermal sinus tumors, however, have been responsive to aggressive chemotherapy. Because of the infrequent occurrence of these tumors, we will not discuss in detail the histologic criteria or chemotherapeutic approaches to this group of tumors. It is recommended that patients with these uncommon lesions be referred to gynecologic oncology centers to facilitate data gathering and controlled clinical trials.

The second large group of ovarian cancers, the gonadal stromal tumors, are tumors of the ovarian mesenchyme or stroma. They may be functioning tumors, which secrete either androgens or estrogens, and they constitute approximately 10 to 13 per cent of all ovarian cancers. As a rule, they are characterized by rather indolent growth patterns and moderate lethality. They are often amenable to repeated surgical efforts, radiotherapy, or a variety of chemotherapeutic approaches.

TABLE 17-2. *Common Epithelial Carcinoma of Ovary: Prognostic Features*

1. Histology (cell type)
2. Grade of differentiation
3. Stage of disease
4. Spillage or rupture at surgery
5. Surface excrescences of tumor
6. Ascites at the time of initial surgery
7. Treatment program
   a. Adequate surgery
   b. Chemotherapy
   c. Radiotherapy

Chemotherapy is indicated when disease has recurred in a previously irradiated field or when the tumor has spread beyond the abdomen. Responses have been noted to melphalan alone but combination therapy improves response rates. A frequently used combination is known as VAC. The VAC regimen consists of vincristine given at a dosage of 1.5 mgm/m^2 I.V. weekly for 8 to 12 weeks (weekly dose not to exceed 2.5 mgm), actinomycin-D 0.5 mgm/day I.V. for 5 days repeated every 6 weeks for 1 to 2 years, and cyclophosphamide 5 to 7 mgm/kg/day I.V. for 5 days repeated every 4 weeks for 2 years. This regimen is also quite useful for germ cell tumors of the ovary.

The final group of ovarian cancers, the common epithelial tumors of the ovary, are cancers which are derived from the surface epithelium of the ovary and, as a group, represent the single most common ovarian cancers. This group constitutes approximately 85 per cent of all cancers and is responsible for more deaths than any other gynecologic cancer. This group includes the serous carcinomas, the mucinous carcinomas, the endometrioid carcinomas, the clear-cell carcinomas and solid or undifferentiated carcinomas of the ovary. In addition, the Brenner tumor of the ovary is usually classified as an epithelial tumor, but it is a rare cancer.

A major problem in the treatment of the common epithelial tumors of the ovary is the fact that these tumors are usually diagnosed at an advanced stage.[11] Approximately 75 per cent of all women with common epithelial cancers of the ovary will be either Stage III or Stage IV at the time of diagnosis.[8] Efforts at early diagnosis of these tumors have generally been frustratingly unsuccessful. An important advent, however, has been the concept of the palpable postmenopausal ovary syndrome. By this we mean that when an ovary is palpable in a woman who is two years or more beyond the menopause, there is an increased likelihood of an ovarian cancer. Furthermore, there is an increased likelihood of early diagnosis of the cancer when this principle is utilized routinely. A laparoscopy to evaluate the ovary may be indicated in such cases and if the degree of suspicion is high or is confirmed by laparoscopy, an exploratory laparotomy for purposes of histologic confirmation may be indicated.

To administer chemotherapy in ovarian cancer most appropriately, the prognostic features of the common epithelial tumors of the ovary listed in Table 17-2 must be understood.[21] The most important of these are the histologic cell type, stage of disease and histologic grade of the tumor. The current International Federation of Obstetrics and Gynecology staging criteria for ovarian cancer are stated in Table 17-3.

It is important to understand the role of histologic cell type as an independent variable in prognosis of the common epithelial tumors of the ovary. As a general rule, the worst prognosis is associated with the solid or undifferentiated ovarian cancers, followed in order by the serous, mucinous, endometrioid and clear-cell cancers of the ovary.[10] The history of every tumor should be reviewed by the clinician with the pathologist and specific statements regarding the histologic cell type and grade of differentiation of the tumor should be part of every clinical evaluation of an ovarian tumor.

Clinical staging of ovarian cancer has historically been correlated with prognosis and 5-year survival figures. The clinical staging process is subject to extensive variation and inadequacy and a great deal of attention should be paid to a detailed operative note which clearly and extensively defines the sites of tumor involvement with description of tumor volume.

Animal studies using chromium-tagged red cells and carbon particle, as well as the clinical observation of frequent tumor extension to the undersurface of the diaphragm suggests that there is a natural clockwise flow of peritoneal fluid. The result of such flow is

TABLE 17-3. *The International Federation of Obstetrics and Gynecology: Stagegrouping for Primary Carcinoma of the Ovary (to Be Used from January 1, 1975)*

STAGE I	Growth limited to the ovaries
Stage Ia	Growth limited to *one* ovary; no ascites (i) No tumor on the external surface; capsule intact (ii) Tumor present on the external surface or/and capsule ruptured
Stage Ib	Growth limited to *both* ovaries; no ascites (i) No tumor on the external surface; capsule intact (ii) Tumor present on the external surface or/and capsule(s) ruptured
Stage Ic	Tumor either Stage Ia or Stage Ib, but with ascites* present or positive peritoneal washings
STAGE II	Growth involving one or both ovaries with pelvic extension
Stage IIa	Extension and/or metastases to the uterus and/or tubes
Stage IIb	Extension to other pelvic tissues
Stage IIc	Tumor either Stage IIa or Stage IIb, but with ascites* present or positive peritoneal washings
STAGE III	Growth involving one or both ovaries with intraperitoneal metastases outside the pelvis and/or positive retroperitoneal nodes. Tumor limited to the true pelvis with histologically proven malignant extension to small bowel or omentum.
STAGE IV	Growth involving one or both ovaries with distant metastases. If pleural effusion is present there must be positive cytology to allot a case to Stage IV. Parenchymal liver metastases equals Stage IV.
SPECIAL CATEGORY	Unexplored cases which are thought to be ovarian carcinoma

*Ascites is peritoneal effusion which in the opinion of the surgeon is pathological and/or clearly exceeds normal amounts.

Based on findings at clinical examination and surgical exploration. The final histology (and cytology when required) after surgery is to be considered in the staging.

that viable tumor cells may be carried from the pelvis to the upper abdomen. Because of physiologic impediments such as the ligament of Treitz, these tumor aggregates tend to lodge on the undersurface of the diaphragm and the surface of the liver and spleen. Therefore, it is important that careful attention be paid to palpation of the surface of the liver and the undersurface of the diaphragm, and all suspicious areas biopsied for histologic confirmation of tumor.[8]

The peritoneum is richly supplied with lymphatics. These lymphatics drain to the retroperitoneal lymph nodes of the pelvis and abdomen. Ovarian tumor cells may be carried through these lymphatics and lodge in the retroperitoneal lymph nodes, especially the periaortic and abdominal lymph nodes. Metastatic spread to retroperitoneal lymph nodes has been demonstrated in nearly 20 per cent of patients who were thought to have Stage I disease. Accurate clinical staging, therefore, should include palpation and biopsy of the retroperitoneal nodes to confirm or deny metastases.

Recently, the important role of histologic differentiation in predicting prognosis of ovarian cancer independent of other variables has been recognized. Basically, there are two general types of malignant ovarian neoplasms.

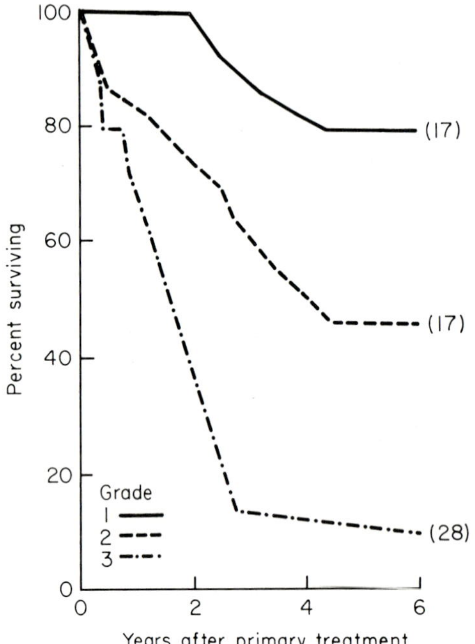

FIG. 17-1. Serous Cystadenocarcinoma, Stage II (62 Cases): Survival By Grade. From Malkasian G D Jr: Histology of epithelial tumors of the ovary: Clinical usefulness and prognostic significance of the histologic classification and grading. Semin Oncol 2(3):191–202, 1975 (with permission).

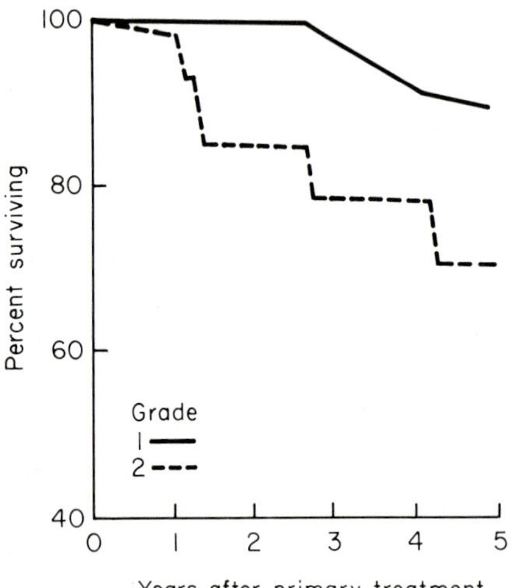

FIG. 17-2. Mucinous Cystadenocarcinoma, Stage 1 (100 Cases): Survival By Grade (Grades 3 And 4, With Only 2 Cases Not Plotted). From Malkasian G D Jr: Histology of epithelial tumors of the ovary: Clinical usefulness and prognostic significance of the histologic classification and grading. Semin Oncol 2(3):191–202, 1975 (with permission).

These are the frankly invasive cancers which can be subdivided according to the degree of differentiation utilizing cellular morphologic criteria, and a separate category of tumors with low potential malignancy or "borderline" ovarian cancers. For purposes of treatment planning, clinical trials and survival analysis, these groups must be clearly separated. The response rate and 5-year survival rate of patients exhibiting a borderline carcinoma is uniformly better stage for stage and cell type for cell type than the frankly malignant cancers. When stage and histologic cell type are controlled, the degree of differentiation becomes an important independent variable pertaining to prognosis and survival. Clinicians are encouraged to evaluate the grade of differentiation of every tumor prior to therapy. The role of histologic grade in serous and mucinous carcinomas is demonstrated in Figures 17-1 and 17-2.

Thus, before making a therapeutic decision, the following should be done.

1. The patient should undergo a surgical exploration for purposes of establishing a diagnosis and the extent of the disease.
2. At the time of exploration, careful attention should be paid to the undersurface of the diaphragm, the surface of the liver and the retroperitoneal nodes and the findings recorded.
3. Ascitic fluid or peritoneal washings should be collected and sent for cytologic evaluation.
4. Every effort, short of compromise of the GI or GU systems, should be made to remove as much tumor as possible, as the amount of residual tumor following surgery plays an important role in chemotherapeutic efficacy.[22]

Radiation therapy has long been a mainstay in the therapeutic approach to ovarian carcinoma. Large fields and higher radiation dosage have increased survival. Fuks and Bagshaw report, however, that 20 per cent of patients staged initially as I, 60 per cent of patients staged as II, and 90 per cent of patients staged as III succumb to their disease.[26] The historical standard for chemotherapy has been the various alkylating agents with a preference toward melphalan or cyclophosphamide. Experience with these agents is great

TABLE 17-4. *Single Agent Chemotherapy in Stage III/IV Ovarian Carcinoma*

Agent	No. patients treated	Responses No. of Patients	%
Alkylaters			
Cyclophosphamide (conventional dose)	335	144	43
Cyclophosphamide (intensive therapy)	36	22	61
Chlorambucil	388	196	51
Triethylene Thiophosphamide	337	162	48
Nitrosoureas	26	3	12
Non-Alkylating			
Hexamethylmelamine	53	22	42
Adriamycin	43	15	35
Methotrexate	20	6	30
Platinum compounds	20	5	25
5-Fluorouracil	92	18	20
Vinblastine	10	2	20
6-Mercaptopurine	19	1	5
Vincristine	22	0	0

and clinical familiarity with their toxicities and side effects is widespread. Though the experience is small, adriamycin, hexamethylmelamine, cis-Platinum, and 5-FU have demonstrated efficacy as single-agent drugs.[17] Clinical trials with combination chemotherapy programs emphasizing drugs which do not cross-react in terms of toxicity or point of action within the cell cycle are currently underway and appear quite promising.[9,12]

Common chemotherapeutic agents and the frequency of response rates are presented in Table 17-4.

Demonstration of significant response to single alkylating agents has led to the development of adjuvant programs in lesser disease stages. Smith, Rutledge, and Delclos, reporting on a study comparing radiation versus melphalan in Stage I and II disease, find that 63 per cent of patients are well at 2 years.[27] Sixty three per cent of patients receiving chemotherapy are disease free, however, compared to 45 per cent of those receiving radiation therapy. The Gynecologic Oncology Group has also published preliminary data in Stage I disease suggesting an advantage to adjuvant chemotherapy. The next logical steps are to utilize combined modality approaches and combination chemotherapy programs. The concept of a second-look operation to determine the adequacy of chemotherapy and to confirm histologically the absence of tumor prior to concluding chemotherapy is becoming more and more popular.[5] Smith, Delgado, and Rutledge, in their recent review of the second-look operation in ovarian carcinoma, have established that somewhat more than 30 per cent of patients were alive and well after second-look operation postchemotherapy.[7] Most of the patients who died had gross tumor at the time of the second-look procedure. Eighty-three per cent of those who had no evidence of tumor at second-look operation were alive and well. Those patients who had 10 or more courses of chemotherapy had a markedly improved survival when compared to those with the nine or less courses.

ENDOMETRIAL CANCER

The primary therapy of endometrial cancer is surgery and radiotherapy, either alone or in combination. Chemotherapy is applied

TABLE 17-5. *Carcinoma of the Cervix; Treatment of Patients with "Stage" IIIB & IVA*

	Hydroxyurea & Radiotherapy	Radiotherapy
Number of Evaluable Patients	80	69
Median Survival—All Patients	20.1 months	12.3 months

G.O.G. REPORT 6/75

in endometrial cancer for metastatic disease or recurrent disease that is not amenable to treatment by either surgery or radiotherapy.[14,18]

Hormonal chemotherapy with progestins is successful in approximately 30 per cent of cases of recurrent metastatic cancer. The response rate is greater in patients with well-differentiated lesions and lesions in which the duration of time from original tumor to recurrence is great. It has been felt that pulmonary nodules are more likely to respond than abdominal or pelvic lesions, but this concept has been recently questioned.[15]

There appears to be no difference between the various progestins in terms of therapeutic efficacy. Very high doses must be used, however, and the loading dose prior to maintenance therapy is probably worthwhile. Kistner suggests a loading regimen of Depo-Provera 400 mg I.M. daily for 7 days followed by 400 mg. 3 times a week for 2 weeks followed by a maintenance dosage of 400 to 1,000 mg/month.[13] He suggests treatment for a minimum of 12 weeks before deciding if the therapy has failed.

Cytotoxic chemotherapy regimens utilizing adriamycin or MTX have been utilized for patients with recurrent endometrial carcinoma. Results, however, are preliminary and not terribly encouraging.[16]

SQUAMOUS CARCINOMA OF THE CERVIX

Until recently chemotherapy has had little controlled application in cervical carcinoma. The primary treatment approaches have been either surgery or radiotherapy. Each has its advocates and the results in Stage I and II disease are comparable. Trials utilizing combination radiation and radical surgery have been reported. Patients with recurrent disease or Stage IV disease are extremely difficult to cure. Chemotherapeutic agents have been utilized only in small numbers of patients and with uniformly poor results when single-agent treatment has been given. Recent programs utilizing combination chemotherapy have clearly demonstrated responses. Conroy et al[20] and Baker et al[29] have published data suggesting activity in advanced disease with combination of bleomycin and MTX or vincristine, bleomycin and mitomycin-C respectively. Clearly multimodality approaches should be carried out. Wasserman and Carter have published an excellent review and proposed approach using adriamycin, actinomycin, and hydroxyurea to facilitate the effects of radiotherapy.[30] Unfortunately, radiopotentiators generally increase the side effects of radiation as well as the beneficial effects. This is especially true of adriamycin and actinomycin. Table 17-5 relates the recent experience in a clinical trial in which hydroxyurea was used concomitantly with radiotherapy for primary therapy of advanced cervical carcinoma. Hydroxyurea seems to be beneficial in terms of duration of progression-free interval.

A multitude of clinical trials is underway exploring combination chemotherapy, combination chemotherapy and radiotherapy and combination chemotherapy and immunotherapy in gynecologic malignancies. Preliminary results are encouraging, and it would appear that our armamentarium is expanding and will continue to do so in the foreseeable future.[19]

REFERENCES

1. Baggish M S: Gestational trophoblastic neoplasia. Clin Obstet Gynecol, 17:259, 1974
2. Hammond C B, Lewis J L Jr: Gestational trophoblastic neoplasms, in Sciarra J J (ed): Davis' Gynecology and Obstetrics, vol. 1. New York, Harper & Row, 1972, Ch. 37N
3. Hilgers R D, Lewis J L Jr: Gestational trophoblastic neoplasms. Gynecol Oncol 2:460, 1974
4. Hammond C B, et al: Treatment of metastatic trophoblastic disease: Good and poor prognosis. Am J Obstet Gynecol 115:451, 1973
5. Wallach R C, et al: The importance of second look surgical procedures in the staging and treatment of ovarian carcinoma. Semin Oncol 2:243, 1975
6. Curry S L, et al: Hydatidiform mole: Diagnosis, management, and long-term follow-up of 347 patients. Obstet Gynecol 45:1, 1975
7. Smith J P, Delgado G, Rutledge F: Second look operation in ovarian carcinoma postchemotherapy. Cancer 38:1458, 1976
8. Rubin P: Understanding the problem of understaging in ovarian cancer. Semin Oncol 2:235, 1975
9. Young R C, et al: Preliminary trials of chemotherapy in advanced ovarian carcinoma. National Cancer Institute Monograph 42, Symposium on Ovarian Carcinoma, 1975, 145
10. Webb M J, et al: Factors influencing ovarian cancer survival after chemotherapy. Obstet Gynecol 44:564, 1974
11. Day T G Jr, Smith J P: Diagnosis and staging of ovarian cancer. Semin Oncol 2:217, 1975
12. Young R C, DeVita V T: The design of clinical trials in the therapy of ovarian carcinoma. Obstet Gynecol 120:1012, 1974
13. Kistner R W: Chemotherapy for carcinoma of the endometrium. OB/GYN Digest, August 1975, p 26
14. Jones H W: Treatment of adenocarcinoma of the endometrium. Obstet Gynecol Surv 30:147, 1975
15. Rozier J C Jr, Underwood P B Jr: Use of progestational agents in endometrial adenocarcinoma. Obstet Gynecol 44:60, 1974
16. Donovan J F: Non-hormonal chemotherapy of endometrial adenocarcinoma: A review. Cancer 34:1587, 1974
17. Young R C: Chemotherapy of ovarian cancer, past, present. Semin Oncol 2:267, 1975
18. Lucas W E: Causal relationships between endocrine-metabolic variables in patients with endometrial carcinoma. Obstet Gynecol Surv 29:507, 1974
19. Averette H E, et al: Cell kinetics and programmed chemotherapy for gynecologic cancer: One squamous cell carcinoma. Obstet Gynecol 124:912, 1976
20. Conroy J, et al: Low dose bleomycin and methotrexate in cervical cancer. Cancer 37:660, 1976
21. Day T G, Gallagher H S, Rutledge F N: Epithelial carcinoma of the ovary: Prognostic importance of histologic grade. National Cancer Institute Monograph 42, 1975, p 15
22. Griffiths C T: Surgical resection of tumor bulk in the primary treatment of ovarian carcinoma. National Cancer Institute Monograph 42, 1975, p 101
23. Lewis J Jr: Chemotherapy for metastatic gestational trophoblastic neoplasms. Clin Obstet Gynecol 10:330, 1967
24. Lewis J, Ketcham A S, Hertz R: Surgical intervention during chemotherapy of gestational trophoblastic neoplasms. Cancer 19:1517, 1966
25. Smith J P: Trophoblastic Disease: Diagnosis and management in endocrine and nonendocrine hormone producing tumors. Chicago Year Book Med Publ, 1973
26. Fuks Z, Bagshaw M A: The rationale for radiotherapy with curative intent in ovarian carcinoma. Int J Radiat Oncol Bio Phy 1:21–32, 1975
27. Smith J P, Rutledge F N, Delclos L: Results of chemotherapy as an adjunct to surgery in patients with localized ovarian cancer. Semin Onc 11(3):277–281,
28. Hreschehysyn M M: Preliminary report on the results of the Gynecol Oncol Group trials on ovarian cancer. J Natl Cancer Inst Monograph 42:155–165, 1975

20. Conroy J F, et al: Cancer 37:660, 1976

29. Baker L H, Opinari M I, Izbicki R M: Phase 2 study of mitocyn-C, vincristine, and bleomycin in advanced squamous cell carcinoma of uterine cervix. Cancer 38:2222–2224, 1976
30. Wasserman T H, Carter S K: The integration of chemotherapy into combined treatment of solid tumors. VIII Cervical cancer. Cancer Treat Rev 4:25–46, 1977
31. Hammon C B, Parker R T: Diagnosis and treatment of trophoblastic disease. A report from the Southern Regional Center. Obstet Gynecol 120:14, 1974

Sigmund Benham Kahn

18
Chemotherapy of Head and Neck Cancer

Of the almost 700,000 new cancer patients that will be diagnosed during 1977, over 40,000 will have one form of cancer of the head and neck.[1] Since there are more than 20 different neoplasms that arise above the clavicle, however, relatively few patients with a single type and stage of tumor will be available for study. If one limits discussion to lesions of the buccal cavity, pharynx and larynx, nearly 24,000 new cases will be seen and about 8300 of this group will die. Within the newly diagnosed group, however, are 4100 patients with cancer of the lip (a highly curable lesion), and a goodly number of anterior mouth lesions that are also readily controlled. Thus, approximately 15,000 patients yearly may require some form of chemotherapy for head and neck cancer since these patients have disease that may not be cured by X-ray therapy or surgery.

Because head and neck cancers are quite dissimilar from the standpoint of histology, presentation, lymph node involvement, natural history and response to therapy, in this review we will exclude management of: (1) brain bumors, (2) tumors of the eye, (3) lymphomas, (4) melanomas, and (5) thyroid cancer. These tumors are covered by other authors in this book. This chapter will analyze the results of the chemotherapeutic management of cancer of the oral and pharyngeal cavities, that is, the lip, oropharynx, tongue, nasopharynx and larynx. Rarer tumors like sarcomas or tumors of the parotid and salivary glands will be mentioned only in passing since the data are meager.

Problems and Definitions

Because of the diverse types of head and neck neoplasms where natural histories differ so markedly, specific analysis of the usefulness of cancer chemotherapy in a single tumor type is difficult. Most reports in the literature are uncontrolled and involve small numbers of patients. The only proper method of assessing the value of chemotherapy of head and neck cancer would be a controlled randomized study of adequate numbers of patients stratified according to primary site, stage and mode of primary therapy. Unfortunately, only a few randomized studies have been done. Most of the other data that are available for review are reports of groups of patients who are, for the most part, unrandomized and unstratified according to site and stage. Often, responses to chemotherapy have been compared to historical controls. Indeed, response to therapy is defined as a greater than 50 per cent reduction in tumor size. This is at best a one log or less reduction in tumor bulk and represents at most three or fewer tumor doublings. Since most cancers are in their thirtieth doubling at diagnosis, and near their fortieth doubling at death, these results can hardly be called dramatic.[2]

Important to any evaluation of the efficacy of cancer chemotherapy of head and neck tumors are the following:

1. Most patients with carcinoma of the lip, oropharynx and larynx are heavy smokers, and many are alcoholics.[3] Thus, their nutritional status is poor, and they are not likely to report to the physician when their tumor burden is small.
2. Almost all patients with head and neck cancer have been treated with irradiation or surgery or both prior to the initiation of chemotherapy.[4]
3. Often used surgical procedures are mutilating and serve to impair further an already precarious physical status.
4. Many patients are referred for chemotherapy following failure of surgery or irradiation to control the primary process, and at this time tumor burdens are large and tumor growth is often in the plateau phase.[5]
5. Sensitivity to chemotherapy of tumors arising from various sites in the head and neck differs. It is generally conceded that well-differentiated squamous cell lesions are more likely to respond than are more undifferentiated tumors.[5]
6. While the TNM staging system has been fairly well defined for head and neck lesions,[6] many reports do not state the stage clearly. The reader has great difficulty finding patients of similar stage in order to draw adequate comparisons. Indeed, most of the patients in any individual report have had marked differences in tumor bulk, making comparisons among studies impossible.
7. Some studies[7,8] have suggested that patients with better immune systems, as measured by clinical testing, have a better response rate than do patients with a poor immune system. There is little data prospectively acquired to verify this hypothesis, but it may be important.
8. The skill of the therapist is of great importance in obtaining a response. There is no doubt that appropriate support of patients undergoing chemotherapy for head and neck cancer may be as important in yielding success as is the selection of a specific agent.

Criteria of Response

In all of the reported studies the criteria of an objective response was a 50 per cent reduction in tumor nodules as measured in two perpendicular dimensions. This response is labelled significant partial remission (PR). While there have been very few reports of complete remissions utilizing drugs, a complete remission (CR) would be defined as a complete disappearance of a tumor nodule. It should be recalled that a 50 per cent reduction in tumor diameter may represent no more than a one log reduction in tumor volume. (Reduction of the diameter of a sphere by one-half reduces the volume to one-eighth). This represents about three doublings; while a 99 per cent reduction in tumor burden is six doublings. The median duration of response following a 50 per cent (estimate one log) reduction in tumor size induced by a single drug treatment has been no more than 3 to 6 months. This response agrees with kinetic data indicating a doubling time of many squamous cell carcinomas of about 1 to 2 months.[2]

Single Agent Treatment

In a recently published compendium of single-agent treatment of various tumors[9] in head and neck cancer, only bleomycin and MTX were found to have definite activity following adequate evaluation. 5-FU and adriamycin were thought to have some activity on adequate trial, but the activity was not clearly established. Many other cancer chemotherapeutic agents have either not been evaluated or have been found to have no activity. Indeed, of 29 agents listed, 20 have never been evaluated, two had no activity, three had inadequate evaluation and the other four had some activity under adequate testing.

MTX has had the most trials. More than

200 patients from different institutions have been reported as having responded to this drug, but complete remissions occur in fewer than 10 per cent of patients. The schedule that has yielded the best results with minimum toxicity is the intermittent dosage program of 30 to 40 mg/m^2 once or twice a week.[5] The dose-limiting toxicity of MTX is bone marrow aplasia and gastrointestinal ulceration.[10] Nutritional status, liver function and renal function are critical factors in any program that utilizes MTX, and it is unfortunate that many patients with head and neck cancer have impaired liver function and poor nutritional status. Larger doses of methotrexate, that is, 120 to 1,000 mg/m^2 by I.V. infusion followed by leukovorin rescue (i.e. 9–15 mg/m^2 q 6h x 2–3 days) have been stated to yield less mucosal toxicity.[11] Randomized studies comparing the high-dose MTX-leukovorin rescue program with the intermittent lower dose methotrexate program have not yielded significant differences in response.[5,11]

Bleomycin, a drug which is usually administered in dosages of 10 to 30 mg/m^2/week has also been evaluated. Toxicity is not related to the bone marrow but rather to pulmonary fibrosis. The total dosage of about 300 mg/m^2 should not be exceeded. In a controlled clinical trial the Medical Research Council Working Party of the United Kingdom failed to demonstrate any better response utilizing bleomycin when compared to other agents.[12]

Adriamycin has been reported to yield some activity, but the response rate is less than 25 per cent.[9,13] The dosage of this drug is 50 to 90 mg/m^2 I.V. every 3 to 4 weeks. Cardiac toxicity is a much dreaded complication. Total dosages in excess of 400 mg/m^2 should not be exceeded. Adriamycin is also marrow toxic, causes alopecia and seems to potentiate irradiation. Patients who have had prior irradiation often develop a severe mucositis when adriamycin is given. Bleomycin shares in this radio-sensitizing potential. The final shortcoming of both bleomycin and adriamycin is their expense.

The nitrosourea, CCNU, has also been reported to yield a 10 to 30 per cent response rate when used alone. Actually, substantial tumor regression occurred in less than 20 per cent of patients.[14]

In brief, except for MTX, no other agent used alone seems to have yielded significant control of recurrent head and neck cancer. It should be stressed that in all of these studies the duration of the response has usually lasted only about 8 to 12 weeks.

A summary of single-drug usage and effectiveness is given in Table 18-1.

Combination Chemotherapy

A number of investigators have reported on multiple drug chemotherapy of head and neck cancer (Table 18-2). The combination of cyclophosphamide, oncovin, me-CCNU and bleomycin (acronym: COMB) was evaluated by Livingston, et al. at the MD Anderson Hospital.[15] Thirty-two patients with head and neck cancers derived from various sites, but all with advanced disease, were entered into the study and 31 had adequate trials. Eleven patients responded with a greater than 50 per cent reduction in tumor bulk. There were no complete responses. Marrow suppression was an almost universal phenomenon. Granulocytopenia was noted in about 20 per cent of patients, and many of these patients required hospitalization. Vincristine neuropathy was noted in 11 per cent of patients, and other patients developed a syndrome characterized by anorexia, weight loss and apathy even without other local neuropathic or myelosuppressive signs. There was little evidence of marked prolongation of survival in any of the responding patients, and the responses lasted only a few months. These authors cautioned that the program was fairly toxic and would require modification in order to make it more acceptable for phase III studies.

Donegan and Harris combined intra-arterial FU, MTX and bleomycin for palliation of advanced head and neck cancer.[16] They noted that 13 of 15, or 87 per cent, of their patients had a greater than 50 per cent reduction in tumor volume, and 3 out of the 15 (20 per cent) had complete regression of clinical disease. In this study, regressions lasted up to 15 months. Most of the patients that were treated had squamous cell carcinoma of the mouth or pharynx, but several had undifferentiated carcinomas of the parotid or the nasopharyngeal areas. These authors noted that of the patients who had responses, most had

TABLE 18-1. *Summary of Effectiveness of Single Agent Chemotherapy in Head and Neck Cancer*

Drug Class/Type	Schedule	Reported Response (% of Patients)
1) Antimetabolite		
a. Effective		
Methotrexate[5]	30-40 mg/m² wk P.O. I.V. I.M.	30-40
Methotrexate & leukovorin[11]	100-1000 mg/m² I.V. followed by leukovorin 9-15 mg/m² q 6 h × 48 h	25-35
5-FU[21]	400-600 mg/m² I.V. × 5 or other (variable schedule)	
b. Ineffective or not evaluated[6]		
Ara C[13]	ineffective	—
6 MP	not evaluated	—
6TG	not evaluated	—
2) Antibiotics		
a. Effective		
Adriamycin[13]	60-90 mg/m² q 3 w I.V.	20-30
Bleomycin[12]	10-30 mg/m² q w I.M., sq, I.V.	20-40
b. Ineffective or not evaluated[6]		
Actinomycin D	not evaluated	
Mithramycin	not evaluated	
3) Alkylating Agents		
a. Effective		
None		
b. Ineffective or not evaluated[6]		
Cyclophosphamide	not effective	
Chlorambucil	not evaluated	
Melphalan	not evaluated	
Busulfan	not evaluated	
4) Mitotic Inhibitors		
a. Effective	None	
b. Part of combination—effectiveness uncertain		
Velban[25]		
Vincristine[15]		
5) Miscellaneous Drugs		
a. Effective		
CCNU[14]	70 mg/m² q 6 w po	10-30
b. Ineffective[6]		
Hexamethylmelamine		
DTIC[13]		
Methyl CCNU[14]		
c. Part of combination—effectiveness uncertain		
Hydroxyurea[17]		
d. Not evaluated[6]		
Dibromomannitol		
Procarbazine		
Streptozotocin		

TABLE 18-2. *Dosage Schedules of Drug Combinations for Head and Neck Cancer*

1) COMB[15]

Cyclophosphamide	1000 mg/m^2 I.V.	day 1 & q 6 w
Oncovin	0.75-1.0 mg. I.V.	day 2, then twice weekly
Methyl CCNU	100 mg/m^2 P.O.	day 1 & q 6 w
Bleomycin	30 mg I.V.	day 2 (6 h after oncovin) (repeat twice weekly × 12)

(other schedules changed dosages of Cyclophos., and Bleomycin)

2) COMF[13]

Cyclophosphamide	2 mg/kg/d (100/d max.) P.O.
Oncovin	0.02 mg/kg/wk I.V. (max. 1.0 mg/wk)
Methotrexate	0.5 mg/kg/wk I.V. (max. 25 mg/wk.)
Fluorouracil	10 mg/kg/wk I.V. (max. 500 mg/wk.)

3) BMH[17]
Bleomycin 15 mg/m^2 I.V. over 48 h, rest, 24 h, then Methotrexate—30 mg/m^2 I.V. push, alternate q 2 with Bleomycin, 15 mg/m^2 I.V., over 48 h; rest 24 h, then Hydroxyurea, 2000 mg/m^2 P.O.
Repeat above q 2 weeks for 3 treatments

4) BACON[18]
Day 1
CCNU—65 mg/m^2 P.O. q 8 w
Mechlorethamine—8 mg/m^2 I.V. push q 4 w
Adriamycin—40 mg/m^2 I.V. q 4 w (limit 450 mg/m^2)
Day 2, then weekly × 6 doses
Vincristine 1.0 mg (0.75 mg if age >50 years)
I.V. push in A.M.
Bleomycin—30 mg. I.V. 6-12 h later

5) Low Dose B-M[19]
Bleomycin—10 mg/m^2 sq wkly (total 300 mg/m^2)
Methotrexate—10 mg/m^2 p.o. q 4th d.

6) BDAM (unpublished)
Bleomycin—30 mg/m^2 I.V. over 24 h
DTIC—300 mg/m^2 I.V. push q 24 h × 5 doses
Adriamycin—20 mg/m^2 I.V. daily q 24 h × 3 doses
Methotrexate—20 mg/m^2 I.V. push at the 12th hour of the Bleomycin infusion

*Results of therapy given in text.

squamous cell lesions rather than more undifferentiated lesions, and there were few responses of tumors such as parotid gland cancer.

Costanzi et al reported a program utilizing a bleomycin infusion for 48 hours followed by I.V. methotrexate or oral hydroxyurea.[17] The design of the program was based upon the concept that bleomycin would synchronize the tumor rendering the MTX or hydroxyurea more effective. Thirty-six patients with disseminated carcinoma were treated, and there was a 59 per cent response rate for the patients with carcinoma of the head and neck. The median response time was approximately 2 months. These workers noted that even those patients with prior irradiation had responses. Other reports suggested that prior irradiation might impair the response to chemotherapy.[5]

Dowell et al, reported for the Central Oncology Group, published the results of six-drug programs in advanced head and neck cancer.[13] Protocol one consisted of a combination of cytoxan, oncovin, MTX and 5-FU (COMF), while protocol two evaluated COMF plus prednisone. There were no complete responses in any of these arms. One of 13 patients responded to the four-drug arm, and 2 of 32 responded to the five-drug program with a greater than 50 per cent reduction of tumor bulk. These responses lasted 5 and 6 months respectively. Fifteen other patients had partial responses (that is, less than 50 per cent reduction in tumor bulk) that were not sustained and lasted about 2 months. These workers concluded that approximately one-third of patients may have some response to courses of COMF-P.

Parenthetically, these investigators evaluated 28 other patients who were given repeated courses of adriamycin; 18 patients who were given DTIC; 29 patients who were given cytosine-arabinoside; and 38 patients who were given CCNU. Used alone, CCNU and adriamycin gave partial responses in less than 20 per cent of patients, while DTIC and cytosine arabinoside were ineffective.[13]

Richman et al, reported the results of a randomized study comparing a five-drug chemotherapy program alone versus the same drugs plus immunotherapy with BCG.[18] Thirty-four patients with squamous cell carcinoma of the head and neck were entered, 20 in the chemoimmunotherapy arm, and 14 in the chemotherapy arm. Almost all had been treated previously with surgery or X-ray therapy. The five drugs used were bleomycin, adriamycin, CCNU, vincristine (oncovin) and mechlorethamine (nitrogen mustard) (acronym:BACON). Forty-four per cent of the patients demonstrated an objective response and there were three CRs in the BACON plus BCG group. The percent CR plus PR for each group was 50 per cent utilizing drugs alone, and 40 per cent utilizing drugs plus BCG (no statistical difference). The median length of remission was 30 weeks for BACON plus BCG, 13 weeks for BACON alone ($P = 0.014$). Five of the 34 patients died as a result of chemotherapy. This study suggested that immunotherapy may play a role in prolonging remission (and survival). Again, toxicity of the drug combinations may preclude general usage.

An as yet unevaluated program for the treatment of squamous cell carcinoma of the head and neck is low-dose bleomycin and MTX. This protocol was devised and pilot-tested at the Hahnemann Cancer Institute.[19] The patients treated had Stage IV carcinoma of the cervix, a tumor with different biology than head and neck disease, but of squamous cell origin similar to many head and neck cancers. Twenty patients were evaluated and 50 per cent had an objective response. The program was unique in that the dosages of bleomycin and MTX were rather low and toxicity was minimal. The bleomycin was given subcutaneously in a dosage of 10 mg/m^2 weekly, while the MTX dosage was 10 mg/m^2 q 4 days P.O. (20 mg/m^2/week). Whether or not this program will be successful in carcinoma of the head and neck remains to be seen, but personal experience with individual patients has yielded some regressions. The chief limitation of a program utilizing bleomycin and MTX is: (1) expense, (2) mucositis in areas previously irradiated and (3) the necessity for weekly injections. It is interesting to note that Livingston et al, in their four-drug COMB program outlined above,[15] felt that higher weekly doses of bleomycin, i.e., 35 to 40 mg./week as opposed to 15 mg./week, increased the response.

Another protocol that is being pilot-tested at the Hahnemann Cancer Institute utilizes bleomycin, DTIC, adriamycin and MTX (BDAM). A twenty-four hour bleomycin infusion is followed by sequential doses of adriamycin, DTIC and MTX. A number of responses in squamous cell carcinoma of the lung have been seen, but there has been little experience with head and neck patients. As mentioned above, Costanzi et al[17] reported success with the bleomycin infusion technique and these data, coupled with low but significant responses to adriamycin and more frequent responses to MTX, suggest that the BDAM program might be of value in a phase II trial against head and neck cancer.

An outline of the dosage schedules for the drug programs listed above is given in Table 18-2.

Intra-arterial Therapy

In the preceding edition of this book, Strawitz outlined a method of infusion therapy for various organ systems and noted that the use of nitrogen mustard intra-arterially in certain patients with head and neck cancer might help control locally recurrent disease.[20] No well-controlled studies, however, comparing the systemic to intra-arterial drug administration in head and neck cancer have been published. Reports of treatment by intra-arterial infusion of drugs, however, suggest that in selected individuals, responses may be rather dramatic and complete.

The rationale behind intra-arterial therapy is the fact that a larger dosage of drug can be administered to the tumor than can be delivered were the drug given by the intravenous route. For drugs with very short half-lives, for example, nitrogen mustard, the total dosage could be delivered via the intra-arterial catheter directly to the tumor's blood supply. Because of the short half-life, very little would leak into the systemic circulation. Other agents, however, like MTX or cyclophosphamide with long half-lives in the circulation would not remain isolated within the head and neck region and would leak into the systemic circulation. The dosage to the tumor in the head and neck, however, would still be higher than to most other parts of the body. Intra-arterial MTX might have a special advantage in that rather high doses could be infused into the head and neck, while the marrow and GI tract could be "rescued" from the toxic effects of these large dosages by the use of an I.M. leucovorin factor. The disadvantages of intra-arterial treatment include the necessity for a surgical procedure, hospital admission, and the risks of bleeding, sepsis and thrombosis. From a theoretical point of view, intra-arterial chemotherapy ought to be evaluated in the management of head and neck cancer since these tumors usually remain localized, and many of the tumor recurrences occur within easily infused areas.

In the last few years a number of reports indicating the efficacy of intra-arterial chemotherapy have appeared. Donegan and Harris' report was mentioned above.[16] Benson reported on the use of cryosurgery and a combination of intra-arterial MTX plus systemic citrovorum rescue, or intra-arterial 5-FU in the primary management of head and neck cancer.[21] Thirty-nine patients were entered, 8 died without recurrence, 18 are alive without disease, and 13 others recurred. He concluded that chemotherapy and surgery combined offered more to the patient than other forms of treatment. Unfortunately in this study, there was no prospective comparison of this treatment with others, and it should be mentioned that the technique of cryosurgery is not readily available.

In 1975 a symposium on the use of intra-arterial chemotherapy was held in Europe. Although none of the workers reported the results of controlled randomized experiments evaluating the efficacy of these techniques, investigators in France, Italy, Greece and Yugoslavia were enthusiastic about the use of intra-arterial MTX (some with CF rescue),[22,23] bleomycin and MTX,[24] MTX, Velban and bleomycin,[25] used alone or in combination with X-ray therapy. The Yugoslavian report was notable in that 6 of 6 patients treated with intra-arterial MTX, Velban and bleomycin responded, and there were five complete remissions.[25] Complications occurred in all series, but in general were minimal. As expected, marrow suppression and cerebrovascular accidents were the most frequent adverse effects.

Combination of Chemotherapy with X-ray or Surgery

There is unanimous agreement that surgery and X-ray therapy are the prime treatments of head and neck cancer. Most head and neck cancers are responsive to irradiation, and modern surgical techniques have been developed to extirpate even large lesions. The needs of surgery, however, are for the development of better maxillo-facial prosthetics. Cancer in the posterior regions of the mouth and throat and the nasopharynx is not amenable to curative surgical excision, while radiotherapy is successful in controlling many of these lesions.[26] Even in the best hands, however, more than 50 per cent of patients with advanced stages of squamous cell carcinoma may succumb to their disease and, while lymphoepitheliomas of the nasopharynx may respond to irradiation, 3-year survival is less than 30 per cent.[27] Because of the high risk of local recurrence and systemic metastases for patients with T3 and T4 disease, adjunctive chemotherapy has been proposed.[5] The rationale for the early use of chemotherapy resides in the fact that patients with small tumor burdens have better tolerance to chemotherapy, and their tumor kinetics are such as to yield increased cell kill as compared to the time when they have bulky disease.[28] The studies mentioned above, describing the success of the combination of intra-arterial chemotherapy with surgery or X-ray therapy, support this contention.[9,16,21,22] Lustig et al, however, reported the results of adjuvant MTX in combination with radiotherapy in advanced head and neck tumor. These workers reported the results of a 10-year follow-up. In one group oral MTX was given to patients prior to irradiation therapy, while the second group received intravenous MTX followed by irradiation, and the third group received radiotherapy alone. There was no significant increase in survival utilizing the drugs and irradiation, but it was concluded that the administration of chemotherapy tended to delay the appearance of distant metastases. Bertino et al, suggested that utilizing high-dose MTX with leucovorin rescue after irradiation yielded as good a response as drugs given before irradiation.[5]

In the overall analysis, however, most studies utilizing chemotherapy preceded by or followed by irradiation therapy have yielded some improvement in short-term control but no significant increase in long-term survival. In most reports the drugs used were single agents such as MTX or 5-FU, and none utilized the combinations of agents reported above.

In brief, there seems to be enough evidence to suggest that the use of adjuvant chemotherapy following primary treatment of advanced head and neck lesions ought to be evaluated.[27] The most rational approach might be to use a combination of drugs[25] rather than a single agent. Whether or not intra-arterial therapy will be more effective than intravenous or oral treatment remains to be determined.

Other Tumors

There are few reports detailing responses to chemotherapy of other tumors of the head and neck.[30] Isolated reports of responses to drugs in patients with ameloblastic sarcoma[31] have appeared. In some reports the response to therapy was dramatic. The usual combinations of standard chemotherapy were used.[30]

A notable report by Kagan et al, outlined the pattern of recurrences for malignant parotid tumors in 130 patients (none had benign mixed tumors).[32] This was a retrospective study. Fifty-six patients suffered recurrences. Thirty patients had adenocarcinoma and 26 had squamous cell carcinoma. The average survival was about 4 years from first recurrence with a median of about 2 years from the time of recurrence. Fourteen of the 56 patients had irradiation therapy at the time of recurrence, however, and are still alive without evidence of disease. These authors suggested that postoperative adjuvant radiation might play a role in the management of carcinoma of the parotid in order to prevent recurrence and thus improve survival. By analogy, perhaps adjuvant chemotherapy may be of use in the management of malignant tumors of the parotid and other sites.

Supportive Care

Patients with advanced head and neck cancer require much specialized care. Their nutritional status is precarious and their addiction to alcohol and tobacco makes them at particular risk for pulmonary infection. Their social status, while variable, is not usually associated with emotional support by family members. Mutilating surgery and protracted irradiation therapy programs further depress them emotionally, making their total care difficult.

These factors suggest the need for specialized teams to formulate decisions and carry out care. Intravenous or per oral hyperalimentation programs, rehabilitation specialists and psycho-social support teams are required. For this reason it is suggested that patients with these cancers be treated in centers that are equipped to handle their multiple problems.

CONCLUSIONS

The story of chemotherapy of head and neck cancer is not a bright one, but, on the other hand, encouraging results have appeared in recent years.[30] The literature is replete with reports of the success of one particular form of treatment or another, but few conclusions can be drawn from unrandomized and uncontrolled experiments. It is difficult to make recommendations from review of the literature. Patients with advanced disease have a number of variables that influence response. These include histopathology, stage, site of origin, prior treatment, nutritional status and even immune status. Supportive care may be as critical in obtaining a response as is the selection of agents. Multiple drug chemotherapy seems more effective than any drug used alone. The use of multiple drug adjuvant chemotherapy offers an exciting prospect for the future. In view of the multiple problems that these patients have, special centers possessing the appropriate team of supportive personnel are recommended.

REFERENCES

1. Cancer Facts and Figures. New York, American Cancer Society, 1977
2. Steel G G: Cytokinetics of neoplasia, in Holland J F, Frei E III (eds): Cancer Medicine, Philadelphia, Lea Febiger, 1973, pp 125-140
3. Shedd D P: Cancer of the head and neck, in Holland J F, Frei E III (eds): Cancer Medicine. Philadelphia, Lea Febiger, 1973, pp 1437-1450
4. Wang C C: Radiation therapy for head and neck cancer. Cancer 36:748-751, 1975
5. Bertino J R, Boston B, Capizzi R L: The role of chemotherapy in the management of cancer of the head and neck: A review. Cancer 36:752-758, 1975
6. American Joint Committee for Cancer Staging and End Results Reporting: Clinical Staging system for carcinoma of the oral cavity (1967), hypopharynx (1965), larynx (1972). Chicago, Am Joint Comm for Cancer Staging & End Results Reporting
7. Eilker F R, Morton D L, Ketcham A S: Immunologic abnormalities in head and neck cancer. Am J Surg 128:534, 1974
8. Bosworth J L, Ghossein N A, Brooks T L: Delayed hypersensitivity in patients treated by curative radiotherapy. Cancer 36:353-358, 1975
9. Committee for Radiation Oncology Studies: Radiation therapy and chemotherapy. Cancer 37:2093-2107, 1976
10. Chabner B A, Myers C E, Coleman C N, et al: The clinical pharmacology of antineoplastic agents. N Eng J Med 292:1107-1113,3, 1975
11. Levitt M, Mosher M B, DeConti R C, et al: Improved therapeutic index of methotrexate with leucovorin rescue. Cancer Res 33:1729-1734, 1973
12. Report of Medical Research Council Working Party on Bleomycin. Bleomycin in advanced squamous cell carcinoma: A random controlled trial. Br Med J 1:188-190, 1976
13. Dowell K E, Armstrong D M, Aust J B, et al: Systemic chemotherapy of advanced head and neck malignancies. Cancer 35:1116-1120, 1976
14. Slavik M: Clinical studies with nitrosureas in various solid tumors. Cancer Treat Rep 60:795-800, 1976
15. Livingston R B, Einhorn L H, Bodey, G P, et al: COMB (cyclophosphamide, oncovin, methyl-CCNU, bleomycin) a four drug combination in solid tumors. Cancer 36:327-332, 1975
16. Donegan W L, Harris P: Regional chemotherapy with combined drugs in cancer of the head and neck. Cancer: 1479-1483, 1976
17. Costanzi J J, Lankas D, Gagliano R G, et al: Intravenous bleomycin infusion as a potential synchronizing agent in human disseminated malignancies. Cancer 38:1503-1506, 1976
18. Richman S P, Livingston R B, Gutterman J V, et al: Chemotherapy versus chemoimmunotherapy of head and neck cancer: Report of a randomized study. Cancer Treat Rep 60:535-539, 1976
19. Conroy J F, Lewis G C, Brady L W, et al: Low dose bleomycin and methotrexate in cervical cancer. Cancer 37:660-664, 1976
20. Strawitz J G: Cancer chemotherapy using isolation perfusion, in Brodsky I, Kahn S B (eds): Cancer Chemotherapy II. New York, Grune & Stratton, 1972, pp 443-451
21. Benson J W: Combined chemotherapy and cryosurgery for oral cancer. Am J Surg 130:596-600, 1975
22. Richard J, Schwaab G, Eschwege F: Results

of intra-arterial infusion in combination with irradiation and surgery in the treatment of cancer of the head and neck. Panminerva Medica 17:308-310, 1975

23. Cerra R, Parisi V, Mastro A A et al: Loco-regional selective chemotherapy in advanced neoplasia of the head and neck. Panminerva Medica 17:315-318, 1975
24. Broussard-Legrand: Our experience of intra-arterial chemotherapy in head and neck tumors. Panminerva Medica 17:319-322, 1975
25. Anersperg M, Vs-Krasnec M, Erjavec M, et al: Combined intra-arterial infusional chemotherapy of advanced head and neck tumors. Panminerva Medica 17:326-328, 1975
26. Hoppe R T, Gaffinet D R, Bugshaw M P: Carcinoma of the nasopharynx. Cancer 37:2605-2615, 1976
27. Urdaneta N, Fischer J J, Vera R, et al: Cancer of the nasopharynx, Cancer 37:1707-1712, 1976
28. Kahn S B: The biologic clock in cancer chemotherapy, in Lowenthal D T, Major D A (eds): Clinical Therapeutics. New York, Grune & Stratton, 1977, (in press)
29. Lustig R A, DeMare P A, Kramer S: Adjuvant methotrexate in the radiotherapeutic management of advanced tumors of the head and neck. Cancer 37:2703-2708, 1976
30. Grant H R: Chemotherapy for head and neck tumors. J Laryngol Otol 90:443-440, 1976
31. Goldstein G, Parker F P, Fitzhugh G S: Ameloblastic sarcoma. Cancer 37:1673-1678, 1976
32. Kagan A R, Nussbaum H, Handler S, et al: Recurrences from malignant parotid salivary gland tumors. Cancer 37:2600-2604, 1976

Robert E. Bellet, Michael J. Mastrangelo
David Berd, and Edward Lustbader

19
Chemotherapy of Malignant Melanoma

In our experience, approximately 50 per cent of all melanoma patients present with or subsequently develop surgically incurable metastatic disease. Furthermore, recent epidemiologic studies have reported a rising incidence of primary cutaneous malignant melanoma.[1-3] Consequently, the chemotherapy of malignant melanoma is gaining greater clinical importance.

A substantial number of published clinical trials have dealt with the chemotherapy of metastatic malignant melanoma. This volume of data has been the subject of several analyses[4-8] of the relative merits of various single and multiple drug regimens. Ideally, an assessment of this type should be based on a multivariate analysis which considers a diversity of factors relating to the *efficacy* of the drug regimens and to the *reliability* of the clinical trials. Factors relating to the *efficacy* of drug regimens include: (1) overall (complete and partial) response rate, (2) complete response rate, (3) response duration, (4) effect on survival, (5) toxicity, (6) patient and physician convenience and (7) cost. In comprehensive reviews, generally only one of these factors is considered: overall response rate. The reasons for this rather limited analysis are primarily the failure of authors to include the needed data and the complexity of assessing multiple variables. This review will likewise analyze only overall response rate as a measure of the *efficacy* of drug regimens.

Factors relating to the *reliability* of an individual drug trial include: (1) sample size, (2) clinical profile of treated patients (especially their similarity to metastatic melanoma patients in general), (3) dose, schedule, and route of administration (especially how closely these approximate the standard method of administering the drug or combination) and (4) the method of selection of subjects, i.e., random assignment to study and control groups, treatment of all patients with the test regimen, or treatment of only selected patients. In most reviews of melanoma chemotherapy, and indeed of the chemotherapy of other solid tumors, none of these factors is analyzed. This review will differ from previous reviews in that it will analyze one of these *reliability* factors: sample size.

The critical importance of sample size is demonstrated by a discussion of the concepts of *observed response rate* and *true response rate*. The observed response rate is the ratio

Supported by U.S.P.H.S. grants CA-13456, CA-06551, CA-06927 and RR-05539 from the National Institutes of Health and by an appropriation from the Commonwealth of Pennsylvania.

TABLE 19-1. *The Distribution of Clinical Trials Comprising the Data Base*

Phase I		5
Broad Based	5	
Melanoma Oriented	0	
Phase II		104
Broad Based	73	
Melanoma Oriented	31	
Phase III		13
Broad Based	1	
Melanoma Oriented	12	
Reviews		6
Total		128

of the number of responding patients to the total number of evaluable patients, expressed as a percentage. The traditional assessment of relative therapeutic efficacy has involved simply a ranking of treatment regimens from the highest to the lowest observed response rates. The observed response rate, however, is only an estimate of what we will refer to as the true response rate. The true response rate is a statistical concept defined as the response rate that would result if a clinical trial were conducted in which all melanoma patients in the statistical universe were treated with a specific drug regimen. Such a trial is, of course, impossible. Instead, clinical trials must be conducted with smaller numbers of patients and therefore result in observed (or estimated) response rates. The accuracy with which the observed response rate approximates the true response rate is principally a function of sample size. As the treatment population increases, the observed response rate approaches the true response rate.

Our goals are several. The observed response rates of single agents that have been evaluated in more than 10 patients with metastatic malignant melanoma will be analyzed and the likelihood of the hypothesis that the true response rates of these single agents equal or exceed specified values will be assessed. We will then use these likelihoods (probabilities) to classify single agents as active, inactive or of indeterminate activity. Multiple drug regimens which do not contain an active component will also be assessed in this fashion. Multiple drug regimens which contain an active component will be compared to the active component and classified as having superior, inferior or indeterminate activity.

DATA BASE

Data for analysis were garnered from a literature search conducted for the years 1950 to 1977. This search yielded 232 references pertaining to the chemotherapy of metastatic malignant melanoma. The minimum acceptable response criterion was a 50 per cent decrease in the sum of the products of the perpendicular diameters of all measured lesions for at least 1 month. All studies failing to use this response criterion were rejected. Also rejected were Phase I and II trials in which the dosage of the cancer chemotherapeutic agent was not within a currently acceptable effective range. On the basis of these stringent response criteria and dosage requirements, 128 articles and abstracts were accepted for evaluation. The distribution of the data base is presented in Table 19-1. The majority of reports were broad-based Phase II studies; only 31 melanoma oriented Phase II studies were included.

SINGLE AGENT CHEMOTHERAPY

Materials & Methods

The observed response rate (ORR) (expressed as a percentage) for each single agent was derived by dividing the number of patients exhibiting objective response (partial and complete) by the total number of evaluable patients. The "probability" (Appendix I A) that the true response rate (TRR) for a single agent is equivalent to or exceeds a specified response rate ($s\%$) was determined using the following formula[9]:

$$p = \sum_{i=0}^{r} \binom{n}{i} (x)^i (1-x)^{n-i}$$

p = probability of a TRR $\geqslant$ a specified response rate ($s\%$)
x = $s\%$ expressed as a decimal
r = number of objective responders
n = number of evaluable patients
i = counter

TABLE 19-2. *Single Agents Tested for Antitumor Activity in More than 10 Evaluable Melanoma Patients*

Drug*	Ref.	Drug*	Ref.
Alkylating Agents		Spindle Inhibitors	
Thio-TEPA	10,11	VCR	45–49
TEPA	12–14	VLB	50–58
L-PAM	10,15,16	TMCA	59–61
Leukeran	17		
HN_2	18	Unknown or Misc. Action	
CTX	10,19–26	DBD	62,63
Antimetabolites		TIC-MUST	64,65
		BCNU	66–69
MTX	27,28	CCNU	69–75
ARA-C	29–31	MeCCNU	76–81
5-FU	10,32	DTIC	69,81–95
6-MP	33–35	HU	10,56,96–103
		ICRF-159	104
Antibiotics		HXM	105
		STREPTZ	106,107
ADRIA	36,37	PREGNANE	108,109
ACT-D	38,39		
MITO-C	40–42		
BLEO	43,44		

Total drugs tested = 28

*See appendix II for list of drug abbreviations; Ref. = reference(s).

Response data for each single agent, which when pooled yielded a minimum of 10 evaluable patients, were analyzed in this fashion and the individual drugs "arbitrarily" categorized (Appendix I B) as follows:

1. Active—agents with demonstrated therapeutic benefit:
   Effective—a single agent with at least a 95 per cent probability of having a TRR equal to or greater than 20 per cent.
   Useful—a single agent with at least a 95 per cent probability of having a TRR equal to or greater than 10 per cent.
2. Indeterminate—agents requiring additional study to more precisely define therapeutic merit:
   Potentially Useful—a single agent with an 80 to 94.9 per cent probability of having a TRR equal to or greater than 10 per cent.
   Probably Not Useful (as single agents)—a single agent with a 50 to 79.9 per cent probability of having a TRR equal to or greater than 10 per cent.
3. Inactive—a single agent with a less than 50 per cent probability of having a TRR equal to or greater than 10 per cent.

Results

The single agents which have been tested for objective tumor regression in more than 10 evaluable malignant melanoma patients are listed in Table 19-2. Drugs evaluated for response in 10 or fewer patients are listed in Table 19-3 and drugs that have not as yet been tested in malignant melanoma patients are presented in Table 19-4. Only agents listed in Table 19-2 will be considered in this analysis.

The pooled response data for each single agent listed in Table 19-2 were subjected to analysis to identify those agents which are therapeutically *effective*: at least a 95 per cent probability of a TRR equal to or greater than

TABLE 19-3. *Single Agents Tested for Antitumor Activity in 10 or Fewer Evaluable Melanoma Patients*

Agent	Evaluable Patients	Objective Responders	References
Procarbazine	10	1	110–112
5-Azacytidine	6	2	113–114
Alanine mustard	6	0	115
VP-16	2	0	116
Isophosphamide	1	0	117

20 per cent. The results of this analysis are presented in Table 19-5. Only one drug, DTIC, is in this category. The 278 objective responses reported in 1188 evaluable patients yields an ORR of 23.4 per cent. Statistical analysis reveals a 99.7 per cent probability that the TRR for DTIC is equal to or greater than 20 per cent. It can be estimated with 95 per cent probability that the TRR for DTIC is 23.4 ± 2.4 per cent. As there are no other drugs presently in this category, DTIC emerges as the most effective single agent in the treatment of malignant melanoma and thus can serve as a benchmark for other single and multi-drug therapy regimens.

In an effort to identify other drugs with antitumor activity, the response data for the remaining 27 single agents were then analyzed to determine (for each agent) the probability of a TRR equal to or greater than 10 per cent. The results of this analysis are presented in Table 19-6. The following single agents were identified as clinically *useful:* BCNU, MeCCNU, Thio-TEPA.

The drugs TMCA, TEPA, L-PAM, DBD, MITO-C and MTX were classified as *potentially useful.* Eight drugs were identified as *probably not useful* as single agents (Table 19-6). Finally, 10 drugs were determined to have had adequate trials and to be *inactive* on the basis of a low probability (<50 per cent) of having TRR $\geq$ 10 per cent.

COMBINATION CHEMOTHERAPY

Materials & Methods

Combination drug regimens can be divided into two categories: (1) regimens that include one or more agents that we have classified as active, i.e. *effective* or *useful*, when used singly and (2) regimens that do not contain active components. The antitumor activity of the first type of regimen can be determined in two ways. The first and simplest is a randomized, prospective trial in which the drug combination is compared with its active component. This comparison is ideally made in a randomized, prospective Phase III trial of adequate sample size to distinguish 5 or 10 per cent (e.g., a 20 per cent response rate versus 25 or 30 per cent) improvements in the ORR for the combination over the concur-

TABLE 19-4. *Single Agents Not Tested for Antitumor Activity in Melanoma Patients*

Busulfan	Cyclocytidine	Ftorafur
6-Thioguanine	Fluorocyclocytidine	Thalicarpine
Mithramycin	Piperazinedione	Gallium nitrate
Daunomycin	Diglycoaldehyde	D-Tetrandrine
DDP	Baker's antifol	S-Tritylcysteine
Chromomycin A_3	Cytembena	Pyrazofurin
Yoshi 864	Asaley	Galactitol

TABLE 19-5. *Assessment of Single Agents for Therapeutic Effectiveness in the Treatment of Melanoma*

Agent	Evaluable Patients	Objective Responses	ORR (%)	Probability of TRR ≥ 20%
DTIC	1188	278	23.4	99.7
Thio-TEPA	24	5	20.8	65.6
TEPA	16	3	18.8	59.8
DBD	18	3	16.7	50.1
MTX	13	2	15.4	50.1
L-PAM	24	4	16.7	46.0
STREPTZ	19	2	10.5	23.7
BCNU	140	24	17.1	23.3
VCR	26	3	11.5	20.7
TIC-MUST	26	3	11.5	20.7
CTX	32	4	12.5	20.4
ARA-C	27	3	11.1	18.2
LEUKERAN	22	2	9.1	15.4
MITO-C	65	9	13.8	13.7
TMCA	90	13	14.4	11.5
VLB	58	7	12.1	8.4
MeCCNU	158	24	15.2	7.6
5-FU	20	1	5.0	6.9
6-MP	29	2	6.9	5.2
ICRF-159	20	0	0.0	1.2
HXM	42	2	4.8	0.6
HN_2	25	0	0.0	0.4
CCNU	153	17	11.1	0.3
HU	86	7	8.1	0.2
BLEO	40	1	2.5	0.1
ADRIA	32	0	0.0	0.1
ACT-D	30	0	0.0	0.1
PREGNANE	155	11	7.1	0.1

ORR = observed response rate; TRR = true response rate

rently determined ORR for the active single component. Both figures (5 and 10 per cent) are arbitrary. Five per cent was selected as the minimum improvement in response rate which would justify subjecting patients to the additional toxicity, inconvenience, and/or cost of combination drug therapy. When adequate data from randomized trials are not available (as most frequently they are not) one can assess the probability that the ORR for a combination drug regimen reflects a TRR that is 5 or 10 per cent higher (e.g., a 20 per cent response rate versus 25 or 30 per cent) than the historically determined ORR for its best component.

The combination drug regimens containing active components are "arbitrarily" classified as follows:

1. Superior Activity
   a. *Effective*—a combination with at least a 95 per cent probability of having a response rate ≥ 10 per cent better than the concurrently or historically determined ORR for the most active component.
   b. *Useful*—a combination with at least a 95 per cent probability of having a response rate ≥ 5 per cent better than the concurrently or historically determined ORR for the most active component.

TABLE 19-6. *Analysis of Single Agent Response Data to Determine the Probabiliy of a True Response Rate ≥ 10%*

Status	Agent	Evaluable Patients	OR	ORR(%)	Probability of TRR ≥ 10%
1	BCNU	140	24	17.1	99.6
	MeCCNU	158	24	15.2	98.6
	Thio-TEPA	24	5	20.8	97.2
2	TMCA	90	13	14.4	93.7
	TEPA	16	3	18.8	93.2
	L-PAM	24	4	16.7	91.5
	DBD	18	3	16.7	90.2
	MITO-C	65	9	13.8	88.9
	MTX	13	2	15.4	86.6
3	CTX	32	4	12.5	78.9
	VLB	58	7	12.1	78.0
	VCR	26	3	11.5	74.1
	TIC-MUST	26	3	11.5	74.1
	CCNU	153	17	11.1	73.1
	ARA-C	27	3	11.1	71.8
	STREPTZ	19	2	10.5	70.5
	LEUKERAN	22	2	9.1	62.0
4	6-MP	29	2	6.9	43.5
	5-FU	20	1	5.0	39.2
	HU	86	7	8.1	36.2
	HXM	42	2	4.8	19.5
	ICRF-159	20	0	0.0	17.6
	PREGNANE	155	11	7.1	14.0
	BLEO	40	1	2.5	8.1
	HN_2	25	0	0.0	7.2
	ACT-D	30	0	0.0	4.2
	ADRIA	32	0	0.0	3.4

OR = objective responses; ORR = observed response rate; TRR = true response rate.

STATUS: 1 = Clinically Useful (≥ 95% probability of TRR ≥ 10%)
2 = Potentially Useful (80-94.9% probability of TRR ≥ 10%)
3 = Probably Not Useful (50-79.9% probability of TRR ≥ 10%)
4 = Inactive (less than 50% probability of TRR ≥ 10%)

2. Indeterminate Activity
   a. *Potentially More Useful*—a combination with an 80 to 94.9 per cent probability of having a response rate ≥ 5 per cent better than the concurrently or historically determined ORR for the most active component.
   b. *Probably Not More Useful*—a combination with a 50 to 79.9 per cent probability of having a response rate ≥ 5 per cent better than the concurrently or historically determined ORR for the most active component.
3. Inferior Activity
   a. *Inactive*—a combination with a less than 50 per cent probability of having a response rate ≥ 5 per cent better than the concurrently or historically determined ORR for the most active component.

The second type of combination drug regimen (one that does not contain an active component) is analyzed and categorized, as were single agents, on the basis of the probability that the TRR equals or exceeds a specified

TABLE 19-7. *Randomized Prospective Trials of DTIC-containing Combination Regimens versus DTIC Alone*

Author	Regimen	Evaluable Patients	Objective Responses	ORR (%)	Prob.
Costanza[84]	DTIC	51	9	17.6	—
	DTIC+BCNU	61	12	19.7	0.35
ECOG #1672[81]	DTIC	79	12	15.2	—
	DTIC+MeCCNU	74	14	18.9	0.42
	MeCCNU	77	12	15.6	0.22
Carter[95]	DTIC	47	8	17.0	—
	DTIC+CCNU+VCR	61	11	18.0	0.30
	DTIC+BCNU+VCR	59	13	22.0	0.50
	DTIC+BCNU+HU	55	6	10.9	0.05

ORR = observed response rate; Prob. = probability that the ORR of the combination drug regimen (or MeCCNU) is at least 5% better than that of DTIC alone (test for the difference in proportions).

response rate. The activity categories have been previously described.

Results

Of the 22 combination drug regimens that have been tested for objective evidence of antitumor effect in melanoma patients, 15 have contained DTIC. The randomized prospective trials of DTIC containing regimens against DTIC alone are presented in Table 19-7. In no case was there a 95 per cent probability that the ORR for the combination was 5 or 10 per cent better than the ORR for DTIC alone. Even the largest trial, however, ECOG #1672, could only be reasonably expected to detect a minimum difference of 20 per cent.* The difficulty in distinguishing small but clinically meaningful differences in response rates with controlled trials of modest size is illustrated in Appendix III. Because of this limitation, all 15 combinations were analyzed as if they had been tested only in uncontrolled trials (Table 19-8).

No regimen achieved the criteria for *superior activity: effective*. Only the first combination (DTIC + BCNU + VCR + HU) can be classified as having *superior activity:useful*.

*This and other sample size calculations[9] assume that: (1) the TRR of the regimens are in the 15-25 per cent range, (2) 0.05 is the p value for significance and (3) the experiment should have an 80 per cent chance of success.

The results for combination #2 (DTIC + BCNU + ACT-D) are indeterminate but the regimen is classified as *potentially more useful* than DTIC alone. The remaining 13 combinations have a low probability (< 50 per cent) of having a TRR ≥ 5 per cent better than the 23.4 per cent ORR of DTIC alone and by our definition are *inferior* to DTIC alone.

Several DTIC-containing combinations have been tested against each other and none has emerged as superior (Table 19-9).

Only one multi-drug regimen (BCNU + VCR) contained BCNU as its most active component (Table 19-10). This combination has a 72 per cent probability of being ≥ 5 per cent better than BCNU alone and is *probably not more useful* than BCNU alone. Nonetheless, two Phase III studies have been conducted comparing BCNU + VCR and DTIC alone. Neither demonstrated a significant difference (Table 19-9), but the sample sizes precluded a reasonable expectation (≥ 80%) of detecting a difference smaller than 30 per cent. Three combinations have been evaluated which contain MeCCNU as their most active component (Table 19-10). Only MeCCNU + VCR has a reasonable probability (86.2 per cent) of being *more useful* than MeCCNU alone.

Only three combination regimens have been studied which contain no single agent shown to be *effective* or *useful* in the treatment of malignant melanoma by our criteria (Table 19-11). Of interest, the combination of VLB + PROCARB + ACT-D can be classified

TABLE 19-8. *Combination Chemotherapy With Regimens Containing DTIC*

Regimen	Evaluable Patients	OR	ORR(%)	Prob of TRR ≥ 28.4%*	Ref.
1. DTIC+BCNU+VCR+HU	68	27	39.7	98.4	118
2. DTIC+BCNU+ACT-D	36	12	33.3	80.2	119
3. DTIC+VCR+CTX	20	5	25.0	47.9	120
4. DTIC+BCNU+VCR	304	84	27.6	41.1	83,95,119, 121–123
5. DTIC+BCNU+VCR+PROCARB	25	6	24.0	40.7	124
6. DTIC+CCNU	29	7	24.1	39.2	125
7. DTIC+BCNU+HU	119	30	25.2	25.4	95,118
8. DTIC+PROCARB	45	10	22.2	22.9	83
9. DTIC+ADRIA	27	5	18.5	17.9	125
10. DTIC+HU	28	5	17.9	15.1	125
11. DTIC+ACT-D	69	14	20.3	8.4	126
12. DTIC+BCNU	61	12	19.7	8.2	84
13. DTIC+CCNU+VCR	61	11	18.0	4.5	95
14. DTIC+MeCCNU	74	14	18.9	4.3	81
15. DTIC+VCR	77	11	14.3	0.3	73,78,127

OR = objective responses; ORR = observed response rate; TRR = true response rate; Ref = reference(s); *28.4% = the ORR for DTIC + 5%.

TABLE 19-9. *Miscellaneous Randomized Prospective Trials of Combination Chemotherapy Regimens*

Author	Regimen	Evaluable Patients	Objective Responses	ORR (%)	Prob.
Ahmann[73]	CCNU	26	1	3.8	0.84
	DTIC+VCR	29	5	17.2	
Ahmann[78]	MeCCNU	19	5	26.3	0.50
	DTIC+VCR	19	4	21.1	
Ahmann[127]	MeCCNU+CTX	28	1	3.6	0.39
	DTIC+VCR	29	2	6.9	
Costanzi[118]	DTIC+BCNU+HU	64	24	37.5	0.37
	DTIC+BCNU+HU+VCR	68	27	39.7	
Beretta[119]	DTIC+BCNU+VCR	54	14	25.9	0.60
	DTIC+BCNU+ACT-D	36	12	33.3	
Pugh[75]	CCNU	97	10	10.3	0.85
	CCNU+VCR	87	18	20.7	
Gerner[125]	DTIC+CCNU	29	7	24.1	0.55
	DTIC+HU	28	5	17.9	
	DTIC+ADRIA	27	5	18.5	0.34
Moon[90]	DTIC	46	12	26.1	0.74
	BCNU+VCR	51	8	15.7	
Bellet[93]	DTIC	36	8	22.0	0.41
	BCNU+VCR	36	9	25.0	

Prob. = probability that the ORR's differ by at least 5% (test for the difference in proportions); ORR = observed response rate.

TABLE 19-10. *Combination Chemotherapy Regimens Containing MeCCNU or BCNU as Most Active Component*

Regimen	Evaluable Patients	OR	ORR (%)	Prob of TRR ⩾ 20.2%*	Ref.
MeCCNU+VCR	22	6	27.3	86.2	128
MeCCNU+CTX+VCR+BLEO	39	7	17.9	45.6	129
MeCCNU+CTX	40	4	10.0	7.2	127,130
				Prob of TRR ⩾ 22.1%**	
BCNU+VCR	126	30	23.8	72.0	90,93,131–133

*20.2% = ORR for MeCCNU + 5%; **22.1% = ORR for BCNU + 5%; OR = objective responses; ORR = observed response rate; TRR = true response rate; Ref. = reference(s).

as *active:effective* (a 97.0 per cent probability of having a TRR ⩾ 20 per cent). The combination of CCNU + VCR is classified as *active:useful*. The evaluation of 5-FU + CTX + MTX + VCR is indeterminate but indicates *potential usefulness*.

CONCLUSIONS

Of the single chemotherapeutic agents tested in metastatic melanoma, only DTIC is classified as *effective* by our criteria. BCNU, MeCCNU and Thio-TEPA have been designated as *useful*. Six other drugs (TMCA, TEPA, L-PAM, DBD, MITO-C, and MTX) are *potentially useful*. Of the combination regimens containing DTIC, none has been shown to be superior to DTIC alone in randomized, controlled trials, but the design (i.e., small sample size) of these trials precluded the detection of small but clinically meaningful differences in response rates. Uncontrolled studies indicate that DTIC + BCNU + VCR + HU is superior to DTIC alone and that the data for DTIC + BCNU + ACT-D are inconclusive. All other DTIC combinations are inferior to DTIC alone. The only other combination including a *useful* drug that may be superior to that drug alone is MeCCNU + VCR which we classify as *potentially more useful*. Of three drug combinations not incorporating active agents, VLB + PROCARB + ACT-D is *effective*, CCNU + VCR is *useful*, and 5FU + CTX + MTX + VCR is *potentially useful*.

In summary, our analysis has indicated which single agents and combinations have the best chance of being therapeutically active in patients with metastatic malignant melanoma. Perhaps more significantly, it has categorized a large number of regimens that are almost certainly *ineffective* or not superior to single agents alone. In addition, it has indicated a number of regimens of indeterminate activity which are worthy of further trial. Finally, our analysis has demonstrated that listing single agents and combinations in or-

TABLE 19-11. *Combination Chemotherapy Regimens Which Do Not Contain Active Single Agents*

Regimen	Evaluable Patients	OR	ORR (%)	Prob of TRR ⩾20%	Prob of TRR ⩾10%	Ref.
VLB+PROCARB+ACT-D	13	5	38.5	97.0	99.9	134
CCNU+VCR	87	18	20.7	62.5	99.9	75
5-FU+CTX+MTX+VCR	26	4	23.8	38.3	88.8	135–137

OR = objective responses; ORR = observed response rate; TRR = true response rate; Ref. = reference(s).

der of overall response rate—the traditional method of reviewing the chemotherapy of a cancer—may lead to unwarranted conclusions.

Current Therapy—Recommendations

DTIC is presently the drug of first choice in the treatment of patients with metastatic malignant melanoma. A nitrosourea (BCNU or MeCCNU or CCNU + VCR) constitutes second line treatment. Third line treatment is problematic; the clinician can choose from among the following: (1) Thio-TEPA or one of the *potentially useful* single agents (Table 19-6), (2) a combination regimen which does not contain either DTIC or a nitrosourea (Table 19-11, #1 or #3) administration of an untried agent (Tables 19-3 and 19-4).

APPENDIX I

Definition of Terms

(A) TRR is the true (but unknown) response rate of a given single or multiple drug regimen and s is a specified rate that the TRR will be compared against. To be logically correct, the probability that the TRR is equivalent to or exceeds s is either 0 or 1. That is, either the TRR is, or is not, greater than or equal to s. However, the TRR is unknown, and, with the observation of r responders in n patients, we can evaluate the hypothesis that the TRR $\geq s$ by computing the probability, p, of r or fewer responses. If p is sufficiently small, for example, $p < 0.05$, we can sensibly reject the hypothesis that the TRR $\geq s$ in favor of the hypothesis that the TRR $< s$. In this sense, p is a measure of the likelihood of the hypothesis that the TRR $\geq s$. We have taken the liberty, in this paper, of dropping the phrase "likelihood of the hypothesis" and simply state that p is the probability that the TRR $\geq s$.

(B) The definitions of "effective," "useful," etc. also take a liberty in technical precision. To be perfectly precise, for instance, an effective single agent is a drug with at least a 95% likelihood of the hypothesis that the TRR $\geq s$. We have substituted the word "probability" for the phrase "likelihood of the hypothesis" and state that an effective drug has at least a 95% probability of a TRR $\geq s$.

APPENDIX II

Drug Abbreviations Used

DTIC	Imidazole Carboxamide	6-MP	6-Mercaptopurine
DBD	Dibromodulcitol	HXM	Hexamethylmelamine
MTX	Methotrexate	HN_2	Nitrogen Mustard
L-PAM	Melphalan	HU	Hydroxyurea
STREPTZ	Streptozotocin	BLEO	Bleomycin
TMCA	Trimethylcolchicinic Acid	ADRIA	Adriamycin
		ACT-D	Actinomycin-D
VCR	Vincristine	PROCARB	Procarbazine
TIC-MUST	NSC-82196	6-TG	6-Thioguanine
CTX	Cyclophosphamide	DDP	*Cis*-diammine-dichloroplatinum
ARA-C	Cytosine Arabinoside		
MITO-C	Mitomycin-C	PREGNANE	Pregnanetrione
VLB	Vinblastine		

APPENDIX III

Tables of Probabilities of Demonstrating Specific Differences in True Response Rates (TRR) for Various Sample Sizes

1) 25 patients per arm

TRR Regimen #1	TRR Regimen #2 15%	20%	25%	30%	
10%	0.14	0.26	0.44	0.55	Probability of showing differences in TRR's
15%	—	0.12	0.23	0.35	
20%	—	—	0.11	0.20	

2) 50 patients per arm

TRR Regimen #1	TRR Regimen #2 15%	20%	25%	30%	
10%	0.19	0.44	0.63	0.81	Probability of showing differences in TRR's
15%	—	0.17	0.35	0.56	
20%	—	—	0.15	0.31	

3) 75 patients per arm

TRR Regimen #1	TRR Regimen #2 15%	20%	25%	30%	
10%	0.24	0.53	0.79	0.93	Probability of showing differences in TRR's
15%	—	0.20	0.46	0.71	
20%	—	—	0.18	0.41	

4) 100 patients per arm

TRR Regimen #1	TRR Regimen #2 15%	20%	25%	30%	
10%	0.28	0.63	0.88	0.97	Probability of showing differences in TRR's
15%	—	0.24	0.55	0.82	
20%	—	—	0.21	0.50	

Alpha, that is the probability of demonstrating a significant difference when none exists, is 0.05.

From Brownlee K A: Statistical Theory and Methodology in Science and Engineering. New York, John Wiley and Sons, 1960, p104

Example: The probability is 0.14 of finding a difference between two treatment regimens with TRR's of 10% and 15% if 25 patients per arm are used in a randomized prospective trial with alpha equal to 0.05.

References

1. Magnus K: Incidence of malignant melanoma of the skin in Norway 1955–1970. Cancer 32:1275, 1973
2. Elwood J M, Lee J A H: Recent data on the epidemiology of malignant melanoma. Semin Oncol 2:149, 1975
3. Cosman B, Heddle S B, Crikelair G F: The increasing incidence of melanoma. Plast Reconstr Surg 57:50, 1976
4. Luce J K: Chemotherapy of malignant melanoma. Cancer 30:1604, 1972
5. Comis R L, Carter S K: Integration of chemotherapy into combined modality therapy of solid tumors. IV. Malignant melanoma. Cancer Treat Rev 1:285, 1974
6. Cohen S M: Malignant melanoma, in Greenspan E M (ed): Clinical Cancer Chemotherapy. New York, Raven Press, 1975, p 235
7. Luce J K: Chemotherapy of melanoma. Semin Oncol 2:179, 1975
8. Aust J B: Melanoma and chemotherapy, in Ariel I M (ed): Progress in Clinical Cancer, vol. VI. New York, Grune & Stratton, 1975, p 199
9. Brownlee K A: Statistical Theory and Methodology in Science and Engineering. New York, Wiley, 1960, p 104
10. Larsen R R, Hill G J: Improved systemic chemotherapy for malignant melanoma. Am J Surg 122:36, 1971
11. Gumport S L, Wright J C, Golomb F M: The treatment of advanced malignant melanoma with triethylene thiophosphormide (ThioTEPA or TSPA). Ann Surg 147:232, 1958
12. Sykes M P, Karnofsky D A, Philips F S, et al: Clinical studies on triethylene phosphoramide and diethylenephosphoramide, compounds with nitrogen-mustard-like activity. Cancer 6:142, 1953
13. Farber S, Appleton R, Downing V, et al: Clinical studies on the carcinolytic action of triethylenephosphoramide. Cancer 6:135, 1953
14. Tullis J L: Triethylenephosphoramide in the treatment of disseminated melanoma. JAMA 166:37, 1958
15. Clifford P, Clift R A, Gillmore J H: Oral melphalan therapy in advanced malignant disease. Br J Cancer 17:381, 1963
16. Holland J F, Regelson W: Studies of phenylalanine nitrogen mustard (CB 3025) in metastatic malignant melanoma of man. Ann NY Acad Sci 68:1122, 1958
17. Moore G E, Bross I D J, Ausman R, et al: Effects of chlorambucil (NSC-3088) in 374 patients with advanced cancer. Cancer Chemother Rep 52:661, 1968
18. Brindley C O, Salvin L G, Potee K G, et al: Further comparative trial of triethylene thiophosphoramide and mechlorethamine in patients with melanoma and Hodgkin's disease. J Chron Dis 17:19, 1964
19. Buckner C D, Rudolph R H, Fefer A, et al: High-dose cyclophosphamide therapy for malignant disease: Toxicity, tumor response, and the effects of stored autologous marrow. Cancer 29:357, 1972
20. Bergsagel D E, Levin W C: A prelusive clinical trial of cyclophosphamide. Cancer Chemother Rep 8:120, 1960
21. Haar H, Marshall G J, Bierman H R, et al: The influence of cyclophosphamide upon neoplastic diseases in man. Cancer Chemother Rep 6:41, 1960
22. Gottlieb J A, Mendelson D, Serpick A A: An evaluation of large intermittent intravenous doses of cyclophosphamide (NSC-26271) in the treatment of metastatic malignant melanoma. Cancer Chemother Rep 54:365, 1970
23. Korst D R, Johnson F D, Frenkel E P, et al: Preliminary evaluation of the effect of cyclophosphamide on the course of human neoplasms. Cancer Chemother Rep 7:1, 1960
24. Shnider B I, Gold G L, Hall T, et al: Preliminary studies with cyclophosphamide. Cancer Chemother Rep 8:106, 1960
25. Rundles R W, Laszlo J, Garrison F E, et al: The antitumor spectrum of cyclophosphamide. Cancer Chemother Rep 16:407, 1962
26. Mullins G M, Colvin M: Intensive cyclophosphamide (NSC-26271) therapy for solid tumors. Cancer Chemother Rep 59:411, 1975
27. Sullivan R D, Miller E, Zurek W Z, et al: Reevaluation of methotrexate as an anticancer drug. Surg Gynecol Obstet 125:819, 1967
28. Vogler W R, Huguley C M, Kerr W: Toxicity and antitumor effect of divided doses of methotrexate. Arch Intern Med 115:285, 1965
29. Burke P J, Owens A H, Colsky J, et al: A clinical evaluation of a prolonged schedule of cytosine arabinoside (NSC-63878). Cancer Res 30:1512, 1970
30. Frei E, Bickers J N, Hewlett J S, et al: Dose schedule and antitumor studies of arabinosyl cytosine (NSC-63878). Cancer Res 29:1325, 1969
31. Hart J S, Ho D H, George S L, et al: Cytokinetic and molecular pharmacology studies of arabinosylcytosine in metastatic melanoma. Cancer Res 32:2711, 1972
32. Moore G E, Bross I D J, Ausman R, et al: Effects of 5-fluorouracil (NSC-19893) in 389 patients with cancer. Cancer Chemother Rep 52:641, 1968
33. Regelson W, Holland J F, Gold G L, et al: 6-

Mercaptopurine (NSC-755) given intravenously at weekly intervals to patients with advanced cancer. Cancer Chemother Rep 51:277, 1967
34. Fink D J, Foye L V: 6-Mercaptopurine (NSC-755) given intermittently in high doses: Phase II study. Cancer Chemother Rep 54:31, 1970
35. Moore G E, Bross I D J, Ausman R, et al: Effects of 6-mercaptopurine (NSC-755) in 290 patients with advanced cancer. Cancer Chemother Rep 52:655, 1968
36. O'Bryan R M, Luce J K, Talley R W, et al: Phase II evaluation of adriamycin in human neoplasia. Cancer 32:1, 1973
37. Sieper W J, Mastrangelo M J, Bellet R E: Phase II study of adriamycin (NSC-123127) in patients with metastatic melanoma. Cancer Chemother Rep 59:1181, 1975
38. Golomb F M, Solowey A C, Postel A, et al: Induced remission of malignant melanoma with actinomycin-D: Immunologic implications. Cancer 20:656, 1967
39. Moore G E, DiPaolo J A, Kondo T: The chemotherapeutic effects and complications of actinomycin D in patients with advanced cancer. Cancer 11:1204, 1958
40. Whittington R M, Close H P: Clinical experience with mitomycin C (NSC-26980). Cancer Chemother Rep 54:195, 1970
41. Godfrey T E, Wilbur D W: Clinical Experience with mitomycin C in large infrequent doses. Cancer 29:1647, 1972
42. Moore G E, Bross I D J, Ausman R, et al: Effects of mitomycin C (NSC-26980) in 346 patients with advanced cancer. Cancer Chemother Rep 52:675, 1968
43. Blum R H, Carter S K, Agre K: A clinical review of bleomycin: A new antineoplastic agent. Cancer 31:903, 1973
44. Clinical Screening Co-operative Group of the European Organization for Research on the Treatment of Cancer: Study of the clinical efficiency of bleomycin in human cancer. Br Med J 2:643, 1970
45. Costa G, Hreshchyshyn M M, Holland J J: Initial clinical studies with vincristine. Cancer Chemother Rep 24:39, 1962
46. Gubisch N J, Norena D, Perlia C P, et al: Experience with vincristine in solid tumors. Cancer Chemother Rep 32:19, 1963
47. Shaw R K, Bruner J A: Clinical evaluation of vincristine (NSC-67574). Cancer Chemother Rep 42:45, 1964
48. Reitemeier R J, Moertel C G, Blackburn C M: Vincristine (NSC-67574) therapy of adult patients with solid tumors. Cancer Chemother Rep 34:21, 1964
49. Smart C R, Ottoman R E, Rochlin D B, et al: Clinical experience with vincristine (NSC-67574) in tumors of the central nervous system and other malignant diseases. Cancer Chemother Rep 52:733, 1968
50. Frei E, Franzino A, Shnider B I, et al: Clinical studies of vinblastine. Cancer Chemother Rep 12:125, 1961
51. Armstrong J G, Dyke R W, Fouts P J, et al: Hodgkin's disease, carcinoma of the breast, and other tumors treated with vinblastine sulfate. Cancer Chemother Rep 18:49, 1962
52. Acute Leukemia Group B, Eastern Cooperative Group: Neoplastic disease: Treatment with vinblastine. Arch Intern Med 116:846, 1965
53. Bond W H, Rohn R J, Bates L H, et al: Treatment of neoplastic diseases with an improved oral preparation of vinblastine sulfate. Cancer 19:213, 1966
54. Hodes M E, Rohn R J, Bond W H, et al: Vincaleukoblastine: A summary of two and one-half years' experience in the use of vinblastine. Cancer Chemother Rep 16:401, 1962
55. Hill J M, Loeb E: Treatment of leukemia, lymphoma, and other malignant neoplasms with vinblastine. Cancer Chemother Rep 15:41, 1961
56. Falkson G, van Dyk J J: The chemotherapy of malignant melanoma. S Afr Med J 42:89, 1968
57. Wright T L, Hurley J, Korst D R, et al: Vinblastine in neoplastic disease. Cancer Res 23:169, 1963
58. Smart C R, Rochlin D B, Nahum A M, et al: Clinical experience with vinblastine sulfate (NSC-49842) in squamous cell carcinoma and other malignancies. Cancer Chemother Rep 34:31, 1964
59. Johnson F D, Jacobs E M: Chemotherapy of metastatic malignant melanoma: Experience with 73 patients. Cancer 27:1306, 1971
60. Stolinsky D C, Jacobs E M, Bateman J R, et al: Clinical trial of trimethylcolchicinic acid methyl ether *d*-tartrate (TMCA; NSC-36354) in advanced cancer. Cancer Chemother Rep 51:25, 1967
61. Stolinsky D C, Jacobs E M, Braunwald J, et al: Further study of trimethylcolchicinic acid, methyl ether, *d*-tartrate (TMCA; NSC-36354) in patients with malignant melanoma. Cancer Chemother Rep 56:263, 1972
62. Andrews N C, Weiss A J, Ansfield F J, et al: Phase I study of dibromodulcitol (NSC-104800). Cancer Chemother Rep 55:61, 1971
63. Phillips R W, Brook J: Clinical experiences with dibromodulcitol (NSC-104800) in solid tumors. Cancer Chemother Rep 55:567, 1971
64. Falkson G, Van der Merwe A M, Falkson H C: Clinical experience with 5-[3,3-bis(2-chloroethyl)-1-triazeno] imidazole-4-carbox-

amide (NSC-82196) in the treatment of metastatic malignant melanoma. Cancer Chemother Rep 56:671, 1972

65. Bagley C M, Canellos G P, Young R C, et al: Clinical trials with 5-[3,3-bis(2-chloroethyl)-1-triazeno] imidazole-4-carboxamide (NSC-82196) given intravenously. Cancer Chemother Rep 56:387, 1972
66. Lessner H E: BCNU [1,3,bis(2-chloroethyl)-1-nitrosourea]: Effects on advanced Hodgkin's disease and other neoplasia. Cancer 22:451, 1968
67. Ramirez G, Wilson W, Grage T, et al: Phase II evaluation of 1, 3-bis (2-chloroethyl)-1-nitrosourea (BCNU; NSC-409962) in patients with solid tumors. Cancer Chemother Rep 56:787, 1972
68. DeVita V T, Carbone P P, Owens A H, et al: Clinical trials with 1, 3-bis(2-chloroethyl)-1-nitrosourea, NSC-409962. Cancer Res 25:1876, 1965
69. Hill G J, Ruess R, Berris R, et al: Chemotherapy of malignant melanoma with dimethyl triazeno imidazole carboxamide (DTIC) and nitrosourea derivatives (BCNU, CCNU). Ann Surg 180:167, 1974
70. DeConti R C, Hubbard S P, Pinch P, et al: Treatment of advanced neoplastic disease with 1-(2-chloroethyl)-3-cyclohexyl-1-nitrosourea (CCNU; NSC-79037). Cancer Chemother Rep 57:201, 1973
71. Hoogstraten B, Gottlieb J A, Caoili E, et al: CCNU (1-[2-chloroethyl]-3-cyclohexyl-1-nitrosourea, NSC-79037) in the treatment of cancer: Phase II study. Cancer 32:38, 1973
72. Perloff M, Muggia F M, Ackerman C: Role of nitrosourea (CCNU, NSC-79037) in advanced nonhematologic cancer. Cancer Chemother Rep 58:421, 1974
73. Ahmann D L, Hahn R G, Bisel H F: A comparative study of 1-(2-chloroethyl)-3-cyclohexyl-1-nitrosourea (NSC-79037) and imidazole carboxamide (NSC-45388) with vincristine (NSC-67574) in the palliation of disseminated malignant melanoma. Cancer Res 32:2432, 1972
74. Broder L E, Hansen H H: 1-(2-chloroethyl)-3-cyclohexyl-1-nitrosourea (CCNU, NSC-79037): A comparison of drug administration at four-week and six-week intervals. Eur J Cancer 9:147, 1973
75. Pugh R P, Jacobs E M, Bateman J R, et al: CCNU vs. CCNU + vincristine in disseminated melanoma. Proc Am Soc Clin Oncol 16:246, 1975
76. Firat D, Tekuzman G: Treatment of solid tumors and lymphomas with methyl-CCNU (NSC-95441): A phase II study. Cancer Chemother Rep 59:1021, 1975
77. Tranum B L, Haut A, Rivkin S, et al: A phase II study of methyl CCNU in the treatment of solid tumors and lymphomas: A Southwest Oncology Group study. Cancer 35:1148, 1975
78. Ahmann D L, Hahn R G, Bisel H F: Evaluation of 1-(2-chloroethyl)-3-(4-methylcyclohexyl)-1-nitrosourea (Methyl-CCNU, NSC-95441) versus combined imidazole carboxamide (NSC-45388) and vincristine (NSC-67574) in palliation of disseminated malignant melanoma. Cancer 33:615, 1974
79. Young R C, Canellos G P, Chabner B A, et al: Treatment of malignant melanoma with methyl CCNU. Clin Pharmacol Therap 15:617, 1974
80. Gottlieb J A, McCredie K B, Hersh E M, et al: Initial clinical studies with 1-(2-chloroethyl)-3-(4-methyl-cyclohexyl)-1-nitrosourea (Methyl CCNU). Proc Am Assoc Cancer Res 13:79, 1972
81. Eastern Cooperative Oncology Group Protocol #1672, (Personal communication)
82. Gerner R E, Moore G E: Study of 5-(3,3-dimethyl-1-triazeno) imidazole-4-carboxamide (NSC-45388) in patients with disseminated melanoma. Cancer Chemother Rep 57:83, 1973
83. Einhorn L H, Burgess M A, Vallejos C, et al: Prognostic correlations and response to treatment in advanced metastatic melanoma. Cancer Res 34:1995, 1974
84. Costanza M E, Nathanson L, Lenhard R, et al: Therapy of malignant melanoma with an imidazole carboxamide and bis-chloroethyl nitrosourea. Cancer 30:1457, 1972
85. Cowan D H, Bergsagel D E: Intermittent treatment of metastatic malignant melanoma with high-dose 5-(3,3-dimethyl-1-triazeno) imidazole-4-carboxamide (NSC-45388). Cancer Chemother Rep 55:175, 1971
86. Burke P J, McCarthy W H, Milton G W: Imidazole carboxamide therapy in advanced malignant melanoma. Cancer 27:744, 1971
87. Carter S K, Friedman M A: 5-(3,3-dimethyl-1-triazeno) imidazole-4-carboxamide (DTIC, DIC, NSC-45388)—A new antitumor agent with activity against malignant melanoma. Eur J Cancer 8:85, 1972
88. Wagner D E, Ramirez G, Weiss A J, et al: Combination phase I-II study of imidazole carboxamide (NSC-45388). Oncology 26:310, 1972
89. Gottlieb J A, Serpick A A: Clinical evaluation of 5-(3,3-dimethyl-1-triazeno) imidazole-4-carboxamide in malignant melanoma and other neoplasms: Comparison of twice-weekly and daily administration schedules. Oncology 25:225, 1971
90. Moon J H, Gailani S, Cooper M R, et al: Com-

parison of the combination of 1,3-bis (2-chloroethyl)-1-nitrosourea (BCNU) and vincristine with two dose schedules of 5-(3,3-dimethyl-1-triazeno) imidazole-4-carboxamide (DTIC) in the treatment of disseminated malignant melanoma. Cancer 35:368, 1975

91. Luce J K, Thurman W G, Isaacs B L, et al: Clinical trials with the antitumor agent 5-(3,3-dimethyl-1-triazeno) imidazole-4-carboxamide (NSC-45388). Cancer Chemother Rep 54:119, 1970
92. Vogel C L, Comis R, Ziegler J L, et al: Clinical trials of 5-(3,3-dimethyl-1-triazeno) imidazole-4-carboxamide (NSC-45388) given intravenously in the treatment of malignant melanoma in Uganda. Cancer Chemother Rep 55:143, 1971
93. Bellet R E, Mastrangelo M J, Laucius J F, et al: Randomized prospective trial of DTIC (NSC-45388) alone versus BCNU (NSC-409962) plus vincristine (NSC-67574) in the treatment of metastatic malignant melanoma. Cancer Treat Rep 60:595, 1976
94. Nathanson L, Wolter J, Horton J, et al: Characteristics of prognosis and response to an imidazole carboxamide in malignant melanoma. Clin Pharmacol Therap 12:955, 1971
95. Carter R D, Krementz E T: DTIC and combination therapy for metastatic melanoma: A COG cooperative study. Proc Am Assoc Cancer Res 16:16, 1975
96. Slack N H, Jones R: Single reversal trial of hydroxyurea (NSC-32065) in 91 patients with advanced cancer. Cancer Chemother Rep 54:53, 1970
97. Cole D R, Beckloff G L, Rousselot L M: Clinical results with hydroxyurea in cancer chemotherapy: Preliminary report. NY State J Med 65:2132, 1965
98. Creasey W A, Capizzi R L, DeConti R C: Clinical and biochemical studies of high-dose intermittent therapy of solid tumors with hydroxyurea (NSC-32065). Cancer Chemother Rep 54:191, 1970
99. Bolton B H, Kaung D T, Lawton R L, et al: Hydroxyurea (NSC-32065): A phase I study. Cancer Chemother Rep 39:47, 1964
100. Cassileth P A, Hyman G A: Treatment of malignant melanoma with hydroxyurea. Cancer Res 27:1843, 1967
101. Gottlieb J A, Frei E, Luce J K: Dose-schedule studies with hydroxyurea (NSC-32065) in malignant melanoma. Cancer Chemother Rep 55:277, 1971
102. Nathanson L, Hall T C: Phase II study of hydroxyurea (NSC-32065) in malignant melanoma. Cancer Chemother Rep 51:503, 1967
103. Lerner H J, Beckloff G L, Godwin M C: Hydroxyurea (NSC-32065) intermittent therapy in malignant diseases. Cancer Chemother Rep 53:385, 1969
104. Bellet R E, Catalano R B, Danna V G, et al: A study of the antitumor (phase II) and immunosuppressive effects of ICRF-159 (NSC-129943) in patients with metastatic melanoma. J Clin Pharmacol 16:433, 1976
105. Blum R H, Livingston R B, Carter S K: Hexamethylmelamine: A new drug with activity in solid tumors. Eur J Cancer 9:195, 1973
106. du Priest R W, Huntington M C, Massey W H, et al: Streptozotocin therapy in 22 cancer patients. Cancer 35:358, 1975
107. Schein P S, O'Connell M J, Blom J, et al: Clinical antitumor activity and toxicity of streptozotocin (NSC-85998). Cancer 34:993, 1974
108. Ramirez G, Weiss A J, Rochlin D B, et al: Phase II study of 6α-methylpregn-4-ene-3, 11, 20-trione (NSC-17256). Cancer Chemother Rep 55:265, 1971
109. Johnson R O, Bisel H, Andrews N, et al: Phase I clinical study of 6α-methylpregn-4-ene-3, 11, 20-trione (NSC-17256). Cancer Chemother Rep 50:671, 1966
110. De Vita V T, Serpick A, Carbone P P: Preliminary clinical studies with ibenzmethyzin. Clin Pharmacol Therap 7:542, 1966
111. Brunner K W, Young C W: A methylhydrazine derivative in Hodgkin's disease and other malignant neoplasms. Ann Intern Med 63:69, 1965
112. Backhouse T W, Sicher K: Initial experience with methylhydrazine, a new cytotoxic agent. Clin Radiol 17:132, 1966
113. Weiss A J, Stambaugh J E, Mastrangelo M J, et al: Phase I study of 5-azacytidine (NSC-102816). Cancer Chemother Rep 56:413, 1972
114. Bellet R E, Mastrangelo M J, Engstrom P F, et al: Clinical trial with subcutaneously administered 5-azacytidine (NSC-102816). Cancer Chemother Rep 58:217, 1974
115. Wilson W L, Hurley J D, Mrazek R G: Phase II study of alanine mustard (NSC-17663). Cancer Chemother Rep 54:361, 1970
116. Falkson G, van Dyk J J, van Eden E B, et al: A clinical trial of the oral form of 4′-dimethyl-epipodophyllotoxin-β-D ethylidene glucoside (NSC-141540) VP 16-213. Cancer 35:1141, 1975
117. Bremner D N, McCormick J S, Thomson J W W: Clinical trial of isophosphamide (NSC-109724): Results and side effects. Cancer Chemother Rep 58:889, 1974
118. Costanzi J J, Vaitkevicius V K, Quagliana J M, et al: Combination chemotherapy for disseminated malignant melanoma. Cancer 35:342, 1975

119. Beretta G, Bajetta E, Tancini G: Controlled study with imidazole carboxamide (DTIC), bis-chloroethyl-nitrosourea (BCNU) and vincristine (VCR) versus actinomycin D (Act. D), DTIC, BCNU in metastatic malignant melanoma. Eleventh International Cancer Congress 3:541, 1974
120. Gardere S, Hussain S, Cowan D H: Treatment of metastatic malignant melanoma with a combination of 5-(3,3-dimethyl-1-triazeno) imidazole-4-carboxamide (NSC-45388), cyclophosphamide (NSC-26271), and vincristine (NSC-67574). Cancer Chemother Rep 56:357, 1972
121. Beretta G, Bajetta E, Bonadonna G, et al: Polichemioterapia con 5-(3,3 dimetil-1-triazeno) imidazole-4-carboxamide (DTIC; NSC-45388), 1,3-bis (2-cloroetil)-1-nitrosourea (BCNU; NSC-409962) e vincristina (NSC-67574) nel melanoma in fase metastatizzata. Tumori 59:239, 1973
122. Luce J K, Torin L B, Price H: Combination dimethyl triazeno imidazole carboxamide (NSC-45388; DIC), vincristine (NSC-67574; VCR) and 1,3-bis(2-chloroethyl)-1-nitrosourea (NSC-409962; BCNU) chemotherapy of disseminated malignant melanoma. Proc Am Assoc Cancer Res 11:50, 1970
123. Cohen S M, Greenspan E M, Ratner L H, et al: Combination chemotherapy of malignant melanoma with imidazole carboxamide, BCNU and vincristine. Cancer 39:41, 1977
124. van Dyk J J, Falkson G: A clinical trial of procarbazine plus vincristine plus bis-chloroethyl-nitrosourea plus imidazole carboxamide dimethyl triazeno in metastatic malignant melanoma. Med Pediat Oncol 1:107, 1975
125. Gerner R E, Moore G E, Dickey C: Combination chemotherapy in disseminated melanoma and other solid tumors in adults. Oncology 31:22, 1975
126. Gerner R E, Moore G E, Didolkar M S: Chemotherapy of disseminated malignant melanoma with dimethyl triazeno imidazole carboxamide and actinomycin D. Cancer 32:756, 1973
127. Ahmann D L, Hahn R G, Bisel H F et al: Comparative study of Methyl-CCNU (NSC-95441) with cyclophosphamide (NSC-26271) and 5-(3,3-dimethyl-1-triazeno) imidazole-4-carboxamide (NSC-45388) with vincristine (NSC-67574) in patients with disseminated malignant melanoma. Cancer Chemother Rep 59:451, 1975
128. Bellet R E, Mastrangelo M J: Unpublished data
129. Livingston R B, Einhorn L H, Bodey G P, et al: COMB (cyclophosphamide, oncovin, methyl-CCNU, and bleomycin): A four drug combination in solid tumors. Cancer 36:327, 1975
130. Murphy W K: Phase I-II study of combination chemotherapy with cyclophosphamide (CTX) and methyl CCNU. Proc Am Soc Clin Oncol 16:253, 1975
131. Moon J H: Combination chemotherapy in malignant melanoma. Cancer 25:468, 1970
132. Marsh J C, DeConti R C, Hubbard S P: Treatment of Hodgkin's disease and other cancers with 1,3-bis(2-chloroethyl)-1-nitrosourea (BCNU; NSC-409962). Cancer Chemother Rep 55:599, 1971
133. Stolinsky D C, Pugh R P, Bohannon R A, et al: Clinical trial of BCNU (NSC-409962) combined with vincristine (NSC-67574) in disseminated gastrointestinal cancer and other neoplasms. Cancer chemother Rep 58:947, 1974
134. Perlin E, Engeler J, Reid J W, et al: Treatment of malignant melanoma with vinblastine (NSC-49842), procarbazine (NSC-77213), and actinomycin-D (NSC-3053). Cancer Chemother Rep 59:767, 1975
135. Coltman C A, Costanzi J J, Dudley G M, et al: Further clinical studies of combination chemotherapy using cyclophosphamide, vincristine, methotrexate and 5-fluorouracil in solid tumors. Am J Med Sci 261:73, 1971
136. Hanham I W F, Newton K A, Westbury G: Seventy-five cases of solid tumors treated by a modified quadruple chemotherapy regime. Br J Cancer 25:462, 1971
137. Shnider B I, Baig M, Serpick A, et al: Combination therapy with 5-fluorouracil, cyclophosphamide, vincristine, and methotrexate. J Clin Pharmacol 15:69, 1975

Bruce I. Shnider
Benedicta Ordona Meneses

20 Chemotherapy of Soft Tissue Sarcomas

The soft tissue sarcomas are tumors of mesenchymal origin that may develop at any site in the body. They include tumors that arise from fibrous and adipose tissue, blood vessels, lymphatic structures, fascia, synovial structures, nerves and smooth and striated muscles. They are rare tumors that account for about 2.1 per cent of all cancer deaths. Although they can appear localized, an accurate appraisal of their extent may be difficult because these tumors extend along muscle bundles, fascial planes and nerve sheaths beyond the palpable mass and this accounts for the frequent recurrence after a simple excision. They metastasize to regional lymph nodes and through the hematogenous route to the lungs, bone marrow, liver and bones, but rarely to the brain. With the advent of newer combinations of chemotherapeutic agents used in conjunction with surgery and radiation therapy and the resulting prolongation of the survival time, however, the number of patients that relapse with cerebral metastases is increasing.

Table 20-1 shows the histologic classification of soft tissue sarcomas and this discussion of the chemotherapy of soft tissue sarcomas will be limited to those that are listed in this table. These neoplasms are subclassified according to their metastatic potential in Table 20-2. Those with high metastatic potential are the undifferentiated fibrosarcoma and liposarcoma, rhabdomyosarcoma, malignant hemangioendothelioma and lymphaniosarcoma, synovial cell sarcoma and malignant mesenchymoma. The soft tissue sarcomas that

TABLE 20-1. *Soft Tissue Sarcomas*

(1) Fibrous tissue
- Fibrosarcoma
- Dermatofibrosarcoma protuberans

(2) Adipose tissue
- Liposarcoma

(3) Muscle tissue
- Leiomyosarcoma
- Rhabdomyosarcoma

(4) Vascular tissue
- Malignant hemangioendothelioma
- Malignant hemangiopericytoma
- Kaposi's sarcoma
- Lymphangiosarcoma

(5) Primitive mesenchyme—Myxoma

(6) Other sarcomas
- Synovial sarcoma
- Malignant mesenchymoma
- Malignant mesothelioma
- Chondrosarcoma
- Carcinosarcoma

From Shnider B I: Sarcomas. Lawyers Med J 7:45–64, 1978 (with permission).

TABLE 20-2. *Soft Tissue Sarcomas*

Malignant (with high metastatic potential)
- Undifferentiated fibrosarcoma and liposarcoma
- Rhabdomyosarcoma
- Malignant hemangioendothelioma and lymphangiosarcoma
- Synovial sarcoma
- Malignant mesenchymoma

Less Malignant (spread by infiltrative growth or, infrequently metastasize)
- Skin fibrosarcoma
- Myxoma
- Differentiated liposarcoma
- Kaposi's sarcoma
- Hemangiopericytoma (malignant)

From Shnider B I: Sarcomas. Lawyers Med J 7:45–64, 1978 (with permission).

spread by infiltrative growth or infrequently metastasize are dermatofibrosarcoma protruberans, myxoma, Kaposi's sarcoma and malignant hemangiopericytoma.

The earlier treatment of soft tissue sarcomas has been disappointing (Table 20-3) because of their tendency to metastasize early and widely. The curative approach to soft tissue sarcomas requires that the treatment be early, aggressive, accurate and adequate. A wide local excision has been considered adequate for localized tumors that were minimally aggressive but more extensive surgery becomes necessary for tumors that have a tendency to infiltrate locally or metastasize

TABLE 20-3. *5-Year Survival with Soft Tissue Sarcomas*

Type	Per cent
Rhabdomyosarcoma	20.8-35
Liposarcoma	25-40
Synovial sarcomas	27.5-37
Fibrosarcoma	48
(Desmoid variety)	95
Dermatofibrosarcoma	88-96
Neurofibrosarcoma	35.7
Leiomyosarcoma	39.6
Kaposi's sarcoma	45.9

widely. The location of the tumor sometimes may make surgery impossible. When the tumor was bulky or when there was microscopic or gross residual disease after surgery, radiation therapy was added to the treatment program. Chemotherapy was given when recurrence of metastases occurred after surgery and/or radiation therapy.

Of the 40 agents tested in soft tissue sarcomas in the last 25 years only actinomycin-D, MTX, vincristine and cyclophosphamide (Table 20-4) were found in the earlier studies to show promise. These agents had been used in a sufficient number of cases so that a definite conclusion could be made as to their effectiveness. While complete and partial responses occured, the duration of response was of short duration and the patient usually succumbed to the disease. The two newer agents that have been added to this list of active agents are DTIC and adriamycin. Although a study done by the Southwest Oncology Group using DTIC alone gave a response rate of only 17 per cent, it was felt that DTIC was an active drug in the treatment of soft tissue sarcomas because of the advanced nature of the disease of patients entered into the study. The response rate to adriamycin used alone in various soft tissue sarcomas has been reported to range from 27 to 31 percent.

In 1967, Haddy et al[4] gave Cytoxan intravenously to patients with rhabdomyosarcoma (RMS) and noted a response of 50 per cent or better in 6 of 13 patients and a partial response of 25 to 50 per cent tumor regression in 4 patients. Cytoxan was given at 30 mg/kg body weight orally or intravenously on day 1 in three divided doses. Cittadini,[5] Mannheimer,[6] and Sutow[7] treated a group of 45 patients with undifferentiated soft tissue sarcomas and noted over 50 per cent regression in 13 patients and 25 to 50 per cent response in 9 additional patients. The dosage of Cytoxan varied from an initial dose of one gram intravenously followed by oral maintenance of 100 to 200 mg daily to 30 mg/kg/week for a total of 4 weeks by either the intravenous or oral route.

Actinomycin-D has been the most widely used drug in the group of chemotherapeutic antibiotics in the earlier studies. Sagerman et al[8], Burrington,[9] Edland[10] and James et al[11] reported a response rate of approximately 50 per cent in the patients with rhabdomyosarcoma treated with actinomycin-D. Malkasian[12] and Cupps et al[13] found the drug to be fairly effective in the treatment of leiomyosarcoma, fibrosarcoma, liposarcoma and undifferentiated sarcomas and reported a high response rate with remissions lasting from 3 to 10 months. Kyalwazi[14] reported a better than 50 per cent response rate in Kaposi's sarcoma of the florid variety in patients treated with actinomycin-D. Hreschyshyn[15] noted a response in 7 to 20 patients with uterine sarcoma who received actinomycin-D in the standard dose of 75 mcg/kg over a 5-day-period with courses repeated once every 3 to 4 weeks.

Vincristine, a member of the plant alkaloid group, is the only drug in the group that has undergone extensive trial (Table 20-4). Sutow et al[16] and Selawry et al[17] reported 13 complete responses and five partial responses in a group of 32 patients with rhabdomyosarcoma treated with vincristine. The dosage in Sutow's series was 0.02 mg/kg for 5 days, then 0.05 mg/weekly, and in Selawry's series, 0.8 mcg/m^2 to 2.5 mcg/m^2.

The antimetabolites reported as active in the treatment of soft tissue sarcomas are MTX and 5-FU (Table 20-4). Van Dyk et al.[18] and Malkasian et al[12] reported a 70 per cent response rate in patients with leiomyosarcomas treated with 5-FU, but a low response rate was seen in undifferentiated sarcomas treated with this agent or fluorodeoxyuridine. Sullivan et al[19] reported five of 16 undifferentiated sarcomas responding to oral and parenteral MTX.

The use of combination chemotherapy was a natural outgrowth of the demonstrated activity of these drugs in soft tissue sarcomas. The more effective combinations have been those using actinomycin-D plus an alkylating agent and a variety of other compounds with varying activity (Table 20-5). Lawton et al[20] in 1965 reported responses in seven of nine undifferented sarcomas treated with the combination of 5-FU, MTX, vinblastine and hydroxyurea with a mean survival time of 16 months. Malkasian et al[21] using the combination of actinomycin-D, 5-FU, thio-TEPA and Cytoxan reported a response rate of over 50 per cent in seven of 13 leiomyosarcomas.

In all the studies reported, the duration of response in general has not been longer than 12 months. Retreatment with the same therapy or new forms of therapy was not effective.

TABLE 20-4. *Single Agents with Activity in Soft Tissue Sarcomas*

Alkylating Agents	Response Rate
Cyclophosphamide	52%
Chlorambucil	25%
Anti-metabolites	
Methotrexate	30%
DTIC	17%
Plant alkoloids	
Vincristine	55%
Antibiotics	
Adriamycin	31%
Actinomycin-D	50%

RHABDOMYOSARCOMA (RMS)

One of the soft tissue sarcomas found to be sensitive to chemotherapy is rhabdomyosarcoma (RMS). This is particularly true for those occuring in younger patients. Rhabdomyosarcomas may occur in the head and neck region, the trunk, the extremities and in the GU tract. A study of death certificates of 1170 children in the United States by Miller and Dalager[21] revealed that there are two peaks, one soon after birth and the other at age 15 to 19 years. The rank in order of fatal rhabdomyosarcoma by anatomical site under 15 years of age was: head and neck, 43.2 per cent GU tract, 28.6 per cent, trunk, 16 per cent and limbs, 12.2 per cent. Willis[22] feels that a majority of the rhabdomyosarcomas in children and adolescents are derived from embryonic tissue, not from muscle mass, and this causes their responsiveness to therapy.

The chemotherapy for RMS prior to 1965 consisted mostly of single agents. The usual sequence of treatment was biopsy and surgery, followed by radiation therapy and, on recurrence or metastasis, chemotherapy. In 1965 the Children's Cancer Study Group[23] used a combination of vincristine and actinomycin-D in conjunction with surgery and radiation therapy. Patients were treated for 1 year. The recurrence or metastatic rate was 17.6 per cent in the children with localized tumor that could be resected surgically and

TABLE 20-5. *Drug Combinations*

Drug Combinations	Over-All Response Rate	Sarcomas
VAC Vincristine + Actinomycin-D + Cyclophosphamide	65%	Rhabdomyosarcoma (Childhood)
CY-VADIC Cyclophosphamide + Vincristine + Adriamycin + DTIC	73%	Angiosarcoma Fibrosarcoma Leiomyosarcoma Liposarcoma Neurofibrosarcoma Rhabdomyosarcoma Synovial Cell Undifferentiated
Actinomycin-D + 5-FU + Sarcolysin + Cytoxan	42%	Myxosarcoma (response short in duration)
CY-VADACT Cyclophosphamide + Vincristine + Adriamycin + DTIC	70%	Angiosarcoma Fibrosarcoma Leiomyosarcoma Liposarcoma Rhabdomyosarcoma Neurofibrosarcoma Synovial Cell Undifferentiated Sarcomas
Adriamycin + DTIC	42%	Fibrosarcoma Leiomyosarcoma Liposarcoma Neurofibrosarcoma Synovial Cell Undifferentiated Sarcomas Angiosarcoma Rhabdomysarcoma
Adriamycin + DTIC + Vincristine	42%	Angiosarcoma Fibrosarcoma Leiomyosarcoma Liposarcoma Neurofibrosarcoma Rhabdomyosarcoma Undifferentiated Sarcomas
Actinomycin-D + Vincristine	92%	Kaposi's Sarcoma Florid Type (40% relapse rate)

91 per cent in those that had residual microscopic disease.

In 1967 Wilbur et al, at the MD Anderson Hospital, began the use of vincristine, actinomycin-D, and cyclophosphamide (VAC) in conjunction with surgery and radiation therapy in children with RMS. Vincristine was given at 2 mg/m²/wk I.V. for 12 weeks; actinomycin-D at 0.75 mcg/kg for 5 days was given I.V. every 12 weeks; Cytoxan was given at 2.5 mg/kg/day orally for 2 years. Patients who had gross residual disease at the start of therapy were given a more intensive therapy called Pulse VAC. There were 21 of 32 patients who had complete responses and were free of disease 1 to 4 years after completion of chemotherapy. The standard vincristine, actinomycin-D, cyclophosphamide (VAC), and the Pulse VAC treatments are very toxic combinations. The granulocytopenia is profound and the thrombocytopenia is significant. The other side effects observed were due to individual toxicity of the drugs in the combination. These consisted of neurotoxicity due to vincristine, hemmorrhagic cystitis due to Cytoxan and intensified toxicity in patients treated with local radiation therapy due to actinomycin-D. Reduction in dosage was often necessary because of the severity of the toxic reaction or gradual decrease in bone marrow reserve following multiple courses of chemotherapy.

Rivard et al[25] in reviewing the results of treatment in rhabdomyosarcoma of the pelvis in children treated at the Children's Hospital of Los Angeles between 1950 and 1972 showed that the survival was 4.5 times higher in children treated in the intensive VAC chemotherapy group. The median survival of the others who were treated in other therapeutic programs was 6 months, and all died. Those treated with VAC in conjunction with surgery and radiation therapy had a survival time in excess of 22 months. In the intensive chemotherapy group only two died with tumor and both had Stage IV disease at diagnosis. Five of 9 patients were alive between 12 and 60 months with no evidence of disease. The use of chemotherapy prior to surgery and radiation therapy sometimes eliminated the need for surgery because of regression of the tumor mass.

The reported 2 to 5 year survival rate of 100 patients with embryonal rhabdomyosarcoma of the GU tract ranges from 19 to 50 per cent. Ghavimi et al[26] reported on 27 patients with RMS of the GU tract treated between 1960 and 1971 at the Sloan Kettering Cancer Center, where multimodal therapy was used. The multiple drug therapy consisted of actinomycin-D, adriamycin, vincristine and cyclophosphamide in conjunction with radiation therapy following surgery and/or biopsy. Sixty-three per cent of 17 of 27 patients with Stage I or II disease were alive and without evidence of disease for periods ranging from 18 to 129 months.

Donaldson et al.[27] reported a minimal 2-year survival of 74 per cent and local control rate of 89 per cent 14 of 19 in patients with RMS of the head and neck treated with combination of surgery, radiation therapy and chemotherapy. Fourteen patients were living with no evidence of disease between 2 and 7 years, with mean of 2 years and 11 months and a median of 2 years and 18 months. The drug-related toxicities were bone marrow depression related to the administration of actinomycin-D and cyclophosphamide, neurotoxicity due to vincristine and hemorrhagic cystitis due to cyclophosphamide. Severe oral, dental, soft tissue and bone complications occurred. Some of the complications were seen early and some occurred late. "Recall phenomenon" was observed in patients who previously had radiation therapy and were treated with actinomycin-D.

Kaposi's Sarcoma

Kaposi's sarcoma is a tumor that is common in many parts of Africa and it is the fifth most common tumor in Ugandan men. This tumor is rare in the United States and Europe. It presents as multicentric, red-blue violaceous tumor masses on the skin and sometimes in the internal viscera. Kaposi's sarcoma is extremely sensitive to radiation therapy and chemotherapy. In a randomized study that compared actinomycin-D and cyclophosphamide, actinomycin-D was found to be superior. The overall response rate was 67 per cent but the relapse rate was high.

Vogel et al[29] reported on a randomized

study comparing actinomycin-D against an actinomycin-D and vincristine combination. There were four complete responses and five partial responses of 10 patients treated with acrinomycin-D alone. Of the 14 patients that received the combination, there were 10 complete and three partial responses. The relapse rate reported was 25 and 40 per cent in each group, respectively.

In a later study Vogel et al[30] showed that DTIC could produce a response rate of 50 per cent in patients whose disease was refractory to actinomycin-D. In a Phase II clinical trial of 1,3-BIS (2-chloroethyl) 1-nitrosourea (BCNU) and bleomycin, the same authors[31] reported objective antitumor responses in 9 of 21 patients treated with BCNU and 6 of 10 patients treated with bleomycin. The responses to BCNU were more complete and of longer duration than the responses to bleomycin, although the response rate to bleomycin was 60 per cent. The first 5 patients were treated with BCNU at a dose of 125 mg/m^2/day in 3-day courses and severe toxic effects were seen in 3 patients. There were no drug-related deaths due to septicemia. The toxicity in the remaining patients that were treated with 200 mg/m^2 in a single dose repeated every 6 to 8 weeks was tolerable. Bleomycin was given at a dose of 30 mg every 4 days by rapid I.V. infusion up to a total of 300 mg. There was no hematologic toxicity due to bleomycin. The dermatologic toxicities seen were hyperpigmentation, pruritus, cutaneous ulceration and alopecia. Fever spikes were seen in 9 patients and usually occured within 3 hours of drug administration. There was only 1 patient who received more than 300 mg of bleomycin, and he died of progressive pulmonary fibrosis. There were no radiographic changes seen in the other patients who received bleomycin.

Olweny et al[32] used ICRF 159 (NSC-129943) in a dose of 1gm/m/day orally for 3 days, repeated every 2 weeks, in 18 patients. There was one complete response and 10 partial responses in 18 patients for an overall response rate of 60 per cent. The complete response seen was in a patient who had florid monomorphic disease.

Other Soft Tissue Sarcomas

Starting in 1969, the Southwest Oncology Group (SWOG) and the MD Anderson Hospital[33] have been engaged in a series of protocols using adriamycin alone or in combination with other drugs in an attempt to improve the chemotherapy available for adult patients with soft or bone tissue sarcomas (Table 20-6). The responses obtained with vincristine, actinomycin-D and cyclophosphamide when used alone or in combination were disappointing because the duration of responses were short. The use of the same drugs in combination and in conjunction with surgery and radiation therapy gave better outlook to sarcoma patients in the pediatric age group especially those with rhabdomyosarcoma.

TABLE 20-6. *Soft Tissue Sarcomas. Adriamycin Responses (Adriamycin Alone and in Combination)*

Sarcomas	Evaluable Patients	Complete Response	Partial Response	Response Rates
Angiosarcomas	35	3	17	57%
Chondrosarcoma	29	1	4	17%
Fibrosarcoma	90	9	37	51%
Leiomyosarcoma	147	14	60	50%
Liposarcoma	71	7	28	49%
Neurofibrosarcoma	50	7	15	44%
Rhabdomyosarcoma	69	13	25	55%
Synovial cell sarcoma	25	4	10	56%
Unidifferentiated sarcoma	76	9	27	47%
Total	592	64	223	42.6%

As there were very few drugs that were effective in the treatment of soft tissue sarcomas new drugs were being sequentially evaluated.[33] One of these was 5-(3,3-dimethyl-1-triazeno) imidazole-4-carboxamide (NSC-45388) a chemically synthesized purine analogue. Fifty-three patients who had failed on other drugs were evaluated. There was one complete and eight partial remissions for an overall response rate of 17 per cent. While the result was not encouraging, it was felt that this compound had some activity in patients with metastatic sarcomas and could be considered for use in new combinations.

The next study undertaken by SWOG was a Phase II study involving the use of adriamycin in a dose of 75 mg/m^2 for patients with adequate marrow reserve and 45-60 mg/m^2 for patients with inadequate marrow reserve. Among 49 evaluable patients two complete and thirteen partial responses were seen for an overall response rate of 31 per cent. The survival time for responders and nonresponders was 8 and 4 months, respectively. This was not considered statistically significant so that further trials were undertaken to improve the results. In July 1971 the SWOG[33] using adriamycin at 60 mg/m^2 on day 1 and DTIC at 250 mg/m^2 on days 1 to 5 with courses repeated every 3 to 4 weeks. Two hundred and eighteen patients with sarcomas were evaluated with 25 complete and 67 partial remissions observed for an over all response rate of 42 per cent. Thirty-three per cent of the patients showed no change and 25 per cent had disease progression. Almost all of the sarcomas responded except for chondrosarcoma, mesothelioma and osteogenic sarcomas. The tumors that were particularly responsive were fibrosarcoma, leiomysarcoma, neurofibrosarcoma and rhabdomysarcoma. Those tumors that were located in the head and neck, in the GU tract and in the uterus were more responsive, while those that were in the pelvis, trunk and the GI tract were less responsive. Metastases to the soft tissue, lymph nodes, skin and lung responded better that metastases to the liver, bone and CNS. The median duration of survival for responders was 30 months or better and for partial responders 14 months or better.

An additional study[33] using adriamycin alone was undertaken in 1973 in which the dose-response relationship was explored in a wide variety of tumors including soft and bone tissue sarcomas. Patients with adequate marrow were randomly assigned to get 45, 60, or 75 mg/m^2 every 3 weeks and patients with inadequated marrow reserve were randomly assigned to get 25 or 50 mg/m^2 every 3 weeks. A 31 per cent response rate was obtained in 48 evaluable patients. There was one complete response and 14 partial responses. In addition to duplicating the response rate in the previous study using adriamycin alone, the duration of response was also comparable. This latter study had only 25 per cent of patients who were given prior chemotherapy. In addition, it was observed that the higher the dose, the more likely a response would occur in sarcoma patients.

Due to the higher response rate obtained by combining adriamycin and DTIC, vincristine was added to see if further increase in response rate would occur. Using these three drugs in combination, the SWOG activated its study in 1972. Vincristine was given at 1.5 mg/m^2 on days 1 and 5; Adriamycin was given at 60 mg/m^2 on day 1 and DTIC was given at 250 mg/m^2 from days 1 to 5. Patients with inadequate marrow reserve had a reduction in their adriamycin and DTIC dose to 45 mg/m^2 and 200 mg/m^2, respectively. Of the 107 evaluable patients 9 achieved complete remission and 36 achieved partial remission for an overall response rate of 42 per cent. The median duration of survival was in excess of 30 months for complete responders and in excess of 14 months for partial responders. These were virtually identical to the survival rates seen in their previous study using adriamycin and DTIC in combination.

In 1973 the Department of Therapeutics of the MD Anderson Hospital activated a cooperative study using the combination of cyclophosphamide, vincristine, adriamycin and DTIC.[34] Cyclophosphamide was given at 500 mg/m^2, vincristine at 1.5 mg/m^2 on days 1 and 5 and DTIC at 250 mg/m^2 from days 1 to 5 with courses repeated every 3 weeks. Of 136 patients evaluable, 19 achieved complete remission and 56 achieved partial remission for an overall response rate of 55 per cent. The degree of myelosuppression was more significant with the addition of cyclophosphamide. Twenty-seven per cent of the patients receiving the four drugs had a absolute granulocyte count of 500 cells/mm^3 sometime during the course of their chemotherapy. The duration of myelosuppression was short, so that there were very few episodes of infection and no deaths attributable to infection occurred. Thrombocytopenia was insignificant. Only 5 per cent of the patients had a platelet count of less than 50,000 cells/mm^3 during the study and serious bleeding problems were not observed. One complete and eight partial responders died one year after the close of the study which suggests that the overall survival rates will be improved.

A randomized clinical trial was undertaken by SWOG in 1973 to determine whether DTIC or actinomycin-D would be a more beneficial addition to the three-drug regimen of Cytoxan, vincristine and adriamycin. Vincristine was given I.V. at 1.5 mg/m^2 every week for 7 weeks starting on day 1 and then every 3 weeks. Cytoxan was given I.V. at 500 mg/m^2 on day 2 every 3 weeks. Adriamycin was given at 50 mg/m^2 on day 2 every 3 weeks. Actinomycin-D was given at 0.3 mg/m^2 for 3 days every 3 weeks starting on day 3. DTIC was given I.V. at 250 mg/m^2 daily for 5 days starting on day 1 every 3 weeks. Of the 178 patients on CY-VADIC that were evaluable 13 per cent had complete remission, 33 per cent had partial remission and 27 per cent had stable disease. Of the 175 evaluable patients on CY-VADACT, 12 per cent had CR, 27 per cent PR and 31 per cent, stable disease. The median survival was 10 months in the CY-VADACT groups and 13 months in the CY-VADIC group.

Eilber and his colleagues[35] at the 21st Annual Clinical Conference of The University of Texas System Cancer Center, MD Anderson Hospital in Houston, reported on presurgical treatment of 17 patients with soft tissue sarcomas with intra-arterial adriamycin and radiation. The 17 patients were among 42 with soft tissue sarcomas of the extremity who were treated between 1973 and 1976 by UCLA's Division of Surgical Oncology. Nineteen had surgical resection alone and 6 had radical amputation and adjuvant chemotherapy with adriamycin followed by MTX and leucovorin rescue. Of the 19 patients who had surgical resection alone 31 per cent had local recurrence and 60 per cent had distant metastases. Among the group who had radical amputation followed by adjuvant chemotherapy with adriamycin followed by MTX and leucovorin rescue, 16 per cent had local recurrence and 50 per cent had distant metastases. In the group who had adriamycin prior to radiation therapy 16 or 17 patients had functioning neurologically intact extremities. All 16 patients remained free of local recurrence and distant metastases 4 to 34 months after operation.

Table 20-7 lists the various soft tissue sarcomas responsive to combination chemotherapy, the drug schedules, dosage and response rates reported by a variety of investigators. The results indicated increasing success in the eradication of disease and in the control of local and metastatic recurrence.

Summary

The response rate of adults and children with soft tissue sarcomas has shown a remarkable improvement in the past 5 years. Eradication of disease and prevention of recurrence can be achieved in over 50 per cent of the

TABLE 20-7. *Effective Drug Combinations in Soft Tissue Sarcomas*

Sarcomas	Drugs	Dosage/Schedule	Overall Response Rate	Comments
Rhabdomyosarcoma	Vincristine +	2 mg/m2 I.V. weekly ×12	65%	Childhood rhabdomyosarcoma— in conjunction with surgery and radiation therapy

TABLE 20-7. (continued)

Sarcomas	Drugs	Dosage/Schedule	Overall Response Rate	Comments
	Actinomycin-D +	.075 mg/kg/course-I.V. over 5 days every 3 months		Toxicity significant-most effective for inoperable or metastatic rhabdomyosarcomas of childhood. Median duration of survival 3 years after start of treatment with no evidence of disease(23,24,25,26,27,35)
	Cyclophosphamide	2.5 mg/kg/day orally for 2 years		
	Actinomycin-D +	15 mcg/kg/I.V. for 5 days with 2 weeks drug free interval then	80%	Repeat courses required to obtain maximum remission (39,40)
	Vincristine	.05 mg/kg/week for 6 weeks		
	Actinomycin-D +	15 mcg/kg/day I.V. for 5 days	40%	Mean survival 3 plus years (37,38)
	Mechlorethamine	30 mg single intra-arterial dose		
	Actinomycin-D +	15 mcg/kg/day I.V. for 5 days	55%	Lesions of orbit. 5 patients alive and well (39,40)
	Methotrexate +	1.25 mg qid for 6–10 days orally		
	Cyclophosphamide	Intra-arterial infusion		
Rhabdomyosarcoma	Vincristine +	1.5 mg/m² IV days 1 and 5	67%	1-CR and 4-PR in 9 evaluable patients/ Median survival in excess of 30 months (33)
	Adriamycin + DTIC	60 mg/m² day 1 250 mg/m² days 1–5		
	Cyclophosphamide	500 mg/m² day 1 I.V.	67%	6-CR and 4-PR in 27 evaluable patients/ Median survival in excess of 30 months for CR and 14 months for PR (35)

TABLE 20-7. (continued)

Sarcomas	Drugs	Dosage/Schedule	Overall Response Rate	Comments
	Vincristine	1.5 mg/m² days 1 and 5		
	Adriamycin +	50 mg/m² day 1		
	DTIC	250 mg/m² days 1 to 5		
Rhabdomyosarcoma	Vincristine +	2 mg/m² week I.V.		Modified VAC in conjunction with radiation therapy as primary treatment for unresectable childhood RMS 8 of 9 patients were disease free from 12 to 51 months (median 22 months) (42)
	Actinomycin-D +	225 gamma/m²/d×10 days 12 weeks I.V.		
	Cyclophosphamide	300 mg/m²/d×10 days every 6 weeks I.V.		
Angiosarcoma	Vincristine +	1.5 mg/m² days 1 and 5 I.V.	57%	(33)
	Adriamycin +	50 mg/m² day 1 I.V.		
	DTIC	250 mg/m² days 1 to 5 I.V.		
	Vincristine +	1.5 mg/m² I.V. days 1 and 5	80%	(35)
	Adriamycin +	50 mg/m² day 1 I.V.		
	DTIC +	250 mg/m² days 1 to 5 I.V.		
	Cyclophosphamide	500 mg/m² day 1 I.V.		
	Vincristine	1.5 mg/m² I.V.		In 19 patients conjunction with radiation therapy and surgery CR-17 PR-2 offered as a alternative to radical surgery in growing child (41)

TABLE 20-7. (continued)

Sarcomas	Drugs	Dosage/Schedule	Overall Response Rate	Comments
	Actinomycin-D	0.4 mg/m² I.V.		
	+			
	Cyclophosphamide	300 mg/m² I.V.		
Fibrosarcoma	Vincristine	1.5 mg/m² days 1 to 5 I.V.	60%	1 CR and 5 PR in 10 evaluable patients (33)
	+			
	Adriamycin	50 mg/m² day 1 I.V.		
	+			
	DTIC	250 mg/m² days 1 to 5 I.V.		
	Cytoxan	500 mg/m² day 1 I.V.	57%	(35)
	+			
	Vincristine	1.5 mg/m² days 1 to 5 I.V.		
	+			
	Adriamycin	50 mg/m² day 1 I.V.		
	+			
	DTIC	250 mg/m² days 1 to 5 I.V.		
Lieomyosarcoma	Cytoxan	35–50 mg a day for 4 doses	77%	Exact criteria for response not clear (12)
	+			
	Melphalan	8 mg/day until toxicity		
	+			
	Thio-tepa	45 mg/week I.V.		
	Actinomycin-D	0.25–0.5 mg/day for 5 days I.V.		Cyclic therapy every month. Response criteria is not clear (12)
	+			
	5-Fluorouracil	15 mg/kg/day for 5 days I.V.		
	+			
	Thio-tepa	45 mg for 5 days I.V.		
Liposarcoma	Vincristine	1.5 mg/m² day I.V. day 5	47%	7-PR (33)
	+			
	Adriamycin	50 mg/m² day 1		
	+			
	DTIC	250 mg/m² days 1 to 5		
	Cytoxan	500 mg/m² day 1	60%	(35)
	+			
	Adriamycin	50 mg/m² day 1		
	+			
	Vincristine	1.5 mg/m² days 1 and 5		
	+			
	DTIC	250 mg/m² days 1 to 5		

children afflicted with this disease. In adults, combination chemotherapy has been responsible for better response rates and improved survival. With continuing refinement of dosage, scheduling and intensity of multimodal therapy, we may anticipate achieving a significant number of "cures" in patients with early disease and ultimately in some patients with inoperable and metastatic disease.

References

1. Gercovich F G, Luna M A, Gottlieb J A: Increase incidence of cerebral metastasis in sarcoma patients with prolonged survival from chemotherapy. Cancer 36:1843-1851, 1975
2. Luce J K, Thurman W G, Isaacs B L, et al: Clinical trials with the antitumor agent 5(3,3-dimethyl-triazeno) imidazole-4-carboxamide, NSC-45388. Cancer Chemother Rep 54:119–124, 1970
3. O'Bryan R M, Luce J K, Talley R W, et al: Phase II evaluation of adriamycin in human neoplasia. Cancer 32:1–8, 1973
4. Hardy T B, Nora A H, Sutow W W: Cyclophosphamide treatment for metastatic soft tissue sarcomas. Am J of Dis Child 114:301, 1967
5. Cittadini G: Problem di cancerologia clinica: Lo shock citostatico con ciclofosfamide. Minerva Med 57:1715, 1966
6. Mannheimer E, Karrer K, Boeckl O, Presching A: Hochdosierte zytostatistiche therapie und autologe knochemarks re infusion bei malignen tumoren. Munchen Med. Wochenschr 109:1808, 1967
7. Sutow W W: Cyclophosphamide in Wilm's tumor and rhabdomyosarcoma. Cancer Chemother Rep 51:407, 1967
8. Sagerman R H, Cassady J R, Tritter P: Radiation therapy for rhabdomyosarcoma of the orbit. Trans Acad Ophthalmol Otolaryngol 72:849, 1968
9. Burrington J D: Rhabdomyosarcoma of the paratesticular tissue in children. J Ped Surg 4:503, 1969
10. Edland R W: Embryonal rhabdomyosarcoma. Am J Roentgenol 93:671, 1965
11. James D H Jr, Hustu O, Wrenn E L Jr: Childhood malignant tumors: Concurrent chemotherapy with dactinomycin and vincristine sulfate. JAMA 197:1043, 1966
12. Malkasian G D Jr, Mussey E, Decker D G, Johnson C E: Chemotherapy of gynecologic sarcomas: Cancer Chemother Rep 51:507, 1967
13. Cupps R E, Ahmann D L, Spule E H: Treatment of pulmonary metastatic disease with radiation therapy and adjuvant actinomycin-D; Cancer 24:719, 1969
14. Kyalwazi S K: Kaposi's sarcoma E Afr Med J 46:459, 1969
15. Hreshchyshyn M M: Experiences with chemotherapy in gynecologic cancer N Y State J Med 64:2431, 1964
16. Sutow W W, Berry D H, Haddy T B: Vincristine sulfate therapy in children with metastatic soft tissue sarcoma. Pediatrics 38:465, 1966
17. Selawry O, Holland J F, and Wolman I J: Effect of vincristine on malignant tumors in children. Cancer Chemother Rep 52:497, 1968
18. VanDyk J J, Clarkson B D, Duschinsky R, et al: Clinical evaluation of 5-bromo-5-fluoro-6-methoxy-dihydro-2-deoxyuridine. Cancer Res 27:2129, 1967
19. Sullivan R D, Miller E, Zurek W Z: Re-evaluation of methotrexate as an anticancer drug. Surg Gynecol Obstet 125:819, 1967
20. Lawton R L, Latourette H B, Collier R G: Simultaneous high-energy irradiation and chemotherapy. Arch Surg 91:155, 1965
21. Miller R W, Dalager N A: Fatal rhabdomyosarcoma among children in the United States 1960–1969. Cancer 34:1897, 1975
22. Willis R A: Pathology of Tumors. Third Edition. London, Butterworth, 1960
23. Heyn R M, Holland R, et al: The role of combined chemotherapy in the treatment of rhabdomyosarcoma in children. Cancer 34:2128, 1974
24. Wilbur J R: Combination chemotherapy for embryonal rhabdomyosarcoma. Cancer Chemother Rep 58:281, 1974
25. Rivard G, Ortega J, Hittle R, et al: Intensive chemotherapy as primary treatment for rhadbomyosarcoma of pelvis. Cancer 36:1593, 1975
26. Ghairmi F, Exselby P R, D'Angio G J, et al: Combination therapy of urogenital embryonal rhabdomyosarcoma in children. Cancer 32:1178, 1973
27. Donaldson S S, Castro J R, et al: Rhabdomyosarcoma of head in children. Cancer 31:26, 1973
28. Vogel C L, Templeton C J, Templeton A C, et al: Treatment of Kaposi's sarcoma with actinomycin and cyclophosphamide. Results of a randomized clinical trial. Int J Cancer 8:136–143, 1971
29. Vogel C L, Primack A, Dhru D, et al: Treat-

ment of Kaposi's sarcoma with a combination of act-D and vincristine. Results of a randomized trial. Cancer 31:1382, 1973

30. Vogel L, Primack A, Dhru D, et al: Treatment of Kaposi's sarcoma with combination of actinomycin-D and vincristine. Results of randomized clinical trials. Cancer 31:1382–1389, 1973
31. Vogel C L, Clements D, Wanume A, et al: Phase II clinical trials of BCNU and bleomycin in the treatment of Kaposi's sarcoma. Cancer Chemother Rep 57:325, 1973
32. Olweny C L M, Masaba J P, Sikyewunda W, Toya T: Treatment of Kaposi's sarcoma with ICRF (NSC-129943) Cancer Treat Rep 60:111, 1976
33. Gottlieb J A, et al: Adriamycin (NSC-1231270) used alone and in combination for soft tissue and bone sarcomas. Cancer Chemother Rep 6:271–282, 1975
34. Luce J K, Thurman W G, Isaacs B L, Talley R W: Clinical trials with the anti-tumor agent 5-(3,3,-dimethyl-1-triazeno imidozale 4-carboxamide (NSC-45388). Cancer Chemother Rep 54:119, 1970
35. Gottlieb J A: Improved survival with adriamycin (A) combination in patients with metastic sarcomas. Proc Am Assoc Cancer Res 16:238, 1975
36. Eilber F R, et al: Pre-surgery drug, radiation salvage limbs in sarcomas. Oncology News 3:8, 1977
37. Grosfeld J L, Clatworthy H W Jr, Newton W A Jr: Combined therapy in childhood rhabdomyosarcoma. Ped Surg 4:637, 1969
38. Hayes D M, Mirabal V Q, Patel H R: Rhabdomyosarcoma of the spermatic cord. Surgery 65:845, 1969
39. Nelson A J III: Embryonal rhabdomyosarcoma: Report of twenty-four cases and study of the effectiveness of radiation therapy upon the primary tumor. Cancer 22:64, 1968
40. Pratt C B, et al: Response of childhood rhabdomyosarcoma to combination chemotherapy. Pediatrics 74:791, 1969
41. Holton C P, Chapman K, et al: Extended combination chemotherapy of childhood rhabdomyosarcoma. Cancer 32:1210–1216, 1973
42. Jaffee N, Weinstein H, et al: Primary treatment with VAC and radiotherapy for untreatable rhabdomyosarcomas in children. Proc Am Assoc Cancer Res 17:284, 1976

MILTON H. DONALDSON

21

Recent Developments in Wilms' Tumor and Rhabdomyosarcoma in Children

At the Twenty-second Hahnemann Symposium on Cancer Chemotherapy, Dr. Audrey Evans reviewed "refinements"[1] in the treatment of Wilms' tumors and rhabdomyosarcomas that had occurred in the 5-year period since she reported to the preceding Symposium in 1967.[1] At the time of the last Symposium in 1972, the National Wilms' Tumor Study (NWTS) had not been underway long enough to have reportable data and the Intergroup Rhabdomyosarcoma Study (IRS) was not yet begun. Therefore, it is a privilege to add to the annals of the Hahnemann Symposia a review of the now-completed first phase of the NWTS, and a preliminary report of the IRS. Advances with other pediatric tumors are reported by other participants in this Symposium.

WILMS' TUMOR

Since dactinomycin was first found to be effective against Wilms' tumor in 1956[2,3] numerous studies have confirmed that report.[4,5] Also, in the interim, vincristine has demonstrated its ability to cause significant regression of metastatic lesions of Wilms',[6] as well as dramatic shrinkage of the primary tumor.[7] Dactinomycin caused greater toxicity but vincristine did not seem to enhance the effect of irradiation as did actinomycin. The obvious questions arose: (1) Is one of these agents superior to the other in the treatment of Wilms' tumor, or (2) might combining them produce even better tumor control than either agent alone? and (3) could use of vincristine preoperatively improve the survival of children presenting with metastatic tumor? Desiring to eliminate radiation toxicity, especially long-term growth disturbances, many began to question the necessity of irradiating the "tumor bed" after complete resection of those tumors confined to the kidney.

Together with a classification of tumor extent at diagnosis (called Groupings in this study), these questions were formulated and developed into the National Wilms' Tumor Study which was initiated in 1969.[8] Definitions of the classification were as follows:

Group I. Tumor is limited to the kidney and is completely resected. The surface of the renal capsule is intact. The tumor is not ruptured before or during removal. There is no residual tumor apparent beyond the margins of resection.

*Supported in part by USPHS Grants CA 06927, CA 11796, CA 03735 CA 04646 and CA 12012.

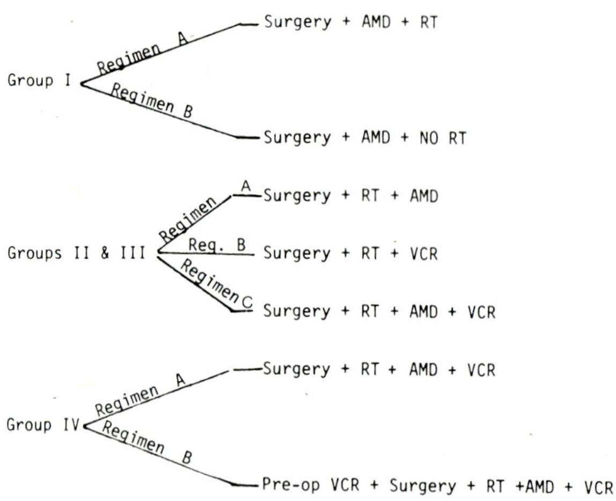

FIG. 21-1. NWTS - I Treatment Schemas.

Group II. Tumor extends beyond the kidney but is completely resected. There is local extension of the tumor, i.e., penetration beyond the pseudocapsule into the perirenal soft tissues, or periaortic lymph node involvement. The renal vessels outside the kidney substance are infiltrated or contain tumor thrombi. There is no residual tumor apparent beyond the margins of resection.

Group III. Residual nonhematogenous tumor confined to the abdomen. Any one or more of the following may occur: (1) The tumor has been ruptured or biopsy performed before or during surgery, (2) There are implants on the peritoneal surfaces, (3) There are involved lymph nodes beyond the abdominal periaortic chains, (4) The tumor is not completely resectable because of local infiltration into vital structures.

Group IV. Hematogenous metastases; deposits beyond Group III (e.g., lungs, liver, bone and brain)

Group V. Bilateral renal involvement either initially or subsequently. (Patients in this group were not included in the study although information on them was gathered.)

The treatment schemas are depicted in Figure 21-1. All patients with Group I tumors underwent nephrectomy and received 5-day courses of dactinomycin (at 1 and 6 weeks and 3,7,9,12 and 15 months from diagnosis); half of them also had irradiation to the "tumor bed", 1800 to 4000 rads depending on age. All patients with Group II and Group III tumors had appropriate surgery and irradiation and were randomized to receive either dactinomycin, vincristine or both. Half of the patients with hematogenous metastases i.e., Group IV tumors, had vincristine prior to surgery, and all received postoperative irradiation and the combination of dactinomycin and vincristine after nephrectomy.

The statistical results of the study[9] are summarized in Table 21-1, with patients in Group I analyzed according to age and treatment regimen. Use of radiotherapy did not significantly improve the proportion of patients either disease free or simply surviving at 2 years, by actuarial analysis, for those under 2 years of age. The older patients in Group I who did not receive irradiation, however, had a poorer disease-free survival than those treated with irradiation, although the projected overall survival rates for both groups of older patients are nearly the same. It is particularly pertinent that of the nine abdominal recurrences in Group I patients, only three were in the site of the primary tumor bed—all occurring in nonirradiated patients who were 35,36 and 63 months of age at the time of their

TABLE 21-1. *Results for Randomized Patients: Modified from D'Angio et al: The treatment of Wilm's tumor. Cancer 38:639, 1976*

Tumor Grouping	Treatment Regimens	No. of Patients	Proportion* NED @ 2 Yrs	Proportion* Alive @ 2 Yrs.
Group I < 2 yrs	A	38	.90	.97
	B	36	.88	.94
Group I ≥ 2 yrs	A	39	.77	.97
	B	41	.58	.91
Groups II & III	A	63	.57	.67
	B	44	.55	.72
	C	59	.81	.86
Group IV	A	13		.83
	B	13		.29

* = Actuarial proportion of patients

original diagnoses. Two of them had distant metastases.

There were so few differences in Groups II and III that their data were combined. No evidence of age effect was noted. The only difference between Group II and Group III was in those on Regimen A, i.e., dactinomycin, where the relapse-free rate was 72 per cent for Group II versus 44 per cent for Group III. There was no explanation for this difference apparent to the NWTS Committee. Certainly, the 81 per cent disease-free and 86 per cent survival rates for those who received both drugs (Regimen C) are superior to the rates for either drug alone.

The analysis for Group IV patients is limited to survival because so many of them had persistent disease postoperatively for indefinite periods. The small numbers randomized was due to the fact that most such patients were operated upon before registration into the study. Even though the survival is much poorer for those receiving preoperative vincristine, the rather select small group precludes unquestioning acceptance of these data for Group IV patients.

The major question about Group I patients in this study was whether irradiation was necessary after nephrectomy if dactinomycin was given at intervals for 15 months. The overall survival rate of 97 per cent for those irradiated versus 92 per cent for the nonirradiated group is not significantly different. The disease-free rate for the non-irradiated Group I patients 2 years or older, however, was barely significantly greater than the rate for those of that age and Group who were irradiated. In addition, only one of the older irradiated patients developed an abdominal recurrence, compared to five such recurrences in the nonirradiated patients. Therefore, the data suggest that irradiation to the primary tumor site in children 2 years or older would offer a lower abdominal recurrence rate. Those younger with a Group I tumor derive no apparent benefit from adding irradiation to the dactinomycin therapy.

The NWTS as originally designed has been completed. The outcomes have stimulated new questions which are now being investigated in NWTS-II. For example, since the toxicity for vincristine and dactinomycin was quite tolerable, that combination is being used for all Group I patients, without irradiation, to determine whether this will sufficiently reduce or eliminate abdominal recurrences. Whether a shorter period of these two drugs will suffice also is being tested by allowing half the patients to stop therapy after 6 months, the others continuing to 15 months. Because adriamycin is known to be effective against Wilms' tumor, it is being combined with vincristine and dactinomycin, with irradiation after nephrectomy, for half of the patients with Group II, III, and IV tumors to determine if it adds to the disease control. The accumulated data for NWTS-II are not yet sufficient to be reported.

Rhabdomyosarcoma

In children, the majority of instances of this tumor are of the embryonal type, or the sarcoma botryoid variant. Until recent years, these tumors were viewed as unresponsive to radiotherapy and chemotherapy and less than half of the resectable lesions were cured. However, since the mid-1960s, much investigation of the treatment has taken place. Review of all that work is beyond the scope of this presentation but two studies are especially worthy of mention.

In 1971, Wilbur et al reported their vigorous use of vincristine, dactinomycin and cyclophosphamide in a regimen called "pulse VAC", with surgery and irradiation used as fully as practical.[10] Only 8 of the 32 patients had fully operable disease and they continue to be well without recurrence at last report. Ten of the 16 with inoperable disease also remain well, with a median time of 65 months, while 4 of 8 with metastatic disease are without evidence of tumor a median time of 74 months. Collectively, 68 per cent of this group of patients are alive with no evidence of disease a median time of over 5 years from the start of therapy which was administered for only 2 years.[11]

Heyn et al, in 1970[12] gave a preliminary report of a study of the Children's Cancer Study Group using vincristine and dactinomycin in 9 week cycles for 1 year in rhabdomyosarcoma patients. The definitive report of this investigation, 4 years later, indicate that 23 of the 28 patients "made grossly tumor free by surgery and radiotherapy" have no evidence of tumor for periods greater than 2 years.[13] A recent personal communication with Heyn revealed that 25 of the original 28 patients are still alive with no evidence of disease.

The early experiences of Wilbur and Heyn and their associates and the successful development of the NWTS stimulated formation of the Intergroup Rhabdomyosarcoma Study (IRS) by the Children's Cancer Study Group (CCSG), the Cancer and Acute Leukemia Group B (CALGB) and the Southwest Oncology Group (SOG) in 1972. The following is a review of the study design and some of the preliminary data as of March 9, 1977.

As in the NWTS, therapy is designed and allocated according to extent of tumor detectable and/or known to be residual after definitive surgery or biopsy. The patients are then grouped as follows:

Group I. Localized disease, completely resected (regional nodes not involved).
- a. Confined to muscle or organ of origin.
- b. Contiguous involvement - infiltration outside the muscle or organ of origin, as through fascial planes.

Group II.
- a. Grossly resected tumor with microscopic residual disease (nodes negative)
- b. Regional disease, completely resected (nodes positive or negative)
- c. Regional disease with involved nodes, grossly resected, but with evidence of microscopic residual disease.

Group III. Incomplete resection or biopsy with gross residual disease.

Group IV. Metastatic disease present at onset.

It is essential that such grouping or staging criteria be adhered to firmly in order to ensure true comparability of patient data between institutions in the IRS, or even subsequently between the IRS data and that of other studies.

Treatment regimens as related to Clinical Groups are depicted in Figure 21-2. The primary therapeutic objectives are:

1. Is irradiation to the primary tumor site necessary in Group I patients?
2. In Group II patients, are two drugs for 1 year (Regimen C) as effective and less toxic than three drugs (Regimen D) for a total of 2 years?
3. Does adriamycin, added to vincristine, dactinomycin and cyclophosphamide (Regimen E) improve disease control and survival more than the latter three drugs without adriamycin (Regimen F)?

All patients in Groups II, III and IV receive irradiation to all areas of known disease or "tumor bed," while in Group I only Regimen

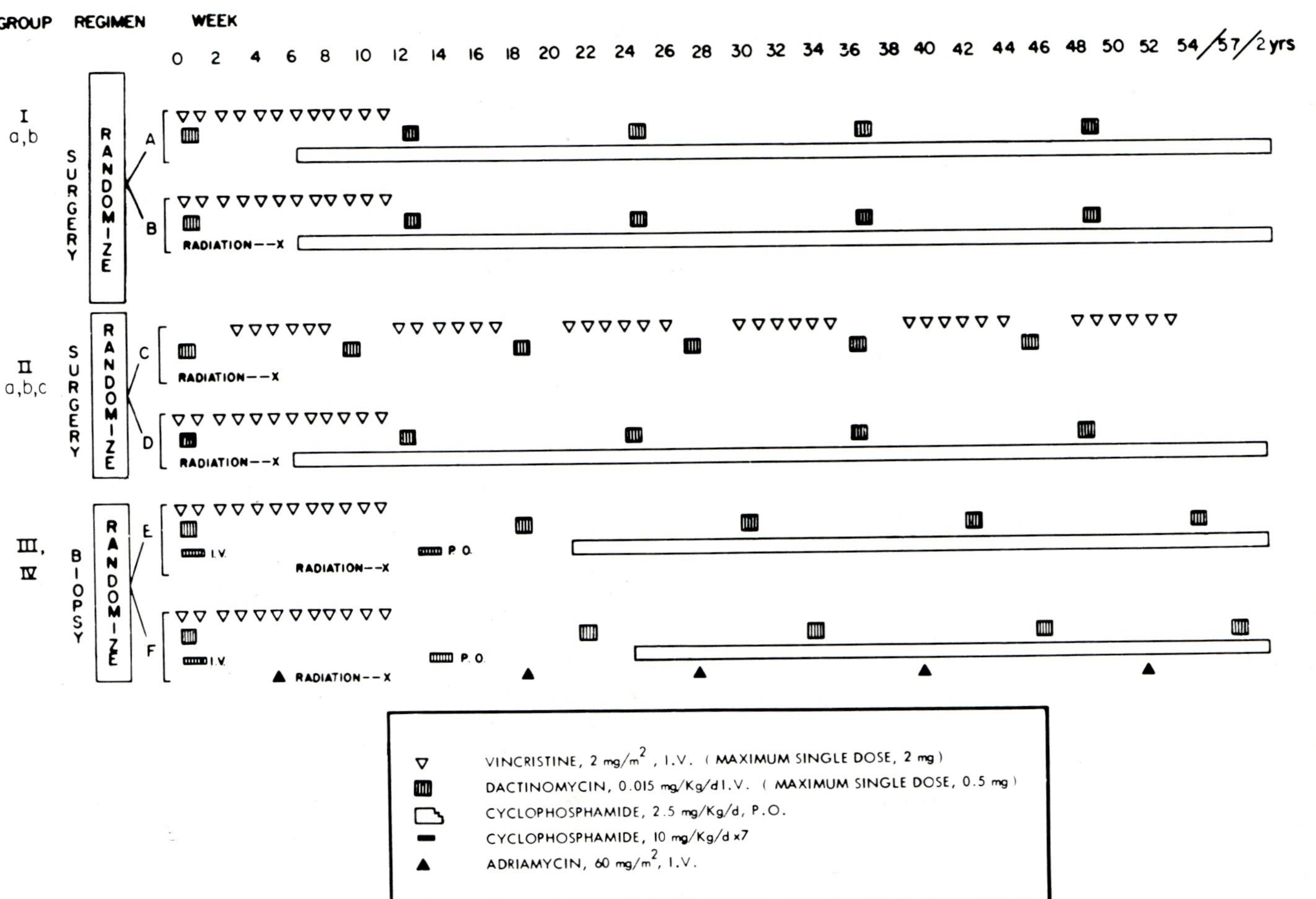

FIG. 21-2. Treatment Schedules for Intergroup Childhood Rhabdomyosarcoma Study.

TABLE 21-2. *Complete responses and ranges of duration by Clinical Group and Treatment Regimen.*

Clinical Stage, Treatment	Number Evaluated	No. CR %	No. Still in CR (%)	Duration of CR (wks.) Range
I - A	34	34 (100)	30 (88)	1 - 190
I - B	22	22 (100)	21 (95)	0 - 199
I - G	8	8 (100)	4 (50)	17 - 170
II - C	47	47 (100)	36 (77)	0 - 189
II - D	54	54 (100)	44 (81)	0 - 195
III - E	85	44 (52)	35 (80)	0 - 191
III - F	80	45 (56)	32 (71)	0 - 159
IV - E	42	18 (43)	6 (33)	3 - 144
IV - F	44	24 (55)	11 (46)	2 - 177
	417			

B patients receive irradiation. Group I extremity tumors, which are amputated, and paratesticular tumors treated by hemiscrotectomy are assigned to Regimen A because there is no "tumor bed" to be irradiated should the patient be randomized to Regimen B; such patients are designated as treated with Regimen G.

Thus far, of the 468 eligible patients randomized on study, 416 (88 per cent) are evaluable in part or fully. Sixty-four (15 per cent) are Group I, 101 (24 per cent) Group II, 165 (40 per cent) Group III and 86 (21 per cent) are Group IV.

Table 21-2 illustrates the complete responses and their ranges of duration according to Clinical Group and treatment regimen. There is no significant difference in the relapse rates of patients on Regimens A (12 per cent) and B (5 per cent). The amputees (Regimen G) have sustained a 50 per cent relapse rate. Over 85 per cent of the patients on Regimens A & B are projected to survive 140 weeks, while the rate for Regimen G amputees is projected to be 50 per cent.

A total of 21 relapses has occurred in Group II patients. The 23 per cent relapse rate for Regimen C is not significantly different from the 19 per cent rate of Regimen D ($p = 0.20$). On Regimen C there have been eight deaths as compared to six on Regimen D, allowing a projection of 75 per cent survival at 120 weeks.

Group III Patients show approximately 50 per cent complete response rate on each regimen, as do the Group IV patients on the four-drug Regimen F. Although the Group IV Regimen E patients achieved only 43 per cent complete response rate, it is not significantly different. Fifty-nine patients of Groups III and IV achieved partial responses but only 29 have not then regressed and, thus, may yet progress to becoming disease free.

Based on the IRS Committee's preference to be 80 per cent confident that there is no more than 30 per cent difference between regimens for each Clinical Group, there yet needs to be a minimum of 7 months' accrual of Group II patients to 2 years' accrual for Group I patients. Obviously, the final outcomes of this study will not be achieved for several years yet.

OTHER CHILDHOOD SOLID TUMORS

In the intervening 5 years since the last Hahnemann Symposium on Cancer Chemotherapy, numerous investigative studies have been conducted about neuroblastoma. Unfortunately, although refinements of therapeutic approaches and greater knowledge of prognostic factors have accrued[14,15] no increase in the cure rate has been achieved for this tumor. On the brighter side, some remarkable results have been achieved with new agents and more aggressive and enlightened usage of already known drugs in the treatment of bone tumors. These are discussed elsewhere in this Symposium, as are similar advances in the treatment of brain tumors and acute leukemias in children. Thus, although much remains to be achieved in the control of pediatric malignancies, several gratifying advancements have occurred in recent years which have resulted in significant improvements in survival for this age group.

References

1. Evans A E: Refinements in the treatment of children with solid tumors, in Brodsky I, Kahn S (eds): Cancer Chemotherapy II. New York, Grune & Stratton, 1967, p 181
2. Farber S, Sears H, Pinkel D: Advances in chemotherapy of cancer in man. Adv Cancer Res 4:1, 1956
3. Farber S, D'Angio G, Evans A E, et al: Clinical studies of actinomycin D with special reference to Wilms' tumor in children. Ann N Y Acad Sci 89:421, 1960
4. Farber S: Chemotherapy in the treatment of leukemia and Wilms' tumor, JAMA 198:154, 1966
5. Fernbach D J, Martyn D T: Role of dactinomycin in the survival of children with Wilms' tumor. JAMA 195:1005, 1966
6. Sullivan M: Curable metastatic tumors of childhood. Tex Med 61:800, 1965
7. Sutow W W, Sullivan M: Vincristine in primary treatment of Wilms' tumor. Tex Med 61:794, 1965
8. D'Angio G: Management of children with Wilms' tumor. Cancer 30:1528, 1972
9. D'Angio G J, Evans A E, Breslow N, et al: The treatment of Wilms' tumor. Results of the national Wilms' tumor study. Cancer 38:633, 1976
10. Wilbur J R, Sutow W W, Sullivan M P, et al: Successful treatment of inoperable embryonal rhabdomyosarcoma. (abstr) Proceedings of the Society for Pediatric Research, 1971, p 90
11. Wilbur J R, Sutow W W, Sullivan M P, et al: Chemotherapy of sarcomas. Cancer 36:765, 1975
12. Heyn R M, Holland R: Treatment of rhabdomyosarcomas in children. For The Childrens Cancer Study Group A. (abstr) Proceedings of American Association Cancer Research, 1970, p 36
13. Heyn R M, Holland R, Newton W A Jr, et al: The role of combined chemotherapy in the treatment of rhabdomyosarcoma in children. Cancer 34:2128, 1974
14. Evans A E, Albo V, D'Angio G J, et al: Cyclophosphamide treatment of patients with localized and regional neuroblastoma. A randomized study. Cancer 38:665, 1976
15. Evans A E, Albo V, D'Angio G J, et al: Factors influencing survival of children with nonmetastatic neuroblastoma. Cancer 38:661, 1976

Norman Jaffe

22
Chemotherapy of Malignant Bone Tumors in Children

During the past 5 years, several reports have demonstrated the potential for an improved prognosis in malignant bone tumors in children. This review examines the role of chemotherapy, with particular emphasis on its integration into a multidisciplinary program.

Principles of Treatment

The immediate objective is to eradicate the primary tumor unless the disease is fairly extensive, when palliation becomes a major consideration. Surgery and radiation therapy constitute the major weapons of primary treatment. Surgical ablation is usually instituted for osteogenic sarcoma, chondrosarcoma and fibrosarcoma. In contrast, radiation therapy is the principal mode of treatment for Ewing's sarcoma. It is also used extensively for palliation.

Surgery and radiation therapy have a limited potential since their major thrust is usually directed against localized disease. The biological behavior of most malignant neoplasms, particularly bone tumors, suggests that microscopic dissemination of disease is present at diagnosis. This dissemination is subclinical and is usually undetectable by currently available techniques. Systemic treatment is required to destroy such micrometastases and is usually attempted through the administration of chemotherapy. This is designated "adjuvant treatment."

The choice of adjuvant treatment is determined by clinical and experimental investigation and past experience. Generally, evidence must be adduced to demonstrate effective destruction of tumor; this is usually obtained in patients with advanced disease. Once satisfactory responses have been achieved, the treatment is administered for eradication of microscopic tumor. The experimental and clinical rationale for this approach constitutes one of the fundamental principles of cancer treatment.

The tactics and strategy governing the effective application of primary and adjuvant therapy are also predicated by a knowledge of the exact diagnosis and the extent of tumor. The former is achieved through pathology expertise and the latter through the following investigations: radiographic examination of the presenting lesion and chest, bone scintigraphy, chest fluoroscopy and laminography

Supported in part by a research grant (CA06516) from the National Cancer Institute and a grant (RR-05526) from the Division of Research, National Institute of Health

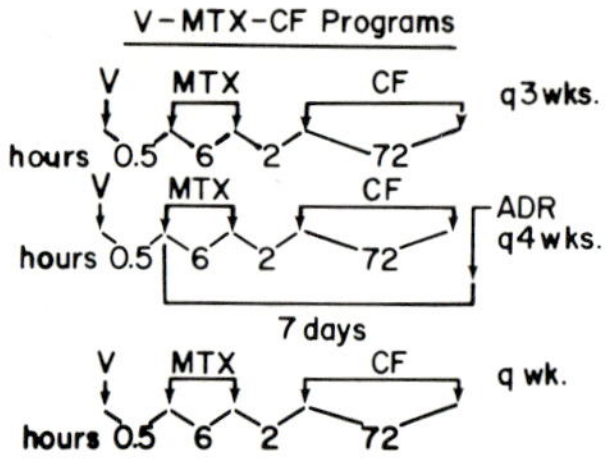

FIG. 22-1. V-MTX-CF Programs

V = vincristine, MTX = methotrexate, CF = citrovorum factor, ADR = adriamycin. The doses are as follows: V: 2 mg/m^2 (maximum 2 mg); MTX: 3, 6 and 7.5 gm/m^2 (1st, 2nd and subsequent doses, respectively. More recently, treatment has commenced with 7.5 gm/m^2); CF: 15 mg q 3 h intravenously for 24 hours and q 6 h for 48 hours, the first oral dose commencing 3 hours after the last intravenous dose; ADR: 75 mg/m^2 (maximum cumulative dose 450 mg/m^2). Modified from Jaffe N: Osteogenic Sarcoma: Advances in treatment. CA 26(6), 1976.

and bone marrow aspirate (if indicated). Special histochemical stains may also be helpful, e.g., to reveal the presence of glycogen in Ewing's sarcoma.

Osteogenic sarcoma and Ewing's sarcoma are the two most common malignant bone tumors encountered in children. An outline of the chemotherapeutic regimens currently employed in these tumors will be provided and the experience will be utilized to plan therapy for the less commonly occurring tumors.

OSTEOGENIC SARCOMA

Two specific chemotherapeutic regimens have demonstrated major activity in osteogenic sarcoma; adriamycin (ADR) and high-dose MTX with citrovorum factor ("citrovorum factor rescue") (V-MTX-CF). Both chemotherapeutic regimens have produced responses in the vicinity of 40 per cent in patients with established disease.[1,2] When employed as adjuvant therapy, 60 to 80 per cent of patients have remained free of pulmonary metastases for variable periods of time.[3,4] The drugs have also been used in combination with cyclophosphamide and phenylalanine mustard with similar results.[5-8]

V-MTX-CF PROGRAMS (FIG. 22-1)

V-MTX-CF constitutes a major component of the therapeutic regimens employed in our clinics. Treatment involves the administration of vincristine, 2 mg/m^2 (maximum 2 mg), followed one-half hour later by MTX (3 to 7.5 gm/m^2) administered intravenously over 6 hours. Two hours later, citrovorum factor is administered as 15 mg q 3 h intravenously for 8 doses followed by 15 mg q 6 h for 8 doses by the oral route. The first oral dose commences 3 hours after the last intravenous dose. In the adjuvant programs, treatment is administered every 3 or 4 weeks if ADR is interposed between courses. A weekly schedule is used for patients with pulmonary metastases or preoperatively in the limb preservation program.[9,10]

Prerequisites for V-MTX-CF treatment comprise a normal creatinine clearance, hemogram, liver function studies and hydration. Patients are hospitalized for a 3-day period for each treatment during which adequate hydration is insured. Throughout each course, daily serum creatinine and MTX levels are obtained. A MTX level in excess of 1×10^{-7} at 72 hours carries the potential for toxicity and requires escalation of the fluid intake to promote MTX excretion.

The utility of V-MTX-CF and V-MTX-CF-ADR as adjuvant treatment has been investigated in 34 patients with "classic" osteogenic sarcoma and local control during the past 5 years. Eleven developed pulmonary metastases and the remainder have remained free of disease for 12^+ to 48^+ months.[11] When compared to an historical group of 78 previously treated similar patients, the difference in the incidence of pulmonary metastases is highly significant ($p < 0.001$) (Fig. 22-2).

A major advance in the application of V-MTX-CF treatment has been the weekly schedule. In contrast to the tri-weekly administration, this schedule produced an 88 per cent response rate in previously untreated patients. In addition, previously treated patients who appeared resistant to the tri-weekly schedule also achieved responses.[10] An example of a response obtained in a patient with pulmonary metastases treated with the weekly schedule is outlined in Figure 22-3.

V-MTX-CF also enhances the tumoricidal

effects of radiation therapy.[12,13] The latter is normally ineffective in eradicating established pulmonary disease.[14] The potentiating effect is more likely to occur if MTX is administered during or juxtaposed to the immediate postirradiation period (within 1 to 2 months). With longer intervals, tumor responses are less impressive. The effect can also be observed in the radiation portals of the skin.[12,13]

Radiation therapy and V-MTX-CF are important components of multidisciplinary treatment. Such treatment has produced cavitation and shrinkage of pulmonary metastases, regression of bulky primary tumors, immediate and sustained responses in cord compression and appreciable relief of bone pain. This approach has also been used with greater frequency to eradicate residual disease after surgical resection of pulmonary metastases. The latter, developing during adjuvant treatment, appear limited and delayed and have encouraged the integrated use of surgery, radiation therapy and V-MTX-CF to render additional patients free of disease.[9] Results achieved with this approach are outlined in Figure 22-4.

Chemotherapy has also affected treatment to the primary tumor. Considerable controversy surrounds the level of amputation in patients with long-bone tumors. Enneking ad-

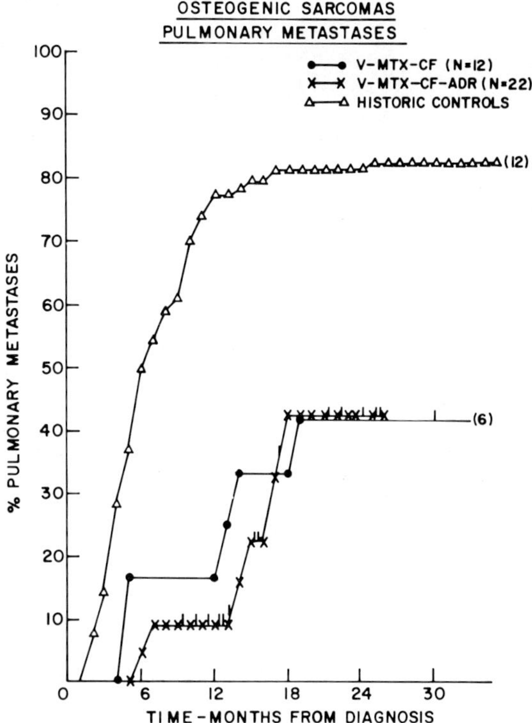

FIG. 22-2. Cumulative Incidence of Pulmonary Metastases in Patients with Local Control of the Primary Tumor Achieved by Amputation. The historic controls represent 78 previously treated patients at the Sidney Farber Cancer Institute and Children's Hospital Medical Center.

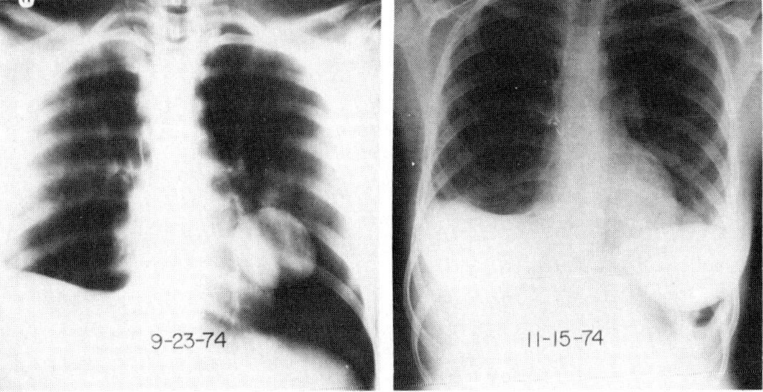

FIG. 22-3. Response in A Patient with Bilateral Pulmonary Metastases Following 8 Weekly V-MTX-CF Courses. The left radiograph is an over-penetrated view demonstrating pulmonary metastases in the left and right lung field. The right radiograph demonstrates complete disappearance of tumor. Patient had previously undergone a right lower lobe lobectomy for removal of a large pulmonary metastasis at another institution. This accounts for the surgical clips visible in the right paravertebral area. From Jaffe N, et al: Weekly high-dose methothrexate-citrororum factor in osteogenic sarcoma. Cancer 39:45–50, 1977 (with permission).

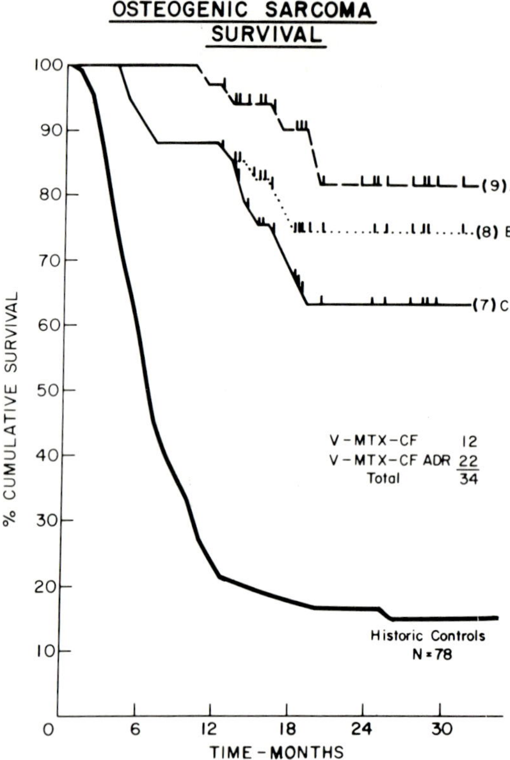

FIG. 22-4. Cumulative Survival in 34 Patients Treated with Adjuvant V-MTX-CF Programs. Curve A represents survival in all patients. Curve B represents survival in patients rendered free of disease by multidisciplinary treatment. Curve C represents survival in patients continuously free of disease.

vocates disarticulation for such tumors because of the possibility of "skip" lesions.[15] Such lesions, however, are generally treated by transmedullary amputation in our clinic provided the bone can be amputated 7 cm above the most reactive site seen on the bone scintigraph leaving the residual stump suitable for a functional prosthesis.[16] Thirty patients have been so treated, all have received adjuvant chemotherapy and none has developed stump recurrences. This may have been due to the operative technique and/or destruction of microscopic disease by chemotherapy. Also, there does not appear to be any difference in the incidence of pulmonary metastases in patients undergoing transmedullary amputation as compared to those undergoing hemipelvectomy or forequarter amputation for removal of the primary tumor.

Effective chemotherapy in osteogenic sarcoma has also provided the impetus to investigate the possibility of limb preservation in selected patients. This involves preoperative treatment with chemotherapy which has produced variable degrees of tumor destruction. Local en bloc resection is then performed and the resected bone is replaced by an internal prosthesis. Pre- and posttreatment angiographic studies related to the procedure are illustrated in Figure 22-5. Initial results reported by Rosen et al. and Jaffe et al. are encouraging but further periods of observation are warranted to determine the potential of such limbs.[10,17] The procedure should only be undertaken in institutions where the necessary resources and commitments are available.

Toxicity

A discussion of the V-MTX-CF programs would be incomplete without due recognition of their potential for serious toxicity.[18] This includes myelosuppression, renal dysfunction, aberrations in liver function studies, stomatitis, convulsions and skin eruptions. Several drug-related deaths have been reported. These programs should only be employed in major centers where the necessary investigative procedures and facilities for supportive care to avoid or treat such complications can be marshalled.

Ewing's Sarcoma

The utility of chemotherapy in Ewing's sarcoma has been reported in a number of studies. Tumor regression and improved survival were demonstrated following the administration of vincristine,[19] cyclophosphamide,[20] actinomycin D,[21] BCNU,[22] mithramycin,[23] daunorubicin[24] and adriamycin.[25] Unfortunately, while chemotherapy appeared effective, no significance in long-term survival was reported.

With increasing experience, combination programs were investigated. Hustu et al. treated 15 patients with localized disease with cyclophosphamide and vincristine for 2 years.[26] Twelve of the 15 patients (80 per cent) survived and 10 patients (67 per cent) re-

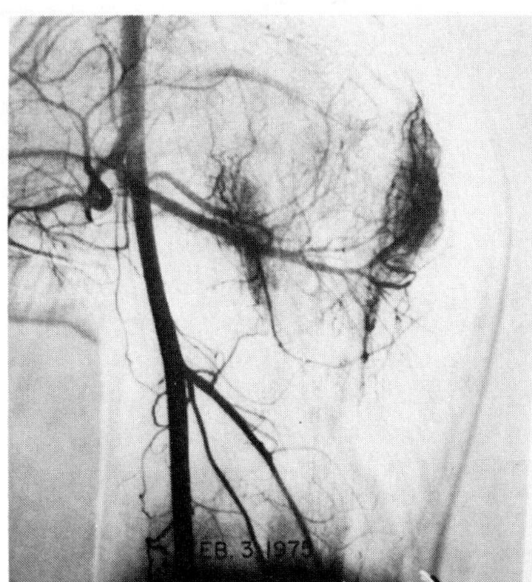

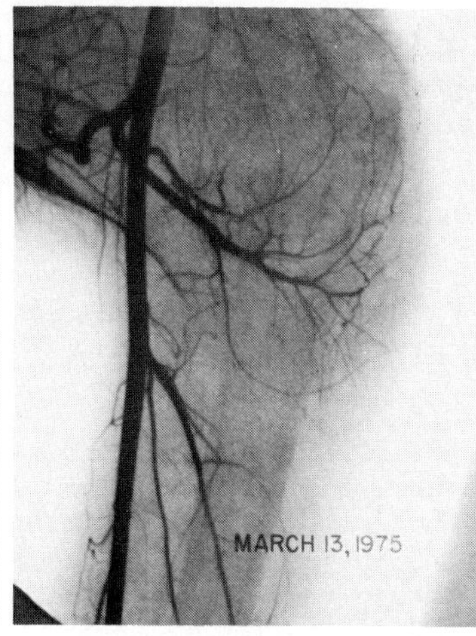

FIG. 22-5. Subtraction Arteriogram in Patient with an Osteogenic Sarcoma of the Humerus. The left radiograph represents the appearance of the tumor prior to initiation of 4 weekly V-MTX-CF courses. Moderate tumor neovascularity is obvious. The right radiograph demonstrates complete disappearance of tumor neovascularity. This was accompanied by reduction in the size of the tumor mass and subjective improvement. From Jaffe N, et al: Weekly high-dose methotrexate-citrororum factor in osteogenic sarcoma. Cancer 39:45–50, 1977 (with permission).

vealed no evidence of active disease from 4^+ to 21^+ months (median 18^+ months). Local control of disease was achieved in 14 of the 15 patients (93 per cent).

Rosen et al. utilizing a combination of vincristine, actinomycin D, cyclophosphamide and adriamycin reported a 79 per cent disease-free survival in 15 of 19 patients with a median of 37 months.[27]. Not all patients in this series presented with localized tumor. Eight had metastases and only two were disease free at the time of the report. This experience led him to conclude that in metastatic disease, the treatment was insufficient to destroy every last tumor cell and that, in patients with localized disease, there is a minority in whom chemotherapy also will not eradicate microscopic disease, but will merely delay the onset of clinical manifestations. More aggressive treatment was, therefore, required to improve the results.

Johnson[28] and Pomeroy and Johnson[29] treated 66 patients with four progressive chemotherapeutic regimens comprising combinations of cyclophosphamide, vincristine, actinomycin D and adriamycin. Some patients also received intrathecal MTX and whole brain irradiation. The overall actuarial survival of nonmetastatic patients was approximately 50 per cent with approximately 40 per cent free of disease. The median survival was over 5 years and over 95 per cent of patients achieved local control.

Fernandez et al. administered cyclophosphamide and vincristine to 19 patients for 1 year after treatment of the primary tumor.[30] The overall survival rate was 58 per cent (11 of 19 patients) with 6 patients (32 per cent) free of disease. Eighteen of the 19 patients had local control of the primary tumor.

At the Sidney Farber Cancer Institute, chemotherapy for Ewing's sarcoma comprises a combination of vincristine, actinomycin D and cyclophosphamide[31] (Fig. 22-6). Therapy is administered as vincristine, 2 mg/m^2 (maximum 2 mg) at weekly intervals for 10 or more doses if tolerated, actinomycin D, 225 μg/m^2 daily for 7 days every 12 weeks and cyclophosphamide, 300 mg/m^2 daily for 7 days every 6 weeks. Actinomycin D is omitted during treatment of large sections of the bowel and cyclophosphamide is omitted if the portal of irradiation encompasses structures adjacent to the bladder. Adequate hydration must also be insured during cyclophosphamide treatment in order to prevent hemorrhagic cystitis. Treatment is interrupted if the white blood count falls below 2,000 or the platelet count

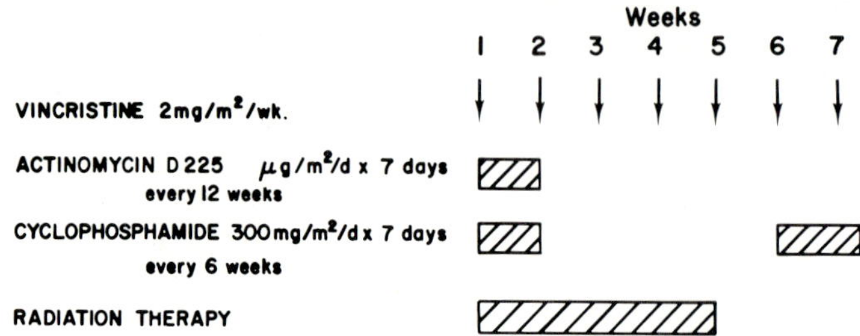

FIG. 22-6. Chemotherapy (VAC) for Ewing's Sarcoma. Vincristine, 2 mg/m² (maximum 2 mg), is administered at weekly intervals for 12 or more doses, if tolerated; actinomycin D, 225 gamma/m²/day, for 7 days every 12 weeks, and cyclophosphamide, 300 mg/m²/day for 7 days every 6 weeks. Treatment is interrupted if the white count falls below 2,000 or the platelet count below 100,000. Modified from Jaffe N: Multidisciplinary treatment for childhood *sarcoma. Am J Surg 133:405–413, 1977 (with permission).*

below 100,000. An example of a complete response obtained with this chemotherapeutic approach in a patient with pulmonary metastases is outlined in Figure 22-7.

In most centers, radiation therapy is administered for treatment of the primary tumor concurrently with chemotherapy. Such combined treatment, however, must be skillfully integrated because of the radiation enhancing effects of certain agents, particularly actinomycin D and adriamycin. This increases the potential for morbidity which may result in severe bone and tissue changes with permanent sequelae.[27] The occurrence of these complications may also be minimized or avoided by utilizing megavoltage irradiation in doses of 5000 to 6000 rad. The initial radiation portal encompasses the entire bone with a generous margin of soft tissue. After approximately 4000 rad have been administered, the portal is progressively narrowed with the final 500 to 750 rad delivered only to the clinically and radiographically abnormal bone and soft tissue. The duration of treatment is approximately 5 to 6 weeks.

The results of treatment with radiation

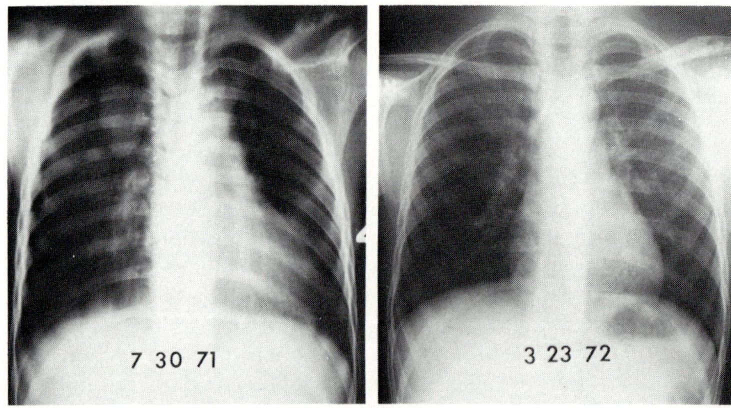

FIG. 22-7. Response to VAC Chemotherapy. The left radiograph demonstrates pulmonary metastases in a patient with Ewing's sarcoma of the left clavicle. Following several cycles of VAC treatment, complete disappearance to tumor was achieved. This is demonstrated in the right radiograph. From Jaffe N: Chemotherapy of osteogenic sarcoma and Ewing's sarcoma: Methods and results. Excerpta Medica International Congress Series no. 354. 6:192–199, 1974 (with permission).

therapy administered to the primary tumor and VAC chemotherapy have recently been reported.[31] Survival in patients with localized disease was 78 per cent in contrast to 27 per cent computed for patients who were previously treated by surgical ablation or radiation therapy and single-agent chemotherapy ($p = 0.002$). All surviving patients also achieved local control of the primary lesions and useful functioning limbs.

In patients with metastatic disease, regression of tumor was achieved with chemotherapy alone. Survival here was also prolonged but all patients eventually developed recurrent tumor and died. It appeared, therefore, that microscopic disease persisted in sites of previous bulk tumor where responses with chemotherapy had been obtained. This experience is similar to that reported by Rosen.[34] To improve the results, combination treatment with radiation therapy and actinomycin D to such areas is currently under investigation. Because of possible myelosuppression, this form of therapy will be extended over several months with radiation therapy coinciding with each cycle of actinomycin D.

Several investigators have suggested that meningeal involvement similar to leukemia may occur in Ewing's sarcoma.[32,33] Pomeroy and Johnson consequently recommend administration of intrathecal MTX and 2000 rad of whole brain irradiation.[29] This phenomenon, however, was not observed in a review of over 80 patients treated at the Sidney Farber Cancer Institute during the past 25 years and conforms with a report by Rosen et al.[34]

The experiences derived from the application of chemotherapy in the two most commonly encountered malignant bone tumors in childhood demonstrate that the skillful and judicious application of effective agents has changed the biological behavior of these tumors. This prompts a recommendation to administer chemotherapy for other less commonly encountered malignant tumors where, because of their rarity, optimum treatment has not been defined. Chemotherapy for non-Hodgkin's lymphoma of bone should comprise agents known to be effective in this disease.[35] Fibrosarcoma and chondrosarcoma should probably be treated in a manner similar to osteogenic sarcoma. Hemangeoendotheliosarcoma, which resembles Ewing's sarcoma, should receive identical treatment. All patients should be approached with curative intent to achieve maximum impact.

References

1. Jaffe N: Recent advances in the chemotherapy of metastatic osteogenic sarcoma. Cancer 30:1627, 1972
2. Cortes E P, Holland J F, Wang J J, et al: Chemotherapy of advanced osteosarcoma. reprinted from vol. 24 of the Colston Papers, Proceedings of the 24th Symposium of the Colston Research Society, London, Butterworth, 1972, p 265
3. Cortes E P, Holland J F, Wang J J, et al: Amputation and adriamycin in primary osteosarcoma. N Engl J Med 291:998, 1974
4. Jaffe N, Frei E III, Traggis D, et al: Adjuvant methotrexate-citrovorum factor treatment of osteogenic sarcoma. N Engl J Med 291:994, 1974
5. Rosen G, Tan C, Sanmaneechai A, et al: The rationale for multiple drug chemotherapy in the treatment of osteogenic sarcoma. Cancer 35:936, 1975
6. Sutow W W, Sullivan M P, Fernbach D J, et al: Adjuvant chemotherapy in primary treatment of osteogenic sarcoma. A Southwest Oncology Group Study. Cancer 36:1598, 1975
7. Sutow W W, Gehan E A, Vietti T J, et al: Multidrug chemotherapy in primary treatment of osteosarcoma. J Bone Jt Surg 58-A:629, 1976
8. Pratt C, Shanks E, Hustu O, et al: Adjuvant multiple drug chemotherapy for osteosarcoma of the extremity. Cancer 39:51, 1977
9. Jaffe N, Traggis D, Cassady J R, et al: Multidisciplinary treatment for macrometastatic osteogenic sarcoma. Br Med J 2:1039, 1976
10. Jaffe N, Frei E III, Traggis D, et al: Weekly high-dose methotrexate-citrovorum factor in osteogenic sarcoma: Pre-surgical treatment of primary tumor and of overt pulmonary metastases. Cancer 39:45, 1977
11. Jaffe N, Frei E III, Watts H, et al: High-dose methotrexate in osteogenic sarcoma: A 5-year experience. Cancer Treat Rep 62:259, 1978
12. Jaffe N, Farber S, Traggis D, et al: Favorable

response of osteogenic sarcoma to high dose methotrexate with citrovorum rescue and radiation therapy. Cancer 31:1367, 1973

13. Rosen G, Tefft M, Martinez A, et al: Combination chemotherapy and radiation therapy in the treatment of metastatic osteogenic sarcoma. Cancer 35:622, 1975
14. Jenkin R D T, Allt W E C, Fitzpatrick P J: Osteosarcoma. An assessment of management with particular reference to primary irradiation and selective delayed amputation. Cancer 30:393, 1972
15. Enneking W F, Kagan A: The implications of "skip" metastases in osteosarcoma. Clin Orthop Related Res 111:33, 1975
16. Jaffe N, Watts H: Multidrug chemotherapy in primary treatment of osteosarcoma. J Bone Jt Surg 58:634, 1976
17. Rosen G, Murphy M L, Huvos A G, et al: Chemotherapy, en bloc resection, and prosthetic bone replacement in the treatment of osteogenic sarcoma. Cancer 37:1, 1976
18. Jaffe N, Traggis D: Toxicity of high-dose methotrexate (NSC-740) and citrovorum factor (NSC-3590) in osteogenic sarcoma. Cancer Chemother Rep 6:31, 1975
19. Sutow W W: Vincristine (NSC-67574) therapy for malignant solid tumors in children (except Wilm's tumor). Cancer Chemother Rep 52:55, 1968
20. Sutow W W, Sullivan M P: Cyclophosphamide therapy in children with Ewing's sarcoma. Cancer Chemother Rep 23:55, 1962
21. Geopfert H, Rochlin D B, Smart C R: Palliative treatment of Ewing's sarcoma. Am J Surg 113:246, 1967
22. Palma J, Gailani S, Freeman A, et al: Treatment of metastatic Ewing's sarcoma with BCNU. Cancer 30:909, 1967
23. Kofman S, Perlia C P, Economou S G: Mithramycin in the treatment of Ewing's sarcoma with radiation therapy and adjuvant chemotherapy. Cancer 27:1051, 1971
24. Sutow W W, Vietti T J, Fernbach D J, et al: Evaluation of chemotherapy in children with metastatic Ewing's sarcoma and osteogenic sarcoma. Cancer Chemother Rep 55:67, 1971
25. O'Bryan R M, Luce J K, Talley R W, et al: Phase II evaluation of adriamycin in human neoplasia. Cancer 32:1, 1973
26. Hustu H O, Pinkel D, Pratt C G: Treatment of clinically localized Ewing's sarcoma with radiotherapy and combination chemotherapy. Cancer 30:1422, 1972
27. Rosen G: Management of malignant bone tumors in children and adolescents, in Belfus, L D (ed): Pediatrics Clinics of North America. Symposium on Pediatric Oncology, 23:183, Philadelphia, Saunders, 1976
28. Johnson R E, Pomeroy T C: Evaluation of therapeutic results in Ewing's sarcoma. Am J Roentgenol 123:583, 1975
29. Pomeroy T C, Johnson R E: Combined modality therapy of Ewing's sarcoma. Cancer 35:36, 1975
30. Fernandez C H, Lindberg R D, Sutow W W, et al: Localized Ewing's sarcoma—Treatment and results. Cancer 34:143, 1974
31. Jaffe N, Traggis D, Sallan S, et al: Improved outlook for Ewing's sarcoma with combination chemotherapy (vincristine, actinomycin D and cyclophosphamide) and radiation therapy. Cancer 38:1925, 1976
32. Marsa G W, Johnson R E: Altered pattern of metastasis following treatment of Ewing's sarcoma with radiation therapy and adjuvant chemotherapy. Cancer 27:1051, 1971
33. Mehta Y, Hendrickson F R: CNS involvement in Ewing's sarcoma. Cancer 33:859, 1974
34. Rosen G, Wollner N, Tan C, et al: Disease-free survival in children with Ewing's sarcoma treated with radiation therapy and adjuvant four-drug sequential chemotherapy. Cancer 33:384, 1974
35. Jaffe N, Buell D, Cassady J R, et al: The role of staging in childhood non-Hodgkin's lymphoma. Cancer Treat Rep 61:1001, 1977

Jeffrey G. Rosenstock

23
Chemotherapy for Brain Tumors and Retinoblastoma

Part I—Brain Tumors

Primary intracranial neoplasms represent a significant portion of the tumors in both adults and children. Although these tumors rarely metastasize, local cure is infrequently achieved. Those patients who are cured often have significant permanent sequelae.

Two recent developments may change the long-term prognosis for the brain tumor patient. Computerized axial tomography (CAT), a noninvasive technique, is quite sensitive and specific in diagnosing intracranial lesions.[1] Earlier diagnosis before significant brain damage has occurred may be a reality. CAT scans may also better evaluate chemotherapeutic agents, especially in those tumors which do not have as uniform and rapid an endpoint as does glioblastoma multiforme. Several chemotherapeutic agents have temporarily improved the clinical status of patients with recurrent tumors.[2] Used as adjunctive therapy, they may extend survival and improve cure rates.

Brain tumors, in contrast to most other tumors, pose a therapeutically different problem for the oncologist. The prevention or treatment of metastases, which is a major part of the therapy in many other tumors, is unnecessary in these locally distorting and invasive tumors. Chemotherapy, however, has proved its ability to control locally such tumors as rhabdomyosarcoma of childhood.[3] Unfortunately in brain tumors, the routine chemotherapeutic agents are often effectively excluded by the blood brain barrier (BBB). With the better understanding of both the pharmacology of some of the agents and of the special physical limitations of intracranial tumors, the goal of long-term quality survival appears to be an obtainable reality.

Tumors of the CNS account for over 8000 deaths a year.[4] This is 3 per cent of the annual number of cancer deaths. In childhood, where malignancy is the second most common cause of death next to accidents, tumors of the CNS are second only to the leukemias in incidence.[5] The improvement in survival rates for children with leukemia is so great that brain tumors may shortly become the leading cause of death among children with malignancies.

The stage is set for new inroads in brain tumor management. The fears of brain damage followed shortly by death need not persist. In a long-term followup study in Denmark, Djerris found that 80 per cent of children who survived their brain tumor were leading normal lives.[6] Earlier diagnosis and more aggressive therapy will extend quality survival.

Supported in Part by USPHS Grant CA 14489

Incidence of Intracranial Tumors

The actual incidence of each type of tumor depends on the data base and the pathologic criteria. Surgical and autopsy series differ markedly from each other, and geographic studies are also different. The range of percentage of patients with metastatic versus primary intracranial tumors varies from series to series. Approximately 50 per cent of intracranial tumors are gliomas and over 50 per cent of gliomas are glioblastoma multiformes. Another 25 per cent of gliomas are also high grade.[7]

In childhood these high-grade gliomas represent a much smaller proportion of intracranial tumors. Medulloblastomas and ependymomas are the two most common locally invasive tumors.[8,9] They represent almost 40 per cent of childhood intracranial tumors.

Evaluation

The newly developed CAT scan allows easy early diagnosis of brain tumors. The CAT scanner has shown excellent sensitivity and specificity. In a study of 63 patients with possible tumor in contrast to those with certain tumors, only one false negative scan appeared.[1] The lowest tomographic cuts allow excellent views of the posterior fossa.[10] Not only does the CAT scan localize the tumor, it also shows the size and position of the ventricles. This helps the surgeon plan the approach and procedure and more accurately defines the fields for the radiotherapist.

The CAT scan is usually used in conjunction with radioisotopic scans as well as with angiography and air studies when indicated. The selection of patients for these further studies can now be done with this simple noninvasive technique, and patients can be evaluated earlier. No longer does a physician have to be certain of the diagnosis of brain tumor before beginning the in-depth evaluation.[10]

Until recently the availability of CAT scanners has been limited. Their precious time has been allocated to diagnosis of intracerebral conditions. Prior to the CAT scanner, it was virtually impossible to document precisely drug responses of recurrent tumors in the patient with brain tumors.[11] A patient's neurologic status may reflect the presence of tumor, but also many other factors, such as radionecrosis, cerebral edema, hemorrhage, hydrocephalus secondary to scarring and transient post radiation encephalopathy may mimic recurrent tumor. Tumor response may not be reflected in the clinical status because the patient may have fixed neurologic deficits from the tumor's destruction or from the surgery.[12] The length of survival in patients with glioblastoma multiforme whose median survival is only 8 months may serve as an end point in measuring drug efficacy, but in slower growing or less common tumors, such as those found in children, the evaluation of drug efficacy is greatly facilitated by CAT scans.

Pharmacologic Principles

The purpose of drugs in treating patients with brain tumors may be three-fold. Each objective has very different pharmacologic restrictions. Drugs can be used to: (1) treat the primary tumor, (2) prevent extension within the cerebral spinal fluid or (3) increase the radiosensitivity.

The justification for using drugs in conjunction with other therapies that have been successful in treating several solid tumors requires that the drug invade the tumor itself and kill the cells which are either in a resting or dividing state. The very specific requirements of delivery of drugs to intracerebral tumors has recently been reviewed.[13] The BBB excludes molecules that are highly ionized, large, or lipophobic. The BBB in tumors as shown by Broder and Rall is less effective at the tumor center, but becomes more and more intact as the tumor-brain interface is approached.[14] In fact, the edema surrounding a tumor may heighten the exclusion of drugs which are not lipophilic. Cerebral metastases have been noted to grow while the primary tumors were responding to chemotherapy.[15] Though brain tumors have very low growth fractions,[16] the more peripheral parts of the tumors have the highest growth fraction.[17,18] Ideally a chemotherapeutic agent should be non-cell cycle specific, of small molecular size, lipophilic, and poorly bound to serum proteins. Local chemotherapy injected into the spinal or ventricular fluid, which are of necessity water soluble, are unable to penetrate deeply into brain tissue. Studies with tritiated thymidine-label MTX demonstrate the limited parenchymal penetration.[19] Such agents may be able to control free-floating cells that can potentially cause drop metastases, as in medulloblastomas. Systemic agents, whether lipophilic or not, that are effective in controlling bone marrow leukemia are unable to control or prevent meningeal leukemia.[20] Children with CNS leukemia, when treated with BCNU which is lipophilic, show no evidence of therapeutic response.[21] Intrathecal MTX will rapidly decrease the number of leukemic cells in the CNS and is an effective method of treating CNS meningeal disease,[21] although very high doses of MTX systemically do not produce CSF levels at a therapeutic level for the very sensitive leukemic cells.[22]

Some investigators have injected MTX directly into cerebrally transplanted ependymoblastomas[23] demonstrating rapid but uneven distribution within the tumors. The levels were much higher than those produced by intravenous injection, but the drug had its greatest concentration at the tumor center and less at the tumor-brain interface. This technique is also limited by difficulties in administration since they require repeated administration. Cell cycle-specific agents would be of limited value by this technique.

Intra-arterial administration has been considered in order to obtain higher concentration to the tumor. The success of such therapy depends on totally isolating the blood supply. Many hemispheric glioblastomas cross the midline. Prolonged catheterization of the vertebral artery for posterior fossa tumors is technically formidable, especially in children where the posterior fossa is most often involved. The higher concentration of the agent must also be acceptable to the surrounding normal tissue. Drugs which are cleared from the sera, degraded or fixed rapidly would have some advantage in being given by arterial perfusion rather than by arterial bolus or intravenous injection.[13] Levin described some advantage for intra-arterial perfusion for the nitrosoureas.[24] In general, clinical studies demonstrated little advantage and have been hampered by technical problems.[25]

Radiotherapy can achieve appreciable cure rates in many patients with certain types of brain tumors, and survival of patients with glioblastoma multiforme is at least slightly extended. In a prospective randomized study of patients with glioblastoma multiforme, Walker and Gehan found a median survival of 4 months with surgery alone against 7.5 months for surgery plus radiation therapy.[26] To improve the results of radiotherapy, radioenhancing agents have been studied.[27] These agents appear to work by increasing the cell-kill of hypoxic cells. Sano treated patients with glioblastoma with intra-arterial 5-bromouridine (5-BUDR) during the 5 weeks of radiotherapy.[28] He concluded this treatment was effective; however, Landolt who used both MTX and 5-BUDR had only equivocal results.[29] A recent randomized study showed no definitive advantage in using oral metronidazole as the radiosensitizer in patients with glioblastomas.[30] In a randomized trial in patients with glioblastoma multiforme treated with 5-FU, which is probably a radiosensitizer, Edland could find no increase in survival.[31] Radiosensitizers may also decrease the therapeutic ratio and increase toxicity to normal tissues.[32] Radioenhancement remains an important area of investigation.

Systemic Chemotherapy

The major thrust of clinical therapeutic trials has been in oral and intravenous administration of chemotherapeutic agents. Glioblastoma multiforme was studied primarily because of its high frequency and short consistent natural history. Evaluation of response in patients with apparent clinical recurrence or in uncontrolled studies is very difficult. Even brain scans and angiograms are notoriously inaccurate.[11,12,33] Evaluation of drug response by CAT scan has yet to be reported. There are several extensive reviews of brain tumors treated by single-agent chemotherapy.[14,34,35,36] Despite the difficulty in evaluating brain tumor response, it is obvious that these tumors are not totally insensitive to chemotherapy.

Mithramycin

Mithramycin is a polycylic antibiotic produced by *Streptomyces plicatus* that acts by binding to DNA and indirectly inhibiting RNA synthesis. It is not cell cycle specific.

Mithramycin comprises few of the pharmacologic properties important in brain tumor therapy. It is readily bound to plasma proteins, has a molecular weight over 1000, and is not significantly lipid soluble. Kennedy noted responses in several patients with glioblastoma as well as inhibition of growth of a mouse glioma.[37,38] The Brain Tumor Study Group has reported a randomized controlled study of mithramycin for patients with glioblastomas.[39] Despite some questions about the study design,[40] the 52 patients in the treatment group did not have a greater median survival than the control. There was a slight trend suggesting that those patients who received the highest doses of radiation and mithramycin had longer survival times, but the numbers in these subgroups were too small for statistical validity. Mealey was also unable to demonstrate clinical benefit in patients treated with mithramycin alone or with vincristine (VCR).[41]

Vincristine

Vincristine (VCR) is an alkaloid derivative from the plant *Vinca rosea*, which exerts its antineoplastic action by inhibiting microtubule formation in the mitotic spindle. Its neurotoxicity instead of hematotoxicity is unusual among antineoplastic agents. This neurotoxicity sometimes makes clinical evaluation of a patient's neurologic status difficult. Because of the lack of cross-toxicity with other antineoplastic agents, this is an excellent drug to use in combination chemotherapy. Although not generally regarded as lipid soluble, it is partially so.[42] Also, its molecular size is close to that which penetrates the BBB. Meningeal extension of parameningeal rhabdomyosarcoma, however, occurs readily in patients who have shown excellent response to systemic vincristine.[43]

Several reports document responses to vincristine alone in both children and adults with recurrent high-grade gliomas.[44,45] A prospective study by Fewer of 81 patients with recurrent primary or metastatic brain tumors treated with BCNU or BCNU and VCR, however showed no enhanced effectiveness with VCR.[33] Its value in high-grade gliomas remains to be firmly established. It is a cell cycle-specific agent, however, that is able to penetrate the BBB and may prove of value in combination chemotherapy with non-cell cycle-specific agents.

Epipodophyllotoxin

The compound 4′-demethyl-epipodophyllotoxin-β-D-thenylideneglucoside (VM-26) is a semisynthetic podophyllotoxin derivative. It appears to act by inhibiting DNA synthesis and arresting cells in metaphase, much like VCR. Its molecular weight is low and it is relatively lipid soluble. It therefore meets the requirements of being a cell cycle-specific agent which can cross the BBB. Also its hematologic toxicity is modest.[46]

Shapiro demonstrated that in mice bearing intracerebral ependymoblastomas, VM-26 was able to reach the tumors, but produced only a 20 per cent increase in survival.[47] Subcutaneously implanted tumors responded better. In the initial Phase I studies of VM-26, responses were noted in 2 patients with malignant astrocytomas.[46] Interestingly, these patients received less than 100 mgm/m^2/week. Sklansky treated 19 patients with primary intracranial tumors with VM-26 at weekly dosages of 100 mgm/m^2 to 130 mgm/m^2, depending on previous therapy.[48] The response rate to VM-26 of 38 per cent was comparable to other agents tried. Several of the patients had shown prior progressive disease while receiving nitrosoureas. This suggests little, if any, cross reactivity and these two agents may well work together. A recent study using VM-26 in combination with adriamycin and CCNU reported 31 responses in 43 patients with progressive or inoperative malignant gliomas.[49]

Procarbazine

Procarbazine is a methylhydrazine which is rapidly oxidized from its original salt into a lipid soluble azo intermediate which readily crosses the BBB.[50] It has been effective in several animal and human tumors and is apparently especially effective against intracerebral L1210 leukemia. In a Phase II study of procarbazine in 29 patients, Kumar found that the overall response was 48 per cent, though patients with glioblastoma had a slightly lower response rate. Those patients who had previously failed therapy with nitrosourea showed no response to the procarbazine, suggesting cross-resistance.[50] Currently, procarbazine is included in several prospective protocols for malignant gliomas.

Nitrosoureas

The nitrosoureas are the most important family of drugs in brain tumor chemotherapy. These compounds are nonionized, lipid soluble with molecular weights around 200.[51] Being alkylating agents, they assert their activity on both resting and dividing cells. They are among the most active agents screened against the murine ependymoblastoma.[52] The pharmacologic differences between the three nitrosoureas (BCNU, 1-(2-chloroethyl)-3-cyclohexyl-1-nitrosourea (CCNU) and 1-(2-chloroethyl)-3-(4-methylcyclohexyl)-1-nitrosourea)(MeCCNU) that have had the most clinical evaluation have recently been reviewed.[51] Their molecular weights are comparable. Only BCNU is even marginally water soluble. Though agents must be lipid soluble to cross the BBB, the intracellular fluid as well as the extracellular fluid through which the drug must traverse is aqueous. The clinical trials with BCNU and CCNU have consistently shown response rates approaching 50 per cent in patients with glioblastomas while their response to MeCCNU has been somewhat lower.[53]

Wilson et al[2] reviewed their single-agent chemotherapy results. Of 40 patients with high-grade astrocytoma treated with BCNU alone, there were 20 responders; while only 6 out of 12 patients treated with BCNU and VCR responded. Three of these patients treated with BCNU for recurrent disease are disease free at 30, 36, and 37 months, suggesting occasional long-term response.[54] These results are consistent with those of other investigators. These responses tend to require several weeks with a maximum response after one to two cycles. The length of remission tended to be less than 6 months and recurrences were unresponsive to further therapy.[55] Levels of toxicity with CCNU also seemed to be acceptable.

These single-agent studies have prompted investigators to try combination chemotherapy to improve the 30 to 50 per cent response rates noted with single agents. As noted earlier, the combination of BCNU and VCR was no better, and possibly worse than BCNU alone.[33,2] BCNU with procarbazine also showed no improvement over either agent alone,[56] although there was some suggestion that the combination extended survival. The best combination tested for recurrent malignant gliomas has been CCNU, procarbazine and VCR. Eighteen out of 24 patients with malignant gliomas on this regimen showed significant responses.[57]

The goal of all these Phase II studies is to identify active agents that, when used as adjunctive therapy, could significantly extend survival and possibly increase the cure rate. Several studies comparing supportive care, radiotherapy, chemotherapy with single or multiple agents and chemotherapy plus radiotherapy have been reported (Table 23-1). The results are somewhat discouraging. Almost 450 patients have been treated on these protocols with approximately 250 receiving adjunctive chemotherapy. Walker, reporting for the Brain Tumor Study Group, showed that supportive care or BCNU alone was inferior to radiotherapy. The BCNU-radiotherapy group had a median survival of 41 weeks compared to 28 weeks for the radiotherapy recipients alone.[26] Interestingly, Shapiro in a smaller study found chemotherapy with BCNU and VCR without radiotherapy to be no worse than radiotherapy plus BCNU and VCR.[58] As noted earlier, the combination of BCNU and VCR may have been less effective than BCNU alone.[33] Some form of antagonism or, more likely, noncomparable groups could account for the differences between these two prospective randomized studies.

Three prospective studies with CCNU have been reported. Reagan randomized 63 patients into three groups. One group received CCNU alone, one group radiotherapy, and the third group received both modalities.[59] The two groups who received radiotherapy had comparable survival which was superior to CCNU alone. Weir, in a slightly smaller study that was similarly designed except for more frequent doses of CCNU, found similar results. He did feel that those patients who received combined therapy had a longer disease-free interval.[60] The EORTC study comparing CCNU and radiotherapy against radiotherapy alone did not show the disease-

TABLE 23-1. *Response of Patients with High-Grade Astrocytoma: Prospective Controlled Studies*

Regimen	No. Patients	Results	Reference
Radiotherapy	16	No difference	74
Radiotherapy plus BCNU, CCNU or MeCCNU	17		
BCNU & VCR	16	No difference	58
Radiotherapy + BCNU + VCR	17		
CCNU	22	Radiotherapy	
Radiotherapy	22	±CCNU better	59
Radiotherapy + CCNU	19	than CCNU alone	
Radiotherapy	15	No significant	60
CCNU	13	difference	
Radiotherapy + CCNU	13		
Radiotherapy + CCNU		CCNU did	61
Radiotherapy + CCNU for recurrence	81-total	not increase disease-free survival	
MeCCNU	4	55 week median	75
DTIC	2	survival	
DTIC + MeCCNU	9		
Control (historical)	15	35 week median survival	
Supportive therapy	total 180	Medial survival	26
BCNU		17 weeks	
Radiotherapy		20 weeks	
BCNU + Radiotherapy		28 weeks	
		41 weeks	

free interval to be extended, but did demonstrate CCNU useful in treating the recurrences in those who had been initially treated with radiotherapy alone.[61]

These studies at best show a slightly improved length of survival for patients on chemotherapy, but the increases, if any, are neglible. Even if the median length of survival is unchanged, one could hope that at least a few patients would have greatly extended survival, but this does not seem to occur. Further studies with single- and multiple-agent chemotherapy are in progress, and possibly these studies will be more encouraging.

Brain Tumors in Children

Both the distribution of types and the natural histories of brain tumors in childhood vary from those in adults. Malignant astrocytoma and medulloblastoma each make up 20 per cent of childhood intracranial tumors. Approximately 10 per cent of intracranial tumors in this age group are ependymomas.[8,9] Both medulloblastoma and ependymoma have cure rates, with radiotherapy, of 30 to 40 per cent.[62,63,64] The time pattern of recurrence of both these tumors following radiotherapy is very different from that of malignant high-grade astrocytoma. The median survival for patients with medulloblastoma is greater than 2 years.[62] Survival is 12 months for all patients with ependymoma and much greater for those surviving surgery and radiotherapy.[63,64] In both types of tumors, there are recurrences after 2 years and even after 5 years. Medulloblastomas, and to a lesser degree ependymomas, readily spread via the spiral fluid, and, therefore, radiation fields often encompass the spinal canal as well as the intracranial contents in order to eradicate any microscopic

TABLE 23-2. *Response of Patients with Recurrent Medulloblastoma to Various Chemotherapeutic Agents*

Drug	# Patients	# Responses	Reference
VCR	1	1	69
VCR	1	1	70
VCR	2	2	71
VCR	4	3	45
VCR	1	1	14
VCR + other therapy	9	VCR increase length of response	72
CCNU	1	1	73
CCNU	1	0	55
CCNU	1	1	2
BCNU	3	1	33
Procarbazine	4	3	2
Procarbazine, CCNU, VCR	12	7 + 4 probable responses	57
Methotrexate (Intrathecal)	9	9	14
Methotrexate (Intra-arterial)	3	3	14
VM-26	1	1	48

drop metastases.[62,65] Among ependymomas there are differing grades of malignancy histologically. The clinical significance is unclear; the primary site may well be of greater clinical prognostic value.[63,64]

Reports of individual cases and of small series of patients with recurrent medulloblastomas treated with chemotherapy suggest that this tumor is sensitive to several chemotherapeutic agents. (Table 23-2). MTX given into the spinal or ventricular fluid often gives rapid clinical improvement,[66,67] but can cause local toxicity especially if given into ventricles when the outflow is blocked.[68] Vincristine, while not very effective in adult intracranial tumors, has been described by several investigators as giving responses often lasting greater than one year.[44,45,69,70,71] Responding patients may take several weeks to show any clinical improvement. Mealey, in a recent review of his experience with medulloblastoma, showed a much longer response lasting up to 18 months in patients with recurrent tumors who received both chemotherapy (especially vincristine) and radiotherapy instead of radiotherapy alone.[72] Unfortunately, 28 out of 29 patients who had recurrences died. There are reports of two responses in 6 patients treated with nitrosoureas.[57,55,2,58,73] Three out of 4 patients treated with procarbazine have responded.[2] Gutin's eleven responses among 12 patients treated with a three-drug regimen of VCR, CCNU and procarbazine may suggest that multiple-agent chemotherapy may be better than single agent at least for this tumor.[57]

The response to chemotherapy in recurrent ependymomas is even more difficult to evaluate. Too few patients have been reported to determine the effectiveness of the single agents used in the other tumors. Interestingly, both Rosenblum and Calogero each describe patients whose responses lasted 20+ and 36+ months, respectively.[54,55]

Presently, randomized prospective trials have been started to evaluate multiple-agent chemotherapy in extending the disease-free interval in children with several different types of tumors, but it is too early to draw any conclusions.

Conclusion

Brain tumor therapy is entering a new era. Surgery no longer presents untoward hazards. Early diagnosis before overwhelming damage has occurred is a reality. Chemotherapeutic agents can improve the status of patients with recurrent tumors. The early trials in adults with adjuvant therapy have had discouraging results. The goal of greatly lengthened quality survival has not yet been achieved. The mechanism to evaluate new agents, along with the better understanding of the pharmocodynamics involved, is now available in addition to several proven agents. The time cannot be too distant when our goals for quality long-term survival will be achieved.

Part II—Retinoblastoma

Retinoblastoma is a rare tumor of childhood, representing 3 per cent of childhood tumors. Fortunately, greater than 80 per cent of the patients can be expected to survive.[76] Of the patients who succumb, about 70 per cent die from spread outside the CNS and 30 per cent due to intracranial extension.[77] The Staging System developed at the Institute of Ophthalmology of the Presbyterian Hospital, Columbia University, correlates an inverse prognosis with increasing volume of tumor.[78]

Several chemotherapeutic agents are effective in palliating metastatic disease. The most extensively used agent was triethylene melamine (TEM).[79] Patients with extensive primary tumors were treated for a period with radiotherapy and adjuvant intra-arterial or intramuscular TEM to try and enhance local control and decrease CNS and blood-born spread. Though never tested in a randomized fashion, this therapy has fallen into disfavor.[80]

Several other agents have been studies. Cyclophosphamide gave good responses in greater than 50 per cent of the patients with hematogenous metastases while only 2 out of 8 children given vincristine responded.[81,82] More recently, adriamycin has been shown to be effective in Phase II studies.[83]

None of these agents is known to control or prevent intracranial extension of retinoblastoma. MTX given intrathecally can temporarily control arachnoid seeding.[84]

A control trial of chemotherapy of children with extensive primary disease is presently underway, but results are unavailable as yet.

References

1. Gawler J, du Boulay G, Bull J W, et al: A comparison of computer assisted tomography (EMI scanner) with conventional neuroradiologic methods in the investigation of patients clinically suspected of intracranial tumor. J Can Assoc Radiol 27:157–169, 1976
2. Wilson C B, Gutin P, Boldrey E B, et al: Singe-agent chemotherapy of brain tumors. Arch Neurol 33:739–744, 1976
3. Voute P A, Vos A: Combination chemotherapy as primary treatment in children with rhabdomyosarcoma. Proc Am Assoc Cancer Res 18:327 (abstr 244), 1977
4. Silverberg E: Cancer Statistics, CA 27:26–41, 1977
5. Young J L Jr, Miller R W: Incidence of malignant tumors in children. J Pediatr 86:254–258, 1975
6. Gjerris F: Clinical aspects and long-term prognosis of intracranial tumours in infancy and childhood. Dev Med Child Neurol 18:145–159, 1976
7. Zimmerman H M: Brain tumors: Their incidence and classification in man and their experimental production. Ann NY Acad Sci 159:337–359, 1969
8. Gjerris F, Klee J G, Klinken L: Malignancy grade and long-term survival in brain tumours of infancy and childhood. Acta Neurol Scand 53:61–71, 1976
9. Schoenberg B S, Schoenberg D G, Christine B W, et al: The epidemiology of primary intracranial neoplasms of childhood. Mayo Clin Proc 51:51–56, 1976
10. Wilson C B: Diagnostic procedures. Semin Oncol 2:9–10, 1975
11. Koo A H, Fewer D, Wilson C B, et al: Lack of correlation between clinical and angiographic findings in patients with brain tumors under BCNU chemotherapy. J Neurosurg 37:9–14, 1972
12. Crafts D, Wilson C B: Differential diagnosis of tumor regrowth. Semin Oncol 2:15–17, 1975
13. Blasberg R G: Pharmacodynamics and the blood-brain barrier. J Natl Cancer Inst, (in press)
14. Broder L E, Rall D P: Chemotherapy of brain tumors. Prog Exp Tumor Res 17:373–399, 1972
15. Benjamin R S, Wiernik P H, Bachur N R: Adriamycin chemotherapy—Efficacy, safety, and pharmacologic basis of an intermittent single high-dosage schedule. Cancer 33: 19–27, 1974

16. Hoshino T, Barker M, Wilson C B, et al: Cell kinetics of human gliomas. J Neurosurg 37:15–26, 1972
17. Barendsern G W, Broerse J J: Experimental radiotherapy of a rat rhabdomyosarcoma with 15 MeV neutrons and 300 KV x-rays. I. Effects of single exposures. Eur J Cancer 5:373–391, 1969
18. Tannock I F: The relation between cell proliferation and the vascular system in a transplanted mouse mammary tumour. Br J Cancer 22:258–273, 1968
19. Rieselbach R E, DiChiro G, Freireich E J, et al: Subarachnoid distribution of drugs after lumbar injection. N Engl J Med 267:1273–1278, 1962
20. Evans A E, Gilbert E S, Zandostra R: The increasing incidence of central nervous system leukemia in children. Cancer 26:404–409, 1970
21. Sullivan P, Vietti T J, Haggard M E, et al: Remission maintenance therapy for meningeal leukemia: Intrathecal methotrexate vs. intravenous bis-nitrosourea. Blood 38:680–688, 1971
22. Shapiro W R, Young D F, Mehta B M: Methotrexate: Distribution in cerebrospinal fluid after intravenous, ventricular and lumbar injections. N Engl J Med 293:161–166, 1975
23. Tator H, Wassenaar W: Intraneoplastic injection of methotrexate for experimental brain-tumor chemotherapy. J Neurosurg 46:165–174, 1977
24. Levin V A: A pharmacologic basis for brain-tumor chemotherapy. Semin Oncol 2:57–61, 1975
25. Madoc-Jones H, Mauro F: Site of action of cytotoxic agents in the cell cycle, in Sartorelli A C, Johns D G (eds): Handbook of Experimental Pharmacology New Series. New York, Springer Verlag, 1974, p 205
26. Walker D, Gehan E A: An evaluation of 1-3 bis (2-chloroethyl)-1-nitrosourea (BCNU) and irradiation alone and in combination for the treatment of malignant glioma. Proc Am Assoc Cancer Res 13:67 (abstr 267), 1972
27. Adams G E: Chemical radio-sensitization of hypoxic cells. Br Med Bull 29:48–53, 1973
28. Sano K, Hoshino T, Nagai M: Radiosensitization of brain tumor cells with a thymidine analogue (bromouridine). J Neurosurg 28: 530–538, 1968
29. Landolt A M: Resultate der postoperativen behandlung des glioblastoma multiforme mit einer strahlensensibilisierenden substanz (5-bromo-2′-deoxyuridin). Acta Neurochir (Wien) 24:263–268, 1971
30. Urtasun R, Pierre B, Chapman J D, et al: Radiation and high-dose metronidazole in supratentorial glioblastomas. N Engl J Med 294:1364–1367, 1976
31. Edland W, Javio M, and Ansfield F J: Glioblastoma multiforme: An analysis of the results of postoperative radiotherapy alone versus radiotherapy and concomitant 5-fluorouracil. Am J Roentgenol Radium Ther Nucl Med 111:337–342, 1971
32. Rosenstock J G: Unpublished material
33. Fewer D, Wilson C B, Boldrey E B, et al: Clinical experience with carmustine (BCNU) and vincristine. JAMA 222:549–552, 1972
34. Goldsmith A, Carter S K: Glioblastoma multiforme—A review of therapy. Cancer Treat Rev 1:153–165, 1974
35. Shapiro W, Ausman J: Recent advances in neurology, in Plum F (ed): Contemporary Neurology Series, vol. 6. Philadelphia, Davis, 1969, p 149
36. Wilson C, Hoshino T: Current trends in the chemotherapy of brain tumors with special reference to glioblastomas. J Neurosurg 31:589–603, 1969
37. Kennedy B J, Brown J H, Yarbro J W: Mithramycin (NSC-24559) therapy for primary glioblastomas. Cancer Chemother Rep 48:59–63, 1965
38. Kennedy B J, Yarbro J W, Kickertz V, et al: Effect of mithramycin on mouse gliomas. Cancer Res 28:91–97, 1968
39. Walker M D, Alexander E Jr, Hunt W E, et al: Evaluation of mithramycin in the treatment of anaplastic glioma. J Neurosurg 44:655–667, 1976
40. Kennedy B J: Chemotherapy of brain tumors, in Brodsky I, Kahn S B (eds): Cancer Chemotherapy II. New York, Grune & Stratton, 1972, pp 221-229
41. Mealey J Jr, Chen T T, Pedlow E: Brain tumor chemotherapy with mithramycin and vincristine. Cancer 26:360–367, 1970
42. Creasey W A: Biochemical effects of vinca alkaloids-IV: Studies with vinleursine. Biochem Pharmacol 18:227–232, 1969
43. Tefft M, Fernandez C, Donaldson M, et al: Incidence of meningeal involvement by rhabdomyosarcoma of the head and neck in children. Proc Am Assoc Cancer Res 18:4 (abstr 13), 1977
44. Alfra D: Vincristine therapy in malignant glioma recurrences. Neurochirurgia 16: 189–198, 1973
45. Rosenstock J G, Evans A E, Schut L: Response to vincristine of recurrent brain tumors in children. J Neurosurg 45:135–140, 1976
46. Muggia G M, Selawry O S, Hansen H H: Clinical studies with a new podophyllotoxin derivative, epipodophyllotoxin, 4′ demethyl-9 (4,6-0-2-thenylidine-β-D-glucopyranoside) (NSC-122819). Cancer Chemother Rep 55:575–581, 1971

47. Shapiro W R: The chemotherapy of intracerebral vs subcutaneous murine gliomas. Arch Neurol 30:222–226, 1974
48. Sklansky B D, Mann-Kaplan R S, Reynolds A F Jr, et al: 4′-demethylepipodophyllotoxin-β-D-thenylidene-glucoside (PTG) in the treatment of malignant intracranial neoplasms. Cancer 33:460–467, 1974
49. Pouillart P, Mathe G, Thy T H, et al: Treatment of malignant gliomas and brain metastases in adults with a combination of adriamycin, VM 26, and CCNU. Cancer 38:1909–1916, 1976
50. Kumar A R V, Renaudin J, Wilson C B, et al: Procarbazine hydrochloride in the treatment of brain tumors. J Neurosurg 40:365–371, 1974
51. Walker M D, Hilton J: Nitrosourea pharmacodynamics in relation to the central nervous system. Cancer Treat Rep 60: 725 – 728, 1976
52. Geran R I, Congelton G F, Dudeck L E, et al: A mouse ependymoblastoma as an experimental model for screening potential antineoplastic drugs, part 2. Cancer Chemother Rep 4:53–87, 1974
53. Walker M D, Weiss H D: Chemotherapy in the treatment of malignant brain tumors. Adv Neurol 13:149–190, 1975
54. Calogero J, Crafts D C, Wilson C B, et al: Long-term survival of patients treated with BCNU for brain tumors. J Neurosurg 43:141–196, 1975
55. Rosenblum M L, Reynolds A F Jr, Smith K A, et al: Chloroethylcyclohexyl-nitrosourea (CCNU) in the treatment of malignant brain tumors. J Neurosurg 39:306–314, 1973
56. Levin V A, Crafts D C, Wilson C B, et al: BCNU (NSC-77213) treatment for malignant brain tumors. Cancer Treat Rep 60:243–249, 1976
57. Gutin P H, Wilson C B, Kumar A R V, et al: Phase II study of procarbazine, CCNU and vincristine combination chemotherapy in the treatment of malignant brain tumors. Cancer 35:1398–1404, 1975
58. Shapiro W R, Young D F: Treatment of malignant glioma: A controlled study of chemotherapy and irradiation. Arch Neurol 33:494–500, 1976
59. Reagan T J, Bisel H F, Childs D S, et al: Controlled study of CCNU and radiation therapy in malignant astrocytoma. J Neurosurg 44:186–190, 1976
60. Weir B, Band P, Urtasun R, et al: Radiotherapy and CCNU in the treatment of high-grade supratentorial astrocytomas. J Neurosurg 45:129–134, 1976
61. EORTC Brain Tumor Study Group. Effect of CCNU on survival, rate of objective remission and duration of free interval in patients with malignant brain glioma—First evaluation. Eur J Cancer 12:41–45, 1976
62. Bloom H J G: Concepts in the natural history and treatment of medulloblastoma in children. CRC Crit Rev Clin Radiol Nucl Med 2:89–143, 1971
63. Dohrmann G J, Farwell J R, Flannery J T: Ependymomas and ependymoblastomas in children. J Neurosurg 45:273–283, 1976
64. Liu H M, Boggs J, Kidd J: Ependymomas of childhood. Childs Brain 2:92–110, 1976
65. Phillips T L, Sheline G E, Boldrey E: Therapeutic consideration in tumors affecting the central nervous system: Ependymomas. Radiology 83:98–105, 1964
66. Newton W A, Sayers M D, Samuels L D: Intrathecal methotrexate therapy for brain tumors in children. Cancer Chemother Rep 52:257–261, 1968
67. Norrell H, Wilson C: Brain tumor chemotherapy with methotrexate given intrathecally—A new technique. JAMA 201:93–95, 1967
68. Shapiro W R, Chernik N L, Posner J B: Necrotizing encephalopathy following intraventricular instillation of methotrexate. Arch Neurol 28:96–102, 1973
69. Crist W M, Ragab A H, Vietti T J, et al: Chemotherapy of childhood medulloblastoma. Am J Dis Child 130:639–642, 1976
70. Lampkin B C, Mauer A M, McBride B H: Response of medulloblastoma to vincristine sulfate: A case report. Pediatrics 39:761–763, 1967
71. Lassman L P, Pearce G W, Gang J: Effect of vincristine sulfate on the intracranial gliomata of childhood. Br J Surg 53:774–777, 1966
72. Mealey J Jr, Hall P V: Medulloblastoma in children: Survival and treatment. J Neurosurg 46:56–64, 1977
73. Shapiro W R: Chemotherapy of primary malignant brain tumors in children. Cancer 35:965–972, 1975
74. Brisman R, Housepian E M, Chang C, et al: Adjuvant nitrosourea therapy for glioblastoma. Arch Neurol 33:745–750, 1976
75. Taylor S G, Nelson L, Baxter D, et al: Treatment of grade III and IV astrocytoma with dimethyl triazeno imidazole carboxamide (DTIC, NSC-45388) alone and in combination with CCNU (NSC-79037) or methyl CCNU (MeCCNU, NSC-95441). Cancer 36:1269–1276, 1975
76. Editorial: Problems of Retinoblastoma. Br Med J 1:67, 1972

77. Taktikos A: Investigation of retinoblastoma with special reference to histology and prognosis. Br J Ophth 50:225–234, 1966
78. Ellsworth R M: The practical management of retinoblastoma. Trans Am Ophth Soc 67:462–534, 1969
79. Hyman G A, Feind C R, Spalter H F, Finkel M D: Chemotherapy of retinoblastoma. Cancer 17:992–996, 1964
80. Thompson R W, Small R C, Stein J J: Treatment of retinoblastoma. Am J Roentgenol Radium Ther Nucl Med 114:16–23, 1972
81. Lonsdale D, Berry D H, Holcomb T M, et al: Chemotherapeutic trials in patients with metastatic retinoblastoma. Cancer Chemother Rep 52:631–634, 1968
82. Skeggs D B L, Williams I G: The treatment of advanced retinoblastoma by means of external irradiation combined with chemotherapy. Clin Radiol 17:169–172, 1966
83. Tan C, Etcubanas E, Wollner N, et al: Adriamycin—An antitumor antibiotic in the treatment of neoplastic diseases. Cancer 32:9–17, 1973
84. Wolff J A, Pratt C B, Sitarz A L: Chemotherapy of metastatic retinoblastoma. Cancer Chemother Rep 16:155, 1962

PART III

Bone Marrow Physiology and Supportive Care

ALLAN J. ERSLEV

24
Chemotherapy and Erythropoiesis

Bone marrow suppression is the most serious of the many toxic side effects of chemotherapeutic agents and blood counts are generally used as a guide to steer chemotherapy along the narrow path between toxicity and tolerance. Because of the long life-span of red cells, platelet and white cell counts are usually used to assess bone marrow activity. Serial determinations of reticulocytes, however, will provide crucial information of the effect of chemotherapy on erythropoiesis and, indirectly, on bone marrow function in general.

NORMAL ERYTHROPOIESIS

The sustained production of mature red blood cells depends on the capacity of a pool of self-perpetuating erythropoietin-responsive stem cells to differentiate to proerythroblasts and, in turn, of the capacity of these proerythroblasts to divide and mature. The differentiation of erythroid stem cells to proerythroblasts is the last of a series of differentiations beginning with the fertilization of the egg cell. This step wise differentiation results in the formation of increasingly specialized stem cells and continues until the stem cells have become unipotential and committed to a single mature cell line. In the human embryo unipotential stem cells committed to the red cell line first appear in the yolk sac 15 to 20 days after gestation.[1] From that time on they serve as a self-perpetuating source of nucleated red cells adjusting their number and the rate of their differentiation to the demand of the body. They are small mononuclear cells, indistinguishable from lymphocytes, but capable of responding to erythropoietin with multiplication and differentiation to proerythroblasts.

Erythropoietin is a hormone produced in response to cellular hypoxia by the liver or reticuloendothelial system in the fetus[2] and by the kidney in the adult.[3] It acts on erythropoietin-responsive stem cells by generating a cytoplasmic RNA presumably necessary for blast transformation and early erythroid differentiation.[4] Subsequent maturation and multiplication of nucleated red cells appear to proceed independently of erythropoietin and are only affected by local microenvironmental factors and the supply of B_{12}, folic acid, iron and needed metabolic building blocks (Fig. 24-1). The nucleated red cells develop in close physical proximity of a reticular cell, forming an "erythroid island,"

Supported in part by NIH Grant 4612 and 6374

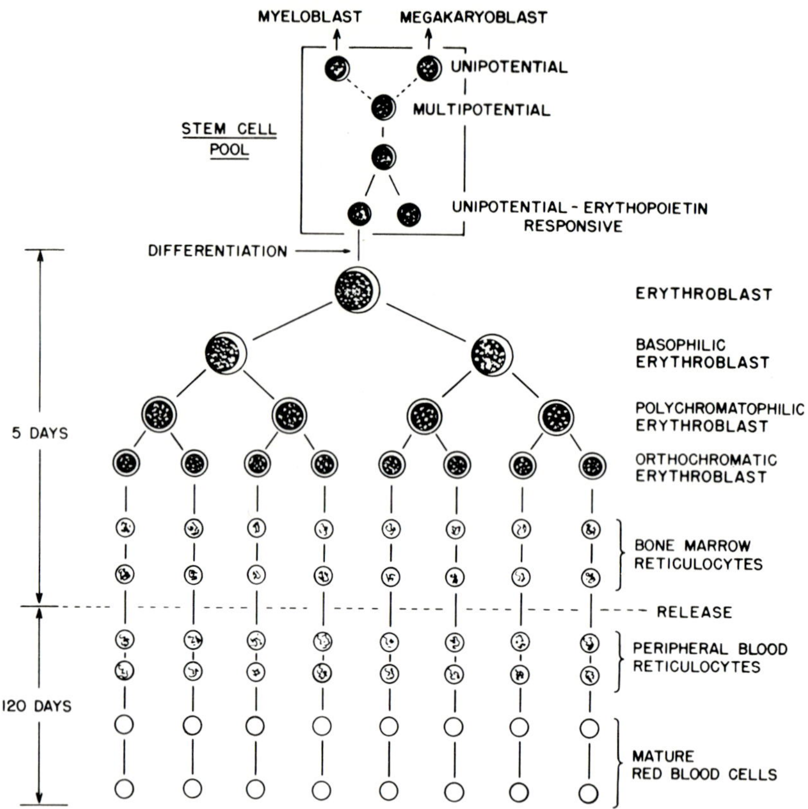

FIG. 24-1. A cellular flow chart showing the differentiation, multiplication and maturation of erythroid cells from multipotential stem cells to mature red blood cells.

with the reticular cells serving both as a mechanical and metabolic support.[5] After three to five divisions, fully hemoglobinized erythroblasts lose their nuclei by squeezing through narrow openings in the basement membrane of the bone marrow sinusoids. The timing of this bone marrow release may be affected in part by erythropoietin,[6] but the possible relationship between bone marrow storage or bone marrow transit time and erythropoietin concentration is still not clear.

The continuous erythropoietin-dependent differentiation of erythroid stem cells would deplete the stem cell pool unless erythropoietin, directly or indirectly, causes a compensatory multiplication.[7] It has been difficult, however, to construct a kinetic model that can account for both erythropoietin-induced stem cell replacement and erythropoietin-induced stem cell differentiation. An unequal mitotic division with one daughter cell becoming a proerythroblast and the other remaining a stem cell would be a possible, but not attractive possibility. It seems more likely that the loss of a stem cell through differentiation generates a cell-mediated stimulus for division to another member of the stem cell pool (Fig. 24-2). A further complication is that studies based on the tritiated thymidine suicide technique suggest that erythropoietin-responsive stem cells will divide and multiply even in the absence of erythropoietin.[8] Since the size of the stem cell pool remains fairly constant, this observation would suggest a continuous production of stem cells which either become differentiated by erythropoietin or die.[5]

The erythropoietin-responsive stem cell pool may be self-perpetuating for life or may need replenishment from time to time from a

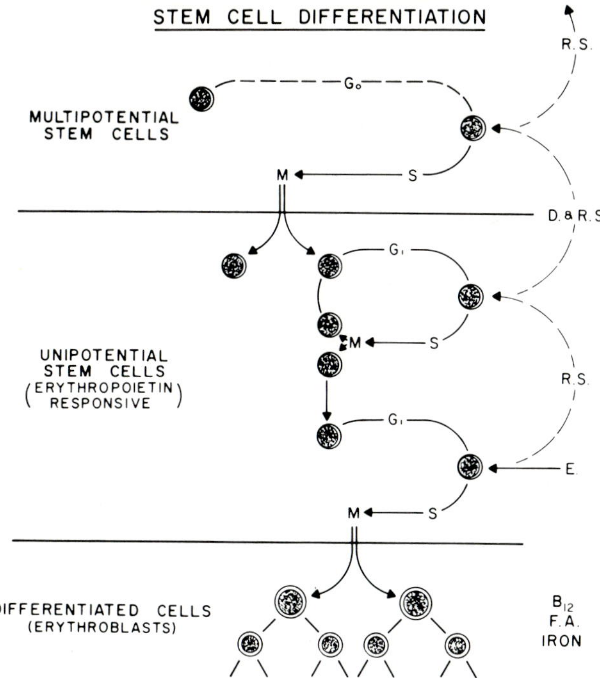

FIG. 24-2. One hypothesis explaining stem cell differentiation and renewal would envision that erythropoietin (E) acts on an erythropoietin-responsive, unipotential stem cell causing it to enter the synthetic phase (S), leading to mitosis (M) and the production of two proerythroblasts. The loss of an erythropoietin-responsive stem cell leads in turn to local cell-cell recruitment signals (R.S.), resulting in the mitotic division of another unipotential stem cell with restoration of the stem cell pool.

In case of depletion of the unipotential stem cell pool, differentiation and recruitment signals (D. & R.S.) will be generated and act on a dormant multipotential stem cell (Go), causing it to differentiate, enter mitotic divisions and replenish the erythropoietin responsive stem cell pool.

pool of earlier multi- or pluripotential stem cells. This pool, committed to forming unipotential stem cells with myeloid, erythroid or megakaryocytic potentials, is believed to be dormant but capable of reactivation and differentiation in response to cell-mediated signals generated by depletion or injury of unipotential stem cells (Fig. 24-2).[9] The process of reactivation and differentiation has been studied in the spleen of radiated mice after a transfusion of bone marrow cells from an isologous donor.[10] Dormant multipotential stem cells lodged in the spleen will become metabolically and mitotically active and will, over a period of 3 to 4 days, build up pools of unipotential stem cells. At that point, poietins and the immediate microenvironment will interact to cause differentiation into specific cell lines resulting in the formation of bone marrow colonies. Erythropoietin-responsive stem cells will become differentiated primarily on the surface of the spleen, while the microenvironment in the center of the spleen or in the bone marrow is far less receptive for erythroid differentiation despite the presence of both specific stem cells and erythropoietin. These latter areas, however, are readily colonized by stem cells forming myeloid and megakaryocytic cells.

Proximal to the multipotential stem cells are stem cells supporting total bone and bone marrow development. These cells are probably even more dormant and inactive, but the existence of pathologic conditions such as myelosclerosis, myelofibrosis and extramedullary bone and bone marrow formation suggest that they also can be activated when appropriately stimulated.

Measurements of Erythropoiesis

The effect of chemotherapeutic agents on erythropoiesis, from the level of multipotential stem cell to the release of reticulocytes from the marrow, can be evaluated by a number of clinical and experimental techniques.

1. Hemoglobin concentration, red blood cell count and hematocrit provide basic information about erythropoietic function. Hemolysis and blood loss may, of course, tax the compensatory capacity of a normal bone marrow, but since normal erythropoietic activity can increase about tenfold, severe anemia is usually a sign of absolute or relative erythropoietic failure.
2. Serial reticulocyte counts are a valuable index of the rate of red cell production. If they remain "normal," or low, despite anemia erythropoietic failure is present.
3. Bone marrow examination with determination of morphologic and numerical changes in the erythroblastic series are, of course, essential in the evaluation of the effect of chemotherapeutic agents on erythropoiesis. Morphologically, the megaloblastic changes frequently observed after the use of chemotherapeutic agents reflect impaired DNA and RNA synthesis. Numerically, an erythroid hypoplasia usually reflects stem cell injury. A bone marrow aspirate, however, measures only the composition of a tiny part of an organ weighing more than 1500 gm and it may not always be representative of the whole bone marrow.
4. Ferrokinetic techniques, measuring radioactive iron clearance, plasma iron turnover and red cell iron utilization, give data reflecting the total mass and effectiveness of erythropoietic tissue.
5. Erythropoietin titres in plasma may provide information about renal production of erythropoietin and about the size or functional capacity of the erythropoietin-responsive stem cell pool.
6. Responsiveness to erythropoietin in an experimental animal given a chemotherapeutic agent will also measure potential damage to the pool of erythropoietin-responsive stem cells.
7. Erythroid colony formation in plasma clots or methylcellulose is a recently developed technique which measures the number of erythropoietin-responsive stem cells (CFU-E) in a bone marrow sample.[11] In the presence of erythropoietin, small colonies of early erythroblasts can be observed and enumerated after 2 days of incubation. They grow in size and after 2 to 4 additional days of incubation, appear as large colonies (16 to 64 cells) of hemoglobinized erythroblasts. Clusters of individual colonies can often be observed after 7 to 10 days of incubation and may reflect the progeny of single, more primitive erythropoietin-responsive stem cells (burst-forming units, or BFU-E)[12] Enumeration of CFU-E and BFU-E in cultures of bone marrow from animals pretreated with chemotherapeutic agents will provide information about potential damage to the erythroid stem cells and can be compared to potential damage to the myeloid stem cells as determined in agar cultures (CFU-C).
8. The development of bone marrow colonies in the spleen of radiated and bone marrow transfused mice depends on the number of multipotential stem cells present in the donor marrow (CFU-S). The composition of the splenic colonies, whether erythroid, myeloid or megakaryocytic, depends primarily on the microenvironment and on the presence of poietins in the host and are of less importance than the number of colonies. Determination of erythroid repopulating ability (ERA) by measuring ^{59}Fe incorporation into circulating red cells derived from the erythroid component of these colonies also depends on many other factors distal to the multipotential stem cells. Similarly, the granulocytic repopulating ability (GRA) is only a moderately specific test of multipotential stem cells. All these tests are used extensively to assess the effect of chemotherapeutic agents on the multipotential bone marrow stem cells, but only the

basic enumeration of bone marrow colonies (CFU-S) can be considered accurate.

Effect of Chemotherapeutic Agents on Erythropoiesis

Chemotherapeutic agents are often divided into two main groups, cell-cycle- and non-cell-cycle-dependent. The synthetic analogues, for example, are most effective on dividing, cycling cells while the alkylating agents act on macromolecules in both resting and dividing cells. It is not always possible, however, to appreciate this difference since cells presumed dormant may become activated during treatment. Consequently, chemotherapeutic agents are better divided according to their metabolic action as specified by biochemical and biologic studies succinctly summarized by Calabresi and Parks[13] and by Marsh.[14] Unfortunately, species differences in metabolic handling of these agents are so great that it is difficult to predict from animal studies their hematopoietic effects in humans. Even clinical studies of the effect of chemotherapeutic agents on the bone marrow are difficult to interpret, since changes in maturation and proliferation of differentiated cells may obscure specific effects at the stem cell level. In general, a primary effect on differentiated erythroid cells leads to megaloblastosis and a hyperplastic, ineffective bone marrow; a primary effect on erythropoietin-responsive stem cells leads to isolated erythroid hypoplasia and anemia; and a primary effect on multipotential stem cells leads to bone marrow hypoplasia and pancytopenia.

Alkylating Agents

A number of compounds have the capacity to form highly reactive alkyl-ions capable of combining with and altering certain subunits of key macroglobules. The attachment, for example, of monofunctional alkyl-ions to the guanine of DNA will cause disruptive steric and charge changes, and the attachment of bifunctional alkyl-ions will cause the formation of intra- and intermolecular cross linkages. Although this may occur in all cells, both resting and dividing, it appears that cytotoxicity is mainly observed when cells containing alkylated DNA are stimulated to divide, hence the special sensitivity of bone marrow and gastrointestinal epithelium.[15] The dormant multipotential stem cells of bone marrow may initially be protected from the cytotoxic action of alkylating agents. When activated by recruitment signals from depleted marrow, however, they become extremely sensitive and often have a slower rate of regeneration than their more differentiated progeny. Despite the common biochemical action, the alkylating agents have developed therapeutic specialization because of differences in stability, gastrointestinal absorption, cellular penetration and intracellular activation.

Nitrogen Mustard. This parent compound of most alkylating agents is extremely unstable in solution and needs to be given intravenously shortly after having been dissolved. It has an immediate effect on function and viability of bone marrow cells, and a single injection of nitrogen mustard will result in measurable decreases in circulating granulocytes, thrombocytes and lymphocytes lasting up to 3 weeks. It damages all erythroid precursor cells regardless of phase, but actively proliferating cells appear to be more sensitive than resting cells.[16] The apparent sensitivity of multipotential stem cells may, in part, lie in delayed recovery rather than in early cytotoxicity. In rats, erythropoietin-responsive stem cells have been reported to be quite resistent to HN_2,[17] but that has not been observed in other species.

Cyclophosphamide. Cyclophosphamide can be given by mouth since it is biologically inert until converted to active short-lived metabolites by a hepatic cytochrome oxidase. In rats and mice, nucleated red cells appear to be more sensitive than stem cells,[18] but the early pancytopenia observed in humans suggests that here the stem cell effect may be dominant.

Chlorambucil. Chlorambucil ionizes slowly and can be given by mouth, but it does not need preliminary activation in order to exert its alkylating action. It is the slowest acting and least toxic of the therapeutically useful alkylating agents and suppression of stem cells and nucleated red cells is usually brief and easily managed.

Melphalan. Melphalan is a nitrogen mustard linked to the amino acid, phenylalanine. This combination was designed to provide melphalan with enhanced cellular penetration of cells engaged in active protein synthesis. This goal was presumably achieved since melphalan appears to affect plasma cells preferentially. Its affect on erythropoietic cells is similar to that of other mustards with stem cells affected in approximately the same way as differentiated erythroid cells.

Busulfan. This compound differs significantly in action from that of other alkylating agents.[19] Its myelotoxic action is primarily directed against granulopoietic and thrombopoietic cells. Furthermore, and more importantly, it appears to suppress resting cells far more than dividing cells, a unique reverse proliferation dependency.[20] Consequently, the slowly proliferating multipotential stem cells are particularly affected and may stay suppressed long after the erythropoietin-responsive stem cells and the nucleated red cells have recovered.

Bischloroethylnitrosourea (BCNU). BCNU and the closely related CCNU are lipid-soluble alkylating compounds with a delayed and often capricious effect on bone marrow function. The nadir of cytopenia may not occur until 4 to 6 weeks after the administration of a single dose as compared to the 1 to 3 week nadir observed after most nitrogen mustards. Otherwise, the effect on erythropoietic cells appears the same with stem cells suppressed about the same as nucleated red cells and with multipotential stem cells regenerating more slowly than the erythropoietin-sensitive stem cells.

Synthetic Metabolic Analogues

Competitive inhibition of the synthesis of DNA and other nucleic acid macromolecules can be achieved by a number of synthetic analogues. These compounds are usually cycle- and proliferation-dependent and have a greater suppressive effect on differentiated erythroid cells than on their stem cells. The characteristic megaloblastic changes usually observed early after treatment suggest the presence of imbalanced DNA-RNA synthesis with DNA suppressed preferentially.[22]

Folic Acid Analogues. The antifolic acid agent most widely used is methotrexate (MTX). It apparently acts by inhibiting dihydrofolate reductase, rendering this key enzyme unavailable for the transformation of folic acid to the tetrahydrofolic acid needed for DNA synthesis. RNA synthesis is unaffected, resulting in macrocytosis and megaloblastic changes of differentiated erythroid cells. Suppression of stem cells is less pronounced and erythroid or bone marrow aplasia first occurs after administration of large doses of MTX.[23]

Purine Analogues. The most commonly used inhibitors of purine synthesis are 6-mercaptopurine (6-MP), thioguanine (6-TG) and azathioprine (Imuran). These compounds inhibit the de novo synthesis of adenine and guanine, as well as their later incorporation into DNA, RNA and other purine-containing macromolecules.[24] The megaloblastic changes observed after administration of purine analogues are usually not as pronounced as after folic acid analogues are given, and stem cell suppression with bone marrow hypoplasia also appears to be less severe and less sustained.

Pyrimidine Analogues. 5-fluorouracil (5-FU) and floxuridine (FUdR) block the synthesis of thymidylic acid, presumably by inhibiting thymidylate synthetase, while 6-azouridine (6-AzUR) appears to block de novo synthesis of uridylic acid.[24] Both compounds initially produce mild megaloblastic anemia with later stem cell suppression and bone marrow aplasia.[25]

Cytosine arabonoside (Ara-C) is also a pyrimidine analogue, but its mode of action appears to be different from the uracil analogues. It has been suggested that it inhibits the conversion of cytidylate to desoxycytidylate,[26] but this action, which would make it a specific DNA inhibitor, has not been confirmed. Another mode of action that has been suggested is that it inhibits DNA polymerase.[27]

TABLE 24-1. *Chemotherapy and Erythropoiesis*

	Proliferation Dependency	Differentiated Erythroid Cells	Erythropoietin-responsive stem cells	Multipotential stem cells
I. *Alkylating Agents*				
Nitrogen mustard	++	+++	++	++
Cyclophosphamide	++	++	++	++
Chlorambucil	++	+	+	+
Melphalan	++	++	++	++
Busulfan	(-)	+	+	+++
BCNU, TCNU	++	++	++	++
II. *Synthetic Analogues*				
Folic acid analogues				
MTX	++++	++++	+++	++
Purine analogues				
6 MP	++++	+++	++	+
6 TG	++++	+++	++	+
Azathioprine	++++	+++	++	+
Pyrimidine analogues				
5-FU	+++	+++	++	+
FuDR	+++	+++	++	+
Ara-C	+++	+++	++	+
Hydroxyurea	++++	++++	+++	++
Procarbazine	++	+++	++	+
III. *Vinca Alkaloids*				
Vinblastine	++++	++	+	+
Vincristine	++++	(+)	(+)	(+)
IV. *Antibiotics*				
Actinomycin D	++	++++	++	++
Daunorubicin	++	++	+++	++
Bleomycin	(+)	(+)	(+)	(+)
L-asparaginase	(+)	(+)	(+)	(+)

Hydroxyurea. Hydroxyurea, a synthetic urea analogue, was by chance found to have chemotherapeutic actions, presumably by inhibiting the reductive conversion of ribonucleotides to desoxyribonucleotides and thereby inhibiting the synthesis of DNA. It is cycle-dependent and in tissue culture has been shown to delay entry of G_1 cells into the drug-sensitive S-phase, resulting in partial synchronization of cells.[29] As anticipated, cycling nucleated red cells are most vulnerable and megaloblastic changes are seen early.

Procarbazine. Procarbazine, a monoamine oxidase inhibitor, has been found to be an effective chemotherapeutic agent, but its mode of action is not clear.[30] It may act as an alkylating agent with its effect on bone marrow stem cells being equal to or greater than its effect on differentiated erythroid cells.

Vinca Alkaloids

Vinblastine is an alkaloid derived from the periwinkle plant. It selectively suppresses the synthesis of microtubules and effectively impairs mitotic division, platelet contraction, granulocyte mobility and other processes that are dependent on microtubules.[31] Because of its effect on spindle formation, it is highly cycle-dependent although it is also somewhat cytotoxic to resting cells. Erythroid suppression is usually mild and transient.[32]

Vincristine is also extracted from the periwinkle plant, and it also has a profound suppressive effect on microtubule formation. Despite its stathmokinetic effect on dividing cells, it has little inhibiting action on bone marrow cells and hematologic toxicity is rare.

Antibiotics

Actinomycin D, an antibiotic derived from a species of *Streptomyces*, has the capacity to bind to DNA and thereby impair DNA-directed RNA synthesis.[33] It is not particularly cycle-dependent, although, as is the case for the alkylating agents, cells in active proliferation are more sensitive than resting cells. The erythroid cells appear particularly vulnerable to the action of actinomycin D, and complete erythroid aplasia can be observed in experimental animals at a time when granulo- and thrombopoiesis still are ongoing. This difference in sensitivity has been related to a specific block of erythropoietin-induced stem cell differentiation.[34]

Daunorubicin and its hydroxyl derivative Adriamycin are also *Streptomyces*-derived antibiotics, and are also bound to DNA causing inhibition of its template function.[35] They can produce severe stem cell cytotoxicity with occasionally irreversible bone marrow failure. Unlike actinomycin D, they have not been shown to specifically suppress erythroid activity.

Bleomycin is another *Steptomyces* antibiotic which causes damage to DNA strands, but remarkably enough has very little, if any, hematologic toxicity.

L-asparaginase is derived from *E-coli*. It reduces the concentration of blood asparagine and presumably yields its chemotherapeutic action by depriving tumor cells of asparagine.[36] It is not cycle-dependent and its action on normal bone marrow cells is minimal.

Conclusion and Summary

Normal erythropoietic function is reviewed and the suppressive effect on this function by commonly used chemotherapeutic agents is tabulated. Although certain general metabolic actions of chemotherapeutic agents can be recognized to cause predictable effects on multipotential stem cells, erythropoietin-responsive stem cells and differentiated erythroid cells, many variables exist. Among these variables are dose frequency, route of administration, species tested and proliferative state of the erythropoietic cells. Since almost all chemotherapeutic agents are proliferation-dependent, the state of stem cell proliferation, as determined by the presence or absence of recruitment signals, will to a considerable extent determine the ultimate erythropoietic cytotoxicity. Consequently, the summary in Table 24-1 of the effect of chemotherapeutic agents and erythropoiesis is tenuous and should be considered a guide rather than a statement of fact.

References

1. Hesseldahl H, Larsen F J: Hemopoiesis and blood vessels in human yolk sac. An electron microscopic study. Acta Anato 78:274, 1971
2. Zanjani E D, Peterson E N, Gordon A S, et al: Erythropoietin production in the fetus: Role of the kidney and maternal anemia. J Lab Clin Med 83:281, 1974
3. Erslev A J: The renal biogenesis of erythropoietin. Am J Med 58:25, 1975
4. Piantadosi C A, Dickerman H W, Spivak J L: Sequential activation of splenic nuclear RNA polymerases by erythropoietin. J Clin Invest 57:20, 1976
5. Erslev A J, Weiss L: Structure and function of the bone marrow, in Williams W J, Beutler E, Erslev A J, Rundles R W (eds): Hematology, 2nd ed. New York, McGraw-Hill, 1977, p 57
6. Le Blond P F, Chamberlain J K, Weed R J: Scanning electron microscopy of erythropoietin-stimulated bone marrow. Blood Cells 1:639, 1975
7. Reissmann K R, Somorapoompichit S: Effect of erythropoietin on proliferation of erythroid stem cells in the absence of transplantable colony-forming units. Blood 36:287, 1970
8. Stohlman F Jr: Regulation of red cell production, in Greenwalt T J, Jamieson G A (eds): Formation and Destruction of Blood Cells, Philadelphia, J B Lippincott, 1970, p 65
9. McCulloch E A, Till J E: Cellular interactions in the control of hemopoiesis, in Stohlman F J (ed): Hemopoietic Cellular Proliferation, New York, Grune & Stratton, 1970, p 15
10. Lewis J P, Passovoy M, Freeman M, et al: The

repopulation potential and differentiation capacity of hematopoietic stem cells from the blood and bone marrow of normal mice. J Cell Physiol 71:121, 1968.

11. Stephenson J K, Axelrod A A, McLeod D L, et al: Induction of colonies of hemoglobin-synthesizing cells by erythropoietin in vitro. Proc Natl Acad Sci 68:1542, 1971
12. Heath D S, Axelrad A A, McLeod D L, et al: Separation of the erythropoietin-responsive progenitors BFU-E and CFU-E in mouse bone marrow by unit gravity sedimentation. Blood 47:777, 1976
13. Calabresi P, Parks R E Jr: Chemotherapy of neoplastic diseases, in Goodman L S, Gilman A (eds): The Pharmacologic Basis of Therapeutics, New York, MacMillan, 1975, p 1248
14. Marsh J C: The effects of cancer chemotherapeutic agents on normal hematopoietic precursor cells: A review. Cancer Res 36:1853, 1976
15. Connors T A: Mechanism of action of 2-chloroethyl amine derivatives, sulfur mustards, epoxides and aziridines, in Sarterelli A C, Johns D G (eds): Antineoplastic and Immunosuppressive Agents, part II. Berlin, Springer-Verlag, 1975, p 18
16. Blackett N M, Adams K: Cell proliferation and the action of cytotoxic agents on haemopoietic tissue. Br J Haematol 23:751, 1972
17. Millar J L, Blackett N M: The effect of various cytotoxic agents on the erythroid precursors in rat bone marrow. Br J Haematol 26:535, 1974
18. Canstable T B, Blackett N M: Effect of cytotoxic agents on the maturing granulocytic and erythroid cells of rats. J Natl Cancer Inst 50:515, 1973
19. Dunn C D R: The chemical and biologic properties of busulfan (Myleran). Exp Hematol 2:101, 1974
20. Josvasen N, Bøyum A: Haemopoiesis in busulphan-treated mice. Scand J Haematol 11:78, 1973
21. Reissmann K R, Udupa K B, Kawada K: Effects of erythropoietin and androgens on erythroid stem cells after their selective suppression by BCNU. Blood 44:649, 1974
22. Beck W S: General considerations of megaloblastic anemias, in Williams W J, Beutler E, Erslev A J, Rundles R W (eds): Hematology 2nd ed. New York, McGraw-Hill, 1977, p 300
23. Ernest P, Killmann S A: Perturbation of generation cycle of human leukemic myeloblasts in vivo by methotrexate. Blood 38:689, 1971
24. Elion G B, Hitchings G H: Metabolic basis for the action of analogs of purines and pyrimidines. Adv Chemother 2:91, 1965
25. Brennan M J, Vaitkevicius V K, Rebuck J W: Megaloblastic anemia associated with inhibition of thymine synthesis: Observations during 5-fluorouracil therapy. Blood 16:1535, 1960
26. Creasey W A, Deconti R C, Kaplan S R: Biochemical studies with 1-β-p-arabinofuranosyltosine in human leukemic leukocytes and normal bone marrow cells. Cancer Res 28:1074, 1968
27. Furth J J, Cohen S S: Inhibition of mammalian DNA polymerase by the 5′-triphosphate of 1-β-p-arabinofuranosylcytosine and the 5′-triphosphate of 9-β-p-arabinofuranosylcytosine. Cancer Res 28:2061, 1968
28. Frenkel E P, Arthur C: Induced ribotide reductive conversion by hydroxyurea and its relationship to megaloblastosis. Cancer Res 27:1016, 1967
29. Bhuyen B K, Fraser T J, Gray L G, et al: Cell-kill kinetics of several S-phase-specific drugs. Cancer Res 33:888, 1973
30. Reed D J: Procarbazine, in Sartorelli A C, Johns D G (eds): Antineoplastic and Immunosuppressive Agents, part II. Berlin, Springer-Verlag, 1975, p 747
31. Creasey W A: Vinca alkaloids and colchicine, in Sartorelli A C, Johns D G (eds): Antineoplastic and Immunosuppressive Agents, part II. Berlin, Springer-Verlag, 1975, p 670
32. Twentyman P R, Blackett N M: Red cell production in the mouse following treatment with vinblastine. Blood 38:583, 1971
33. Reich E: Biochemistry of actinomycins. Cancer Res 23:1428, 1963
34. Reissmann K R, Ito K: Selective eradication of erythropoiesis by actinomycin D as the result of interference with hormonally controlled effector pathway of cell differentiation. Blood 28:201, 1966
35. Pigram W J, Fuller W, Hamilton L D: Stereochemistry of intercalation: Interaction of daunomycin with DNA. Nature (New Biol) 235:17, 1972
36. Tallal L, Tan C, Oellgen H, et al: *E coli* L-asparaginase in the treatment of leukemia and solid tumors in 131 children. Cancer 25:306, 1970

Robert A. Joyce
Dane R. Boggs

25
Chemotherapy and Leukokinetics

Most chemotherapeutic agents used in the treatment of malignant neoplastic diseases are also fairly nonspecific cell poisons. They are most particularly damaging to the cellular compartments which are active in the production of new cells such as the lining cells of the gut and the cells of the hematopoietic system. All such chemotherapeutic agents, therefore, have a predictable dose-related hematopoietic toxicity. In other chapters in this volume, the effect of chemotherapeutic agents on platelets and their precursors, and upon red cells and their precursors, are considered. In this section we will consider the effect of chemotherapy upon blood neutrophils and the stem cells for the hematopoietic system and give brief consideration to this effect upon leukocytes.

Some understanding of normal cell kinetic patterns is essential for the intelligent use of chemotherapy. The pattern of proliferation, time required for cell production, cell distribution and life span of hematopoietic cells are subjects quite germane to the design of chemotherapy trials. From an understanding of the physiology of these cellular systems, the seemingly mysterious "delayed" toxicity of some drugs begins to make sense. For instance, after a single dose of a cell-poisoning drug, neutropenia should not develop for a week or more if the marrow is normal. The duration of the neutropenia will be dependent upon whether the agent is cycle-active or non-cycle-active in nature. This discussion is designed to provide the reason for this type of statement and is divided into the following parts: Normal stem cell kinetics, normal neutrophil kinetics, the effects of chemotherapeutic agents upon these classes of cells, methods of predicting the degree of normal cell toxicity induced by chemotherapy agents and the chemotherapeutic effects on other leukocyte systems.

Normal Stem Cell Kinetics

Since the hematopoietic cells of the blood are constantly being lost and must be replaced, the replacement system (stem cell system) for normal hematopoietic tissue must have two distinguishing characteristics: (1) a stem cell must be capable of self replication and (2) it must also be capable of differentiation into more mature cells. In a stem cell compartment of stable size, for each cell that differentiates, another stem cell must be produced by self-replication in order to maintain compartment size.[1]

Pluripotential Stem Cells

There is now excellent evidence in man and in the mouse that there is a single cellular compartment capable of giving rise to megakaryocytes, red cell precursors, neutrophil precursors and eosinophil precursors. Evidence for this cell in man comes primarily from chromosome studies in patients with chronic myelocytic leukemia, since the typical form of this disease in most patients is manifested by a chromosome defect with translocation of a portion of chromosome number 22 most often to chromosome number 9.[2] Whang and co-workers[3] found this chromosome defect, not only in neutrophil precursors, but also in erythrocytic precursors and probably in megakaryocytes. The absence of this defect in other cells, such as lymphocytes, clearly indicates that it is not an inherited chromosome defect. Furthermore, the presence of this defect in these three cell lines of bone marrow origin suggests that the defect arises in a cell which is a common stem cell for these three precursors. In paroxysmal nocturnal hemoglobinuria, there is also evidence for a common defect in neutrophils, platelets and erythrocytes.[4] Demonstrations of a single glucose-6-phosphate dehydrogenase gene expression in granulocytes, red cells and megakaryocytes of heterozygotes with chronic myelocytic leukemia,[5] idiopathic myelofibrosis[6] and polycythemia vera[7] have contributed additional evidence for the existence of pluripotential stem cells common to these cell lines. Thus, in these diseases it seems reasonable to suggest that difficulty began in a single stem cell, that this stem cell was pluripotential for neutrophils, erythrocytes and megakaryocytes, and that this single abnormal cell successfully competed with normal hematopoietic stem cells, thus repopulating the bone marrow.

Similarly, if the mouse's hematopoietic system is severely damaged by irradiation, regeneration of the system is primarily from a pluripotential hematopoietic stem cell. Till and McCulloch[8] demonstrated that if mice were lethally irradiated and injected with syngeneic bone marrow, macroscopic nodules were present on the spleen some 10 days later. Examination of these nodules revealed them to be composed of erythrocytic, neutrophilic or megakaryocytic tissue, or all three. Later studies from their laboratory clearly demonstrated that the nodules began from a single cell, and that these colonies were indeed clones.[9] Thus, in the mouse, a method is available to study this pluripotential hematopoietic stem cell known as the colony-forming unit cell (CFU cell).

There are two general methods by which spleen colonies may be studied in the mouse. The first is the above-mentioned transplantation method, in which tissue from spleen, bone marrow, washings from the peritoneal cavity, buffy coat cells from the blood, or fetal liver are transplanted into a lethally irradiated recipient.[10] The recipient spleen forms colonies from the transplanted material. In the second, or endogenous spleen colony method, the mouse is sublethally irradiated so that it's colony-forming cell compartment is severely reduced, but not eliminated, and the hematopoietic system is regenerated from these surviving cells. In this circumstance, colonies are also available on the spleen some 10 days after irradiation, and the number of colonies is inversely proportional to the dosage of whole body irradiation delivered to the animal.

The CFU cell system is probably at rest in the ordinary steady state. For instance, Becker and co-workers[11] exposed cells to suicidal doses of tritiated thymidine prior to cell transplant and produced little, if any, decrease in the number of colony-forming cells noted in the recipient. This would suggest that this cell is either in a state of G_0 generative cycle, or else is in an exceedingly long generative cycle equivalent to G_0 state. If extremely severe damage ($\geq$ 700 rads whole-body irradiation) is induced in the stem cell compartment of the mouse, there is evidence that regeneration may be from a stem cell more primitive than the CFU cell. In this circumstance, cytogenic evidence suggests that lymphocytes are also derived from such a stem cell.[12] Indirect evidence for such a primitive stem cell population in man is provided by recent reports of lymphoblastic transformation in some patients with blast crisis of chronic myelocytic leukemia.[13-15] Thus, we have evidence that there are concatenated stem cell systems of increasing maturity. It is apparent that since severe damage to this system is required before the stem cell (also pluripotential for lymphocytes) comes into play, this cell, like the CFU cell, must be in a G_0 state or in an exceptionally long generative cycle.

Alternatively, the CFU cell might be the most primitive hematopoietic stem cell in the adult and be pluripotent for lymphocytes as well.[15]

Pattern of Regeneration of Depleted Stem Cell Compartments in the Mouse

Our laboratories have studied the rate of regeneration of colony-forming unit cells after this compartment is damaged by irradiation.[10,16,17] Because of a variety of difficulties attending the transplant system,[10] we have chosen to restrict our studies to regeneration of endogenous colonies. Mice were given a single dose of whole-body irradiation to reduce the stem cell compartment. At intervals of 1, 2, 3, and 4 or more days thereafter, a second dose of whole-body irradiation was given and the number of spleen colonies was measured 10 days after the second irradiation. In this system, spacing the second irradiation at increasing intervals would have no influence upon the number of colonies until regrowth of the colony-forming system occurred. That is, if there is no regrowth for the first 3 days, animals given an initial 350 rads followed by 350 rads on days 1, 2, or 3 should have the same number of colonies 10 days later. Conversely, if the colony-forming compartment were growing during the interval between the first and second irradiation, the number of colonies present would increase as the irradiation was spaced farther apart. Irradiation kills cells in an exponential fashion, so that the compartment is reduced by a fixed percentage rather than by an absolute number of cells.[18] The summation of a number of such studies is illustrated in Figure 25-1. In 11 experiments in which the initial irradiation was 300 rad or more, there was a rapid increase in colonies, indicating that regrowth began almost immediately following reduction of the compartment. The mean colony doubling time in these experiments was 16 hours. When the initial irradiation dose was 200 rads or less, however, a much slower doubling time was observed.

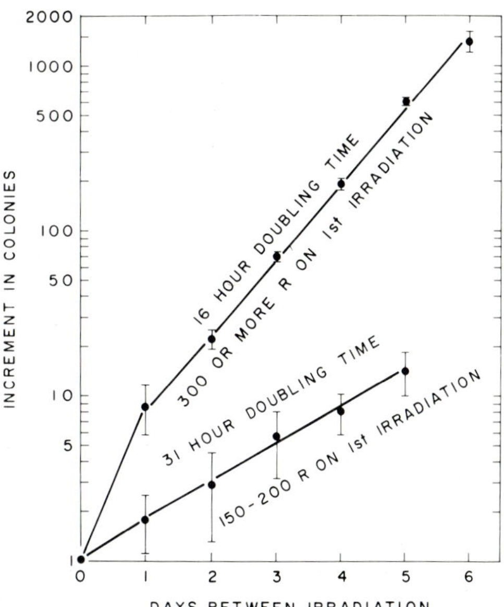

FIG. 25-1. Recovery of the pluripotential hematopoietic stem cell compartment following whole-body irradiation. Mice were given two irradiation exposures at varying intervals. The number of colonies present on the spleen was measured 10 days after the second irradiation.

These studies suggest that the severely reduced compartments (300 rads or more) regrew at a faster rate than the less severely damaged compartments (200 rads or less). One explanation for such a difference was to suggest that differentiation was still occurring from the compartment which was not too severely damaged, whereas, with greater damage, compartment regrowth had to precede the onset of differentiation.

In order to further investigate this hypothesis, studies of the time of onset of differentiation following whole-body irradiation in relation to dose of irradiation were carried out by exposing groups of mice to various levels of whole-body irradiation. Each day thereafter, a subgroup was injected with radioactive iron and then killed to determine when an increased rate of uptake of radioactive iron into marrow, spleen and red blood cells occurred. The results of one such experiment are shown in Figure 25-2. Note that in this figure, the group given 200 rads had an increasing iron uptake as soon as the value could be measured, suggesting erythropoiesis was never completely interrupted. With 400

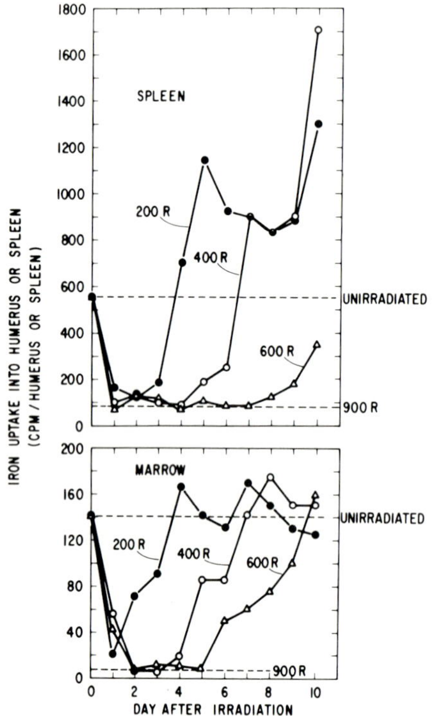

FIG. 25-2. The relation of dose of whole-body irradiation to time of resumption of erythropoiesis. Mice were exposed to varying levels of irradiation, and at daily intervals thereafter groups were injected with radioactive iron and then killed, and iron uptake into spleen (upper figure) and marrow (lower figure) was determined.

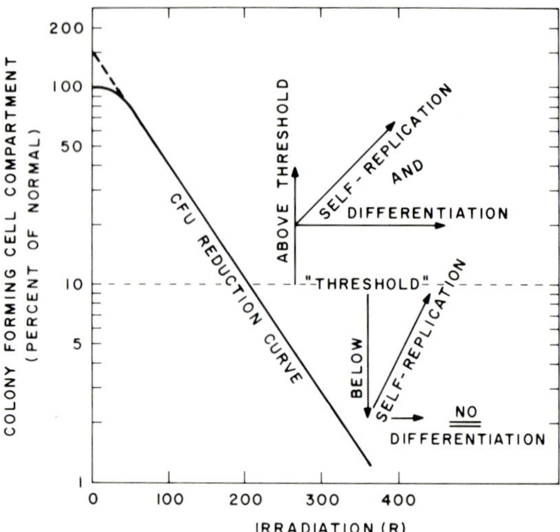

FIG. 25-3. A suggested model for hematopoietic recovery following irradiation. A "threshold" is suggested below which stem cell replication without differentiation is also occurring, so that the doubling time for self-replicating stem cells slows. The threshold is placed at 10 per cent of normal since that is the approximate reduction obtained by 200 rads (see text).

rads there was a period during which no increase was observed, followed by a rapidly increasing iron uptake, and after 600 rads an even longer period of basal iron uptake was observed. In all such experiments, as the dose of irradiation was increased, there was a longer period during which iron uptake remained at a baseline level before it suddenly increased.

A summation of all such experiments suggested that erythropoiesis is interrupted at approximately 200 rads and that for each further increase of 100 rads of whole-body irradiation, there is a lag of approximately 1.6 days before erythropoiesis begins. These data tend to support the previous suggestion that in a severely damaged system, repopulation of the stem cell compartment must precede significant differentiation. This model for recovery of a damaged stem cell compartment is illustrated in Figure 25-3.

If strong stimuli for differentiation (bleeding or endotoxin injection) are introduced immediately following irradiation, an abortive wave of differentiation follows.[19] If administration of these stimuli is delayed for more than a day, however, they are ineffective. Thus, whatever the mechanism is that protects the reduced stem cell compartment from differentiating, it comes into play rapidly.

Radiation survival is primarily dependent upon regeneration of neutrophils and megakaryocytes, since the usual cause of hematopoietic postirradiation death is infection due to neutropenia or bleeding due to thrombocytopenia. We carried out further experiments in order to determine if cells differentiated into these three compartments at a fixed rate or whether the compartment was subject to competing stimuli. In these experiments the rate of erythropoietic demand was changed by inducing polycythemia either by hypertransfusion or in posthypoxic mice; or by accelerating the demand for erythropoiesis by bleeding mice or injecting erythropoietin.[20] In such animals the total number of neutrophils and neutrophil precursors in the humerus was

TABLE 25-1. *Effect of Altered Rates of Erythropoiesis on Marrow Granulocytes After 400 Rads Whole Body Irradiation*

Procedure	Absolute Number of Granulocytes Per Humerus* (% of Control)
Increased Erythropoiesis	
Bleeding + 400 rads	52
Erythropoietin + 400 rads	80
Decreased Erythropoiesis	
Hypertransfusion + 400 rads	170
Hypoxia + 400 rads	235

*Absolute number of granulocytes was determined 10 days after irradiation; control animals had an average of 3×10^6 cells/humerus.

measured at 7 and 10 days following irradiation and the results are summarized in Table 25-1.

In the animals in which demands for erythropoiesis were virtually absent due to the presence of plethora, a larger than normal number of neutrophils and neutrophil precursors was present. Conversely, when an unusual demand for erythropoiesis was superimposed, as represented by the bled or erythropoietin treated mice, a reduced number of neutrophils and neutrophil precursors was observed. These results are compatible with the hypothesis that output from the stem cell compartment is subject to competing demands and that there is a possibility of experimental manipulation of the output of the various differentiated compartments.

Committed Stem Cell

If we are to assume that the CFU cell in the normal state is in a virtual state of G_0, then some other source for the constant replacement of blood cells must be found. There are studies to suggest that this source is stem cells, which are more mature and more differentiated than the CFU cell, and perhaps unipotential for a single cell line. There is evidence for the separation of a cell that can give rise to granulocytes from the CFU cell. If mouse bone marrow,[21] human bone marrow[22] or peripheral blood[23] is cultured in semisolid medium with a proper feeder layer or conditioned media, colonies of granulocytic and mononuclear cells arise from marrow or peripheral blood. When marrow from the WWv mouse with a known severe defect in the CFU cell compartment is used for transplantation experiments, no macroscopic spleen colonies are observed and only very tiny microscopic colonies can be seen. When its marrow is placed in a soft gel medium in vitro, however, a normal concentration of colonies of normal size is observed.[24] This strongly suggests that in this animal the more mature stem cell that gives rise to granulocytes is intact, while the CFU cell compartment is faulty, thus providing direct evidence for two distinct compartments. Similar data have been reported for erythrocyte progenitor cells that arise from the CFU cell. These progenitor cells have been studied in semisolid medium containing erythropoietin and have been separated into two populations based on different erythropoietin responsiveness, in vitro growth characteristics and sedimentation velocity properties.[25]

Stem Cell Model

Figure 25-4 depicts a proposed model for the stem cell system.[1] In normal circumstances, red cells, platelets and neutrophils are maintained in balance by mature, perhaps even unipotent, stem compartments. If these compartments are damaged or if there is an unusual demand for cells, these more mature compartments are replenished by the multipotent CFU cell compartment which is ordinarily at rest. When both of these compartments are severely damaged or are under conditions of extreme stress, a still more primitive compartment is brought into play, which is also capable of feeding the lymphocyte compartment. Under normal steady-state

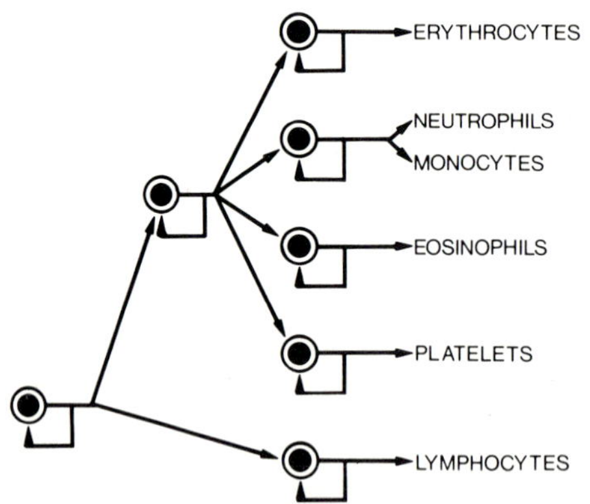

FIG. 25-4. A possible model of the hematopoietic stem cell system. Each cell portrayed is a stem cell, i.e., capable of self-replication as well as differentiation. The myeloid system is shown as normally maintained by three specialized stem cells. There is a cell pluripotent for lymphocytes and myelocytes, but its exact relation to the cell pluripotent for all myeloid tissue is uncertain. As discussed in the text, the exact structure of the entire system is unclear. From Boggs, D R, Winkelstein A: White Cell Manual; ed 3. Philadelphia, F A Davis, 1975 (with permission).

conditions, the lymphocyte constitutes its own stem cell compartment since these cells are capable of division, giving rise to more lymphocytes. It is apparent that the exact structure of the stem cell compartments is not presently known, but from the information available we can make certain generalizations which may be of some use in designing chemotherapeutic experiments, as will be discussed later.

NORMAL NEUTROPHIL KINETICS

Blood Neutrophil Compartment[26,27]

In a normal steady state, the blood neutrophil compartment is maintained by the inflow from the bone marrow balancing the outflow to tissues and body cavities (Fig. 25-5). The average neutrophil spends only 10 hours in the blood and loss from the blood is a random function. That is, the neutrophil that has just entered the blood from the marrow is as likely to leave on its first circulatory circuit as is one which has been around for many hours. This rapid rate of turnover indicates that on

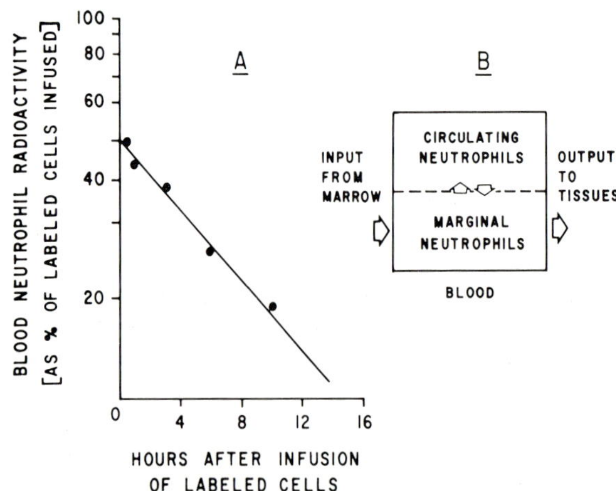

FIG. 25-5. Blood neutrophil kinetics. The curve of radioactivity (5-A) is that obtained after infusion of autologous neutrophils labeled with radioactive diisopropylfluorophosphate. From Boggs, D R, Winkelstein A: White Cell Manual, ed 3, Philadelphia, F A Davis, 1975 (with permission).

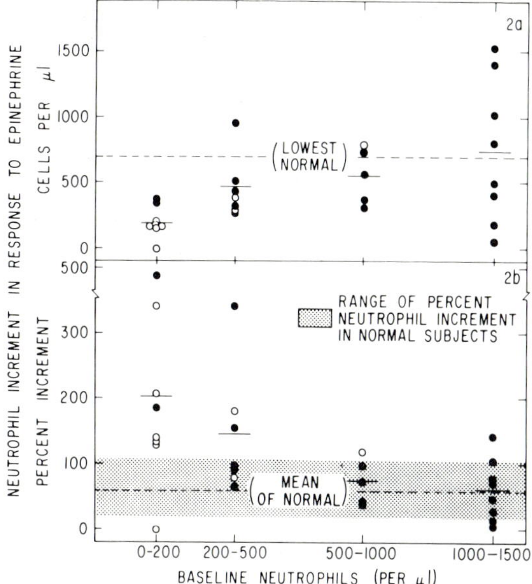

FIG. 25-6. A. Maximum neutrophil increments in response to epinephrine infusion from 28 studies of 26 patients with neutropenia. Open circles indicate patients with palpable splenomegaly. Horizontal bars represent mean increment of each group. Dotted line represents the lowest neutrophil increment in response to epinephrine of 12 normal subjects. B. Maximum per cent increment of neutrophils following epinephrine infusion. Shaded area represents range of neutrophil increment of the 12 normal subjects; and the dotted line, the mean increment of that group. From Joyce R A, Boggs D R, Hasiba U, et al: Marginal neutrophil pool size in normal subjects and neutropenic patients as measured by epinephrine infusion. J Lab Clin Med 88:614, 1976 (with permission).

the average the mass of blood neutrophils is replaced two and one-half times each day. Recently published data[28] have suggested that the granulocyte turnover rate may be modestly overestimated by the above techniques but in any event, the turnover is quite brisk.

The determination of the concentration of neutrophils in venous blood samples can be somewhat misleading since in normal circumstances approximately one-half of blood neutrophils are marginated on the walls of capillary or postcapillary venules. Thus, one underestimates the number of neutrophils in the blood by such a concentration determination. This underestimation is greater when neutropenia is present. We have studied the maximal blood neutrophil increment following epinephrine infusion as a measure of the marginal neutrophil pool in neutropenic subjects (Fig. 25-6). Although absolute neutrophil increments were greater in those less severely neutropenic, there was a significant enhancement of the per cent of neutrophil increase in the neutropenic patients as compared to normal subjects. In addition, there was an inverse correlation between the blood neutrophil concentration and the per cent increment following epinephrine, indicating an inverse relationship between the sizes of the circulating and marginal neutrophil pools as neutropenia becomes more profound.[29]

Neutropenia can be brought about by one of three mechanisms, or combinations of these mechanisms: (1) decreased production with reduced outflow from the bone marrow, (2) increased destruction of neutrophils so that marrow production is overwhelmed, or (3) an increase in the proportion of marginated neutrophils. Since increased margination does not require any change in inflow from the bone marrow, the number of immature neutrophils in the blood does not change. One of the most useful determinations in explaining the change in neutrophil concentration of the blood is a ratio of band to segmented neutrophils. If there is a sudden inflow from the bone marrow, the band-segmented ratio will increase. Thus, if neutropenia is accompanied by little or no increase in band: segmented ratio, it is not considered as functionally severe as neutropenia, in which almost all neutrophils of the blood are bands.

Marrow Neutrophil Compartment

Morphological examination of the bone marrow reveals a continuum of neutrophil maturation in which, for functional descriptive purposes, three subcompartments may be distinguished (Fig. 25-7). The production pool consists of those cells capable of undergoing mitosis: myeloblasts, promyelocytes and myelocytes. The postmitotic maturation pool consists of metamyelocytes, bands and segmented neutrophils. A further subdivision of the maturation pool separates the effective storage pool (marrow granulocyte reserve of Craddock[30]) of band and segmented neutrophils from the metamyelocytes which are not

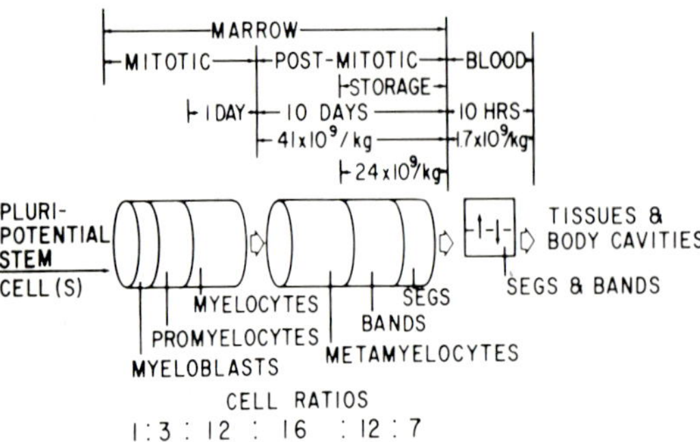

FIG. 25-7. A model of the total neutrophil system. From Boggs D R, Winkelstein A: White Cell Manual, ed 3. Philadelphia, F A Davis, 1975 (with permission).

readily released into the blood. In the average normal subject there are at least 15 times as many band and segmented neutrophils in the bone marrow as there are in the blood. This reserve can be released to the blood upon demand, and such demand is probably controlled by a circulating humoral releasing factor.[31] Therefore, this storage pool constitutes an effective means of rapidly delivering a large number of neutrophils to a site of infection, and can supply the blood with extra cells until production has time to catch up to increasing demands. With a normal marrow structure and even with extreme neutropenia, it is unusual for cells less mature than a band to be released to the blood. Thus, with neutropenia due to increased peripheral cell loss, we see a preserved production pool as well as metamyelocytes, but very few bands and segmented neutrophils are seen in the marrow. This is the circumstance often termed "maturation arrest," a misnomer in the authors' opinion.[32] An explanation for this morphological picture that seems more reasonable than "arrest" is that, with the increased demands for cells in the blood, as is assumed to occur with most instances of neutropenia, as soon as a neutrophil matures to the band stage it is released to the blood and the storage pool is completely exhausted.

In the average normal subject, a period of approximately 11 days is required for a myelocyte to divide, mature into a segmented neutrophil and enter and then leave the blood. It must be realized, however, that much of this time is spent within the storage pool. If there is an increased demand for cells or if the storage pool is attenuated, then the time required for a myelocyte to mature and enter the blood can be markedly reduced.

The exact structure of the production compartment is as yet undetermined. For instance, it is possible that the myeloblast, or for that matter the promyelocyte or myelocyte, is capable of acting as a stem cell. Bainton,[33] however, has published data on dilution of primary granules in cells in the mitotic compartment that suggest that neither the promyelocyte nor the myelocyte self replicates under ordinary circumstances. Conversely, it is possible that the stem cell is as yet unidentified and that all of these compartments are merely doubling compartments. The generation time for the normal myelocyte is probably of the order of 24 hours. Increased production is probably accomplished by a combination of decreasing generation time, "skipped division" and increasing feed in from the stem cell compartment.

The normal site of production for neutrophils is the production pool of the bone marrow (Fig. 25-7). After the last mitosis at the myelocyte stage, a further period of maturation occurs. Normally the mature cells spend a significant length of time in the storage pool of the bone marrow. From this, they are released to the blood for a brief transit and then migrate out of the blood vessels into tissues and body cavities. Here, they presumably provide a cleansing function by phagocytic activities, as well as being immediately available for migration from the blood into beginning inflammatory exudates. The "functional home" of the neutrophil is clearly beyond the blood in tissues, body cavities and beginning exudates. In the absence of a normal number of neutrophils available for migration into such sites, infections are more frequent and are abnormally severe, since they cannot be contained and localized by the rapid entrance of neutrophil into exudates.

Effect of Chemotherapeutic Agents on Stem Cells and Neutrophils

The ideal cancer chemotherapy agent would be one that did not affect normal cells, but would either kill neoplastic cells or lead

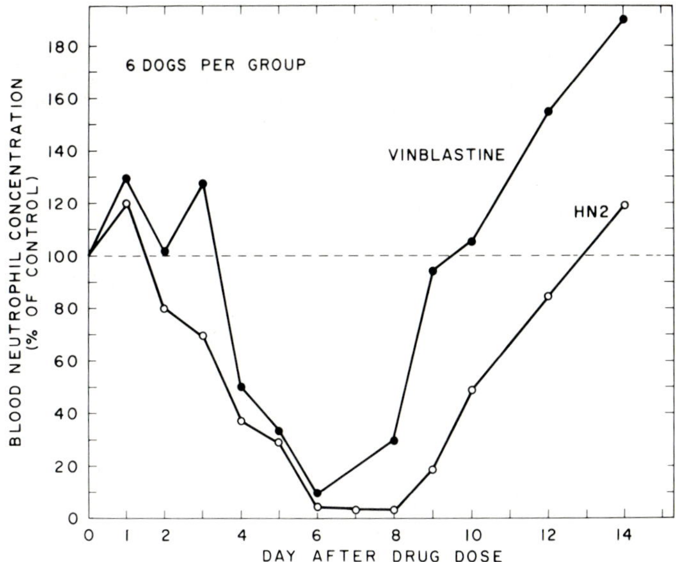

FIG. 25-8. The differing effects of a single dose of vinblastine or nitrogen mustard upon blood neutrophil concentration. Adapted from Boggs D R: The kinetics of neutrophilic leukocytes in health and in disease. Semin Hematol 4:359 1967 (with permission).

to a decrease in their production. Although a few agents such as certain hormones, vincristine, asparaginase and bleomycin[34] have minimal affect upon normal hematopoietic cells, the majority of chemotherapeutic agents have a straight dose-related hematopoietic toxicity. Certain patients are sensitive to even the agents enumerated above. For instance, we have observed a few patients whose normal bone marrow cells were eradicated by a single dose of asparaginase; other investigators have made similar observations.[35]

To understand the effects of chemotherapeutic agents upon hematopoietic cells, it is important to know whether they are cycle-active or non-cycle-active. A cycle-active drug affects only cells which are in an active generative cycle. Most of these act as inhibitors of DNA synthesis, such as hydroxyurea, or as mitotic inhibitors, such as vinblastine. Non-cycle-active agents, such as x-irradiation and various alkylating agents, will damage cells in an active mitotic cycle but will also have severe effects upon potentially dividing cells. Still other agents, such as 6-MP and cyclophosphamide, have effects which are intermediate between the two, but are probably more active upon cells that are in a generative cycle.[36] Actually, there may be no such thing as a truly cycle-independent antitumor agent; all may be more or less active in specific stages of the cell cycle. For example, cells in DNA synthesis appear to be relatively protected from damage by irradiation.

This distinction between cycle-active or non-cycle-active becomes most important when it is remembered that the normal pluripotential stem cell compartment is not in a generative cycle. Thus, in the purest type of system which one can devise, namely, a single dose of a cycle- or non-cycle-active agent, quite different effects upon normal cell level are observed. The neutrophil concentration following a single dose of vinblastine sulfate (cycle-active) or a single dose of nitrogen mustard (non-cycle-active) to normal dogs is shown in Figure 25-8. Both of these agents led to comparable degrees of neutropenia; however, the neutropenia due to nitrogen mustard was of longer duration, and recovery was significantly slower than that due to vinblastine. Vinblastine, a cycle-active agent, would not be expected to significantly damage the pluripotential stem cell compartment if given in a single dose. Therefore, regeneration of identifiable compartments could be

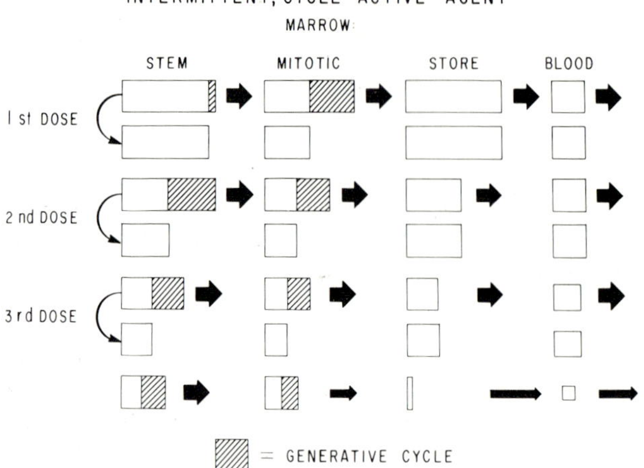

FIG. 25-9. The effect of repeated doses of a cycle-active agent on the neutrophil system. The drug is assumed to act only on cells in DNA synthesis (shaded area of compartments). From Boggs D R, Winkelstein A: White Cell Manual, ed 3. Philadelphia, F A Davis, 1975 (with permission).

accomplished very rapidly from this intact back-up system. This was evidenced by study of the bone marrow of such dogs, in which a return of myeloblasts, promyelocytes and myelocytes occurred quickly and the neutropenia was quite brief.[37] Conversely, nitrogen mustard would damage the pluripotent stem cell compartment. Before the mature compartment could fully recover, therefore, a certain amount of self-replication would be demanded in the stem cell compartment and, thus, a slower recovery would be expected.

The above difference in drug effect on neutrophil kinetics is not limited completely to effects on the proliferating compartments.[37] Note the difference in pattern of onset of neutropenia between these two drugs (Fig. 25-8). With vinblastine sulfate, neutrophil levels were maintained for 3 days, but more gradually developing neutropenia occurred with nitrogen mustard. Kinetic study of these two situations indicated that after administration of vinblastine sulfate, the storage pool of the marrow was able to feed into the blood at a regular rate until it was exhausted, whereas feed-in from the storage pool was gradually reduced by nitrogen mustard. A possible explanation for these two differences is that nitrogen mustard also damages the structural characteristics of the marrow as well as the proliferation compartments, leading to a damaged output from the storage pool system.

The difference in activity of these two drugs in single doses in dogs is also supported by human chemotherapeutic studies. Vinblastine can be given every 7 to 10 days without producing progressive toxicity in most patients, suggesting that the damage can be repaired in man within this time. This is reasonable considering the time parameters of the marrow neutrophil system. Conversely a much longer period of some weeks is required between dosages of nitrogen mustard if repair of the system is to occur. If nitrogen mustard is given at 7- to 10-day intervals, at a dose that will induce a degree of neutropenia comparable to that after vinblastine, the neutrophil system may become exhausted. This presumably reflects repetitive damage to the pluripotential stem cell pool.

The use of drugs in a single dose is not the ordinary circumstance in which we administer chemotherapy. The effect on neutrophils and stem cells of regularly repeated dosages is much more complex. We have attempted to illustrate this in a theoretical situation in Figure 25-9, showing the effect of giving a repeated single dose of a DNA-inhibiting cycle-active agent upon the stem cell system, the marrow mitotic pool, the marrow storage pool and the blood neutrophil compartment. This theoretical dose of drug is sufficient to destroy any cells that are in an active generative cycle. It is assumed that DNA synthesis accounts for one-half of the cycle.

With the first dose, the stem cell compartment is only very slightly reduced, since only a small proportion is in DNA synthesis. The marrow mitotic pool is reduced by half, since half of it is in DNA synthesis. Neither the marrow storage pool nor the blood is immediately affected. By the time the second dose is administered, the stem cell pool has hypertrophied slightly in response to the damage in the more mature compartments. Half of it is now in DNA synthesis and, with the second dose, half of it is destroyed. Again the marrow mitotic pool is reduced by half, and since it had not fully regenerated, it is smaller than after the first dose. The marrow storage pool again is not affected by the second dose, but is smaller than normal because of reduced feed-in from the marrow mitotic pool and continued output to the blood. Since significant storage remains, the blood has not been affected. By the time of the third dose, some regeneration has ocurred in the stem cell compartment, but it is not back to normal, and half is still in DNA synthesis. Therefore, it is again reduced by half and the same is true for the marrow mitotic pool. Again, because of continued normal feed-in to the blood and subnormal feed-in from the marrow mitotic pool, the marrow storage pool is now quite small. It is still maintaining the blood at a near-normal size, however. By the time the next dose is due, disaster has struck. There is severe neutropenia, since the storage pool has become completely exhausted and feed-in into the blood is markedly reduced.

If we are correct in our hypothesis that a severely reduced stem cell pool will not differentiate until it is reconstituted to a certain size, it is possible that feed-in from that pool to the marrow mitotic pool would cease at some point in Figure 25-9, and a still longer delay would be required before recovery of blood cells occurred.

The main practical point to be considered from this type of kinetic diagram is the insensitivity of the blood neutrophil level to the degree of damage occurring in the system.

It cannot be emphasized too strongly that the last compartment in which damage appears is the blood compartment. By the time neutropenia appears, severe damage to the entire system has occurred.

If the time between dosages of the drug shown in Figure 25-9 were lengthened until complete repair, and even over-shoot in the stem cell and marrow mitotic compartment, had occurred between dosages, neutropenia would not develop or would at most be transient. The storage pool serves as an effective buffer between the production compartment and the blood. The question that remains is whether or not a spaced dose of chemotherapeutic agents can be found that will avoid serious long-term damage to the neutrophil system, but will still have effective antitumor activity. As previously noted, the ideal chemotherapeutic agent is one that affects tumor cells, but not normal cells. Lacking such agents, we can exploit studies of differences in generative times of tumor cell populations and normal cell populations.

Various studies suggest that many tumor cell populations in man have a slower generative cycle than do normal hematopoietic cells.[38] In this case these differences can be exploited, even if they are slight, by properly timed doses of cell-killing chemotherapy. A theoretic graph of the effect of such timing is illustrated in Figure 25-10.

In Figure 25-10, we have assumed that we are dealing with a normal hematopoietic cell population with a generation time (in this case considered synonomous with the doubling time) of 24 hours. Generation and doubling times are the same, assuming there is no cell loss in the compartment and all cells are in cycle. In this system, the tumor which we are attacking has a longer generation and doubling time (36 hours) than the normal cell compartment (24 hours). We are administering a non-cycle-active drug which will reduce both the normal cell population and the tumor cell population to 10 per cent of its original value with each dose, i.e., the tumor and normal cell populations are equally damaged. By timing the dosage to approximately 3.5 days, the normal cell population returns to base line levels between doses. The tumor cell population, however, with its slower growth rate, does not attain these levels. Yet the proportional reduction with each dose leads to a pro-

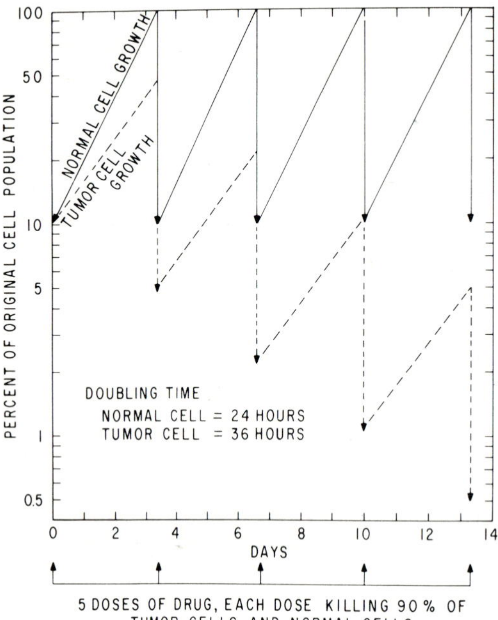

FIG. 25-10. Differential effect of an antitumor agent given in repeated dosages on normal cells and tumor cells (see text).

gressive decrease in total tumor cell population. By these means the normal cell population is never reduced to more than 10 per cent of its starting value, whereas following the fifth dose, the tumor cell population is reduced to less than 1 per cent of its original value. This type of therapy has been effective in murine leukemia[39] and may form the basis for the effectiveness of certain intermittent therapeutic regimens in man. It must be remembered, however, that a number of assumptions, all of which are unproven, are built into this type of theoretic design:

1. The normal hematopoietic system can repair itself from chemotherapeutic damage with equal facility following an infinite number of dosages. Studies attempting to exhaust the recovery potential of the murine hematopoietic system are equivocal in their results,[40] but most investigators have the clinical impression that in man the more exposure to chemotherapeutic agents the patient has, the less capable is his bone marrow of recovery.
2. The rate of tumor cell growth remains constant for various sizes of tumor cell populations. There is now evidence in certain murine tumors and in human myeloma[41] that this is a false assumption and that tumor cell growth slows as tumor mass increases. Growth rate thus analyzed using Gompertzian kinetics[42] is not constant, suggesting that as tumor size is reduced, rate of regrowth may accelerate and equal or exceed that of normal tissue.
3. The overall assumption that a tumor can be destroyed simply by killing the cells composing it.

However, this type of consideration gives strong emphasis to efforts designed to measure not only normal cell generation and doubling times but tumor cell generation and doubling times in man.

Methods of Predicting Degree of Hematopoietic Toxicity

Normal stem cell assays in man are still in their infancy and at the present time are limited to assaying what are probably committed stem cells for granulocytic and mononuclear cells[23] and erythropoietin-responsive red cells precursors.[43] As more thorough and sophisticated assays for this class of cell become available, however, it may be the most important means of determining how susceptible a patient may be to the hematological ravages of chemotherapy.

At present there are methods available for determining the relative size of the neutrophil system at the beginning of chemotherapy or during courses of chemotherapy. As should be evident from the preceding discussion of normal neutrophil kinetics and of the effect of chemotherapy on neutrophils, merely measuring the concentration of neutrophils in venous blood samples is entirely unsatisfactory as a means of assessing the size of the neutrophil system. If a careful look at a blood smear is coupled with blood neutrophil concentration measurements, a bit more information can be obtained. If the predominant cell on blood smears is a band rather than a segmented neutrophil, then in all probability the marrow storage pool is markedly reduced in size and the patient is likely to develop severe neutropenia even at chemotherapeutic dosages calculated to be benign.

Perhaps the most widely used methods of assessing the size of the marrow neutrophil storage pool are measuring the blood neutrophil response after the injection of endotoxin, corticosteroids or etiocholanolone.[44,45] If there is an existing storage pool that is functionally normal, there will be an increase in concentration of blood neutrophils following the injection of one of these drugs. The primary disadvantage of these techniques, however, is that they do not measure the size of the storage pool. If there is no response, one can be relatively certain that the store is functionally absent. There is no guarantee, however, that a store significantly reduced in size would not feed out enough neutrophils to provide a normal blood neutrophil rise in response to these agents. Thus, these crude tests can determine if there is or is not a storage pool, but they can give little assessment of its size.

Careful examination of a marrow aspirate probably gives as much, if not more, information as the above tests and is probably less traumatic to the patient than repeated venipunctures required. If the store is absent, it is visually absent; that is, the marrow has very few bands and segmented neutrophils. If the patient is not anemic, the myeloid to erythroid ratio gives futher semiquantitative information. Alternatively, marrow storage pool size may be estimated from marrow mass calculations based on plasma iron turnover. Finch and co-workers[46] have demonstrated that, in the absence of marked iron overload and with the exception of the patient who is producing few or no red cells, there is a fairly good correlation between plasma iron turnover and the marrow nucleated red cell mass. Using this estimate of total nucleated red cell precursors and the myeloid to erythroid ratio of a marrow aspirate, a rough quantitation of marrow neutrophil mass can be computed. In a recent study of neutropenic patients, however, estimates of the storage pool were compared based on blood neutrophil concentration, M:E ratio, marrow differential counts, and marrow mass measurements derived from plasma iron turnover and M:E ratio. The marrow differential count was the most predictive of marrow reserve. All patients who responded normally to endotoxin had >25 per cent of marrow neutrophils and neutrophil precursors that were band and segmented forms while, with one exception, subnormal responders to endotoxin had fewer than 25 per cent.[47]

The coupling of a needle biopsy of the marrow with examination of a smear from a marrow aspirate gives additional information. In a good biopsy specimen, if the cellular portion of the marrow exceeds or is equal to the fat spaces, then one can be reasonably assured that a normal marrow mass is present. The major problem in interpreting marrow biopsies, however, is whether this small sample is representative of the entire marrow. There is reasonably good evidence that cell ratios are constant from one portion of the active marrow to another in man, with the exception of diseases such as multiple myeloma. There are no studies which assure us that the overall cellularity of the marrow, as measured by biopsy, is similar from one site to another, however.

Chemotherapeutic Effects on Other Leukocytic Systems

The effect of chemotherapeutic agents upon lymphocytes and monocytes, and perhaps upon eosinophils and basophils, is unquestionably of significant consequence to the patient. We have not, however considered these cells in detail for two reasons: (1) the kinetics of these cell types in man are as yet only partially understood and (2) there are no reliable means of measuring the effect of chemotherapy upon these cellular systems. Some brief consideration concerning the lymphocytic and monocytic systems, however, is certainly justified.

Monocytes are excellent phagocytes moving into the tissues from blood, and there becoming macrophages. Monocytes arise from the bone marrow from as yet unidentified precursors[48] and probably have a common origin with the neutrophil.[26] In addition to the role of killing offending organisms, they play a role in the development of the immune response. Antigen is processed by macrophages, and a product of this processing, whether antigen or a related product, stimulates antibody formation by the lymphocytic system.[1] Most chemotherapeutic agents, if delivered in sufficient dosage, reduce the number of monocytes, but the clinical consequence of this effect has not been clearly delineated.

In an oversimplified view[1] the function of the lymphocyte is to form humoral antibodies, represented by circulating immunoglobulins, and cell-bound antibodies, such as those involved in skin hypersensitivity reactions and in tissue transplantation rejection. Generalizing from studies in animals, one can state that the lymphocytes that are produced in the bone marrow migrate through the thymus where they are acted upon either by thymic lymphocytes or by thymic factors. These modified immunocytes thereafter move into peripheral lymphocyte tissues where they form the functioning immunocyte system.

Most small lymphocytes of the blood are cells with an exceedingly long life-span.[49] Actually, "life-span" is a misnomer, since the lymphocyte is capable of being its own stem cell and producing two identical progenitors by cell division. As judged by chromosomal studies in patients subjected to irradiation, however, the average intermitotic interval for the small blood lymphocyte is probably 2 years or more.[49] Blood lymphocytes, particularly thymic-derived lymphocytes, constantly recirculate, leaving the blood through specialized postcapillary endothelial networks in lymph nodes where they make up the cuff of small lymphocytes surrounding the germinal follicles of the node. Leaving the nodes, they are picked up by lymphatics and reenter the blood through the thoracic duct.

The recirculation of lymphocytes can be modified by a variety of means. A decrease in the concentration of blood lymphocytes accompanies almost any stressful phenomenon and follows almost all varieties of chemotherapy as an acute response. There is little or no evidence to suggest that this transient type of lymphopenia represents either a decrease in lymphocyte production or an increase in lymphocyte destruction. It may represent simply a redistribution of lymphocytes. Any factor that induces a change in the recirculatory pattern of this cell will produce a profound effect upon blood lymphocyte concentration, since the overwhelming majority of small lymphocytes are not in the blood, but are in the recirculatory phase in the tissues. For this reason, interpretation of lymphopenia, as such, is exceedingly difficult.

Many chemotherapeutic agents lead to reduced antibody formation and, indeed, this characteristic has been utilized in employing these agents for immune suppression in nonmalignant diseases. Antibody production by lymphocytes, whether of the cell-bound or humoral variety, probably depends on some variation of the following: Antigen with or without modification by macrophages stimulates the small lymphocyte to proliferate into a blast-like stage. The cell divides and produces progeny capable of producing antibody to the offending antigen. If of a cell-bound nature, the cell remains a lymphocyte in morphologic appearance and carries the antibody. If of a humoral nature, the cell converts to a plasma cell that produces and releases immunoglobulins. If this is a new antigen in the experience of the host, this new information is coded into a previously uncommitted immunologically competent small lymphocyte. If the host has prior experience with the antigen, a small lymphocyte carrying the memory for antibody production to that antigen is stimulated. The first, or primary, response is a more delayed response than the secondary antibody response. In either event, cell proliferation is probably required, and all chemotherapeutic agents that reduce capacity for cell proliferation in all probability have some influence upon the potential immune response. Quantitation of this effect in man lags behind our understanding of the effects of chemotherapy upon the neutrophil system. This lag in understanding does not necessarily imply a difference in the importance of the two mechanisms.

It may prove that chemotherapeutic damage to the immune system is of greater long-range importance than is damage to the neutrophil system. As a theoretical example, let us consider the possibility that the normal immune system is in the process of trying to contain and banish the offending tumor that has invaded its province. By administering overly vigorous chemotherapy, we may not only reduce the size of existing tumor tissue, but also reduce the ability of the immune system to cope with tumor tissue. Perhaps the occasional apparent cures resulting from chemotherapy[50] represent reduction of tumor size to a level that the host can control, rather than killing all cells by chemotherapy per se.

Chemotherapy is a two-edged sword with respect to the treatment of cancer. If it is ever to be considered curative, it must reduce the tumor cell population either to zero or to a degree where the host is able to manage the cancer with its own defense system. If reduction of the tumor cell population to zero is the aim, then enough normal cells must be preserved to allow the host to survive, and of course, the inciting factor leading to the original malignant proliferation must have disappeared for the cancer to be cured. Alternatively, if one assumes that at least certain patients have developed some degree of resistance to their own tumor, and that they can be helped by reducing the tumor population to the point that they can handle it themselves, then severe damage to the immune system must be avoided.

References

1. Boggs D R, Winkelstein A: White Cell Manual. ed 3, Philadelphia, F A Davis, 1975
2. Rowley J: A new consistent chromosomal abnormality in chronic myelogenous leukaemia identified by quinacrine fluorescence and Giemsa staining. Nature 243:290, 1973
3. Whang J, Frei E III, Tjio J H, et al: The distribution of the Philadelphia chromosome in patients with chronic myelogenous leukemia. Blood 22:664, 1963
4. Aster R H, Enright S E: A platelet and granulocyte membrane defect in paroxysmal nocturnal hemoglobinuria: Usefulness for the detection of platelet antibodies. J Clin Invest 48:1119, 1969
5. Fialkow P J, Lisker R, Detter J, et al: 6-phosphogluconate dehydrogenase: Hemizygous manifestation in a patient with leukemia. Science 163:194, 1969
6. Jacobson R, Fialkow P J: Idiopathic myelofibrosis: Stem cell abnormality and probable neoplastic origin. Clin Res 24:439(A), 1976
7. Adamson J W, Fialkow P J, Murphy S, et al: Polycythemia vera: Stem-cell and probable clonal origin of the disease. N Engl J Med 295:913, 1976
8. Till J E, McCulloch E A: A direct measurement of the radiation sensitivity of normal mouse bone marrow cells. Radiat Res 14:213, 1961
9. Becker A J, McCulloch E A, Till J E: Cytological demonstration of the clonal nature of spleen colonies derived from transplanted mouse marrow cells. Nature 197:452, 1963
10. Boggs D R, Chervenick P A: Hematopoietic stem cells. In Greenwalt T J, Jamieson G A, (eds): Formation and Destruction of Blood Cells. Philadelphia, Lippincott, 1970, pp 240–255
11. Becker A J, McCulloch E A, Siminovitch L, Till J E: The effect of differing demands for blood cell production on DNA synthesis by hematopoietic colony-forming cells of mice. Blood 26:296, 1965
12. Wu A M, Till J E, Siminovitch L, McCulloch E A: Cytological evidence for a relationship between normal hematopoietic colony-forming cells and cells of the lymphoid system. J Exp Med 127:455, 1968
13. McCaffrey R, Harrison T A, Packman R, Baltimore D: Terminal deoxynucleotidyl transferase activity in human leukemia cells and in normal human thymocytes. N Engl J Med 292:775, 1975
14. Sarin P S, Anderson P N, Gallo R C: Terminal deoxynucleotidyl transferase activities in human blood leukocytes and lymphoblast cell lines: High levels in lymphoblast cell lines and in blast cells of some patients with chronic myelogenous leukemia in acute phase. Blood 47:11, 1976
15. Boggs D R: Hematopoietic stem cell theory in relation to possible lymphoblastic conversion of chronic myeloid leukemia. Blood 44:449, 1974
16. Chervenick, P A, Boggs D R: Pattern of hematopoietic stem cell repopulation. Clin Res 17:114, 1969
17. Chervenick P A, Boggs D R: A kinetic model of hematopoietic stem cell repopulation and differentiation. J Clin Invest 48:47A, 1969
18. Marsh J C, Boggs D R, Bishop C R, et al: Factors influencing hematopoietic spleen colony formation in irradiated mice. I. The normal pattern of endogenous colony formation. J Exp Med 126:835, 1967
19. Boggs S S, Chervenick P A, Boggs D R: The effect of post-irradiation bleeding or endotoxin in proliferation and differentiation of hematopoietic stem cells. Blood 40:375, 1972
20. Chervenick P A, Boggs D R: The effect of altered rates of erythropoiesis on granulocytopoiesis. J Clin Invest 47:19A, 1968
21. Bradley T R, Metcalf D: The growth of mouse

bone marrow cells in vitro. Aust J Exp Biol Med Sci 44:287, 1966
22. Pike B L, Robinson W A: Human bone marrow colony growth in agar-gel. J Cell Physiol 76:77, 1970
23. Chervenick P A, Boggs D R: In vitro growth of granulocytic and mononuclear colonies from blood of normal individuals. Blood 37:131, 1971
24. Bennett M, Cudkowicz G, Foster R S, Metcalf D: Hematopoietic progenitor cells of W anemic mice studied in vivo and in vitro. J Cell Physiol 71:211, 1968
25. Heath D S, Axelrod A A, McLeod D L, Shreeve M M: Separation of the erythropoietin-responsive progenitor BFU-E and CFU-E in mouse bone marrow by unit gravity sedimentation. Blood 47:777, 1976
26. Athens J W: Blood: Leukocytes. Ann Rev Physiol 25:195, 1963
27. Boggs D R: The kinetics of neutrophilic leukocytes in health and in disease. Semin Hematol 4:359, 1967
28. Dancey J T, Deubelbeiss K A, Harker L A, Finch C A: Neutrophil kinetics in man. J Clin Invest 58:705, 1976
29. Joyce R A, Boggs D R, Hasiba U, Srodes C H: Marginal neutrophil pool size in normal subjects and neutropenic patients as measured by epinephrine infusion. J Lab Clin Med 88:614, 1976
30. Craddock C G, Perry S, Lawrence J S: The dynamics of leukopenia and leukocytosis. Ann Intern Med 52:281, 1960
31. Boggs D R, Chervenick P A, Marsh J C, et al: Neutrophil releasing activity in the plasma of dogs injected with endotoxin. J Lab Clin Med 72:177, 1968
32. Joyce R A, Boggs D R, Chervenick P A: Neutrophil kinetics in hereditary and congenital neutropenias. N Engl J Med 295:1385, 1976
33. Bainton D F, Ullyot J L, Farquhar M G: The development of neutrophilic polymorphonuclear leukocytes in human bone marrow: Origin and content of azurophil and specific granules. J Exp Med 134:907, 1971
34. Boggs S S, Sartiano G P, DeMessa A: Minimal bone marrow damage in mice given bleomycin. Cancer Res 34:1938, 1974
35. Ho D H, Whitecar J P, Luce J K, Frei E: L-asparagine requirement and the effect of L-asparaginase on the normal and leukemic human bone marrow. Cancer Res 30:466, 1970
36. Bruce W R, Meeker B E, Valeriote F A: Comparison of the sensitivity of normal hematopoietic and transplanted lymphoma colony-forming cells to chemotherapeutic agents administered in vivo. J Nat Cancer Inst 37:233, 1966
37. Boggs D R, Athens J W, Cartwright G E, Wintrobe M M: The different effects of vinblastine sulfate and nitrogen mustard upon neutrophil kinetics in the dog. Proc Soc Exp Biol Med 121:1085, 1966
38. Mauer A M, Fisher V: Characteristics of cell proliferation in four patients with untreated acute leukemia. Blood 28:428, 1966
39. Simpson-Herren L, Harris H: Kinetic parameters and growth curves for experimental tumor systems. Cancer Chemother Rep 54:143, 1970
40. Boggs D R, Marsh J C, Chervenick P A, et al: Factors influencing hematopoietic spleen colony formation in irradiated mice. III. The effect of repetitive irradiation upon proliferative ability of colony-forming cells. J Exp Med 126:871, 1967
41. Sullivan P W, Salmon S E: Kinetics of tumor growth and regression in IgG multiple myeloma. J Clin Invest 51:1697, 1972
42. Laird A K: dynamics of relative growth. Growth 29:249, 1965
43. Iscove N N, Sieber F, Winterhalter K H: Erythroid colony formation in cultures of mouse and human bone marrow: Analysis of the requirement for erythropoietin by gel filtration and affinity chromalography on agarose-concanavalin A. J Cell Physiol 83:309, 1974
44. Wolff S M, Rubenstein M, Mulholland J H, Alling D W: Comparison of hematologic and febrile response to endotoxin in man. Blood 26:190, 1965
45. Dale D C, Fauci A S, Guerry D, Wolff S M: Comparison of agents producing a neutrophilic leukocytosis in man. J Clin Invest 56:808, 1975
46. Finch C A, Deubelbeiss K, Cook J D, et al: Ferrokinetics in man. Medicine 49:17, 1970
47. Joyce R A, Boggs D R: Visualizing the marrow granulocyte reserve. Clin Res 24:312(A), 1976
48. Volman A, Gowans J L: The origin of macrophages from bone marrow in the rat. Br J Exp Pathol 46:62, 1965
49. Ford W L, Gowans J L: The traffic of lymphocytes. Semin Hematol 6:67, 1969
50. Burchenal J D: Long term survivors in acute leukemia. Cancer Res. 25:1491, 1965

Jack Levin

26 Chemotherapy and Thrombopoiesis

The effects of various drugs on thrombopoiesis can be better understood by first considering the physiologic mechanisms that produce and maintain normal levels of circulating platelets. Platelets are nonnucleated, but are structured pieces of megakaryocytes that enter the circulation after the megakaryocytes mature and demarcation of their cytoplasm into platelets has occurred. Studies of the kinetics of platelet production indicate that cells recognized as megakaryocytes do not replicate, and that the megakaryocyte pool is maintained by the entry of new cells from a yet unidentified population of precursor cells.[1,2] DNA synthesis, however, in immature megakaryocytes (endoreduplication) results in polyploid cells.[3-6] Recognizable megakaryocytes usually contain a multilobed (or segmented) nucleus[2-4, 7-9] and have ploidy levels of 8N, 16N, or 32N (diploid cells are 2N), based on measurements of DNA content.[1,3-5,10-12] Megakaryocytes, at any level of ploidy, are capable of undergoing cytoplasmic maturation with subsequent production of platelets.[1,2,4,5,8-10] The nonreplicating, but polyploid nature of megakaryocytes makes them unique elements of the bone marrow.

Many experimental studies in rodents and dogs have demonstrated that the production of platelets by megakaryocytes normally reflects the level of circulating platelets. Thrombocytopenia produced either by exchange transfusion or by administration of platelet antiserum is followed by an increased production of platelets; subsequently platelet levels rise to greater than normal ("rebound thrombocytosis").[13-17] Increased platelet production is associated with an increase in the number and size of megakaryocytes,[7,16,18-21] their rate of maturation,[15,18,22,23] and the influx of precursor cells into the pool of identifiable megakaryocytes.[15,18,19,22] Conversely, thrombocytosis produced by hypertransfusion of platelets is followed by rebound thrombocytopenia, which has been interpreted as secondary to suppression of platelet production.[24-27] Reduction of the number of megakaryocytes 3 to 4 days after the induction of thrombocytosis,[25] and a decrease in the number and size of megakaryocytes after 4 to 10 days of thrombocytosis[7,28] also suggests decreased thrombopoiesis. Furthermore, the fact that platelet

Carried out under Contract COO-3014-19 between the U.S. Energy Research and Development Administration and the Johns Hopkins University, and supported in part by Graduate Training Grant No. TI-AM-5260 from the National Institute of Arthritis, Metabolism, and Digestive Diseases, National Institutes of Health, Bethesda, Maryland.

production is suppressed in these circumstances has been suggested by decreases in the rate at which radioactively labeled platelets appear in the circulation after the administration of $Na_2{}^{35}SO_4$ or selenomethionine-^{75}Se(^{75}SeM), isotopes that are incorporated into the cytoplasm of megakaryocytes.[29] It appears that thrombopoiesis is not totally suppressed by sustained thrombocytosis,[30] just as erythropoiesis is not uniformly suppressed by polycythemia.[31,32]

Both stimulation and suppression of thrombopoiesis in rats after the production of thrombocytopenia or thrombocytosis, respectively, are detectable only after a delay of approximately 18 to 24 hours.[16,19,21,23,25] Adjustment in the rate of thrombopoiesis apparently occurs at the level of megakaryocytic precursors or Stage I megakaryocytes,[7,16,19,20,28] and subsequently a population of megakaryocytes that has been altered in number, ploidy, size and rate of maturation can be identified in the bone marrow. Maximal rebound thrombocytosis or rebound thrombocytopenia, after the induction of thrombocytopenia or thrombocytosis, occurs approximately 6 days after alteration of the platelet levels of rabbits and rats.[16,17,25,27] This period of time is that which is required for two consecutive populations (cohorts) of megakaryocytes to enter the marrow pool, mature, and release platelets.[33,34]

Limited but similar data have been obtained in humans. The administration of ^{3}H-thymidine to one patient resulted in a gradual increase of the fraction of labeled megakaryocytes in the marrow, with the maximum labeled fraction (50 per cent) occurring at 6 days.[24] The administration of $Na_2{}^{35}SO_4$ or ^{75}SeM to humans resulted in the gradual appearance of labeled platelets in the circulation, with maximum levels reached approximately 6 to 9 days after the isotope was administered.[35-37] This is compatible with the initial incorporation of $Na_2{}^{35}SO_4$ or ^{75}SeM into the cytoplasm of megakaryocytes, maturation of these cells, and then the release of labeled platelets into the circulation. Harker demonstrated alterations in the number and size of megakaryocytes in abnormal hematologic states characterized by thrombocytopenia or thrombocytosis; he has shown a correlation between megakaryocyte mass and platelet turnover,[38,39] except in states of ineffective thrombopoiesis. The average megakaryocyte volume in patients with idiopathic thrombocytopenic purpura was increased, and the magnitude of change was inversely related to the platelet count.[39] In contrast, patients with reactive thrombocytosis had megakaryocytes that were smaller in volume than normal cells,[38] However, Kinet-Denoel et al [10] and Penington and Weste[41] did not observe increased ploidy in the megakaryocytes of patients with idiopathic thrombocytopenic purpura, and Lagerlöf[11] noted normal or increased ploidy in patients with reactive thrombocytosis.

The observations suggest that there is an effective feedback mechanism by which the rate of thrombopoiesis is affected by the level or mass of circulating platelets. Odell et al[19,21] and Ebbe et al[23,42] have suggested that the time lag between the change in platelet levels and the detection of altered megakaryocytopoiesis reflects either mechanisms effective at the level of precursor cells, or a delay in the production of a humoral substance (thrombopoietin) responsible for altered thrombopoiesis, or both. Recent studies in animals and humans have provided evidence for such humoral regulators of platelet production.[27,43-48]

Agents Which Produce Thrombocytopenia

There are many mechanisms by which therapeutic agents cause thrombocytopenia. The varied group of substances utilized as antitumor drugs usually act by directly depressing bone marrow functions and, in particular, thrombopoiesis. This is presumably the result of depression, not only of cells identifiable as megakaryocytes, but also of megakaryocytic precursors. These toxic effects often provide opportunities to confirm data obtained from experimental studies of platelet production or to learn new facts about thrombopoiesis in man.

Antitumor Agents

Acute thrombocytopenia produced by antitumor agents often is followed by rebound thrombocytosis with platelet levels occasionally exceeding 1,000,000/mm^3.[49] The administration of cytosine arabinoside by acute intravenous injection is followed by maximal thrombocytopenia 12 days later and by maximum rebound thrombocytosis at 22 days.[50] Folic acid antagonists produce maximal thrombocytopenia 9 to 15 days after administration, with a subsequent rebound thrombocytosis.[51,52] Rebound thrombocytosis, after therapy with amethopterin was started, reached a maximum at about 18 to 22 days, or 7 to 10 days after thrombocytopenia.[52] In contrast, a large dose of mechlorethamine (nitrogen mustard), a non-cycle-active agent, although producing maximal thrombocytopenia at 10 to 15 days, was not associated with rebound thrombocytosis.[53] Non-cycle-active agents injure cells regardless of their stage in the mitotic cycle (including resting phase, or nonproliferating cells). Cycle-active (or cycle-dependent) drugs are antimetabolic agents that exert their primary effects on cells in a specific stage of the generation cycle.

The data strongly suggest that these agents damage megakaryocytic precursors and megakaryoblasts, thus decreasing the input of new platelets into the circulation. Maximal depression of platelet levels, 10 to 15 days after administration of drug, is compatible with estimations of the life span of human platelets.[54,55] Rebound thrombocytosis, approximately 10 days after thrombocytopenia, supports the concept of a feedback mechanism in humans, and possibly represents the response to thrombocytopenia of a cohort of megakaryocytes that have been synchronized, as suggested by Lampkin et al.[56,57]

Some drugs apparently suppress myelopoiesis and thrombopoiesis equally, but this is not always the case. Large dosages of mechlorethamine have produced similar degrees of depression of these hematopoietic elements,[53] as has total-body irradiation.[58] However, the administration of small doses of mechlorethamine on alternate days produced thrombocytopenia in only 20 per cent of cases, whereas anemia and leukopenia occurred in 58 to 87 per cent of the patients studied.[59] Cyclophosphamide, another non-cycle-active agent, produces relatively less thrombocytopenia than leukopenia,[60,61] but, paradoxically, may produce rebound thrombocytosis.[62]

In general, cycle-active agents seem to depress both erythroid and myeloid elements to a significantly greater degree than they do platelet precursors. A striking example of the disparity of the effects of cytosine arabinoside on white blood cells and platelets has been reported by Burke et al,[50] who observed maximal platelet depression at the same time relative leukocytosis occurred, followed by rebound thrombocytosis concomitant with maximal leukopenia. Frei et al[49] reported greater depression of white blood cells than of platelets in 88 patients given cytosine arabinoside in 1-, 2- or 4-day infusions (Table 26-1). Single doses of cytosine arabinoside caused slight leukopenia without thrombocytopenia, whereas the same total amount administered in divided daily dosages produced greater thrombocytopenia with little additional leukopenia (Table 26-2).[63] Similarly, mithramycin produced platelet counts of less than $100{,}000/mm^3$ in only 1 of 23 patients who received 50 $\mu g/kg$ on alternate days, although 52 per cent of patients who received this drug daily (many were administered similar total dosages) developed thrombocytopenia.[64]

Adriamycin, a biosynthetic analogue of Daunorubicin, is another drug that can produce leukopenia as a major side effect in the absence of simultaneous thrombocytopenia.[65] Wang et al[66] reported a frequency of severe leukopenia (white blood cell count less than $2000/mm^3$) of 30 per cent, while severe throm-

TABLE 26-1. *Effect of Cytosine Arabinoside Upon White Blood Cells and Platelets (222 Trials)*

Incidence of Depression			
White Blood Cells/mm³		Platelets/mm³	
3,000-5,000	<3,000	50,000-200,000	<50,000
35	31	26	13

Modified from Frei E III, Bickers J N, Hewlett J S, et al: Dose schedule and antitumor studies of arabinosyl cytosine (NSC-63878). Cancer Res 29:1325, 1969.

Cytosine arabinoside was administered by a single rapid intravenous injection or in a continuous infusion lasting 24, 48, or 96 hours. Hematopoietic suppression increased as the duration of administration was lengthened, and marked leukopenia was more common than thrombocytopenia.

TABLE 26-2. *Effect of Cytosine Arabinoside Upon White Blood Cells and Platelets (8 Trials)*

	Maximal Depression	
	Daily	Single Dose
WBC/mm^3	3,850	4,790
Platelets/mm^3	72,300	237,200

Modified from Talley R W, Vaitkevicius V K: Megaloblastosis produced by a cytosine antagonist 1-β-D-arabinofuranosyl-cytosine. Blood 21:352, 1963.

Cytosine arabinoside (maximal total dose 50 mg/kg) was administered either daily for 4-10 days, or in a single dose. Repeated daily doses produced significant thrombocytopenia.

bocytopenia (platelet count less than 50,000/mm^3) occurred in only 12 per cent. Another study also documented that thrombocytopenia occurred less frequently than leukopenia.[67]

Combination chemotherapy also can be associated with less thrombocytopenia than leukopenia. Following the administration of chemotherapy regimens designated MABOP, MOPP, ABVD, CVP, ABP, and BACOP, the frequency of thrombocytopenia ranged from 11 per cent (ABVD) to 30 per cent (ABP), whereas leukopenia occurred in 27 per cent (BACOP) to 81 per cent (MABOP) of patients.[68,69] The combination of adriamycin and NSC-45388 produced marked leukopenia but infrequent thrombocytopenia.[70] Even following the combination of cyclophosphamide, vincristine, adriamycin and NSC-45388, although levels of granulocytes of less than 1000/mm^3 were produced in 56 per cent of the patients, platelet counts of less than 50,000/mm^3 occurred in only 5 per cent.[70] Similarly, CHOP-Bleo produced more severe leukopenia than thrombocytopenia.[71] A good example of the relative resistance of megakaryocytes and their precursors to combination chemotherapy that produces marked myelosuppression is demonstrated in Table 26-3, that summarizes the relative effects of three different combination schedules upon white blood cells and platelets.[72]

Vincristine, administered intravenously once weekly, produced leukopenia in 25 per cent of the cases, but no instances of thrombocytopenia attributable to the drug were recorded.[73] Experimental studies by Morse and Stohlman demonstrated that doses of vincristine that severely depress erythropoietic activity cause little change in the rate of thrombopoiesis.[74] These studies showed no significant changes in the differential counts or morphology of megakaryocytes in rats given vincristine, despite concomitant depopulation of marrow erythroid elements. Other studies utilizing the same dose of vincristine (0.3 mg/kg) in the same strain of rats, however, demonstrated production of moderate thrombocytopenia and a 40 per cent decrease in numbers of megakaryocytes.[75] Nevertheless, both investigations were compatible with continued entry of precursor cells into the megakaryocytic pool and indicated that vincristine did not halt differentiation of committed stem cells into megakaryocytic precursors. The authors therefore concluded that there were different immediate precursor cells for the differentiated erythroid and megakaryocytic compartments. This is supported by observations that preparations of erythropoietin do not produce thrombocytosis.[18,26] In addition, physiologically increased levels of thrombopoietin (produced by thrombocytopenia) do not stimulate erythropoiesis, and physiologically increased levels of erythropoietin (produced by hypoxia) do not stimulate thrombopoiesis.[76,77] Amphotericin B also produces anemia without apparent concomitant thrombocytopenia.[78,79]

Lindell and Zajicek[80] and Simpson[81] demonstrated that maximal reduction in the number of megakaryocytes in femurs of rats that had received total-body irradiation did not occur until 5 to 7 days after irradiation, suggesting that the damage had occurred to megakaryocyte precursors and not primarily to cells that already were in the pool of recognizable megakaryocytes. Furthermore, irradiation of one femur produced the same changes in that area as when animals received total-body irradiation, indicating that during the period of observation the irradiated marrow had not been recolonized by stem cells from nonirradiated areas of the body.[80] Odell et al[82] reported that the proliferating diploid precursors of megakaryocytes of mice were sensitive to irradiation, in contrast to recognizable megakaryocytes that were radioresis-

TABLE 26-3. *Relative Effects of Combination Chemotherapy upon White Blood Cells and Platelets*

	White blood cell nadir (WBC/mm^3)					Platelet nadir (platelets/mm^3)		
Treatment Schedule*	>4100	3000-4100	2000-3000	1000-2000	<1000	>130,000	75,000-130,000	<75,000
ADR+VCR+MTX	1/23**	3/23	11/23	7/23	1/23	17/23**	2/23	4/23
5-FU+CTX+PRED	3/14	2/14	5/14	4/14	—	13/14	1/14	—
5-FU+CTX+PRED+CAL	6/12	2/12	1/12	1/12	2/12	11/12	—	1/12

Modified from Eagan R T, Ahmann D L, Edmonson J H, et al: Controlled evaluation of the combination of adriamycin (NSC-123127), vincristine (NSC-67574), and methotrexate (NSC-740) in patients with disseminated breast cancer. Cancer Chemother Rep 6:339, 1975.

*ADR = adriamycin; VCR = vincristine; MTX = methotrexate; 5-FU = 5-fluorouracil; CTX = cyclophosphamide; PRED = prednisone; and CAL = calusterone.

**No. of patients with hematologic toxic reaction/No. of patients treated

tant. He also suggested that the time of the nadir of megakaryocyte counts indicated that cell death from radiation might not occur until the second or third division after exposure, and that some megakaryocytic cells would be spared by entering the phases of endomitotic development of polyploidy. In studies of the effects of X-rays on cultured HeLa S3 cells, Tolmach et al[83] observed that although all cells completed the division immediately subsequent to irradiation, 25 per cent were permanently arrested in the second postirradiation mitosis and died. They concluded that lethal damage was preferentially expressed during mitosis, although DNA synthesis also was inhibited.

It is interesting that shortly following total-body or wide field irradiation, the number of platelets either temporarily increases[58,81,84] or a relative 'peak' is observed that interrupts the decrease in platelet counts.[82,84] Odell et al[82] demonstrated that the relative peak observed in mice was preceded by an increase in megakaryocytes, and concluded that this phenomenon was caused by a temporary arrest of platelet production by mature megakaryocytes, along with continued entry of young megakaryocytes into the recognizable megakaryocyte population.

Ebbe and Stohlman have demonstrated that the induction of acute thrombocytopenia either immediately before or after exposure to irradiation partially protects mice against the thrombocytopenic effects of 200 to 400 rads of total-body irradiation.[42] Elson reported that production of thrombocytopenia with a rapidly acting nitrogen mustard partially protects animals against the thrombocytopenic effects of subsequently administered busulfan.[58] Both groups[42,58] concluded that bone marrow stimulation, before the maximal depressive action of busulfan or irradiation, had been protective.

Nitrosoureas (BCNU, CCNU, and methyl-CCNU) produce an unusual pattern of delayed hematologic toxicity. Following the intravenous administration of BCNU (for a 5-day period) or the oral administration of one dose of CCNU or methyl-CCNU, maximum thrombocytopenia occurred at 4 weeks and persisted for 6 to 16 days.[85,86] Although the overall frequency of leukopenia and thrombocytopenia were similar, in some instances severe thrombocytopenia (counts less than 50,000/mm^3) appeared to be more common than severe leukopenia (counts less than 2000/mm^3).[86] Busulfan also may produce severe thrombocytopenia many months after its discontinuation.[87]

Low doses of vincristine and vinblastine may produce thrombocytosis *without* prior thrombocytopenia. This was observed in 13 of 40 cases after weekly intravenous injections of vincristine,[73] and also has been reported by Hwang et al[88] and Robertson and McCarthy.[89] There did not appear to be a significant interval between the time drug therapy was started and the development of thrombocytosis; ces-

TABLE 26-4. *Production of Acute Thrombocytopenia without Suppression of Thrombopoiesis*

Agent	Mechanism	Reference No.
Quinidine*	Immunologic	122,123
Blood Transfusion	Immunologic (post-transfusion purpura)	102,138
Blood transfusion	Intravascular coagulation (hemolytic transfusion reaction)	146,147
Infection	Intravascular coagulation (? endotoxin)	142,143
Malignancy	Intravascular coagulation	143
Blood transfusion	Dilution of circulating platelets	151
Ristocetin	Direct toxic effect on circulating platelets	152

*Many other drugs also produce thrombocytopenia by this mechanism (see text).

sation of the drug seemed to be associated with an immediate drop in the platelet count to pretreatment levels. Thrombocytosis has also been observed in rats after the administration of vincristine.[89-92] Mechanisms that account for these changes are unclear, but it has been suggested that certain dose levels may stimulate thrombopoiesis, even without preceding thrombocytopenia.[90-94]

Another agent has been shown to result in cyclic changes in levels of some circulating blood cells. Kennedy has reported that patients treated with hydroxyurea may show oscillatory changes in levels of circulating white blood cells and platelets;[95] no changes were observed either in reticulocyte counts or hemoglobin levels. These observations support the suggestion of Morley et al[96,97] that the kinetics of normal marrow function may be cyclic and provide additional evidence that committed stem cells of the three hematopoietic cell lines differ significantly from each other.

Other Agents

There are other mechanisms by which drugs or other agents produce thrombocytopenia without suppressing platelet production by megakaryocytes (Table 26-4). Many drugs, including quinidine, quinine, novobiocin, digitoxin, stibophen, cephalothin, chlorothiazide, rifampicin and apronalide (Sedormid), have been shown to produce thrombocytopenia secondary to an antigen-antibody reaction.[98-109] More recent reports, confirmed by in vitro studies, indicate that acetylsalicylic acid, methicillin, ethchlorvynol and iopanoic acid can produce immunologically mediated thrombocytopenia.[110-113] Although immunologic mechanisms seem likely for the isolated thrombocytopenia that has been reported following administration of gold,[114,115] levodopa[116] or methyldopa,[117,118] they have not yet been clearly demonstrated.

The prerequisite components for this phenomenon include the drug, a plasma protein with which the drug binds, antibody to the drug-protein complex, and platelets. Platelets usually are involved only secondarily by providing a surface to which the antigen-antibody complex can adhere.[102,119] Rechallenge of sensitive individuals with offending drugs results in recurrent thrombocytopenia.[102,103,105,107,120,121] Agglutination and lysis of platelets from the patient or from normal donors, inhibition of clot retraction, release of platelet factor 3, stimulation of lymphocytes and complement fixation often can be demonstrated in vitro in the presence of the drug and serum from an affected person that contains the antibody.[99,102,103,106,107,108,120-131] The nature of the antibody appears to be the main factor in determining whether thrombocytopenia, leukopenia or hemolytic anemia is produced in the susceptible patient.[102] Drug-dependent antibodies that are associated with thrombocytopenia usually, but not always, are IgG immunoglobulins.[102,109,132,133] The antibody shows a striking specificity for the drug against which it is active, since quinine cannot be substituted for quinidine,[123] digitoxigenin nor digoxin for digitoxin,[103] chlorothiazide for hydrochlorothiazide,[133] nor diphenhydramine for chlorpheniramine.[134] In one case, thrombocytopenic purpura was produced by nitroglycerin, but not by closely related erythroltetranitrate.[135] Immune thrombocytopenia, secondary to circulating antibody to a metabolic product of a drug but not to the drug itself, has been reported.[136,137] In rare instances, the production of antibodies against *donor* platelets can result in delayed thrombocytopenia (posttransfusion purpura), that takes places when antigen-antibody complexes containing donor platelets or fragments thereof, adhere to platelets of the recipient.[102,138,139] In contrast to the thrombocytopenia that occurs after administration of drugs that depress bone marrow function, drug-induced, immunologically mediated thrombocytopenia is not dose-related, occurs unpredictably after a variable period of exposure to the drug, is usually of sudden onset and is not associated with leukopenia or anemia. In rare instances, however, hemolytic anemia or leukopenia also has been produced concomitantly,[140,141] although not necessarily by the same antibody (vide supra and Ref. 102).

Infection (usually with gram-negative organisms),[142,143] malignancy,[144,145] and hemolytic reactions to blood transfusion[146,147] can result in intravascular coagulopathy that produces both thrombocytopenia and hypofibrinogenemia. Endotoxin or red cell stroma may be the precipitating triggers of the first and last examples,[143,146,147] but the mechanism by which some tumors produce intravascular coagulopathy remains unclear. The production of a thromboplastic substance by tumor cells has been suggested as a possible cause.[143] In other instances, turbulent blood flow in vascular tumors is believed to result in sequestration and destruction of platelets sufficient to produce systemic thrombocytopenia.[148,149] Heparin has been reported to produce thrombocytopenia, often in association with elevated levels of fibrinogen-fibrin degradation products and moderately reduced levels of fibrinogen.[150] These laboratory abnormalities are compatible with the presence of intravascular coagulopathy, but the mechanism remains unknown. Recovery occurred within 5 days of cessation of administration of heparin. Contaminants in some preparations of heparin may be responsible for these effects. The rapid transfusion of large volumes of blood that do not contain viable platelets can produce thrombocytopenia by diluting circulating platelets.[151] Ristocetin, an antibiotic, produces thrombocytopenia in man and rabbits by a direct, dose-related effect on circulating platelets.[152] Lysis of platelets can be demonstrated in vitro by adding the drug to saline suspensions of platelets.[152] Ingestion of alcohol can produce thrombocytopenia, probably as the consequence both of a direct toxic effect on circulating platelets with a resultant shortened platelet survival[153-155] and by depression of thrombopoiesis.[155,156] It also has been suggested that mithramycin (NSC-24559) causes qualitative changes in circulating platelets (and damages the terminal vascular bed) in addition to thrombocytopenia, secondary to hematopoietic depression.[157-159]

The different mechanisms by which thrombocytopenia can be produced without depressing thrombopoiesis should be considered when evaluating any patient who is receiving antitumor agents. Thrombocytosis can be present in patients with malignant disease before therapy.[160-162] The mechanism of thrombocytosis in malignant disease is not understood, and it is not known whether such patients are more resistant to the production of thrombocytopenia by antitumor agents. Harker and Finch[38] have demonstrated overproduction of platelets in patients with thrombocytosis associated with myeloproliferative disorders, suggesting a defective feedback mechanism.

Discussion

The effects of antitumor agents on thrombopoiesis in man and animals strongly support the concept of a feedback mechanism responsive to levels of circulating platelets. Rebound thrombocytosis may be due in part to synchronization of megakaryocytes stimulated by the state of thrombocytopenia during stages of DNA synthesis. Megakaryocytes that mature during a period of thrombocytopenia have increased ploidy and cytoplasmic mass, and probably produce more platelets per megakaryocyte.[3,7,16,20,21,28,38,39] The time required for the development of thrombocytopenia and rebound thrombocytosis after the administration of antitumor agents provides additional evidence that the life-span of platelets in man is approximately 10 days. A similar or perhaps shorter period is required for megakaryoblasts to develop into platelet-producing, mature megakaryocytes.

The dissociation between the production of reticulocytopenia, leukopenia and thrombocytopenia by antitumor agents[49,66,70,72,73,78,95,159,163,164] is most compatible with the existence of biologically different, committed precursors for these three hematopoietic cell lines, with resultant variations in sensitivity to antitumor agents. Such observations also indicate that an important effect of therapeutic doses of most marrow-suppressive drugs is upon committed stem cells, rather than uncommitted or pluripotential stem cells. The administration of ^{75}SeM to rabbits when megakaryocyte function had been severely depressed has provided evidence that megakaryoblasts or their precursors were capable of incorporating and storing this amino acid until function was recovered.[27]

In some studies, single infusions of cytosine arabinoside, a cycle-active drug that blocks DNA synthesis, produced relatively little thrombocytopenia.[49,63] Only megakaryocyte precursors and immature megakaryocytes appear to engage in DNA synthesis;[2,5,21,82] thus, most of the megakaryocyte population escaped damage because the duration of drug effect was not sufficient to significantly alter the input of new cells into the megakaryocyte compartment. When the duration of treatment was extended, however, significant thrombocytopenia occurred.[63]

Another partial explanation for the relative resistance of megakaryocytes to many antitumor drugs is that the thrombopoietin sensitive cell may be in a resting (or nonsynthetic) state, and therefore is not susceptible to the action of ionizing radiation or drugs that cause similar damage.[42,165] Observations that support this concept are the effects on thrombopoiesis of single doses of irradiation or noncycle-active drugs that affect both proliferating and nonproliferating cells and the increased sensitivity of mice to irradiation after the induction of chronic thrombocytopenia, which presumably increases megakaryocyte flux.[42]

Megakaryocytes are unique in that they are polyploid and do not undergo cellular division. This complex state of high ploidy, in addition to an unknown microenvironment,[166] may account for some of the differences observed. Increased ploidy perhaps alters drug uptake. The large amount of DNA present in megakaryocytes may provide these cells with a reserve capability permitting partial inactivation or loss of DNA or synthetic ability, while retaining the potential to produce some platelets.

Thrombocytopenia also can result from the peripheral destruction of platelets, without the suppression of thrombopoiesis (Table 26-4). Some drugs produce thrombocytopenia secondary to an immunologic reaction which includes the production of an antibody against the drug or one of its metabolic products. The resultant damage to platelets causes their removal from the circulation by the reticuloendothelial system. Other mechanisms that result in reduced levels of circulating platelets include intravascular coagulopathy, dilution by administration of large volumes of platelet-poor blood or direct toxic effects on platelets.

References

1. Odell T T Jr, Jackson C W: Megakaryocytopoiesis, in Stohlman F Jr (ed): Hemopoietic Cellular Proliferation. New York, Grune & Stratton, 1970, p 278
2. Ebbe S: Megakaryocytopoiesis, in Gordon A S (ed): Regulation of Hematopoiesis, vol. 2. New York, Appleton-Century-Crofts, 1970, p 1587
3. Odell T T Jr, Jackson C W: Polyploidy and maturation of rat megakaryocytes. Blood 32:102, 1968
4. Paulus J M: DNA metabolism and development of organelles in guinea pig megakaryocytes: A combined ultrastructural, autoradiographic and cytophotometric study. Blood 35:298, 1970

5. Odell T T Jr, Jackson C W, Friday T J: Megakaryocytopoiesis in rats with special reference to polyploidy. Blood 35:775, 1970
6. Garcia A M: Feulgen-DNA values in megakaryocytes. J Cell Biol 20:342, 1964
7. Harker L A: Kinetics of thrombopoiesis. J Clin Invest 47:458, 1968
8. de Leval M: Contribution à l'étude de la maturation des mégacaryocytes dans la moëlle osseuse de cobaye. Arch Biol 79:597, 1968
9. MacPherson G G: Development of megakaryocytes in bone marrow of the rat: An analysis by electron microscopy and high resolution autoradiography. Proc R Soc Lond (Biol) 177:265, 1971
10. Odell T T Jr, Jackson C W, de Leval M, et al: Cytological analysis of megakaryocyte and platelet kinetics, in Paulus J-M (ed): Platelet Kinetics. Amsterdam, North-Holland, 1971, p 183
11. Lagerlöf B: Cytophotometric study of megakaryocyte ploidy in polycythemia vera and chronic granulocytic leukemia. Acta Cytol (Baltimore) 16:240, 1972
12. Penington D G, Streatfield K, Roxburgh A E: Megakaryocytes and the heterogeneity of circulating platelets. Br J Haematol 34:639, 1976
13. Craddock C G, Adams W S, Perry S, et al: The dynamics of platelet production as studied by a depletion technique in normal and irradiated dogs. J Lab Clin Med 45:906, 1955
14. Matter M, Hartmann J R, Kautz J, et al: A study of thrombopoiesis in induced acute thrombocytopenia. Blood 15:174, 1960
15. Odell T T Jr, McDonald T P, Asano M: Response of rat megakaryocytes and platelets to bleeding. Acta Haematol 27:171, 1962
16. Ebbe S, Stohlman F Jr, Overcash J, et al: Megakaryocyte size in thrombocytopenic and normal rats. Blood 32:383, 1968
17. Odell T T Jr, Murphy J R: Effects of degree of thrombocytopenia on thrombocytopoietic response. Blood 44:147, 1974
18. Ebbe S: Megakaryocytopoiesis and platelet turnover. Ser Haematol 1:65, 1968
19. Odell T T Jr, Jackson C W, Friday T J, et al: Effects of thrombocytopenia on megakaryocytopoiesis. Br J Haematol 17:91, 1969
20. MacPherson G G: Changes in megakaryocyte development following thrombocytopenia. Br J Haematol 26:105, 1974
21. Odell T T, Murphy J R, Jackson C W: Stimulation of megakaryocytopoiesis by acute thrombocytopenia in rats. Blood 48:765, 1976
22. Odell T T Jr, Kniseley R M: Thé origin, life span, regulation, and fate of blood platelets, in Tocantins L M (ed): Progress in Hematology, vol. 3. New York, Grune & Stratton, 1962, p 203
23. Ebbe S, Stohlman F Jr, Donovan J, et al: Megakaryocyte maturation rate in thrombocytopenic rats. Blood 32:787, 1968
24. Cronkite E P, Bond V P, Fliedner T M, et al: Studies on the origin, production and destruction of platelets, in Johnson S A, Monto R W, Rebuck J W, et al (eds): Blood Platelets. Boston Little Brown, 1961, p 595
25. Odell T T Jr, Jackson C W, Reiter R S: Depression of the megakaryocyte-platelet system in rats by transfusion of platelets. Acta Haematol 38:34, 1967
26. de Gabriele G, Penington D G: Physiology of the regulation of platelet production. Br J Haematol 13:202, 1967
27. Evatt B L, Levin J: Measurement of thrombopoiesis in rabbits using ^{75}selenomethionine. J Clin Invest 48:1615, 1969
28. Penington D G, Olsen T E: Megakaryocytes in states of altered platelet production: Cell numbers, size and DNA content. Br J Haematol 18:447, 1970
29. Levin J, Evatt B L, Shreiner D P: Measurement of plasma thrombopoiesis stimulating activity using selenomethionine- ^{75}Se: Studies in rabbits and mice, in Baldini M G, Ebbe S (eds): Platelets: Production, Function, Transfusion, and Storage. New York, Grune & Stratton, 1974, p 63
30. Levin J: Humoral control of thrombopoiesis, in Greenwalt T J, Jamieson G A (eds): Formation and Destruction of Blood Cells. Philadelphia, Lippincott, 1970, p 143
31. Stohlman F Jr: Some aspects of erythrokinetics. Semin Hematol 4:304, 1967
32. Schooley J C, Garcia J F: Suppression of erythropoiesis in the plethoric rat by antierythropoietin. Proc Soc Exp Biol Med 133:953, 1970
33. Ebbe S, Stohlman F Jr: Megakaryocytopoiesis in the rat. Blood 26:20, 1965
34. Cooney D P, Smith B A: Maturation time of rabbit megakaryocytes. Br J Haematol 11:484, 1965
35. Vodopick H A, Kniseley R M: Sulfur-35 studies in man: Platelet survival and plasma and urinary radioactivity assayed by beta liquid scintillation spectrometry. J Lab Clin Med 62:109, 1963
36. Najean Y, Ardaillou N: The use of ^{75}Semethionin for the in vivo study of platelet kinetics. Scand J Haematol 6:395, 1969
37. McIntyre P A, Evatt B L, Hodkinson B A, et al: Selenium-75 selenomethionine as a label for erythrocytes, leukocytes, and platelets in man. J Lab Clin Med 75:472, 1970

38. Harker L A, Finch C A: Thrombokinetics in man. J Clin Invest 48:963, 1969
39. Harker L A: Thrombokinetics in idiopathic thrombocytopenic purpura. Br J Haematol 19:95, 1970
40. Kinet-Denoel C, Bassleer R, Andrien J M, et al: Ploidy histograms in ITP, in Paulus J-M (ed): Platelet Kinetics. Amsterdam, North-Holland, 1971, p 280
41. Penington D G, Weste S M: Ploidy histograms in ITP, in Paulus J-M (ed): Platelet Kinetics. Amsterdam, North-Holland, 1971, p 284
42. Ebbe S, Stohlman F Jr: Stimulation of thrombocytopoiesis in irradiated mice. Blood 35:783, 1970
43. Penington D G: Isotope bioassay for "Thrombopoietin." Br Med J 1:606, 1970
44. Harker L A: Regulation of thrombopoiesis. Am J Physiol 218:1376, 1970
45. Shreiner D P, Levin J: Detection of thrombopoietic activity in plasma by stimulation of suppressed thrombopoiesis. J Clin Invest 49:1709, 1970
46. Cooper G W, Cooper B, Chang C-Y: Demonstration of a circulating factor regulating blood platelet production using ^{35}S-sulfate in rats and mice. Proc Soc Exp Biol Med 134:1123, 1970
47. Evatt B L, Shreiner D P, Levin J: Thrombopoietic activity of fractions of rabbit plasma: Studies in rabbits and mice. J Lab Clin Med 83:364, 1974
48. McDonald T P, Cottrell M, Clift R, et al: Purification and assay of thrombopoietin. Exp Hematol 2:355, 1974
49. Frei E III, Bickers J N, Hewlett J S, et al: Dose schedule and antitumor studies of arabinosyl cytosine (NSC-63878). Cancer Res 29:1325, 1969
50. Burke P J, Serpick A A, Carbone P P, et al: A clinical evaluation of dose and schedule of administration of cytosine arabinoside (NSC-63878). Cancer Res 28:274, 1968
51. Holland J F: Symposium on the experimental pharmacology and clinical use of antimetabolites. VIII. Folic acid antagonists. Clin Pharmacol Ther 2:374, 1961
52. Ogston D, Dawson A A, Philip J F: Methotrexate and the platelet count. Br J Cancer 22:244, 1968
53. Sensenbrenner L L, Owens A H Jr: The effects of mechlorethamine on bone marrow function and iron metabolism in man. Johns Hopkins Med J 121:162, 1967
54. Aster R H, Jandl J H: Platelet sequestration in man. I. Methods. J Clin Invest 43:843, 1964
55. Shulman N R, Marder V J, Weinrach R S: Similarities between known anti-platelet antibodies and the factor responsible for thrombocytopenia in idiopathic purpura. Physiologic, serologic and isotopic studies. Ann N Y Acad Sci 124:499, 1965
56. Lampkin B C, Nagao T, Mauer A M: Drug effect in acute leukemia. J Clin Invest 48: 1124, 1969
57. Lampkin B C, McWilliams N B, Mauer A M: Cell kinetics and chemotherapy in acute leukemia. Semin Hematol 9:211, 1972
58. Elson L A: Comparison of the physiological response to radiation and radiomimetic chemicals. Patterns of blood response, in de Hevesy G C, Forssberg A G, Abbatt J D (eds): Advances in Radiobiology. Springfield, C C Thomas, 1957, p 372
59. Dameshek W, Weisfuse L, Stein T: Nitrogen mustard therapy in Hodgkin's disease. Blood 4:338, 1949
60. Mullins G M, Colvin M: Intensive cyclophosphamide (NSC-26271) therapy for solid tumors. Cancer Chemother Rep 59:411, 1975
61. Mullins G M, Anderson P N, Santos G W: High dose cyclophosphamide therapy in solid tumors. Cancer 36:1950, 1975
62. Colvin O M: Unpublished observations
63. Talley R W, Vaitkevicius V K: Megaloblastosis produced by a cytosine antagonist 1-β-D-arabinofuranosyl-cytosine. Blood 21:352, 1963
64. Kennedy B J: Mithramycin therapy in testicular cancer. J Urol 107:429, 1972
65. Hoogstraten B: Adriamycin (NSC-123127) in the treatment of advanced breast cancer: Studies by the Southwest Oncology Group. Cancer Chemother Rep 6:329, 1975
66. Wang J J, Holland J F, Sinks L F: Phase II study of adriamycin (NSC-123127) in childhood solid tumors. Cancer Chemother Rep 6:267, 1975
67. Cortes E P, Holland J F, Wang J J, et al: Adriamycin (NSC-123127) in 87 patients with osteosarcoma. Cancer Chemother Rep 6:305, 1975
68. Bonadonna G, De Lena M, Monfardini S, et al: Combination usage of adriamycin (NSC-123127) in malignant lymphomas. Cancer Chemother Rep 6:381, 1975
69. Skarin A T, Rosenthal D S, Moloney W C, et al: Combination chemotherapy of advanced non-Hodgkin lymphoma with bleomycin, adriamycin, cyclosphosphamide, vincristine, and prednisone (BACOP). Blood 49:759, 1977
70. Gottlieb J A, Baker L H, O'Bryan R M, et al:

Adriamycin (NSC-123127) used alone and in combination for soft tissue and bony sarcomas. Cancer Chemother Rep 6:271, 1975

71. Rodriguez V, Cabanillas F, Burgess M A, et al: Combination chemotherapy ("CHOP-Bleo") in advanced (non-Hodgkin) malignant lymphoma. Blood 49:325, 1977
72. Eagan R T, Ahmann D L, Edmonson J H, et al: Controlled evaluation of the combination of adriamycin (NSC-123127), vincristine (NSC-67574), and methotrexate (NSC-740) in patients with disseminated breast cancer. Cancer Chemother Rep 6:339, 1975
73. Carbone P P, Bono V, Frei E III, et al: Clinical studies with vincristine. Blood 21:640, 1963
74. Morse B S, Stohlman F Jr: Regulation of erythropoiesis. XVIII. The effect of vincristine and erythropoietin on bone marrow. J Clin Invest 45:1241, 1966
75. Ebbe S, Howard D, Phalen E, et al: Effects of vincristine on normal and stimulated megakaryocytopoiesis in the rat. Br J Haematol 29:593, 1975
76. Evatt B L, Spivak J L, Levin J: Relationships between thrombopoiesis and erythropoiesis: With studies of the effects of preparations of thrombopoietin and erythropoietin. Blood 48:547, 1976
77. Shreiner D P, Levin J: The effects of hemorrhage, hypoxia, and a preparation of erythropoietin on thrombopoiesis. J Lab Clin Med 88:930, 1976
78. Brandriss M W, Wolff S M, Moores R, et al: Anemia induced by amphotericin B. JAMA 189:663, 1964
79. Butler W T: Pharmacology, toxicity and therapeutic usefulness of amphotericin B. JAMA 195:371, 1966
80. Lindell B, Zajicek J: The effect of whole-body x-irradiation on the megakaryocytic system in rat femur, in de Hevesy G C, Forssberg A G, Abbatt J D (eds): Advances in Radiobiology. Springfield, C C Thomas, 1957, p 376
81. Simpson S M: Response of megakaryocytes of the 'August' rat to x-irradiation. Int J Radiat Biol 2:181, 1959
82. Odell T T Jr, Jackson C W, Friday T J: Effects of radiation on the thrombocytopoietic system of mice. Radiat Res 48:107, 1971
83. Tolmach L J, Weiss B G, Hopwood L E: Ionizing radiations and the cell cycle. Fed Proc 30:1742, 1971
84. Court Brown W M: Wide field irradiation and the platelet count. Acta Radiologica (Stockholm) 32:407, 1949
85. Ramirez G, Wilson W, Grage T, et al: Phase II evaluation of 1,3-Bis (2-chloroethyl)-1-nitrosourea (BCNU; NSC-409962) in patients with solid tumors. Cancer Chemother Rep 56:787, 1972
86. Moertel C G: Therapy of advanced gastrointestinal cancer with the nitrosoureas. Cancer Chemother Rep 4:27, 1973
87. Galton D A G: Chemotherapy of chronic myelocytic leukemia. Semin Hematol 6:323, 1969
88. Hwang Y F, Hamilton H E, Sheets R F: Vinblastine-induced thrombocytosis. Lancet 2:1075, 1969
89. Robertson J H, McCarthy G M: Periwinkle alkaloids and the platelet-count. Lancet 2:353, 1969
90. Robertson J H, Crozier E H, Woodend B E: The effect of vincristine on the platelet count in rats. Br J Haematol 19:331, 1970
91. Robertson J H, Crozier E H, Woodend B E: Vincristine-induced thrombocytosis studied with ^{75}Se selenomethionine. Acta Haematol 47:356, 1972
92. Choi S, Simone J V, Edwards C C: Effects of vincristine on platelet production, in Baldini M G, Ebbe S (eds): Platelets: Production, Function, Transfusion, and Storage. New York, Grune & Stratton, 1974, p 51
93. Rak K: Effect of vincristine on platelet production in mice. Br J Haematol 22:617, 1972
94. Jackson C W, Edwards C C: Evidence that stimulation of megakaryocytopoiesis by low dose vincristine results from an effect on platelets. Br J Haematol 36:97, 1977
95. Kennedy B J: Cyclic leukocyte oscillations in chronic myelogenous leukemia during hydroxyurea therapy. Blood 35:751, 1970.
96. Morley A: A platelet cycle in normal individuals. Australas Ann Med 18:127, 1969
97. Morley A, King-Smith E A, Stohlman F Jr: The oscillatory nature of hemopoiesis, in Stohlman F Jr (ed): Hematopoietic Cellular Proliferation. New York, Grune & Stratton, 1970, p 3
98. Harrington W J: The purpuras. DM July, 1957, pp 1–51
99. Weintraub R M, Pechet L, Alexander B: Rapid diagnosis of drug-induced thrombocytopenic purpura. Report of three cases due to quinine, quinidine, and dilantin. JAMA 180:528, 1962
100. Huguley C M Jr: Drug-induced blood dyscrasias. DM 1:52, 1963
101. Crosby W H, Kaufman R M: Drug-induced blood dyscrasias. IV. Thrombocytopenia. JAMA 189:417, 1964
102. Shulman N R: A mechanism of cell destruction in individuals sensitized to foreign an-

tigens and its implications in auto-immunity. Ann Intern Med 60:506, 1964

103. Young R C, Nachman R L, Horowitz H I: Thrombocytopenia due to digitoxin. Am J Med 41:605, 1966

104. Sheiman L, Spielvogel A R, Horowitz H I: Thrombocytopenia caused by cephalothin sodium. Occurrence in a penicillin-sensitive individual. JAMA 203:601, 1968

105. Blajchman M A, Lowry R C, Pettit J E, et al: Rifampicin-induced immune thrombocytopenia. Br Med J 3:24, 1970

106. Karpatkin S, Strick N, Karpatkin M B, et al: Cumulative experience in the detection of antiplatelet antibody in 234 patients with idiopathic thrombocytopenic purpura, systemic lupus erythematosus and other clinical disorders. Am J Med 52:776, 1972

107. Gralnick H R, McGinniss M, Halterman R: Thrombocytopenia with sodium cephalothin therapy. Ann Intern Med 77:401, 1972

108. Freedman A L, Brody E A, Barr P S: Immunothrombocytopenic purpura due to quinidine. Report of four new cases with special observations on patch testing. J Lab Clin Med 48:205, 1956

109. Petz L D, Fudenberg H H: Immunologic mechanisms in drug-induced cytopenias, in Brown E B (ed): Progress in Hematology, vol. 9. New York, Grune & Stratton, 1975, p 185

110. Jacobson E S: Fatal immune thrombocytopenia induced by ethchlorvynol. Ann Intern Med 77:73, 1972

111. Garg S K, Sarker C R: Aspirin-induced thrombocytopenia on an immune basis. Am J Med Sci 267:129, 1974

112. Schiffer C A, Weinstein H J, Wiernik P H: Methicillin-associated thrombocytopenia. Ann Intern Med 85:338, 1976

113. Hysell J K, Hysell J W, Gray J M: Thrombocytopenic purpura following iopanoic acid ingestion. JAMA 237:361, 1977

114. Deren B, Masi R, Weksler M, et al: Gold-associated thrombocytopenia. Report of six cases. Arch Intern Med 134:1012, 1974

115. Levin H A, McMillan R, Tavassoli M, et al: Thrombocytopenia associated with gold therapy. Observations on the mechanism of platelet destruction. Am J Med 59:274, 1975

116. Wanamaker W M, Wanamaker S J, Celesia G G, et al: Thrombocytopenia associated with long-term levodopa therapy. JAMA 235:2217, 1976

117. Benraad A H, Schoenaker A H: Thrombopenia after use of methyldopa. Lancet 2:292, 1965

118. Manohitharajah S M, Jenkins W J, Roberts P D, et al: Methyldopa and associated thrombocytopenia. Br Med J 1:494, 1971

119. Shulman N R: Immunoreactions involving platelets. I. A steric and kinetic model for formation of a complex from a human antibody, quinidine as a haptene, and platelets; and for fixation of complement by the complex. J Exp Med 107:665, 1958

120. Day H J, Conrad F G, Moore J E: Immunothrombocytopenia induced by novobiocin. Am J Med Sci 236:475, 1958

121. Kahn H R, Brod R C: Thrombocytopenia due to stibophen. Arch Intern Med 108:496, 1961

122. Larson R K: The mechanism of quinidine purpura. Blood 8:16, 1953

123. Shulman N R: Immunoreactions involving platelets. IV. Studies on the pathogenesis of thrombocytopenia in drug purpura using test doses of quinidine in sensitized individuals; their implications in idiopathic thrombocytopenic purpura. J Exp med 107:711, 1958

124. Ackroyd J F: The pathogenesis of thrombocytopenic purpura due to hypersensitivity to Sedormid (allylisopropyl-acetyl-carbamide). Clinical Science (London) 7:249, 1949

125. Ackroyd J F: The role of complement in Sedormid purpura. Clinical Science (London) 10:185, 1951

126. Bigelow F S, Desforges J F: Platelet agglutination by an abnormal plasma factor in thrombocytopenic purpura associated with quinidine ingestion. Am J Med Sci 224:274, 1952

127. Gynn T N, Messmore H L, Friedman I A: Drug-induced thrombocytopenia. Med Clin North Am 56:65, 1972

128. Deykin D, Hellerstein L J: The assessment of drug-dependent and isoimmune antiplatelet antibodies by the use of platelet aggregometry. J Clin Invest 51:3142, 1972

129. Handin R I, Piessens W F, Moloney W C: Stimulation of nonimmunized lymphocytes by platelet-antibody complexes in idiopathic thrombocytopenic purpura. N Engl J Med 289:714, 1973

130. Dixon R H, Rosse W F: Mechanism of complement-mediated activation of human blood platelets in vitro. Comparison of normal and paroxysmal nocturnal hemoglobinuria platelets. J Clin Invest 59:360, 1977

131. Karpatkin M, Siskind G W, Karpatkin S: The platelet factor 3 immunoinjury technique reevaluated. Development of a rapid test for antiplatelet antibody. Detection in various clinical disorders, including immunologic drug-induced and neonatal thrombocytopenias. J Lab Clin Med 89:400, 1977

132. Eisner E V, Korbitz B C: Quinine-induced thrombocytopenic purpura due to an IgM and an IgG antibody. Transfusion 12:317, 1972
133. Eisner E V, Crowell E B: Hydrochlorothiazide-dependent thrombocytopenia due to IgM antibody. JAMA 215:480, 1971
134. Eisner E V, LaBocki N L, Pinckney L: Chlorpheniramine-dependent thrombocytopenia. JAMA 231:735, 1975
135. Shmushkovich J, Davis E: Thrombocytopenic skin purpura following treatment with trinitrin. Br J Dermatol 67:299, 1955
136. Eisner E V, Shahidi N T: Immune thrombocytopenia due to a drug metabolite. N Engl J Med 287:376, 1972
137. Shulman N R: Immunologic reactions to drugs. N Engl J Med 287:408, 1972
138. Cimo P L, Aster R H: Post-transfusion purpura. Successful treatment by exchange transfusion. N Engl J Med 287:290, 1972
139. Ziegler Z, Murphy S, Gardner F H: Post-transfusion purpura: A heterogeneous syndrome. Blood 45:529, 1975
140. Freedman A L, Barr P S, Brody E A: Hemolytic anemia due to quinidine: Observations on its mechanism. Am J Med 20:806, 1956
141. Castro O, Nash I: Quinidine leukopenia and thrombocytopenia with a drug-dependent leukoagglutinin. N Engl J Med 296:572, 1977
142. Rosner F, Ritz N D: The defibrination syndrome. Arch Intern Med 117:17, 1966
143. Deykin D: The clinical challenge of disseminated intravascular coagulation. N Engl J Med 283:636, 1970
144. Pittman G R, Senhauser D A, Lowney J F: Acute promyelocytic leukemia. Am J Clin Pathol 46:214, 1966
145. Merskey C, Johnson A J, Kleiner G J, et al: The defibrination syndrome: Clinical features and laboratory diagnosis. Br J Haematol 13:528, 1967
146. Krevans J R, Jackson D P, Conley C L, et al: The nature of the hemorrhagic disorder accompanying hemolytic transfusion reactions in man. Blood 12:834, 1957
147. Rock R C, Bove J R, Nemerson Y: Heparin treatment of intravascular coagulation accompanying hemolytic transfusion reactions. Transfusion 9:57, 1969
148. Sutherland D A, Clark H: Hemangioma associated with thrombocytopenia. Am J Med 33:150, 1962
149. Thatcher L G, Clatanoff D V, Stiehm E R: Splenic hemangioma with thrombocytopenia and afibrinogenemia. J Pediatr 73:345, 1968
150. Bell W R, Tomasulo P A, Alving B M, et al: Thrombocytopenia occurring during the administration of heparin. A prospective study in 52 patients. Ann Intern Med 85:155, 1976
151. Jackson D P, Krevans J R, Conley C L: Mechanisms of the thrombocytopenia that follows multiple whole blood transfusions. Trans Assoc Am Physicians 69:155, 1956
152. Gangarosa E J, Johnson T R, Ramos H S: Ristocetin-induced thrombocytopenia: Site and mechanism of action. Arch Intern Med 105:107, 1960
153. Cowan D H, Hines J D: Thrombocytopenia of severe alcoholism. Ann Intern Med 74:37, 1971
154. Haut M J, Cowan D H: The effect of ethanol on hemostatic properties of human blood platelets. Am J Med 56:22, 1974
155. Cowan D H: Thrombokinetic studies in alcohol-related thrombocytopenia. J Lab Clin Med 81:64, 1973
156. Sullivan L W, Adams W H, Liu Y K: Induction of thrombocytopenia by thrombopheresis in man: Patterns of recovery in normal subjects during ethanol ingestion and abstinence. Blood 49:197, 1977
157. Koons C R, Sensenbrenner L L, Owens A H Jr: Clinical studies of mithramycin in patients with embryonal cancer. Bull Johns Hopkins Hosp 118:462, 1966
158. Monto R W, Talley R W, Caldwell M J, et al: Observations on the mechanism of hemorrhagic toxicity in mithramycin (NSC-24559) therapy. Cancer Res 29:697, 1969
159. Kennedy B J: Metabolic and toxic effects of mithramycin during tumor therapy. Am J Med 49:494, 1970
160. Marchasin S, Wallerstein R O, Aggeler P M: Variations of the platelet count in disease. California Med 101:95, 1964
161. Levin J, Conley C L: Thrombocytosis associated with malignant disease. Arch Intern Med 144:497, 1964
162. Davis W M, Mendez Ross A O: Thrombocytosis and thrombocythemia: The laboratory and clinical significance of an elevated platelet count. Am J Clin Pathol 59:243, 1973
163. Levin J, Cluff L E: Endotoxemia and adrenal hemorrhage. J Exp Med 121:247, 1965
164. Burke P J, Owens A H Jr, Colsky J, et al: A clinical evaluation of a prolonged schedule of cytosine arabinoside (NSC-63878). Cancer Res 30:1512, 1970
165. Odell T T Jr, Jackson C W: Megakaryocyte and platelet development and regulation, in Holmes W L (ed): Blood Cells as a Tissue. New York, Plenum, 1970, p 73
166. Stohlman F Jr: Aplastic anemia. Blood 40:282, 1972

Dov Gorshein
Isadore Brodsky

27
Androgens and Cancer Chemotherapy

The role of androgenic hormones in cancer therapy has been increasingly recognized recently.[1] The modes of action may be one or more of the following: (1) Specific anticancer therapy as in hormone-responsive cancer. (2) Anabolic functions. Here androgens are given as adjuvant therapy to diminish or counteract the catabolic effects of the neoplasm. (3) Stimulation of hematopoietic recovery from cytotoxic effects of chemotherapy. Specifically, androgens have been reported to stimulate erythropoietin production, increase the compartment of erythropoietin-sensitive (responsive) cells, shorten the recovery time of myelosuppressive marrow, stimulate granulopoiesis without a concomitant increase in serum levels of colony-stimulating factor and elevate the number of platelets. (4) As cycling agents, some resting cells (G_0) are triggered to enter the cycle following administration of androgens. This is a potential tool for synchronization of tumor cells followed by chemotherapy. (5) Decrease of ineffective erythropoiesis. (6) Possible activation of fibrinolytic pathways in localized areas, thus interfering with metastatic seeding. (7) Possible augmentation of immunocompetence (specifically, proliferation of T-bearing regions in lymphatic tissue). (8) Androgens may be metabolized to derivatives having only one (or some), but not others of the properties already mentioned.

Important complications of androgen therapy include virilization in women, stunted growth in children, fluid retention, acceleration of the leukemic process during androgen administration or after prolonged administration and then discontinuation; jaundice and hepatocellular damage (with oral preparations only) and hepatocellular carcinoma (regression occurs when androgen administration is stopped).

Introduction

The following review describes in some detail the data available on several points mentioned, and summarizes others not yet fully studied.

The molecular structure of steroids was elucidated 100 years ago. A few years later, a crystalline androgenic material was obtained from male urine and was named androsterone. In 1935 testosterone was isolated from the testicular tissue by Laqueur, and shortly thereafter this substance was synthesized commercially. Some 50 androgenic preparations are now commercially available.

Testosterone, the most active androgen

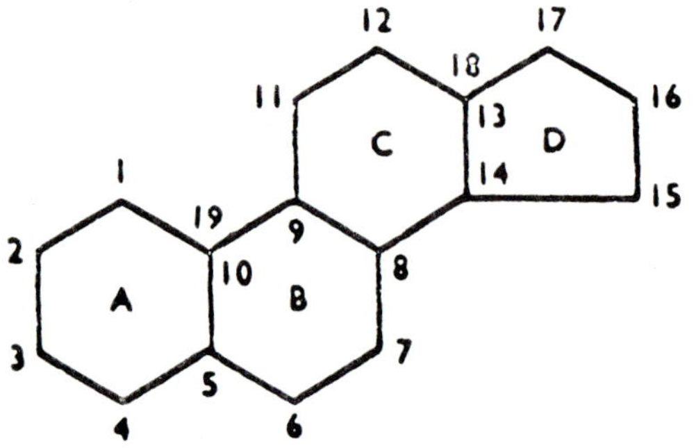

Cyclopentanoperhydrophenanthrene Structure

FIG. 27-1. Depiction of the basic cyclopentanoperhydroxy-phenanthrene structure, showing the numerical position of the carbon atoms and the designation of the rings in alphabetic order.

found in nature, is the dominant androgen secreted by the Leydig cells of the testicles. Precursors of androgens (progesterone, pregnenolone and dehydroepiandrosterone) are secreted by the ovaries and the adrenals, and may be converted into androgens through biosynthetic pathways. The classification of various steroids and their terminology are based on (1) the spatial relation of the hydrogen molecule at the key carbon atom, i.e., alpha (below the ring) or beta (above the ring); (2) hydroxyl (OH) or ketone (C=O) groups; (3) double bonds in the side chain or the ring itself. Figure 27-1 depicts the basic cyclopentanoperhydroxyphenanthrene structure and the numerical position of the carbon atoms and the designation of the rings in alphabetic order.

As mentioned previously, various preparations of androgens are available. The most noticeable difference among them is the C-17 substitution. This is a key position, which confers upon the specific preparation such properties as rate of absorption, duration of action, and anabolic potential. Unfortunately, despite intensive efforts, we have not been successful in separating the anabolic from the virilizing property of the androgenic preparation. Masculinization, therefore, occurs to a certain degree in all women who receive androgens. In addition, the growth of children is stunted. These undesirable side effects led to a search for a basic steroid formula that would retain the desirable properties of the androgenic compounds (e.g., erythropoietic function) and yet be devoid of masculinizing effects.

Specific Anticancer Effect of Androgens

Perhaps the best known use of androgens is in the treatment of breast cancer. Androgens were considered for therapy when it was found that castration inhibits growth of female breast cancer. To date, however, we do not know of any competition for receptor sites between androgens and estrogens, and therefore the mechanism of this anticancer activity in hormone-responsive tumors remains obscure. To suggest an effect of androgen through its capacity to lower gonadotropin level cannot explain regression in advanced cancer, observed in some cases without measurable effect on gonadotropin levels. To further complicate the issue, one knows of the in vivo interconvertibility between female and male sex hormones. Available data indicate that the effectiveness of the androgenic hormone depends on the site of the lesions and, to a limited extent, on the age of the patient.[2-4] Androgenic preparations are effective in breast cancer therapy in premenopausal women, but their use in this age group is limited in view of the unwarranted side effects as well as the feasibility and effectiveness of castration. Oophorectomy, consequently, is used as primary endocrine therapy in estrogen-receptor-positive metastatic breast cancer in premenopausal women. Androgens may be successfully used as a secondary endocrine therapy, for example, as treatment when reactivation of the breast cancer occurs after regression obtained with primary endocrine therapy or when the disease fails to respond.

The status of androgenic therapy in male breast cancer is somewhat confusing. It has been emphasized that the administration of androgenic hormones in male breast cancer is prohibited.[5] A recent report, however, describes a response to calusterone in 2 male patients with breast cancer who failed to respond to other kinds of therapy.[6] In patients who exhibit a favorable response to castration, the use of androgens is contraindicated because of the possible metabolic interconversion into estrogenic compounds. A very distinct group seems to be postmenopausal women with osseous metastases.[3,7] While soft-tissue metastatic lesions seem to respond well to estrogens, osseous metastatic lesions respond to both equally well (approximate response rate of 30 per cent). Symptomatic improvement is noticeable, for example, with relief of pain, weight gain and increased appetite. Unfortunately, one may observe symptomatic improvement following androgenic administration despite obvious progression of the disease. Occasionally, osseous pain is aggravated by the administration of androgenic preparations, necessitating cessation of this therapy. Other complications include hypercalcemia, at times so severe as to require emergency measures. One, therefore, has to closely follow such patients, particularly when therapy is begun.

Anabolic Functions

The growth of neoplastic malignant tissue in the human host results in profound alterations of organs and functions. A syndrome, cachexia, results and is characterized by weakness, anorexia, depletion and redistribution of host components, and deterioration of vital functions. Patients with cancer lose weight because of decreased food intake and poor absorption. Anorexia occurs frequently in patients with cancer and is often one of the initial signs.[8] Such loss of appetite may result from abnormalities in taste, possibly a manifestation of remote effects of cancer.[9] A therapeutic regimen with androgens may seem a logical means to counteract cachexia, but because of the anabolic effects of androgenic preparations, the efficacy of such a regimen is in doubt. Even without regression of metastatic lesions, females with breast cancer who take androgens may live longer than those who do not take them.[5]

Stimulation of Hematopoietic Recovery from Cytotoxic Effects of Chemotherapy

Several reports have shown that 19-nortestosterone decanoate (19-ND) increases erythropoiesis in mice[10,11] and humans.[12] In addition to their ability to increase erythropoietic production,[13] androgens may increase erythropoiesis by direct stimulation of uncommitted G_0 stem cells.[14,15] These elements subsequently trigger a G_1 cycle responsive to erythropoietin.[16] In a murine system wherein erythropoiesis was suppressed by hyperoxia and administration of actinomycin D, the androgenic preparation partially overcame this suppression.

The data of these experiments suggest that 19-ND increases the absolute number of erythroid precursor cells, thus increasing the absolute number of these cells that remain unaffected by the amount of actinomycin injected. Such unaffected cells will mature to normal erythrocytes, thereby maintaining significant erythropoiesis. Actinomycin inhibits DNA-mediated RNA synthesis in G_1 cells, preventing these cells from entering the S-phase of the cell cycle.[17,18] The ability of androgenic administration to partially overcome the suppressive effects of actinomycin is in accord with the recent observations of Byron,[12,19] who demonstrated a stem-cell kill with androgenic steroids by the ^{3}H-thymidine kill technique.

Experimental studies in laboratory animals suggest that the administration of androgenic compounds increases the production of erythropoietin by the kidney. The mechanisms of action of steroids demonstrated in laboratory animals cannot necessarily be extrapolated to the human being. Nevertheless, some data have been duplicated in the prepubertal child and in adults,[20-26] and in human bone marrow cultures.[27-32] In human beings without major hematologic disease, androgens and anabolic steroids increase the excretion of erythropoietin in the urine. This is associated with a moderate rise of the red-cell mass.[20,21]

The adult man excretes more erythropoietin in the urine than does the adult woman;[26] prepubertal boys and girls excrete equal amounts of erythropoietin.[21] The higher levels of erythropoietin in the adult man are seemingly caused by increased androgen production at puberty. It has not been established whether, under normal physiologic conditions, this is due to specific action on the kidney or to the increased muscle mass in men, which has been shown to be related to the level of the circulating red-cell mass.[33] In prepubertal hypopituitary patients treated with human growth hormone, the red-cell mass is increased, as is the urinary excretion of erythropoietin. The red-cell mass continues to increase upon addition of testosterone to the regimen, but not to the degree produced by human growth hormone alone, and the red-cell mass reaches a plateau or declines when human growth hormone is deleted from the regimen, indicating the important role of growth hormone in stimulating erythropoiesis during growth. Similar results following administration of growth hormone have been observed in the hypophysectomized monkey.[34]

In animal experiments, normal mice, mildly plethoric mice,[13,35,36] and hypophysectomized[37] or hypogonadal animals[38] showed increased erythropoiesis after injection of androgenic steroids. The effect was abolished by hypertransfusion[37,39] and by administration of antiandrogens or antisera to erythropoietin.[35,39-41] Stimulation of endogenous erythropoietin by various methods results in peak plasma activity at about 24 hours, followed by an increase of erythropoiesis at 48 to 72 hours. On the other hand, peak plasma concentration of erythropoietin after administration of androgens occurs 72 hours after their injection, and precedes the increase of erythropoiesis observed at 96 to 120 hours.[35]

Erythropoiesis also seems to become refractory to androgen therapy after prolonged treatment of normal animals.[37] A longer interval between initiation of therapy and response is also seen in human beings, in whom several months may be required for an observable effect. This delayed response remains unexplained. It has been suggested that in vivo conversion of the parent compound to more active metabolites is required. Thus the delayed response in the human being could be due to the time required for androgen to alter renal mass or renal metabolism (or both) before sustained increased production of erythropoietin occurs. The response, perhaps due to altered blood/renal oxygen exchange, would be dampened by the rise of the hemoglobin concentration, which increases the oxygen supply to the kidney and thus suppresses the release of erythropoietin. A more recent concept of the mechanism of control of erythropoietin release postulates variations in erythrocyte 2,3-diphosphoglycerate, which is increased by administration of androgens.[42] In fact, further experimentation could indicate that this intraerythrocyte compound plays an important role in the regulation of erythropoietin release.

In view of the very high titers of erythropoietin found in the plasma of patients with severe anemia, it has been difficult to explain increased erythropoiesis entirely on the basis of this increase in erythropoietin production. Some investigators have suggested that, despite remarkably high titers of erythropoietin preceding androgen therapy, the further increase of erythropoietin results in a massive pharmacologic effect on the bone marrow.[24] Current data indicate that the further increase of erythropoietin is not correlated with increased erythropoiesis.[43] The target site of erythropoietin is thought to be the "erythroid-committed" cell, whereas aplastic anemia appears to be the result of disease of the pluripotential stem cell.[44] Thus, even in the presence of high plasma concentrations of erythropoietin, some triggering mechanism would be required to provide cells for the committed compartment upon which erythropoietin could act. Such a mechanism could also account for the failure of some cases of aplasia to respond to androgen therapy. This concept was the basis of the hypothesis that there was a "stem-cell" effect of androgens or their metabolites that could account for the synergistic erythropoietic effect of androgens and erythropoietin.[39,44-49] Recent data support a dual role of androgens in stimulating erythropoiesis, that is, a direct stimulation of bone marrow stem cells (pluripotential?) as well as increased release of endogenous erythropoietin.

Stimulation of heme synthesis and delta aminolevulinic acid synthetase activity, necessary for hemoglobin formation by androgenic metabolites, was first observed in chick blastoderms.[50] The principal induction of heme synthesis occurred under the influence of 5β-H-metabolites. Etiocholanolone, 5β-H metabolite of testosterone, also increased heme synthesis in human marrow cultures, as did testosterone, the parent compound, when added to bone marrow explants.[27] Further data suggested that the pluripotential stem cell was the site of action rather than the pro-

TABLE 27-1. *Results of Tests in Postmenopausal Women with Disseminated Breast Cancer and Primarily Osseous Metastatic Lesions*

	Before Therapy	After 8 Weeks		
		With Chemotherapy	With Chemotherapy and 19-ND	
Hematocrit*	24 ± 4	20 ± 5	27 ± 4	
Iron clearance	160 ± 10	180 ± 20	120 ± 20	P < 0.05
RBC mass†	24 ± 3	22 ± 3	25 ± 4	
Iron incorporation‡	50 ± 5	25 ± 5	45 ± 7	P < 0.05

*Mean ± standard error of the mean (SEM).
†Milliliter per kilogram of body weight.
‡Percentage in 10 days.
Abbreviation: 19-ND, 19-nortestosterone decanoate.

liferating erythroid cell.[30,31] The 5β-H metabolites active in vitro have also been shown to be active in mammals in vivo.[51-53]

It has been demonstrated frequently that the action of erythropoietin is potentiated by testosterone. This effect is dampened and then abolished by increasing the plethora[13,35,39] through the abolition of endogenous erythropoietin. Naets and Wittek[39,48] demonstrated that a more marked erythropoietic response occurred in mice pretreated with androgen and then injected with erythropoietin. They explained the effect on stem-cell induction. Other investigators[13] postulated a summation of endogenous, androgen-induced erythropoietin and injected erythropoietin. Androgen given only 8 hours before hypoxia, however, increased erythropoiesis in plethoric mice, indicating that there was an increase in the number of erythropoietin-responsive cells.[46] Stem-cell depression by estradiol valerate could be compensated for by the administration of testosterone. These reports[39,44-48] suggest that more erythroid-committed stem cells must be present upon which the erythropoietin could act. This has been substantiated by observations in plethoric mice maintained in a hyperoxic environment, which almost completely suppresses erythropoietin production, as compared with the effect of plethora or hyperoxia alone.[11,14,53-57] In this group of experiments 19-ND appeared to provide more cells upon which exogenous erythropoietin could act to increase erythroid differentiation.

The effect of the administration of 19-ND upon granulopoietic recovery of mice made neutropenic by a single dose of BCNU was recently studied by Udupa and Reissmann,[58] who noted a marked enhancing effect. Serum levels of colony stimulating factor (CSF) in the mice treated with BCNU, with or without 19-ND administration, did not differ significantly from those in normal mice. BCNU administration did not alter the CSF increase in response to endotoxic injection whether or not 19-ND was given. Increase in dividing marrow granulocytes in the 19-ND mice was preceded by increase in their marrow colony-forming cells (CFC). They therefore concluded that the acceleration of granulopoietic recovery is not mediated by the serum CSF, but is due to a stimulatory effect of 19-ND on the proliferation of CFC or colony-forming units (CFU), or both.

Reports on the effect of androgens on platelet numbers in patients with cancer are sparse. Calusterone administration has been reported to elevate platelet numbers in patients with breast cancer.[59]

A group of postmenopausal patients with disseminated breast cancer who had primarily (but not exclusively) osseous metastatic lesions received combination chemotherapy with cytoxan, MTX and 5-FU.[12] Six of these received, in addition, 19-ND, 200 mg I.M. weekly, for 8 weeks, but the others did not. The hematocrit levels, RBC mass, iron clearance, and iron incorporation were significantly different in the two groups (Table 27-1).

TABLE 27-2. *Number of Circulating Colony-Forming Cells (CFC) in 6 Patients with Disseminated Breast Cancer*

Normal Value	105 ± 15*
Before androgen therapy	657 ± 157
After androgen therapy	232 ± 41

*Number of colonies, mean ± SEM, in 1 ml of blood.

An interesting finding was a preliminary observation yet unpublished: Granulocytic and mononuclear cell colonies are known to appear in the blood of normal subjects. Their number is increased in patients with myelofibrosis.[60] In a group of 6 patients who had disseminated breast cancer with multiple bone lesions and positive bone marrow involvement, an increase in the number of circulating CFC similarly was found. After 8 weeks of androgenic therapy (without cytotoxic therapy), this number dropped significantly (Table 27-2).

The explanation for this observation is not clear and is open to discussion. The fact, however, that androgenic administration decreases the number of CFS, may suggest a decrease in ineffective or dyspoietic erythropoiesis.

ACTIVITY OF ANDROGENS AS CYCLING AGENTS

Numerous reports have recently supported the concept that androgens have the capacity to trigger cells into cycle. As such enhanced response to erythropoietin is observed in steroid-treated mice, a greater kill is noticed in the suicide high specific activity, thymidine kill technique following androgen administration, etc. The potential of androgens to cycle cells is a double-edged sword and should be studied very carefully. If synchronization could be achieved in a tumor cell population (usually composed partly of G_0 resting cells), then androgen administration could trigger a significant portion into cycle. Cycle-active chemotherapeutic agents given at the appropriate time would then be effective. On the other hand, augmented recovery of myelotoxic effect of chemotherapy, followed by androgen administration, has already been discussed. The issue, then, is how to utilize androgens to synchronize and sensitize tumor cells to chemotherapy, while averting excessively toxic effects on rapidly proliferating tissues (bone marrow).

DECREASE IN INEFFECTIVE ERYTHROPOIESIS

Alexanian et al.[61] reported on patients with aplastic anemia and bone marrow failure who responded favorably to an androgenic preparation. The response to androgen administration in refractory anemia is of interest. The titer of serum erythropoietin in refractory anemia already appears to be very high—50 to 100 times normal,[62] and urinary erythropoietin is increased 1000 times. As these endogenous erythropoietin levels are probably already beyond the point where they are reflected by a comparable marrow output,[63] it is difficult to understand why possible small increases in erythropoietin production would result in a good clinical response. Recently it has been reported that the response was principally mediated by a reduction in ineffective erythropoiesis rather than by elevations of serum erythropoietin titers.[64]

ACTIVATION OF FIBRINOLYTIC PATHWAYS IN LOCALIZED AREAS

This topic has been covered in previous reports by Brodsky.[65] Several other studies support the concept that metastatic implantation depends in part on the intimate interaction between metastatic malignant cells and fibrin. Some trials have been initiated with anticoagulation long-term regimens in an attempt to minimize metastatic seeding. A few years ago, Nilsson and Isacson[66] described the capacity of androgens to enhance the fibrinolytic activity in patients with vascular disease. Abnormally low plasma fibrinolytic activity was found in patients suffering from idiopathic venous thrombosis. It should be mentioned in this regard that often patients with disseminated cancer also suffer from thrombophlebitis. Administration of androgens to the "vascular" patients augmented the fibrinolytic activity of the blood, decreased the fibrinogen level and reduced platelet adhesiveness. However, the other results (euglobulin lysis time, thrombin time, and fibrin degradation products) did not show a significant change.

Still other investigators[67] have reported a significant increase in the plasminogen levels and a decrease in fibrinogen concentration after administration of an 17-alpha alkylated anabolic steroid (for example, oxymetholone or methandrostenolone). The activity is greater than with the non-17 alpha alkylated anabolic steroids. It is not clear whether this increased fibrinolytic activity is related to the hepatotoxicity of oral androgens.

Possible Augmentation of Immunocompetence

This topic has been recently discussed.[63] Androgens, although reducing the lymphatic mass of the thymic cortical region[68] and bone marrow, appear to stimulate proliferation of T-cell bearing regions. Histologic examinations of lymph nodes reveal an increase in the size of lymph follicles along with increased number of plasma cells, whereas thymic and marrow sections show a marked reduction in lymphocytes. The changes seen with androgens gradually occur with long-term use. The slow reduction in marrow and thymic lymphocyte population may be attributed to accelerated migration or increased differentiation. The role of so-called immunologic surveillance in the development of cancer and its function in the propagation of the malignant process are subjects of great interest. Some relation has been reported between the immunologic stimulation capacity of a compound and its antifibrinolytic activity.[69]

Activity of Metabolites of Androgens

The untoward side effects that occur with androgenic therapy resulted in research aimed at finding naturally (or unnaturally) occurring metabolites of testosterone that function effectively by stimulating hematopoietic recovery without also having adverse side effects. Indeed, steroid metabolites with 5-βH configuration have been reported to be capable of stimulating active erythropoietic activity.[12,53,70-73] These metabolites have also been reported to be capable of triggering cells into cycle.[74] In addition, they have the capacity to augment production of erythroid CFU.[75] The steroid metabolite etiocholanolone has recently been reported to augment heme synthesis in malignant marrow.[76] These steroids so far have had only a very limited clinical use,[59] but their potential is promising.

Complications of Androgen Therapy

The virilization occurring with androgen therapy is well recognized, as is the accumulation of fluid and salt retention. Minimal fluid retention was observed in patients receiving 19-ND.[77] In one patient with refractory anemia, acute leukemia developed following cessation of prolonged androgenic therapy.[78] Jaundice and hepatocellular damage occur upon administration of oral alkylated compounds only; such damage has not been observed in patients receiving the injectable preparations. A more recent report describes a possible complication of androgenic therapy, the development of hepatocellular carcinoma. A unique observation is that a noticeable regression may occur when androgenic therapy is stopped.

References

1. Brodsky I, Kahn S B, Conroy J F: The effects of androgens on cancer chemotherapy, in Brodsky I, Kahn S B, Moyer J F (eds): Cancer Chemotherapy II. New York, Grune & Stratton, 1972, p 303
2. Nathanson I: Clinical investigative experience with steroid hormones in breast cancer. Cancer 5:754, 1952
3. Cooperative Breast Cancer Group: Testosterone propionate therapy in breast cancer. JAMA 188:1069, 1964
4. Cooperative Breast Cancer Group: Results of

studies of cooperative breast cancer group: 1961–1963. Cancer Chemother Rep 41 (Suppl): 1, 1964
5. Kennedy B J: Hormonal therapies in breast cancer. Semin Oncol 1:119, 1974
6. Horn Y., Roof B: Male breast cancer: Two cases with objective regressions from calusterone after failure of orchiectomy. Oncology 33:188, 1976
7. Council on Drugs, Subcommittee on Breast and Genital Cancer, Committee on Research, AMA: Androgens and estrogens in the treatment of disseminated mammary carcinoma—Retrospective study of 944 patients. JAMA 172:1271, 1960
8. Costa G: Cachexia and the systemic effects of tumors, in Holland J F, Frei E III (eds): Cancer Medicine. Philadelphia, Lea & Febiger, 1973, p 1035
9. Gorshein D: Posthypophysectomy taste abnormalities: Their relationship to remote effect of cancer. Cancer 39:1700, 1977
10. Gorsheim D, Gardner F H: Comparative study on the erythropoietic function of androgens in mice. Clin Res 17:600, 1969
11. Besa E C, Jepson J H, Gorshein D, et al: The effect of nandrolone decanoate on the stem cell pool. Clin Res 19:725, 1971
12. Byron J W: Effect of steroids on the cycling of haemopoietic stem cells. Nature 228:1204, 1970
13. Fried W, Gurney C W: The erythropoietic stimulating effect of androgens. Ann NY Acad Sci 149:356, 1968
14. Hait W N, Gorshein D, Jepson J H, Gardner F H: Androgen-induced erythropoiesis in the actinomycin-treated hyperoxic mouse. Clin Res 20:488, 1972
15. Gorshein D., Hait W N, Besa E, et al: Rapid cell differentiation induced by nandrolone decanoate. Proc Am Assoc Cancer Res 13:114, 1972
16. Kretchmar A S, McDonald T P, Lange R D: Mode of action of erythropoiesis in polycythemic mice. I. Response in mice treated with 5-fluorouracil. J Lab Clin Med 75:74, 1970
17. Reich E, Franklin R M, Shatkin A J, et al: Effect of actinomycin D on cellular nucleic acid synthesis and virus production. Science 134:556, 1961
18. Sawicki S G, Godman G C: On the differential cytotoxicity of actinomycin D. J Cell Biol 50:746, 1971
19. Byron J W: Effects of steroids and dibutyryl cyclic AMP on the sensitivity of haemopoietic stem cells to ^{3}H-thymidine in vitro. Nature 234:5323, 1971
20. Alexanian R: Erythropoietin and erythropoiesis in anemic man following androgens. Blood 33:564, 1969
21. Jepson J, MacGarry E E: Hemopoiesis in pituitary dwarfs treated with human growth hormone and testosterone. Blood 39:228, 1972
22. Korst D R, Shahidi N T, Rodriques J N (eds): Erythopoietin activity in aplastic anemia before and after and regontherapy, in Proc Thirteenth Congress, International Society of Hematology. Munich, J F Lehmanns, 1970, p 161
23. Mirand E A, Murphy G P, Steeves R A, et al: Erythropoietin activity in anephric, allotransplanted, unilaterally nephrectomized and intact man. J Lab Clin Med 73:121, 1969
24. Rishpon-Meyerstein N, Killiridge T, Simone J, et al: The effects of testosterone on erythropoietin levels in anemic patients. Blood 31:453, 1968
25. Moores R R, Wright C S, Collins L R, et al: Stimulation of erythropoiesis by androgen, in the human. Scand J Haematol 5:415, 1968
26. Alexanian R, Vaughn W K, Ruchel M W: Erythropoietin excretion in man following androgens. J Lab Clin Med 70:777, 1967
27. Reisner E: Measurement of erythropoiesis in vitro by Fe^{59} uptake of marrow, in Abstracts of Twelfth Congress, International Society of Hematology. New York, 1968
28. Jacobson W, Sidman R L, Diamond L K: The effect of testosterone on the uptake of H^3-thymidine by bone marrow of children. Ann NY Acad Sci 149:389, 1968
29. Necheles T F, Rai U S: Studies on the control of hemoglobin synthesis: The in vitro stimulating effect of 5β H steroid metabolites on heme formation in human bone marrow cells. Blood 34:380, 1969
30. Necheles T F: Studies on the control of hemoglobin synthesis: The in vitro relationship between erythropoietin and 5-beta-H steroid induced stimulation of hemoglobin synthesis in human bone marrow cells. Proc Symposium Erythropoieticum, Prague, 1970, no. 29
31. Necheles T F: Studies on the control of hemoglobin synthesis: A mode of erythroid differentiation based upon the in vitro effect of erythropoietin and 5 β H steroids. Blut (in press)
32. Levere R D, Mizognchi H: Effects of certain 5 β steroid metabolites on hemoglobin synthesis in cultured human bone marrow cells, in Necheles T F (ed): Androgens in the Anemia of Bone Marrow Failure. Palo Alto, CA, Syntex Laboratories, 1972
33. Retzlaff J A, Tauxe W N, Keily J M, et al:

Erythrocyte volume, plasma volume and lean body mass in adult men and women. Blood 33:649, 1969

34. Vitale L, Shahidi N T, Kerr G E, et al: The role of growth hormone and thyroxine in erythropoietic restoration in hypophysectomized monkeys. Proc Soc Exp Biol Med 138:418, 1971
35. Gurney C W, Fried W: The erythropoietic effect of androgens in hemopoietic effect of androgens in hemopoietic proliferation, in Stohlman F Jr. (ed): Hemopoietic Cellular Proliferation. New York, Grune & Stratton, 1970, p 133
36. Gordon A S, Mirand E A, Weining J, et al: Androgen action on erythropoiesis. Ann NY Acad Sci 149:318, 1968
37. Meincke H A, Crafts A C: Further observations on the mechanism by which androgens and growth hormone influence erythropoiesis. Ann NY Acad Sci 149:298, 1968
38. Molinari P: Androgens and erythropoiesis in bone marrow. II. Effect of testosterone propionate on Fe^{59} concentration in erythrocytes and bone marrow. Experentia 26:531, 1970
39. Naets J P, Wittek M: The mechanism of action of androgens on erythropoiesis. Ann NY Acad Sci 149:366, 1968
40. Schooley J C: Inhibition of erythropoietic stimulation by testosterone in polycythemic mice receiving anti-erythropoietin. Proc Soc Exp Biol Med 122:402, 1966
41. Mirand E A, Groenewald J H, Kenny G M, et al: The inhibition effect of anti-androgen (SH741) on erythropoietic activity. Experientia 25:1104, 1969
42. Fischer J W, Langston J W: Effects of testosterone, cobalt and hypoxia on erythropoietin production in the isolated dog kidney. Ann NY Acad Sci 149:75, 1968
43. Parker J P, Beirne G J, Desai J N, et al: Androgen-induced increase in red cell 2,3-diphosphoglycerate. N Engl J Med 287:381, 1972
44. Alexanian R, Nadell J, Alfrey C: Oxymetholone treatment for the anemia of bone marrow failure. Blood 3:353, 1972
45. Jepson J H: Current concepts of pathophysiology and treatment of bone marrow failure. Med Clin North Am (in press)
46. Jepson J, Lowenstein L: The effect of testosterone, adrenal steroids and prolactin on erythropoiesis. Acta Haematol 38:292, 1967
47. Jepson J, Lowenstein L: Inhibition of the stem cell action of erythropoietin by estradiol valerate and the protective effect of 17 α-hydroxy progesterone caproate and testosterone propionate. Endocrinology 80:430, 1967
48. Naets G P, Wittek M: Mechanism of action of androgens on erythropoiesis. Am J Physiol 210:315, 1966
49. Jepson J H, McGarry E E: Erythropoietin excretion in a hypopituitary patient: Effects of testosterone and pitressin. Arch Intern Med 122:265, 1968
50. Levere R D, Kappas A, Granick S: Stimulation of hemoglobin synthesis in chick blastoderms by certain 5 β H pregnane steroids. Proc Natl Acad Sci 58:985, 1967
51. Levere R D, Gordon A S, Zanjani E, et al: Stimulation of mammalian erythropoiesis by metabolites of steroid hormones. Trans Assoc Am Physicians 83:150, 1970
52. Gordon A S, Zanjani E D, Levere R D: Stimulation of mammalian erythropoiesis by 5β steroid metabolites. Proc Natl Acad Sci 65:919, 1970
53. Gorshein D, Gardner F H: Erythropoietic activity of steroid metabolites in mice. Proc Natl Acad Sci 65:564, 1970
54. Gorshein D, Jepson J, Hait W N, et al: Rapid stem cell differentiation induced by 19-nortestosterone decanoate. Proc Am Assoc Cancer Res 13:114, 1972
55. Hait W N, Gorshein D, Jepson J H, et al: 19-nortestosterone decanoate induced erythropoiesis in the actinomycin D treated hyperoxic mouse. Biochem Biophys Res Commun 47:426, 1972
56. Jepson J H: Mechanism of action of androgens on erythropoiesis, in Necheles T D (ed): Symposium on the Role of Androgens in the Therapy of the Anemia of Bone Marrow Failure. New York, Grune & Stratton, 1973
57. Jepson J H, Gorshein D, Hait W N, et al: Clearance of plasma radioiron in mice injected with testosterone and exposed to hypoxia. Clinical Research 19:782, 1971
58. Udupa K, Reissman K R: Stimulation of granulopoiesis by androgens without concomitant increase in the serum level of colony stimulating factor. Exp Hematol 3:26, 1975
59. Horn Y, Halden A, Gordan G S: The platelet-stimulating effects of 7-beta, 17-alpha-dimethyltestosterone (calusterone). Blood 40:684, 1972
60. Chervenick P A: Increase in circulating stem cells in patients with myelofibrosis. Blood 41:67, 1973
61. Alexanian R, Nadell J, Alfrey C: Oxymetholone treatment for the anemia of bone marrow failure. Blood 40:353, 1972
62. Napier J A F, Dunn C D R, Ford T W, et al: Pathophysiological changes in serum erythroid stimulating activity. Br J Haematol (in press)

63. Crosby W H: The limits of erythropoiesis: How much can the marrow produce with total recruitment? Blood Cells 1:197, 1975
64. Napier J A F, Cavill I, Dunn C D R, et al: Oxymetholone treatment in aplastic anemia: Changes in erythropoiesis and serum erythropoietin. Br Med J 2:1426, 1976
65. Rigberg S V, Brodsky I: Potential roles of androgens and the anabolic steroids in the treatment of cancer: A review. J Med 6:271, 1975
66. Nilsson I M, Isacson S: Effect of treatment with combined phenformin and ethyloestrenol on the coagulation and fibrinolytic system. J Clin Pathol 25:638, 1972
67. Fearnley G R, Chakrabarti R, Evans J F: Mode of action of phenformin plus ethyloestrenol on fibrinolysis. Lancet 1:723, 1971
68. Frey-Wettstein M, Craddock C G: Testosterone-induced depletion of thymus and marrow lymphocytes as related to lymphopoiesis and hematopoiesis. Blood 35:257, 1970
69. Thornes R D, Smyth H, Browne O, et al: The effects of proteolysis on the human immune mechanism in cancer. J Med 5:92, 1974
70. Gorshein D, Gardner F H: Erythropoietic activity of steroid metabolite in mice. Proc Natl Acad Sci 65:564, 1970
71. Gordon A S, Zanjani E D, Levere R D: Stimulation of mammalian erythropoiesis by 5-βH steroid metabolites. Proc Natl Acad Sci 65:191, 1970
72. Necheles T F, Rai U S: Studies on the control of hemoglobin synthesis: The in vitro stimulating effect of a 5 β-H steroid metabolite on heme formation in human bone marrow cells. Blood 34:380, 1969
73. Dunn C D R, Napier J A F, Ford T W, et al: Oxymetholone and erythropoiesis: Failure to detect an effect in fetal mouse liver cell cultures. (unpublished data)
74. Rao L, Shahidi N: The effect of 11-ketopregnenolone (11-KP) on red cell volume (RCV). Pediatr Res 6:372 (abstr), 1972
75. Singer J W, Adamson J W: Steroids and hematopoiesis. III. The response of granulocytic and erythroid colony-forming cells to steroids of different classes. Blood 48:855, 1976
76. Gorshein D: Effect of a steroid on heme synthesis in marrow cultured from malignant disease. Exp Hematol (in press)
77. Besa E C, Gorshein D, Gardner F H: Androgens and human blood volume changes. Arch Intern Med 133:418, 1974
78. Gorshein D, Besa E C, Gardner F H: Acute myelomonocytic leukemia after cessation of androgen therapy. Ann Intern Med 79:749, 1973

Stephen Bulova

28
Transfusion Therapy in Cancer Patients

The judicious use of blood transfusions is an integral part of the clinical management of patients with malignant disease. Anemia, leukopenia and thrombocytopenia are common problems in cancer patients and must be dealt with according to principles designed to provide optimal supportive care and the most efficient utilization of available resources.

The most common cause of cytopenias in patients with malignant disease is marrow suppression induced by chemotherapeutic agents and radiation therapy. A characteristic of the majority of cancer chemotherapeutic agents is a lack of tumor specificity, and they accordingly have damaging secondary effects on the normal tissues of the host, particularly on the dividing cellular elements in the bone marrow. Marrow suppression, secondary to cytotoxic agents, is the basic dose-limiting factor for the majority of antitumor agents. Cytotoxic drugs are administered by a regimen to ensure effective as well as safe therapy. In fact, one cannot achieve effective drug therapy of cancer without eliciting some degree of bone marrow suppression. The general sequence of marrow suppression due to chemotherapeutic agents is that leukopenia develops first and is followed by thrombocytopenia with anemia occurring later. Recovery proceeds in the same sequence with the return of white cells first, followed by a rise in the platelet count and finally reversal of the anemia.

The dose of chemotherapeutic agent administered is the primary factor responsible for the development of bone marrow suppression. Host factors such as hepatic or renal impairment may alter the metabolism and excretion of a drug, augmenting its adverse action on the marrow. Prior exposure to chemotherapy or radiotherapy are also major host factors determining the effect of drugs as well as the tumor.

Another important factor affecting peripheral blood counts is the presence of bone marrow metastases or the degree of marrow invasion by the tumor. This is most pronounced in neoplasms arising in the marrow such as acute leukemia or multiple myeloma but also becomes a major factor in the later stages of lymphomas and solid tumors. The intent of drug therapy is to destroy tumor in the marrow and provide space for repopulation with normal cellular elements. Myelosuppression invariably develops under these circumstances prior to the regrowth of marrow cells.

Anemia without marrow invasion by tumor or secondary to chemotherapy is a frequent finding in patients with neoplastic disease. This anemia has many labels, including secondary anemia of cancer or anemia of chronic disease, and is a diagnosis of exclusion. It is characterized by a mild to moderate anemia, normocellular marrow, low serum iron and iron binding capacity, increased marrow iron stores, rapid plasma iron clearance and often a shortened red cell survival.[1] To explain some of these findings, Haurani et al[2] have demonstrated impaired reutilization of iron in these patients. This anemia, in itself, is rarely symptomatic, but it provides a lower baseline hematocrit and marrow reserve of erythopoiesis that augments the suppressive effect of chemotherapy, radiation and marrow metastases on the oxygen carrying capacity of the blood.

A less common cause of pancytopenia in patients with cancer is hypersplenism. The enlargement of the spleen that occurs in patients with lymphoproliferative disorders, leukemia and massive hepatic metastases leads to hyperplasia of phagocytic cells, sequestration and subsequent pancytopenia. Any combination of peripheral blood elements may be affected by this process and the clinical evaluation of the role of splenomegaly in depression of any of the peripheral blood elements may be quite difficult.

Gastrointestinal bleeding and blood loss from other sites are common causes for anemia in cancer patients. Autoimmune hemolytic anemia, due to the production of antibody against erythrocytes, may be seen in association with neoplastic diseases, especially those involving the lymphocytic and reticuloendothelial systems.[3] Microangiopathic hemolytic anemia has been described in patients with metastatic adenocarcinoma.[4] Carcinoma of the stomach is the most commonly associated neoplasm, and carcinoma of the breast, prostate, lung, pancreas, gallbladder, and colon and hemangioendothelioma have also been described with this syndrome. The pathophysiology of the hemolysis is thought to involve both contact between red cells and tumor cells within blood vessels, and red cell fragmentation due to intravascular fibrin deposition as a result of intravascular coagulation. It is postulated that intravascular coagulation may be initiated by thromboplastins derived from tumor cells. Disseminated intravascular coagulation (DIC) is also associated with severe sepsis in leukopenic patients. A major clinical problem associated with DIC is bleeding due to thrombocytopenia and deficiency of multiple coagulation factors, primarily fibrinogen, factor V and factor VIII. Anemia and hypoalbuminemia occur in association with malnutrition in patients with advanced malignancy.

Transfusion of blood and its components is often indicated in the supportive treatment of cancer patients. Transfusions of whole blood are indicated only for massive bleeding and blood loss associated with surgical procedures. With the advent of component preparations, the indications for whole blood have decreased markedly. The replacement of the specific blood components that the patient requires provides maximum therapeutic effectiveness and safety of transfusion as well as the most efficient utilization of blood resources.

Red Blood Cells

Red blood cells are prepared from whole blood by removal of the plasma after centrifugation or sedimentation. With slow centrifugation shortly after collection, platelet-rich plasma may be removed from whole blood. The removal of platelets and plasma by either centrifugation or sedimentation has no deleterious effect on the integrity of the oxygen-carrying capacity of red cells. The red cells have the same shelf-life as whole blood (21 days) and an equivalent posttransfusion survival. The plasma may be removed at any time before the expiration date of the blood. If it is removed in a closed system (blood collected in a bag with preattached satellite bags) the shelf-life is unchanged. If the bag is entered to remove the plasma, however, the packed cells only have a shelf-life of 24 hours from the time of entry.[5]

The common symptoms of weakness and lassitude in cancer patients are rarely related to anemia if the hematocrit is greater than 25 per cent and do not respond to transfusions. More specific symptoms such as extreme fatigue, dyspnea or angina may result from the effects of anemia on preexisting pulmonary or coronary artery disease, particularly if the hematocrit is less than 20 per cent, and may be relieved by transfusions. The decision to transfuse red cells for treatment of anemia may be made on a clinical basis. It is not necessary nor indicated to maintain the hematocrit within the normal range. Red cell transfusions are generally indicated to relieve the symptoms that are due to oxygen deprivation, and are usually necessary during and after a course of chemotherapy when erythropoiesis is compromised and the hematocrit cannot sustain itself and falls to symptomatic levels.

Red blood cells are the treatment of choice for symptomatic anemia since they provide the oxygen-carrying capacity of whole blood and minimize side effects such as volume overload and plasma reactions. In the average adult, one unit of packed cells may be expected to cause a rise of 1 gm per cent of hemoglobin, or 3 per cent hematocrit increment.

Nonhemolytic transfusion reactions may be associated with the administration of red blood cells. These reactions may be characterized by fever and chills from antibodies to leukocytes and platelets, or by urticaria due to plasma protein antibodies. Febrile reactions appear to be due primarily to pyrogens released as a result of leukocyte, rather than platelet, destruction. Mild febrile reactions may be suppressed or prevented by the administration of acetaminophen and Benadryl prior to the transfusion. If febrile reactions persist, the patient must be given leukocyte-poor red cells. It is not feasible or practical to provide leukocyte and platelet antigen-matched blood to transfuse red cells. The most effective way to provide leukocyte- and platelet-free red cells is by the administration of frozen deglycerolized cells. Red cells collected in citrate-phosphate-dextrose (CPD) anticoagulant are frozen in the presence of glycerol, which acts as a cryoprotective agent. The cells may be stored for 2 years or longer in this state without deterioration. After the cells are thawed, they are washed free of the glycerol and suspended in saline. The freezing, thawing and washing procedure results in virtually complete removal of leukocyte and platelet material. The red cells remain intact and the procedure ensures at least 70 per cent viability of the transfused cells 24 hours after transfusion. The shelf-life of frozen deglycerolized cells after thawing is 24 hours.[5]

There are several other less effective methods of removing leukocytes. Washing the red cells several times with saline and removing the saline and buffy coat following centrifugation results in removal of 50 per cent to 70 per cent of the leukocytes with some loss of red cells. This is the least effective method and generally does not remove enough leukocytes to prevent febrile reactions. A more effective method of leukocyte removal is by inverted centrifugation. The blood is centrifuged so that the cellular elements are packed against the ports of the bag. The bag is then entered and the red cells are allowed to drain into another bag, leaving the plasma and adjacent buffy coat behind. The drained red cells contain less than 25 per cent of the leukocytes originally present in the blood. Automated cell washers, such as the Haemonetics Model 102 or the IBM 2291, used primarily to wash frozen deglycerolized cells, can also be used to prepare leukocyte-poor blood. The AABB standards, which are an expression of the general effectiveness of leukocyte removal, state that leukocyte-poor red blood cells should contain less than 25 per cent of the leukocytes and platelets originally present and should retain at least 80 per cent of the original red cells.[5] Less than optimal leukocyte removal occurs without the freezing-deglycerolization process.

Platelets

The development of techniques to prepare platelet concentrates has led to the widespread use of platelet transfusions in thrombocytopenic patients. It is possible to harvest viable, functional platelets from whole blood by a variety of methods.

Platelets may be harvested from single units of blood as well as plateletpheresis and the use of continuous centrifugation techniques. The drawing of blood from large numbers of people during short periods of time, such as the visit of a mobile donor unit to a community center or place of employment, makes the harvesting of platelets from single units of blood a feasible and practical way of making large numbers of platelet concentrates available. The blood should remain at room temperature prior to removal of platelets, which must be completed within 4 hours of the time the blood is collected. The blood is centrifuged at slow speed, the platelet rich plasma removed and a platelet concentrate is prepared from further centrifugation of the platelet-rich plasma. The yield of platelets by this method is variable and ranges from 40 to 90 per cent. The AABB standards state that a unit of platelets is defined as the amount of platelets prepared from 1 unit (500 ml.) of whole blood and that 75 per cent of such units should contain at least 0.55×10^{11} platelets. This figure represents a recovery of about 50 per cent from a person with a normal platelet count. Most whole blood is now collected in citrate-phosphate-dextrose (CPD), rather than acid-citrate-dextrose (ACD) anticoagulant. The yield of platelets collected from CPD is lower than from ACD[6] but their viability, function and response to storage is the same with both anticoagulants. For this reason, ACD is used as an anticoagulant when platelets are harvested by pheresis or continuous-flow centrifugation.

In the double plateletpheresis system, immediate harvesting of platelets is carried out from 2 units of blood drawn sequentially and the donor's red cells are promptly reinfused. This procedure requires about 1½ hours and can be repeated using the same donor twice a week. The system is inexpensive, but there is a significant risk of a reinfusion error since the donor is detached from the blood during the platelet separation process.

Newer methods of collection allow the separation of platelets from large volumes of donor blood, whereby the donor is connected to the collection apparatus during the entire procedure. The Haemonetics Model 30, Latham blood processor (Haemonetics Corp., Natick, Mass.) relies on discontinuous-flow centrifugation. Blood is removed from the donor and pumped together with ACD or citrate anticoagulant into a disposable centrifuge bowl that is rotating at a speed of about 4800 rpm. The blood components are continuously separated as the bowl is spinning. When the volume of the blood removed from the donor exceeds the volume of the bowl, the various components—plasma, platelets and granulocytes—overflow the bowl in a sequence that depends on their specific gravity and they can be collected in various containers. The flow in the processor is then reversed and the red cells are returned to the donor. The cycle, or pass, is then repeated to process more blood into its components. Usually, a six-cycle harvest is performed on a donor at a sitting, the amount of blood processed being dependent on the volume of the bowl as well as the hematocrit.

The NCI-IBM Continuous Flow Cell Separator (IBM, Endicott, New York) and the Aminco Celltrifuge (American Instrument Co., Silver Spring, Md.) operate on a continuous-flow principle. The blood is pumped into the top of a revolving bowl and travels to the bottom where the red cells flow to the periphery, the plasma to the top and the leukocytes and platelets to the interface. The leukocytes, platelets, red cells and plasma are removed continuously through separate stationary ports. The red cells and plasma are continuously reinfused into the donor through a second needle in the opposite arm.

The number of platelets collected by either method depends on several variables, including the donor's platelet count and the amount of blood processed. The efficiency of the Haemonetics Model 30 in collecting platelets is 80 to 90 per cent.[7] A six-cycle preparation yields 4 to 7×10^{11} platelets, which compares to about six to twelve units of platelets prepared from single units of whole blood. The process takes about 1½ to 2½ hours and the preparation contains 250 ml of plasma and 3 to 15 ml of red blood cells. The continuous-flow centrifugation (CFC) units harvest platelets with similar efficiency and have a slight advantage in that more blood can be processed since the procedure provides a continuous, uninterrupted, cell separation. The NCI-IBM and Aminco units are more expensive than the Haemonetics unit and are somewhat more complex to operate. The function of platelets prepared by all three of these units is about equal and of good quality.[8,9] Hydroxyethyl starch (HES), which is used in granulocyte separation, slightly impairs the efficiency of platelet separation to about 70 per cent,[7] but has no detrimental effect on platelet function.[10] Thus, platelets may be harvested simultaneously with granulocytes for transfusion.

There is considerable controversy concerning the conditions of platelet storage.

Murphy and Gardner[11] presented evidence of a deleterious effect of refrigerated storage on platelet viability. Studies indicate that platelets stored at room temperature (22° to 24° C) develop a functional lesion that prohibits them from acting effectively in hemostasis for the first few hours, posttransfusion.[12,13] This defect, however, appears to reverse itself in the circulation several hours after transfusion and platelets prepared in this manner provide good hemostastis.[14,15] Becker et al[13] have reported that when stored at 4° C, rather than 24° C, platelets do a better job of reducing the bleeding time in thrombocytopenic patients during the first 4 hour posttransfusion period. Slichter and Harker[9,15] feel that the function and viability of platelets stored at 4° C is impaired to a greater degree than those stored at 24° C, however. Valeri[16] has suggested that patients with dilutional thrombocytopenia, secondary to platelet destruction during extracorporeal circulation, should be treated with platelets stored at 4° C, whereas treatment of thrombocytopenia produced by impaired platelet production may be better treated with platelets stored at 22° C.

Several principles of platelet storage are apparent. The longer the platelets are stored at any temperature, the poorer their function will be. That is, platelets stored for 72 hours under any conditions will not provide as good hemostasis as a 24-hour preparation. Also, the volume of plasma in which the platelets are suspended must be sufficient to preserve metabolic function. The pH of the preparation must not fall below 6.0, or there will be significant impairment of viability and function. Platelets stored at 22° should be gently agitated. The AABB Standards have taken both viewpoints into consideration.[5] The expiration time for platelets is 72 hours, and platelets stored at 22° to 24° must be suspended in a greater volume of plasma than those stored at 4° C.

The indications for platelet transfusions follow a series of guidelines rather than strict criteria. Spontaneous bleeding almost never occurs at platelet counts greater than 50,000 cells/mm^3 unless there is a platelet defect such as that induced by aspirin. The risk of increased bleeding at surgery, however, is considerably increased at platelet counts less than 100,000 cells/mm^3. At platelet counts between 20,000 and 50,000 cells/mm^3 there is a moderate risk of bleeding. At this level, trauma should be avoided and the patient should not take medication that injures platelet function. Prophylactic platelet transfusions are generally not indicated for patients with platelet counts greater than 20,000 cells/mm^3. Platelet transfusions should be given to patients who are actively bleeding due to thrombocytopenia, however. Infection and fever may bring about spontaneous bleeding with a relatively high platelet count. In addition, patients with acute leukemia may have functional defects and bleeding episodes may occur in leukemia patients with platelet counts greater than 50,000 cells/mm^3. In general, however, spontaneous bleeding requiring platelet transfusions tends to occur in patients with platelet counts less than 20,000 cells/mm^3.

It is advocated by many[6,17] that prophylactic platelet transfusions be given to those patients undergoing chemotherapy whose platelet counts fall below 20,000 cells/mm^3 and a period of thrombocytopenia is anticipated. This is particularly true for patients with acute leukemia receiving chemotherapy, who undergo a prolonged period of marrow depression and are particularly susceptible to a critical spontaneous hemorrhage such as an intracranial bleed.

The use of prophylactic platelet transfusions in severely thrombocytopenic patients, with prolonged impairment of marrow function who are not undergoing active chemotherapy, is open to question. Some patients are able to tolerate platelet counts as low as 10,000 cells/mm^3, or less, for long periods of time, requiring platelet transfusions only intermittently for bleeding episodes. Yankee et al,[18] however, have documented the feasibility of a prolonged platelet-transfusion program in patients with aplastic anemia using selected matched donors.

The number of units of platelets and the frequency of transfusions required is variable. Effective prophylaxis may be obtained with 6 to 8 units or one preparation from a cell separator every 2 to 3 days. Daily platelet transfusions, however, may be necessary in patients with fever, infection, bleeding or hepatosplenomegaly. The platelet count should be monitored daily and a goal of greater than 20,000 cells/mm^3 is reasonable.

For the average recipient, the expected increment 20 hours after transfusion is 5000 to 7000 cells/mm^3 per unit of platelets given per square meter of body surface area. Thus, a 1.5 M^2 person receiving 8 units of platelets, or the equivalent, should be expected to have an increment of about 30,000 cells/mm^3 on the day following the transfusion.

In addition to the factors mentioned above, a common cause of refractoriness to platelet transfusions is the development of antibodies in the recipient. HLA antigens are well expressed on platelet membranes and it is estimated that 90 per cent of instances of platelet refractoriness are due to anti-HLA antibodies. The other 10 per cent are probably due to antibodies reactive to platelet-specific antigens. There is no need to transfuse HLA-matched platelets to nonsensitized patients. Many patients respond well to random donors for long periods of time without developing antibodies. It is thought that perhaps patients with leukemia or other types of cancer receiving chemotherapy are immunologically suppressed, and tend not to become sensitized.[19] When antibodies develop, HLA-compatible donors can be used and the antibodies do not impair the response to matched platelets. To give HLA-matched platelets to all patients with thrombocytopenia is a waste of time, effort and resources.

On the other hand, unmatched, incompatible platelets are ineffective in promoting hemostasis in refractory patients.[16] The bleeding time is not shortened unless there is a significant increment in the platelet count. In addition, it has been shown that infusion of incompatible platelets to a refractory patient not only fails to increase the platelet count, but can cause a significant prolonged decrease in the granulocyte count.[20] Yankee et al[21] and Lohrmann et al[22] have demonstrated the feasibility of finding compatible platelets for refractory patients from HLA-type unrelated donors. The genetics of the HLA system is such that siblings have only a 25 per cent chance of being HLA-identical, and parents and their children will generally be mismatched for two of the four major serologic HLA antigens. This indicates that it is very often not possible to find a compatible family member for a refractory patient. The polymorphism of the HLA system is such that 5000 to 10,000 typed donors are required to ensure a reasonable chance of success of finding a compatible donor for a given patient. The task is made somewhat easier by the fact that many HLA antigens are crossreactive. Therefore, complete HLA identity is not required and a mismatched, but crossreactive, antigen would not exclude a donor. Several centers in major metropolitan areas have undertaken the task of HLA-typing large numbers of potential donors so that the feasibility of obtaining HLA-matched platelets is becoming a reality. In addition, the development of cell separators has made possible the preparation of adequate amounts of platelets from HLA-matched donors.

Granulocytes

The advent of granulocyte transfusions has depended on the development of techniques for separating granulocytes from large volumes of blood, since it is not feasible to isolate therapeutic quantities from single units of whole blood. Patients with CML have been used as donors, but they are rarely available, and with recent modifications of cell separation techniques, the preparation of sufficient quantities of granulocytes from normal donors has become possible.

The principles of discontinuous- and continuous-flow cell separation have been described in the platelet section of the chapter and are used to harvest granulocytes. The yield of granulocytes with these techniques, using ACD solution alone is poor, particularly with the Haemonetics unit. The use of hydroxyethyl starch (Volex, McGaw Laboratories, Santa Ana, Calif.) in the cell separator and the pretreatment of the donor with either prednisone, dexamethasone, or etiocholanolone has increased the yield significantly.[25,26,28]

Hydroxyethyl starch (HES) is a rouleaux-producing agent that is derived from waxy sorghum starch and is composed primarily of amylopectin. It is very close in structure to glycogen and is thus free of producing hypersensitivity reactions. About 80 per cent of the HES is excreted within 1 week but approximately 20 per cent remains unaccounted for. Although several studies have demonstrated that HES is safe and does not cause donor reactions,[23,24] its long-term effects are not known. For these reasons, most centers have put an arbitrary limit on the number of times a donor may be exposed to HES. Steroids cause a rise in the granulocyte count and are administered to the donor prior to leukopheresis. Etiocholanolone occasionally causes pain at the injection site and a mild febrile reaction. Prednisone and dexamethasone have no significant side effects in donors, but donor exposure to steroids is limited by most centers because of possible long-term complications.

With HES, the Haemonetics unit can be used to harvest granulocytes with an efficiency of 50 to 70 per cent.[7] The total yield of granulocytes from a six-cycle pheresis using HES is about 1 to 3 × 10^{10} cells and takes 1½ to 2½ hours.[25] The preparation contains about 1 × 10^{11} platelets and is also heavily contaminated with lymphocytes. The NCI-IBM and Aminco units are less efficient than the Haemonetics unit with respect to granulocyte separation, but have the advantage of being able to process more blood. In 2 to 3 hours, either of the CFC units can process 8 to 10 liters of blood, and with HES, yield a preparation with a granulocyte count in the same range as the Haemonetics Model 30.[26] The preparation also contains many platelets and lymphocytes. About 10 to 30 ml. of red cells are also present in granulocyte preparations so that the donor and recipient must be ABO compatible. Donor reactions are rare and mild, and include headache due to volume expansion secondary to HES, and chills due to rapid infusion of processed blood and anticoagulants. Granulocyte function has been shown for many investigators to be unaffected by the centrifugation method of collection, the hydroxyethyl starch and the administration of steroids to donors.[10,27]

Filtration leukopheresis (FL) which was developed by Djerassi,[29] depends on the ability of granulocytes to adhere to nylon fibers from which they can subsequently be eluted. In this system, which requires heparinization of the donor, blood is pumped through one or more nylon filters (Leukopak, Fenwal Laboratories, Morton Grove, Ill.) and back into the donor. About 3 liters of blood is passed through each filter to achieve saturation, and as much as 9 to 15 liters of blood can be processed from a donor in a 3 to 4 hour period. Following the procedure, the granulocytes are eluted from the nylon filters with ACD plasma, concentrated, and infused into the recipient. This setup is considerably less expensive than any of the centrifugation devices and the yield of granulocytes is considerably greater at about 3 to 5 × 10^{10} cells per donation.[30] The purity is also greater, and is almost completely free from the platelets or lymphocytes. HES is not used in filtration leukopheresis, but dexamethasone given to the donor appears to increase the yield.[30,31] Donor reactions have been found by some to be more common with FL than CFC techniques[32] and include shivering and chills. It has been postulated that the interaction of granulocytes with the nylon causes complement activation resulting in transient pulmonary dysfunction in donors.[33] The granulocyte count in donors undergoing filtration leukopheresis declines sharply, followed by a rebound leukocytosis not accounted for on the basis of leukocyte removal, suggesting activation of mediators.[34,35] In contrast, the granulocyte count remains relatively constant in donors undergoing CFC leukopheresis. Premedication with steroids appears to make little difference to changes in donor blood counts following pheresis. There is a mild decrease in the platelet count following leukopheresis and donors undergoing repeated platelet or leukopheresis should have periodic platelet counts performed.

Controversy exists over the degree to which granulocytes prepared by filtration leukopheresis are functionally impaired. Herzig et al[36] noted significant impairment of phagocytosis and bactericidal capacity. Wade et al[27] described an impaired ability to respond to stimulation with latex particles, and Wright et al[37] found impaired chemotaxis, phagocytosis and bacterial killing in granulocytes collected by CFC.[27] On the other hand, Harris et al[38] demonstrated normal phagocytosis, bactericidal capacity and chemotaxis of FL-prepared granulocytes. In addition, the effect of these apparent functional defects on the clinical effectiveness of FL granulocytes is unclear.

The specific indications for granulocyte transfusions are patients with severe granulocytopenia (less than 200 cells/mm^3), with clinical sepsis as determined by fever and preferably a positive culture, and in whom recovery from marrow suppression is not anticipated for more than 3 days. Several controlled studies have demonstrated that granulocytes prepared by either centrifugation or filtration are of significant benefit when transfused to septic granulocytopenic patients.[39,40,41] There were statistically significant survival advantages for those patients receiving granulocyte transfusions. Granulocyte transfusions proved particularly effective in patients with sepsis documented by positive cultures and in patients who had a prolonged (> 10 day) period of profound neutropenia. It is felt that the number of granulocytes transfused should be as many as possible, given daily during the period of granulocytopenia, but there is no conclusive data suggesting that clinical response is related to the number of granulocytes transfused. There has been no clear evidence of superiority of granulocytes prepared by either centrifugation or filtration, although some investigators feel that filtered granulocytes are possibly less effective than an equivalent dose of cells prepared by centrifugation.[31,39] The larger number of granulocytes in a filtered preparation compensates for this deficiency and the clinical effectiveness of filtered granulocytes has been established despite the reported functional impairments.

The granulocyte increment 1 hour posttransfusion varies from 0 to 1000 cells/mm^3. Despite the fact that Graw[42] has demonstrated higher increments with ABO and HLA matched granulocytes, however, the relationship of posttransfusion increment to clinical effectiveness remains unclear. Granulocyte transfusions resulting in 0 increments appear to be effective. Also, the role of HLA matching and presence of granulocyte agglutinins is unclear and remains to be elucidated. Granulocytes have been transfused into patients with preformed antibodies who have been pretreated with steroids with apparent clinical effectiveness.[43]

The occurrence of reactions such as fever and chills is more frequent with granulocytes prepared by filtration.[39,41,42] Mild fever accompanied by chills may occur in 60 per cent of recipients of filtered cells, and high fever, hypotension and respiratory distress have been reported.[44] Slow infusion of filtered granulocytes with temporary interruption of infusion when fever develops, as well as the administration of diphenhydramine, acetaminophen, steroids and, if necessary, demerol, however, controls the reactions effectively and allows the transfusions to proceed to completion.

It is currently accepted that granulocytes should be stored at room temperature and transfused within 24 hours or, preferably, 4 hours after harvest. The AABB as yet has not set standards for storage conditions, temperature, expiration time, yield or cell concentrations of granulocyte preparations, however. The decision to provide granulocyte transfusions should mean commitment to giving daily transfusions to septic, neutropenic patients in whom there is a chance of remission of the primary disease, in addition to appropriate aggressive antibiotic therapy until the infection is under control.

Plasma

The use of plasma in treating cancer patients is limited to the replacement of coagulation factors in patients with severe liver disease who are unresponsive to vitamin K and are actively bleeding. Fresh frozen plasma, which is plasma separated from blood within 4 hours of collection, contains therapeutic quantities of the labile coagulation factors V and VIII, as well as fibrinogen and the vitamin K dependent factors VII, X, IX and prothrombin. The amount of plasma infused depends on the clinical response of the patient, the response of the coagulation assays and the close monitoring of the patient with regard to volume overload. The bleeding associated with disseminated intravascular coagulation (DIC) is generally controlled by treating the primary cause, which is usually sepsis. Chronic disseminated intravascular coagulation associated with certain types of cancer does not usually result in a clinically significant bleeding diathesis, but heparin may be of value in patients with this problem. If bleeding persists in patients who are being adequately treated for the primary cause of DIC, cryoprecipitate and platelets can be of clinical benefit. Cryoprecipitate contains high concentrations of fibrinogen and factor VIII that are consumed in addition to platelets in DIC.

Unless the cause of the DIC is controlled, however, transfusions of these components only adds fuel to the consumptive process.

Albumin, which is prepared as a heat treated hepatitis-free plasma component, is useful in shock, burns, acute liver failure and following surgical procedures or the removal of large amounts of ascites fluid, but has no role in the supportive long-term treatment of patients with hypoalbuminemia due to poor nutrition and chronic inanition.[45]

The use of blood components plays a major role in the supportive treatment of patients with malignancies, and an understanding of the principles of transfusion therapy is essential to optimal patient care and to the effective utilization of blood resources.

References

1. Kremer W B, Laszlo J: Hematologic effects of cancer, in Frei E III, Holland J (eds): Cancer Medicine. Philadelphia, Lea & Febiger, 1973, p 1085
2. Haurani F I, Young K, Tocantins L M: Reutilization of iron in anemia complicating malignant neoplasm. Blood 22:73, 1963
3. Dacie J V: Secondary or symptomatic haemolytic anaemias, in Dacie J V (ed): Haemolytic Anemias Congenital and Acquired, 2nd ed. New York, Grune & Stratton, 1967, p 719
4. Brain M C, Azzapardi J G, Baker L R, et al: Microangiopathic haemolytic anemia and mucin-forming adenocarcinoma. Br J Haematol 18:183, 1970
5. Standards for Blood Banks and Transfusion Services. Committee on Standards—American Association of Blood Banks, Eighth ed. Washington, D C, 1976
6. Hoak J C, Koepke J A: Platelet transfusions. Clin Haematol 5:69, 1976
7. Aisner J, Schiffer C A, Wolff J H et al: A standardized technique for efficient platelet and leukocyte collection using the model 30 blood processor. Transfusion 16:437, 1976
8. Wirman J A, Ruder E A, Smith R T, et al: Functional and ultrastructural status of platelets prepared by the celltrifuge. Transfusion 15:614, 1975
9. Slichter S J, Harker L A: Preparation and storage of platelet concentrates. Transfusion 16:8, 1976
10. Schiffer C A, Aisner J, Schmukler M, et al: The effect of hydroxyethyl starch on in vitro platelet and granulocyte function. Transfusion 15:473, 1975
11. Murphy S, Gardner F H: Platelet preservation. Effect of storage temperature on maintenance of platelet viability—Deleterious effect of refrigerated storage. N Engl J Med 280:1094, 1969
12. Aster R H, Becker G A, Filip D J: Studies to improve methods of short-term platelet preservation. Transfusion 16:4, 1976
13. Becker G A, Tucalli M, Kunicki T, et al: Studies of platelet concentrates stored at 22 C and 4 C. Transfusion 13:61, 1973
14. Valeri C R: Hemostatic effectiveness of liquid and previously frozen human platelets. N Engl J Med 290:353, 1974
15. Slichter S J, Harker L A: Preparation and storage of platelet concentrates. Semin Current Technical Topics, AABB, 1974, pp 87–93
16. Valeri C R: Circulation and hemostatic effectiveness of platelets stored at 4 C or 24 C. Transfusion 16:20, 1976
17. Lokich J J: Managing chemotherapy-induced bone marrow suppression in cancer. Hospital Practice 11(8):61, 1976
18. Yankee R A, Graff K S, Dowling R N, et al: Selection of unrelated compatible platelet donors by lymphocyte HL-A matching. N Engl J Med 288:760, 1973
19. Goldfinger D, McGinniss M H: Rh-incompatible platelet transfusions—Risks and consequences of sensitizing immunosuppressed patients. N Engl J Med 283:942, 1971
20. Herzig R H, Poplack D G, Yankee R A: Prolonged granulocytopenia from incompatible platelet transfusions. N Engl J Med 290:1220, 1974
21. Yankee R A, Grumet F C, Rogentine G N: Platelet transfusion therapy—The selection of compatible platelet donors for refractory patients by lymphocyte HL-A typing. N Engl J Med 281:1208, 1969
22. Lohrmann H P, Bull M I, Decter J A, et al: Platelet transfusions from HL-A compatible unrelated donors to alloimmunized patients. Ann Int Med 80:9, 1974
23. Mishler J M: Hydroxyethyl starch as an experimental adjunct to leukocyte separation by centrifugal means: Review of safety and efficacy. Transfusion 15:449, 1975
24. Mishler J M, Moser A M, Carter J B: The safety of dexamethasone and hydroxyethyl starch in the multiple leukopheresed donor. Transfusion 16:170, 1976

25. Huestis D W, White R F, Price M J, et al: Use of hydroxyethyl starch to improve granulocyte collection in the Latham blood processor. Transfusion 15:559, 1975
26. Mishler J M, Higby D J, Rhomberg W, et al: Hydroxyethyl starch and dexamethasone as an adjunct to leukocyte separation with the IBM blood cell separator. Transfusion 14:352, 1974
27. Wade P H, Skrabut E M, Vinciguerra L, et al: In vitro function of granulocytes isolated from blood of normal volunteers using continuous-flow configuration in the IBM-Aminco celltrifuge and adhesion-filtration leukopheresis using nylon fiber. Transfusion 17:136, 1977
28. Increased granulocyte collection with the blood cell separator and the addition of etiocholanolone and hydroxyethyl starch. Transfusion 14:357, 1974
29. Djerassi I, Kim J S, Mitrabul C, et al: Filtration leukopheresis for separation and concentration of transfusible amounts of normal human granulocytes. J Med 1:358, 1970
30. MacPherson J L, Nushecher J, Bennett J M: The acquisition of granulocytes by leukopheresis: A comparison of continuous flow centrifugation and filtration leukopheresis in normal and corticosteroid-stimulated donors. Transfusion 16:221, 1976
31. Russell J A, Powles R: White cell therapy. Clin Haematol 5:81, 1976
32. Herzig G P, Rost R K, Graw R G Jr: Granulocyte collection by continuous flow filtration leukopheresis. Blood 39:554, 1972
33. Fehr J, Craddock P R, Jacob H S: Complement (C′) mediated granulocyte (PMN and pulmonary dysfunction during nylon fiber leukopheresis). Blood 46:1054, 1975
34. Rubins J M, MacPherson J L, Nusbacher J, et al: Granulocyte kinetics in donors undergoing filtration leukopheresis. Transfusion 16:56, 1976
35. Schiffer C A, Aisner J, Wiernik P H: Transient neutropenia induced by transfusion of blood exposed to nylon fiber filters. Blood 45:141–146, 1975
36. Herzig G P, Root R K, Graw R G Jr: Granulocyte collection by continuous-flow leukopheresis. Blood 39:554, 1972
37. Wright D G, Kauffmann J F, Chusid M J, et al: Functional abnormalities of human neutrophils collected by continous flow filtration leukopheresis. Blood 46:901, 1975
38. Harris M, Djerassi I, Schwartz E, et al: Polymorphonuclear leukocytes prepared by continuous flow filtration leukopheresis: Viability and function. Blood 44:707, 1974
39. Herzig R H, Herzig G P, Graw R G, et al: Successful granulocyte transfusion therapy for gram-negative septicemia. N Engl J Med 296:701, 1977
40. Alavi J B, Root R K, Djerassi I, et al: A randomized clinical trial of granulocyte transfusions for infection in acute leukemia. N Engl J Med 296:706, 1977
41. Higby D J, Yates J W, Henderson E S, et al: Filtration leukopheresis for granulocyte transfusion therapy. N Engl J Med 292:761, 1975
42. Graw R G, Herzig G, Perry S, et al: Normal granulocyte transfusion therapy: Treatment of septicemia due to gram negative bacteria. N Engl J Med 287: 367, 1972
43. Higby D J, Henderson E S: Granulocyte transfusions for infection during neutropenia. Semin Oncol 2:361–368, 1975
44. Schiffer C A, Buckholz D H, Aisner J, et al: Clinical experience with transfusion of granulocytes obtained by continuous flow filtration leukopheresis. Amer J Med 58:373, 1975
45. Tullis J L: Albumin 2. Guidelines for clinical use. JAMA 237:460, 1977

VICTORIO RODRIGUEZ

29
Infections in Cancer Patients During Chemotherapy

Important advances have been made in the management of patients with disseminated malignant diseases during the past 10 years, so that the prognoses of some diseases has improved considerably. Thus, individuals with advanced Hodgkin's disease, diffuse histiocytic lymphoma and acute myelogenous leukemia, among others, achieve a complete remission more frequently and experience prolonged disease-free survival as a result of effective chemotherapy.[1,2,3] These therapeutic advances, however, could not have been accomplished without concomitant progress in the management of complications in these patients. Hence, supportive therapy such as blood component replacement and antiinfective therapy have become an integral part of the modern management of disseminated cancer.

Patients with disseminated cancer, particularly those who have bone marrow involvement, are highly susceptible to the complications of bone marrow failure. The risk of these complications usually increase during periods of chemotherapy until the patients achieve remission of their malignancy. Patients with acute leukemia are highly susceptible to complications such as infection and hemorrhage because of severe and prolonged bone marrow failure. Effective control of most hemorrhagic complications is now possible. Infection, therefore, remains the most important complication. Extensive studies in patients with other forms of disseminated cancer undergoing intensive chemotherapy also indicate that infection is the major cause of morbidity.[4,5] Recent autopsy studies indicate, as well, that infection is the most common cause of death.[6,7,8] The knowledge gained from these studies has identified the most frequent types of infection in these patients and their epidemiologic characteristics. This knowledge has led to the design of studies to improve the therapeutic regimens used for the control of established infection and to attempt the prevention of infections during periods of severe myelosuppression. The application of advances in supportive care used concomitantly with more effective antitumor regimens will hopefully continue to improve the prognosis of patients with cancer.

Supported in part by Contract NO-1-CM-53832 and Grants CA 10376 and CA 10042 from the National Cancer Institute, National Institutes of Health, U. S. Public Health Service, Bethesda, Maryland 20014.

TABLE 29-1. *Episodes of Fever in Acute Leukemia*[9] *During 1966 to 1972*

Number of Patients	494
Number of Hospitalizations	1216
Number of Febrile Episodes	1894
% Episodes Due to Infection	64
% Episodes Due to Noninfectious Cause	1
% FUO	35

FEVER DURING MYELOSUPPRESSION

Fever is a common, early and reliable sign of infection in patients with advanced malignancy and myelosuppression. Fever greater than 101° F, not related to transfusion of blood products, generally heralds the onset of infection and should prompt the physician to initiate thorough diagnostic studies and institute appropriate therapy, particularly in patients with acute leukemia. We have recently concluded a study in acute leukemia that indicates that in these patients, fever is usually due to infection.[9] Four hundred and ninety-four adults with acute leukemia treated at the M. D. Anderson Hospital between 1966 and 1972 were reviewed (Table 29-1). There were a mean of 2.4 febrile episodes per patient and all of the 1894 febrile episodes were analyzed. The patients had fever for 28 per cent of the days spent in the hospital. Sixty-four per cent of the febrile episodes were due to infection and only 1 per cent were due to noninfectious factors identified as the cause of fever, although fevers due to chemotherapy, immunotherapy and blood transfusions were excluded. In 35 per cent of the episodes, the origin of the fever could not be determined (FUO). Fever occurred most often when the patients had severe neutropenia, in spite of the fact that neutropenic patients are unable to mount an adequate inflammatory response. The proportion of febrile episodes due to infection was related to the number of circulating neutrophils. Fevers associated with a high neutrophil count also were most often due to infection, however. The most common types of infection were disseminated infection and pneumonia, which together accounted for 69 per cent of the total episodes of documented infection.

Experiences similar to those in acute leukemia have been described in patients with lymphoma and metastatic carcinoma. During myelosuppressive therapy, most febrile episodes are due to infection.[4,5] Only in a very few patients is fever a result of their underlying disease. Fever, secondary to malignancy, occurs most frequently in patients with lymphoma. In a substantial number of patients, however, no etiologic factor can be recognized as producing fever and these fevers are considered of unknown origin (FUO). Since patients with impaired host defenses often fail to develop other clinical signs of infection, it is likely that a substantial proportion of such FUO episodes are actually due to infection.[9,10] Most physicians have recognized the importance of instituting antibiotics promptly when fever occurs in the neutropenic patient. No uniform criteria exists, however, for the management of those patients with FUO. We recommend instituting broad-spectrum antibiotic therapy in these patients since it is often difficult to differentiate infectious and noninfectious fevers in the neutropenic patient.[10] About two-thirds of patients with FUO become afebrile after initial adequate antimicrobial therapy is begun. This suggests that an unidentified infection may be present and responding and, if not treated sufficiently, may lead to an unnecessary mortality rate. Therefore, these patients should receive antibiotics for about 1 week. One-third of those patients with fever of undetermined origin remain febrile after initiation of antibiotic therapy. In half of these patients, an infection may be subsequently identified. Therefore, those patients who are not responding after 4 days of therapy should be reevaluated and will most likely require a change in antimicrobial therapy.

THE MOST COMMON TYPES OF INFECTION DURING CANCER CHEMOTHERAPY

Bacterial organisms remain the most common pathogens causing infection during cancer chemotherapy in patients with advanced disease. Extensive studies in patients with acute leukemia have indicated that greater than 80 per cent of the infections that occur

TABLE 29-2. *Most Common Types of Organism Causing Infection During Antileukemic Therapy*

1) Bacterial:	Gram-negative bacilli: E. coli, Klebsiella sp., Ps. aeruginosa, Serratia, Enterobacter, Proteus	70%
	Gram-positive cocci: S. aureus, Streptococci	6%
2) Fungal:	Candida, Aspergillus, Mucor	8%
3) Viral:	Herpes, Cytomegalovirus	1%
4) Other:	Pneumocystis, Toxoplasmosis	<1%
5) Multiple Organisms		13%

when the patients are myelosuppressed are due to bacteria.[9] Similarly, studies conducted in patients with Hodgkin's disease, malignant lymphoma and solid tumors treated with intensive combination chemotherapy have also demonstrated that during periods of myelosuppression the pathogens most frequently causing infection are bacteria.[4,5] In a study of the causes of fever in 494 adults with acute leukemia, the most frequent bacterial pathogens were gram-negative bacilli (Table 29-2). Prior to the introduction of effective penicillin therapy, *Staphylococcus aureus* and other gram-positive cocci were frequently seen as cause of morbidity and mortality in such patients. Since the introduction of methicillin and other semisynthetic penicillins, however, the frequency of *Staph. aureus* and other gram-positive cocci as causes of infection in these patients has decreased substantially. During the past 10 years, however, the gram-negative organisms have emerged as the most frequent pathogens. Among these gram-negative organisms, *Pseudomonas sp.* infections used to be the most frequent from 1966 until 1970. Since the introduction of carbenicillin and ticarcillin, however, the mortality rate, and subsequently, the proportion of infections caused by *Pseudomonas* have substantially decreased in major cancer centers.[8,9] Concomitant with this decrease, the incidence of other gram-negative pathogens such as the *Klebsiella-Enterobacter-Serratia* group have become a prevalent problem. In patients with acute leukemia, *E. coli* and *Klebsiella spp.* are the most common cause of gram-negative bacillary infections.[9]

Other bacterial pathogens less frequently seen in these patients are *Salmonella, Citrobacter, Flavobacterium* and *Clostridium spp.* These organisms occur infrequently but they may produce overwhelming infection. Organisms such as *Corynebacterium* and *Bacillus spp.* may be a serious problem because they are usually not recognized as pathogens and also because they are often resistant to available antibiotics. Mycobacterial organisms can also cause infection in myelosuppressed patients. Recent studies on the incidence of mycobacterial infections in cancer patients indicate that they have increased among this population of patients and that as many as 50 per cent are caused by "atypical" organisms.[11]

Fungal infections have been recognized as an emerging problem in cancer patients since the early 1960s[12] and this trend has continued during the past decade. Initially, *Candida albicans* and *Candida sp.* were the most frequent organisms noted during this period. Later, other fungi such as *Aspergillus spp., Phycomycetes, Torulopsis glabrata* and other rare fungi have been reported.[13] Our studies in patients with acute leukemia and other patients with cancer have indicated that the overall incidence of fungal infections is about 20 per cent. *Candida* infections are more prevalent among all types of cancer. In other centers, *Aspergillus* has also become an important pathogen in leukemia patients. Other fungi such as *Cryptococcus neoformans* and *H. capsulatum* are less common.

Viral infections are also of concern among the patients undergoing cancer chemotherapy.[14] Herpes simplex and herpes zoster infections are more frequent in young or very old patients. Among these, herpes zoster occurs commonly in patients with malignant lymphoma, Hodgkin's disease and children with acute leukemia. Recently it has been recognized that the more intense the therapeutic regimen, the greater the susceptibility to viral infections, especially herpes zoster. Studies of patients who have received combination chemotherapy indicate that the incidence of herpes zoster with the potential of dissemination among this population of patients is higher than in those receiving chemotherapy or radiotherapy alone. Other viral infections, such as cytomegalic inclusion disease, multifocal leukoencephalopathy and measles have been described but occur infrequently.[14]

Parasitic infections, specifically *Pneumocystis carinii* pneumonitis and toxoplasmosis appear to be increasing in frequency among patients receiving cancer chemotherapy.[15] In the past, *Pneumocystis carinii* infection occurred mainly in children with continuous myelosuppressive therapy. This infection is being detected more frequently in other cancer patients who are receiving intensive myelosuppressive therapy or extensive radiation. *Toxoplasma gondii* is a parasite which can be pathogenic to debilitated hosts and presents as a disseminated infection in many myelosuppressed patients. This organism, like cytomegalovirus, can be transmitted by blood products that are transfused to the patient; thus, it has the potential of becoming a serious problem. Fortunately, as more and better diagnostic techniques and therapeutic measures become available, the control of opportunistic infection will become a reality.

Antibiotic Therapy of Infections During Cancer Chemotherapy

Important advances have been made in the management of infections in cancer patients through the introduction of new antibiotics. The selection of the appropriate antibiotic is of critical importance in the management of gram-negative bacillary infections. Neutropenia is not only the most important factor responsible for increasing the cancer patient's susceptibility to infection, but it is also an important factor in the outcome of therapy. Several of the antibiotics that appear to be effective in vitro are not very efficacious in the neutropenic patient. The semisynthetic penicillins with antipseudomonal activity and other new aminoglycosides of wide spectrum have been valuable components of therapy developed in recent years.[16]

The introduction of carbenicillin elicited considerable interest because of its activity against *P. aeruginosa* in vitro.[17] Subsequently, ticarcillin was synthesized and found to have a similar spectrum of activity. These drugs are also active in vitro against many isolates of *E. coli* and *Enterobacter spp.* and most isolates of indole negative and indole positive *Proteus spp.* Ticarcillin is about twice as active in vitro as carbenicillin against *P. aeruginosa*.

We have evaluated these drugs alone and in combinations as primary therapy for presumed gram-negative bacillary infections because of the predominance of *Pseudomonas* and *E. coli* infections in our patients (Table 29-3). Carbenicillin has been administered at a rate of 5 gm over a 2-hour period every 4 hours. This schedule of administration maintains a serum concentration of about 150 μg/ml with a peak serum concentration at the end of the infusion of about 200 μg/ml.[18] The drug proved to be very effective against *Pseudomonas* and *Proteus* infections, moderately effective against *E. coli* infections and ineffective against *Klebsiella* and *Serratia* infections.[19] Subsequently, ticarcillin was evaluated as initial therapy during 67 infections in 63 cancer patients. Because this drug was more active in vitro than carbenicillin, we reduced the total daily dosage to 21 gm. Pharmacology studies indicated that serum concentrations of ticarcillin at the end of 6 hours were below the concentration required to inhibit the growth of most organisms.[20] Therefore, we decided to administer 3.5 gm over a 2-hour period every 4 hours. This schedule maintained a serum concentration of about 50 μg/ml with a peak serum concentration of about 200 μg/ml at the end of each infusion. In the 67 infections treated, the overall response rate was 43 per cent.[21] The results with *Pseudomonas* infections were as good as had been achieved with carbenicillin. Ticarcillin was ineffective against *Klebsiella* infections

TABLE 29-3. *Antibiotic Therapy of Infections in Cancer Patients*

Organisms	Carbenicillin		Ticarcillin		Gentamicin		Tobramycin		Amikacin	
	Number	% Responses	Number	% Responses	Number	% Responses	Number	% Responses	Number	% Responses
Pseudomonas	23	91	20	90	22	45	10	40	3	100
Klebsiella-Enterobacter-Serratia	11	0	10	0	42	52	20	55	11	91
E. coli	12	58	11	9	8	75	11	36	7	71
Other gram-negative bacilli	10	40	6	67	6	83	5	80	—	—
Single gram-negative bacilli	48	63	47	49	78	47	46	50	21	86
Total Results	56	57	67	43	122	51	82	54	49	69

TABLE 29-4. *Response to Antibiotic Therapy Related to Neutrophil Count*

Neutrophil/ mm³	Gentamicin*		Tobramycin*		Carbenicillin†		Ticarcillin†	
	Number	% Cure	Number	% Cure	Number	% Cure	Number	% Cure
<100	22	23	21	24	16	75	12	92
101–1000	17	53	10	70	26	88	4	75
>1000	24	79	28	79	9	56	4	100
Decreased	32	31	23	39	29	72	—	—
Increased	31	74	36	69	22	82	—	—

*Gram-negative bacillary infections only.
†Pseudomonas infections only.

and most of the *E. coli* infections. All failures were due to antibiotic resistance. Like carbenicillin, ticarcillin was effective regardless of the patients' neutrophil counts (Table 29-4). Obviously, because of their somewhat limited spectrum of activity, neither of these drugs should be used alone as initial therapy for presumed gram-negative bacillary infection at the present time.

The aminoglycosides have been used extensively because of their broad spectrum of activity. Gentamicin has been evaluated for the treatment of 122 episodes of infection that occurred in 101 cancer patients at our institution.[22] During 55 episodes, the infections failed to respond to prior antibiotic therapy. The total daily dosage of drug was equivalent to 3 mg/kg. The majority of infections were cases of pneumonia, cellulitis, urinary tract infection and septicemia. The most frequent infecting organisms are those listed in Table 29-3. All of the organisms were sensitive to gentamicin in vitro. The overall response rate was 51 per cent and was highest among patients with urinary tract infection and cellulitis. *E. coli* infections responded most frequently and multiple organism infections responded least frequently. Response to gentamicin therapy was related to the patients' neutrophil counts at the onset of their infection (Table 29-4). Only 23 per cent of gram-negative bacillary infections, occurring in patients with less than 100 neutrophils/mm,³ responded. Response was also related to whether the patients' neutrophil counts increased or decreased during their infection. Nephrotoxicity has been observed with gentamicin more often in cancer patients than in other patients. This may be due in part to the fact that these patients often receive multiple courses of nephrotoxic antibiotics or other drugs which may potentiate the nephrotoxicity of gentamicin.

Subsequently, we evaluated tobramycin for the treatment of 82 episodes of infection in 73 cancer patients.[23] During 56 episodes, the infections failed to respond to other prior antibiotic therapy. The dosage of the drug was 50 mg/M² (1.25 mg/kg) every 6 hours intravenously, and the overall response rate was 54 per cent. Two infections were caused by organisms resistant to tobramycin and both failed to respond. Response to tobramycin was also related to the patients' neutrophil counts (Table 29-4). Nephrotoxicity was observed less frequently with tobramycin than with gentamicin, although a higher dosage of the drug was administered.

Amikacin, another new aminoglycoside, is a derivative of kanamycin, but unlike kanamycin, it is active against *P. aeruginosa*. A major advantage of amikacin is its activity against most strains of *Enterobacteriaceae* that are resistant to other aminoglycosides. Amikacin has been effective in 69 per cent of 49 infections in cancer patients.[24] The majority of infections were cases of pneumonia and septicemia, and were caused by *E. coli*, *K. pneumoniae* and *S. marcescens*. These results were especially impressive because all of the patients had neutropenia. The response rate was only 33 per cent among patients with a persistent neutropenia of less than 100/mm³, however. Azotemia occurred in 13 per cent and ototoxicity in 6 per cent of these patients.

The results of these and other studies indicate that the aminoglycoside antibiotics are useful because of their broad spectrum of ac-

TABLE 29-5. *Antibiotic Combinations for Initial Therapy of Infections in the Compromised Host*

	Pseudo-monas	K-E-S	E. Coli	Proteus	Mixed Gram (–)	Staph. Aureus and other Gram (+)
Carb + Ceph	86	33	67	—	80	75
Carb + Ceph	83	90	80	63	—	—
Carb + Kan	87	31	—	—	100	75
Carb + Gent	100	50	25	100	—	50
Carb + Gent	81	—	—	—	—	50
Gent + Ceph	—	90	86	—	—	100
Gent + Chloro	—	60	—	—	40	62
Carb + Ceph + Gent	63	63	80	83	100	—
Carb + Ceph + Gent	58	47	75	—	—	—

tivity. Our most recent data suggest that the results in neutropenic patients can be improved by administering the drugs by continuous, rather than by intermittent, infusion.[25]

A combination of antibiotics should be used to provide optimum therapy for serious gram-negative bacillary infections. A wide variety of antibiotic combinations have been evaluated for the therapy of infections in cancer patients (Table 29-5). Although no regimen is entirely satisfactory as initial therapy for presumed gram-negative bacillary infections, certain recommendations can be made. For patients with adequate neutrophils, an appropriate combination would be a cephalosporin plus an aminoglycoside. If there is reason to suspect an anaerobic infection, however, clindamycin should be substituted for the cephalosporin. For patients with neutropenia, an appropriate combination would be carbenicillin (or ticarcillin), plus a cephalosporin, plus an aminoglycoside. The penicillin or cephalosporin should be eliminated from the regimen once the in vitro antibiotic sensitivities of the etiologic agent are known.

PROPHYLAXIS OF INFECTION DURING CANCER CHEMOTHERAPY

The possibility of preventing infection in cancer patients undergoing chemotherapy has been under investigation for the past decade in our institution.[26] Introduction of the plastic tent isolator made it feasible to protect the patient from nosocomial contamination by providing filtered air and a barrier to the hospital environment and personnel. Subsequently, more sophisticated patient isolators became available with the introduction of the laminar air flow rooms (LAFR). Since a majority of the infections occurring in patients with acute leukemia are caused by their endogenous microbial flora, however, prophylactic antibiotics (PA) have been administered to the patients who entered protected environments (PE).

Our initial study compared the results of antileukemic chemotherapy in 33 patients treated with the PEPA program with the results in two groups of matched controls who were treated concurrently with the same chemotherapeutic regimens.[27] This study demonstrated that patients on the PEPA program had a significantly lower frequency of infectious complications. The frequency of complete remissions was only about 15 per cent higher in the group of the PE, a difference that was not statistically significant. The duration of remission and survival, however, were significantly longer for the patients on the PEPA program. These patients generally received higher doses of antileukemic agents that presumably resulted in a greater reduction in the number of leukemic cells and thus, longer remissions. The encouraging results of

TABLE 29-6. *Major Infections During Remission Induction*

	PE Units In	PE Units Out
Number of Patients	63	82
Percent of Patients with Infection	41	57
Percent of Patients with Fatal Infection	13	28
Total Days	4339	4201
Percent of Days Spent with Infection	9	18
Days Spent with <100 Neutrophils/mm^3	1727	1947
Percent of Days with <100 Neutrophils/mm^3 and Infection	18	28
Days Spent with 101-500 Neutrophils/mm^3	639	760
Percent of Days with 101-500 Neutrophils/mm^3 and Infection	7	15
Days Spent with 501-1000 Neutrophils/mm^3	250	304
Percent of Days with 501-1000 Neutrophils/mm^3 and Infection	10	14

this initial study led us to design a prospectively randomized study of the PEPA program for patients undergoing chemotherapy for acute leukemia. The results in 145 adults with acute leukemia have been recently analyzed.[28] Of the 145 patients entered into this study, 63 were randomized in a PE and 82 outside a PE (Table 29-6). All patients received prophylactic antibiotic regimens. The groups were comparable for those parameters that are prognostic in acute leukemia.

Of the 145 patients, 73 (50 per cent) developed 102 episodes of major infections. Thirty-one (30 per cent) of these infections were fatal. The 145 patients spent a total hospitalization period of 8540 days or an average of 59 days per patient. During 5073 days, the patients had a neutrophil count of less than 500/mm^3, and during 3674 days, or 65 per cent of the time, they had a neutrophil count of less than 100/mm^3. Comparing the 63 patients treated in a PE unit with the 82 patients treated out of a PE unit (Table 29-6), the proportion of patients who developed major infections in a PE was 41 per cent, and outside of the PE the proportion was 57 per cent ($P=0.08$). The rate of fatal infections in a PE was 13 per cent, significantly lower than the 28 per cent rate outside a PE ($P=0.04$). The number of days with infection at less than 100 neutrophils/mm^3, and at 101 to 500 neutrophils/mm^3 was significantly lower inside a PE than outside ($P < 0.01$ for both comparisons). The proportion of patients who survived long enough to receive an adequate trial was higher in the PE (97 per cent) than out of the units (82 per cent). The complete remission (CR) rate was 71 per cent in and 43 per cent out of a PE unit, a statistically significant difference ($P > 0.01$). The median survival time was 72 weeks for patients in a PE, compared with 42 weeks for patients outside a PE, and the difference in survival curves was highly statistically significant ($P < 0.01$). The prophylactic antibiotic regimens were well-tolerated by most patients. Nausea and epigastric discomfort associated with the oral antibiotics were described by one-third of the patients, but they usually subsided in a short time and discontinuation of the antibiotics was not necessary. Acute renal failure occurred in 4 of 90 patients receiving intravenous antibiotics and was attributed to the administration of colistin or amphotericin B. Renal damage was reversible in 3 of the 4 patients.

This prospective randomized study of the PEPA regimen demonstrated statistically significant advantages for risk of fatal infection, higher CR rate and longer survival of patients treated in a PE unit with prophylactic antibiotics as compared with patients treated in a conventional hospital room with the same antibiotic regimens. Several other studies have also demonstrated beneficial effects of protected environment programs for patients undergoing chemotherapy of acute leukemia. Recently we have expanded our program to include patients with advanced malignant lymphoma and solid tumors undergoing chemotherapy. The preliminary results of these studies are also encouraging.[29]

Summary

Important advances made in the management of disseminated malignant disease have been possible with more effective modalities of therapy, including those related to supportive care. Since infection remains the major cause of morbidity and mortality during cancer chemotherapy, its management has become a crucial component of modern cancer therapy. Fever is the major sign of infection in these patients who otherwise are incapable of mounting an inflammatory response to the infection. The diagnosis and management of febrile episodes in these patients is therefore important. Among cancer patients, infections caused by gram-negative organisms are common, particularly those caused by *E. coli*, *Klebsiella* and *P. aeruginosa*. The incidence of gram-positive cocci infections, particularly *Staph. aureus*, has decreased substantially since the introduction of methicillin and other semisynthetic penicillins. Opportunistic infections, such as those produced by *Candida albicans*, *Pneumocystis carinii* and *Toxoplasma gondii* are increasing in frequency. More effective antimicrobial agents have been developed recently and the prompt use of these agents alone or in combination has produced gratifying results. The new semisynthetic penicillins with antipseudomonal activity have been especially effective in the control of *Pseudomonas* infections. The development of antibiotics of wider spectrum of activity such as the aminoglycosides also has contributed to the control of gram-negative infections in these patients. Combination regimens of these agents are indicated as initial therapy of presumed severe infection in myelosuppressed hosts. Newer modalities of preventing overwhelming infection during myelosuppression, such as the use of protected environments, have been demonstrated as a useful tool. Although much remains to be accomplished, present advances have improved the care of the cancer patient.

References

1. DeVita V, Canellos G, Hubbard S, et al: Chemotherapy of Hodgkin's Disease (HD) with MOPP: A 10-Year Progress Report. Proceedings of the 12th Annual Meeting of the American Society of Clinical Oncology, Toronto, May, 1976 (abstr C-131) p 269
2. Rodriguez V, Cabanillas F, Burgess M A, et al: Combination chemotherapy "CHOP-BLEO" in advanced (non-Hodgkin's) malignant lymphoma. Blood 49:325–333, 1977
3. Bodey G P, Coltman C A, Hewlett J S, Freireich E J: Progress in the treatment of adults with acute leukemia. Review of regimens containing arabinosyl cytosine studied by the Southwest Oncology Group. Arch Intern Med 136:1383–1388, 1976
4. Livingston R B, Einhorn L H, Bodey G P, et al: COMB (Cyclophosphamide, oncovin, methyl CCNU and bleomycin): A four-drug combination in solid tumors. Cancer 36:327–332, 1975
5. Bodey G P, Hersh E M, Valdivieso M, et al: Effects of cytotoxic drugs and immunosuppressive agents on the immune system. Postgrad Med 58:67–74, 1975
6. Inagaki J, Rodriguez V, Bodey G P: Causes of death in cancer patients. Cancer 33:568–573, 1974
7. Feld R, Bodey G P, Rodriguez V, Luna M: Causes of death in patients with malignant lymphoma. Am J Med Sci 268:97–106, 1974
8. Chang H Y, Rodriguez V, Narboni G, et al: Causes of death in adults with acute leukemia. Medicine 55:259–268, 1976
9. Bodey G P, Rodriguez V, Chang H Y, Narboni G: Fever and infection in leukemic patients. A study of 494 consecutive patients. Cancer 41:1610–1622, 1978
10. Rodriguez V, Burgess M A, Bodey G P: Management of fever of unknown origin in cancer patients with neoplasms and neutropenia. Cancer 32:1007–1012, 1973
11. Feld R, Bodey G P, Groschel D: Mycobacteriosis in patients in malignant disease. Arch Int Med 136:67–70, 1976
12. Bodey G P: Fungal infections complicating acute leukemia. J Chron Dis 19:667–687, 1966
13. Valdivieso M, Luna M, Bodey G P, et al: Fungemia due to torulopsis glabrata in the compromised host. Cancer 38:1750–1756, 1976
14. Feldman S, Cox F: Viral infections and haematological malignancies, in Bodey G P (ed): Clinics in Haematology, vol. 5. London, Saunders 1976, p 311
15. Hughes W T: Protozoan infections in haematological diseases, in Bodey G P (ed): Clinics

in Haematology, vol. 5. London, Saunders, 1976, p 329
16. Rodriguez V, Bodey G P: Antibacterial therapy—Special considerations in neutropenic patients, in Bodey G P (ed): Clinics in Haematology, vol. 5. London, Saunders, 1976, p 347
17. Bodey G P, Rodriguez V: Advances in the management of pseudomonas aeruginosa infections in cancer patients. Eur J Cancer 9:435–441, 1973
18. Bodey G P, Rodriguez V, Stewart D: Clinical pharmacological studies of carbenicillin. Am J Med Sci. 275:185–190, 1969
19. Bodey G P, Rodriguez V, Luce J K: Carbenicillin therapy of gram-negative bacilli infections. Am J Med Sci 257:408–414, 1969
20. Rodriguez V, Inagaki J, Bodey G P: Clinical pharmacology of ticarcillin (α-carboxyl-3-thienylmethyl penicillin, BRL-2288). Antimicrob Agents Chemother 4:31–36, 1973
21. Rodriguez V, Bodey G P, Horikoshi N, et al: Ticarcillin therapy of infections. Antimicrob Agents Chemother 4:427–431, 1973
22. Bodey G P, Middleman E, Umsawasdi T, Rodriguez V: Infections in cancer patients. Results with gentamicin sulfate therapy. Cancer 29:1697–1701, 1972
23. Valdivieso M, Horikoshi N, Rodriguez V, Bodey G P: Therapeutic trials with tobramycin. Am J Med Sci 268:149–156, 1974
24. Valdivieso M, Feld R, Rodriguez V, Bodey G P: Amikacin therapy of infections in neutropenic patients. Am J Med Sci 270:453–463, 1975
25. Bodey G P, Chang H Y, Rodriguez V, Stewart D: Feasibility of administering aminoglycoside antibiotics by continuous intravenous infusion. Antimicrob Agents Chemother 8:328–333, 1975
26. Bodey G P, Freireich E J: Isolation for the compromised host. JAMA 233:543–545, 1975
27. Bodey G P, Gehan E A, Freireich E J, Frei E III: Protected environment-prophylactic antibiotic program in the chemotherapy of acute leukemia. Am J Med Sci 262:138–151, 1971
28. Rodriguez V, Bodey G P, Gehan E A, et al: Randomized trial of protected environment-prophylactic antibiotics in 145 adults with acute leukemia. Medicine 57:253–266, 1978
29. Rodriguez V, Bodey G P: Effect of protected environments plus oral prophylactic antibiotics (PEPA) on the incidence of infections in cancer patients (PTS) during intensive chemotherapy. Proceedings of the 16th Interscience Conference on Antimicrobial Agents and Chemotherapy, Chicago, October, 1976, (abstr 331)

C. Dean Buckner

30

Marrow Transplantation for Acute Leukemia: Seattle Experience

Marrow transplantation has been utilized to treat refractory patients with AML and ALL who have an identical twin or HLA-matched sibling donors. The basic treatment regimen consisted of total-body irradiation (TBI), preceded in most instances by high dosages of cyclophosphamide (CY), with or without additional chemotherapeutic agents.

Six of 16 patients with hematological malignancy refractory to conventional therapy transplanted from identical twin donors are presently in complete remission 46 to 78 months after transplantation. All six are leading normal lives without maintenance therapy.

One of 6 patients with ALL transplanted from an HLA-matched sibling following TBI alone, is alive 6½ years after transplantation. Relapse of leukemia occurred in the other 5 patients and in 2 of these the relapse was in donor cells.

Thirteen of 100 patients transplanted following CY and TBI are alive 1½ to 5½ years after transplantation, having been off all treatment since day 100 posttransplantation. Four additional patients are alive after grafting, but have had a relapse of their leukemia.

These results are sufficiently encouraging to warrant transplantation earlier in the course of the patient's disease whenever an identical twin or HLA-matched sibling is available as a donor.

Introduction

Marrow transplantation offers the potential of administering larger than normal doses of cytotoxic agents in an attempt to eradicate leukemia. Chemotherapeutic agents and/or TBI can be given in dosages that are potentially lethal to marrow and then reversed by marrow infusion. Thus, with this technique, non-marrow toxicity is the limiting factor to the quantity of cytotoxic agents administered. In addition to the ability to administer high doses of cytotoxic agents, there is theoretical evidence in animal systems that allogeneic marrow transplantation has a specific or nonspecific graft-versus-tumor effect.[1]

The basic immunology of marrow transplantation and clinical results through 1974 have recently been reviewed.[2] The results of allogeneic marrow transplantation in 100 leu-

These investigations were supported by Grant Numbers CA 18029, CA 17117, and CA 15704, awarded by the National Cancer Institute, DHEW, and Contract AI 52515 from the National Institute of Allergy and Infectious Diseases.

kemic patients transplanted following preparation with CY and TBI have recently been reported.[3] This paper will summarize the clinical results of marrow transplantation in acute leukemia in identical twins and in allogeneic recipients transplanted from an HLA-matched sibling.

Materials and Methods

All patients transplanted were felt to have had the maximum benefit of chemotherapy with combinations of drugs. All had donors who were identical twins or HLA-identical with the patient as determined by serologic typing and confirmed by mixed leukocyte culture.[2] Every patient received 1,000 rads of TBI from opposing ^{60}Co sources, calculated as the tissue dose at the midpoint of the abdomen. The dosage rate was 5.5 to 8.0 rad/minute. Most patients received CY 120 mg/kg 3 to 4 days prior to TBI, either alone or with other chemotherapeutic agents. In a few patients, other chemotherapeutic agents were substituted for CY.[3]

Results

Syngeneic Marrow Transplantation for Acute Leukemia

A number of patients with hematologic malignancy have been treated by syngeneic marrow transplantation following high dosages of chemotherapy and TBI with or without immunotherapy. The toxicity and complications of this procedure are minimal with failures almost exclusively limited to recurrence of leukemia. Of the 16 patients reported in 1974,[4] 6 are living and well in complete remission on no maintenance chemotherapy 4 to 6½ years following marrow transplantation (Table 30-1). Over 40 patients with identical twin donors have now been transplanted with results comparable to those published.

Only a small fraction of patients will have an identical twin. The physician must be aware of such cases, however, because of the opportunity to perform relatively uncomplicated marrow transplantation with the potential for extremely long-term benefit.

Allogeneic Marrow Transplantation Using an HLA Identical Sibling as a Marrow Donor

Marrow transplantation for acute leukemia involves chemotherapeutic and irradiation regimens that achieve sufficient immunosuppression to obtain engraftment and eradication of the population of malignant cells. Until recently, marrow transplantation for treatment of these patients was undertaken only after failure of conventional and experimental chemotherapy. As a consequence, most of the patients transplanted were in far-advanced relapse with a heavy body burden of leukemic cells. Despite these obstacles, there are now a number of long-term survivors (Table 30-1). It should be emphasized that these patients have not been on any form of maintenance chemotherapy following transplantation.

Survival

In the Seattle series, 10 patients were prepared for transplantation by the administration of 1,000 rads of TBI[5] and 100 patients were prepared with CY, 60 mg/kg on each of two successive days, followed by TBI.[3] An actuarial analysis of the survival curve of these patients by the method of Kaplan and Meier indicates three periods of interest. The first period concerns the first 120 days following transplantation. There is a rapid loss of patients during this time apparently due to the problems of advanced disease, graft-versus-host disease (GVHD), associated infections and, to a lesser extent, the problems of recurrent leukemia. The second period extends from approximately 120 days to 2 years after grafting. There is a much slower rate of loss of patients during this time and the loss is due primarily to recurrent leukemia. The curve representing the third period, which now extends from 2 to 6½ years, is almost flat with a negligible loss of patients and no recurrent leukemia. This flat portion of the curve, which corresponds to about 15 per cent of the patients, constitutes an operational definition of cure for these patients and it is reasonable to conclude that marrow transplantation can be considered to be curative for some patients even in the end stages of acute leukemia.

TABLE 30-1. *Seattle Marrow Transplant Summary for Acute Leukemia as of February, 1977**

Disease	Donor	Number	No. alive at 1 year	No. now alive	Longest living survivor (years)
ALL**	Twin	6	5	3	6
	HLA matched	52	16	11	6
AML**	Twin	8	3	3	5
	HLA matched	58	10	7	5

* Including only transplants done before 11/75.
** ALL = acute lymphoblastic leukemia; AML = acute myelogenous leukemia.

Causes of Transplant Failure

Table 30-2 presents the causes of death in a group of 100 transplant recipients. These patients received CY and TBI and were transplanted from HLA-matched siblings. The predominant causes of death were recurrent leukemia and interstitial pneumonitis related to GVHD.

Efforts to Eradicate the Leukemic Cell Population

The first 10 patients in Seattle were prepared only with TBI because of our experience with irradiation and marrow transplantation in the dog, because irradiation is known to be effective in destroying leukemic cells and because irradiation penetrates the privileged sites where residual leukemic cells occur. Leukemic relapse occurred in 5 of 6 ALL patients treated with TBI alone and in two instances the relapse was in donor cells. We added two large doses of CY prior to irradiation in an attempt to decrease the relapse rate. In addition, a number of patients received added chemotherapy, principally rubidomycin and cytosine arabinoside, in an effort to achieve maximal cytoreduction of the leukemic cell population. In an analysis of the effects of cytoreduction, we were unable to determine any benefit from the added chemotherapy in addition to CY. Instances of recurrent leukemia continue to be observed despite intensive additional chemotherapy and in certain instances there was a suggestion that adding drugs to CY contributed to an increased morbidity and mortality. There have been no relapses in donor cells since CY was added to the TBI.

Other investigators have utilized vigorous chemotherapy instead of TBI before transplantation. Santos et al employed CY, 50 mg/kg on each of 4 days,[6] and Graw et al utilized the same regimen with 45 mg/kg of CY.[7] These CY regimens were well-tolerated but all patients who survived developed recurrent leukemia. Graw et al developed a BACT regimen consisting of bis-chloroethyl-nitrosourea, cytosine arabinoside, CY and 6-thioguanine.[8] The BACT regimen was very toxic with many early deaths. One patient with end-stage AML, however, is now alive and well 5 years after transplantation.[9]

TABLE 30-2. *Causes of Death in Transplant Recipients*

	Number of Patients
1. Graft rejection	1
2. Infection without a functioning graft	8
3. Absent or mild GVHD, interstitial pneumonia, respiratory failure	8
4. Moderate to severe GVHD, interstitial pneumonia, respiratory failure	26
5. GVHD and infection	8
6. Chronic GVHD	2
7. Recurrent or residual leukemia (complications of disease or therapy)	26
8. Cardiac failure	2
9. Unknown cause	2
Total	83

Gale et al have developed a regimen known as SCARI (6-thioguanine, CY, cytosine arabinoside, rubidomycin, TBI) that employs high-dose chemotherapy followed by TBI.[10] The SCARI regimen has proved to be very toxic for patients over the age of 18 years. Preliminary results are encouraging in that only 2 patients have suffered a relapse of leukemia. The number of patients treated by the SCARI regimen and the duration of the survival is as yet inadequate for a valid comparison with the Seattle regimen.

One approach to increasing the success rate of marrow grafting for patients with acute leukemia involves a resort to marrow transplantation before the patient reaches the end stages of the disease. The obvious advantages of this approach include (1) treatment before the leukemic cell population becomes resistant to therapeutic modalities, (2) treatment at a time when the body burden of leukemic cells is minimal and (3) treatment when the patient is in excellent clinical condition and, therefore, better able to tolerate the transplantation regimen. In January 1976, we initiated a protocol which involves CY plus TBI and marrow transplantation for patients with AML in the first remission and for patients with ALL in the second or subsequent remission. It is too early to evaluate this series of patients except to say that the early posttransplantation course has been relatively benign.

REFERENCES

1. Bortin M M: Graft versus leukemia, in Bach F H, Good R A (eds): Clinical Immunobiology, vol. 2. New York, Academic Press, 1974, p 287
2. Thomas E D, Storb R, Clift R A, et al: Bone-marrow transplantation. N Engl J Med 292:832, 895, 1975
3. Thomas E D, Buckner C D, Banaji M, et al: One hundred patients with acute leukemia treated by chemotherapy, total body irradiation, and allogeneic marrow transplantation. Blood 49:511, 1977
4. Fefer A, Einstein A B, Thomas E D, et al: Bone-marrow transplantation for hematologic neoplasia in 16 patients with identical twins. N Engl J Med 290:1389, 1974
5. Thomas E D, Buckner C D, Rudolph R H, et al: Allogeneic marrow grafting for hematologic malignancy using HL-A-matched donor-recipient sibling pairs. Blood 38:267, 1971
6. Santos G W, Sensenbrenner L L, Anderson P N, et al: HL-A-identical marrow transplants in aplastic anemia, acute leukemia, and lymphosarcoma employing cyclophosphamide. Transplant Proc 8:607, 1976
7. Graw R G Jr, Yankee R A, Rogentine G N, et al: Bone marrow transplantation from HL-A-matched donors to patients with acute leukemia. Transplantation 14:79, 1972
8. Graw R G Jr, Lohrmann H-P, Bull M I, et al: Bone-marrow transplantation following combination chemotherapy immunosuppression (BACT) in patients with acute leukemia. Transplant Proc 6:349, 1974
9. Bleyer W A, Blaese R M, Bujak J S, et al: Long-term remission from acute myelogenous leukemia after bone marrow transplantation and recovery from acute graft-versus-host reaction and prolonged immunoincompetence. Blood 45:171, 1975
10. Gale R P, Feig S, Opelz G, et al: Bone marrow transplantation in acute leukemia using intensive chemoradiotherapy (SCARI-UCLA). Transplant Proc 8:611, 1976

PART IV

Hematologic Neoplasms

Mortimer J. Lacher

31
Hodgkin's Disease

Introduction

It should be more and more clear that Hodgkin's disease is a systemic disorder that rarely, if ever, actually exists as a unifocal lesion. We may occasionally define it as unifocal by anatomical criteria, but ultimately the definition of Hodgkin's disease will depend on other factors such as the identification of tumor specific antigens,[1,2] immune system defects or aberrations,[3,4,5] and changes and activation of the complement system.[6,7] Hodgkin's disease is a complex disorder of the lymphoid system that exists diffusely spread throughout the body. The manifestations of Hodgkin's disease may result in local swellings of particular lymph nodes and some patients may even appear to be cured by radiation therapy and/or chemotherapy. Hodgkin's disease is in the process of being redefined, however, and its systemic nature is becoming more apparent.[8,9] In fact, even after the symptoms and overt signs of the disease are suppressed, the more subtle manifestations linger on. These manifestations are associated with persistent alterations in delayed hypersensitivity and persistent T-cell abnormalities, and are still poorly understood.

Patients with apparent complete clinical remission, who have not had any therapy for years, relapse. Patients with no apparent "active" disease still have disordered T cells.[11] It is this phenomenon of persistent systemic deficiency or aberration beyond the morphological and anatomical delineation that gives further credence to thinking of Hodgkin's disease as a chronic disorder with a high potential for relapse, even though initially effective treatment may be associated with long survival.[10]

In addition, as high-dose radiotherapy was applied to all major lymph node chains in a local and prophylactic manner, it became obvious that the failure to cure these patients depended on the fact that radiation alone could not eliminate the Hodgkin's tumor in areas outside of these major lymph node chains.[12,13] The lung and liver, especially, have remained vulnerable to recurrences.

Staging laparotomy, done primarily to effect analysis of the spleen, proved that occult Hodgkin's disease could readily be discovered in 30 to 40 per cent of patients who seemed to have the disease restricted above the diaphragm.[14,15,16,17,18]

These discoveries over the past 10 years

Supported in part by the M.J. Lacher Fund of Memorial Hospital, New York, N.Y.

have fortunately been paralleled by the fortuitous empirical successful application of single and multi-drug chemotherapy that has resulted[19-25] in a remarkable increase in life expectancy in all classes of patients with Hodgkin's disease.[26]

The presumption that Hodgkin's disease is a systemic disorder has led to a drastic change in the approach to primary treatment. This is a result of an attempt to more thoroughly eliminate both the gross occult manifestations of the Hodgkin's tumor at the point of initial diagnosis. Because of this, we are now applying more radiation treatment to more extended areas of accessible nodal aggregates and then sequentially applying chemotherapy to attack the less obvious residual tumor in areas not encompassed by the radiation treatment. In patients with primary gross manifestations of tumor outside of nodal aggregates, chemotherapy has become the recommended primary therapy. If the refinements of single- or multi-drug chemotherapy ultimately achieve their anticipated success, then chemotherapy alone will become the primary treatment for all stages of Hodgkin's disease.

No matter who the expert is who recommends radical radiotherapy, radical chemotherapy or combinations of these treatments for all patients with Hodgkin's disease as primary treatment, in every audience there is a physician who is familiar with at least 1 patient who received minimal treatment and enjoyed long survival. Needless to say, if we could properly identify such a patient, we would definitely give lesser therapy to that individual. Unfortunately, the state of the art has not been reached where that can be accomplished. We are now, in fact, in a period of giving more treatment to everyone in all stages of presentation. Furthermore, we are all aware of the potential dangers of employing more extensive initial treatment. At this point in time, therefore, the various complications of survival must be dealt with as the anticipated alternative to earlier deaths.

The ultimate measure of the cure of Hodgkin's disease will eventually be defined in a precise metabolic manner, and not by the crude estimation of the disappearance of gross lymph node swellings. The precedent for this has already been set in one malignancy that can be successfully cured by chemotherapy. The classical histologic subdivision of gestational trophoblastic disease (hydatidiform mole, chorioadenoma destruens, invasive mole, and choriocarcinoma) is of little use today, as treatment is monitored by alternate means (measurement of human chorionic gonadotrophin or the B-subunit) and the therapy and prognosis is the same for all histological categories.[27] The measurement of human chorionic gonadotrophin serves as a marker for diagnosis and for the end point of treatment as well as a sign of relapse. It is anticipated that in the very near future, comparable markers will be found to guide us in the identification and treatment of patients with Hodgkin's disease.

Histologic Diagnosis

The use of the Lukes and Butler histologic classification scheme[28] was a radical change from the old Jackson and Parker scheme,[29] but it is not an improvement.

The history of the development of the current histologic classification deserves some comment. Lukes and Butler developed their classification in response to their desire to relate histologic types of Hodgkin's disease to the stage of disease (extent of recognizable tumor) at onset, and to prognosis. In 1966 Lukes and Butler described six groups of histological subtypes of Hodgkin's disease: (1) lymphocytic and/or histiocytic (L and H), diffuse, (2) lymphocytic and/or histiocytic (L and H), nodular, (3) mixed, (4) nodular sclerosis, (5) diffuse fibrosis and (6) reticular.[28] They also declared the existence of a new entity that they called nodular sclerosing Hodgkin's disease, that was said to have a remarkably high incidence of primary mediastinal involvement (as Stage I or localized tumor in the mediastinum). They believed that nodular sclerosing Hodgkin's disease represented a "regional expression of Hodgkin's disease in the mediastinum," with an extraordinarily good prognosis. It was their belief that their new histological classification created "an effective basis for prognostication." Their implied hope was that their classification would ultimately lead to a solution to the still unsettled nature of the basic process of Hodgkin's disease. Subsequently, at the Rye conference, a committee of experts[30] "deliberated at length" and decided to adjust the Lukes and Butler classification to make it more acceptable by simplifying it into more readily useable terms that "clearly convey a histological connotation." They recommended four histological subsets, now well-known as: (1) lymphocytic predominant, (2) nodular sclerosis, (3) mixed cellularity and (4) lymphocytic depletion (includes diffuse fibrosis and reticular types of Lukes and Butler and the sarcoma type of Jackson and Parker).

It was the contention of Lukes and Butler and the Rye Conference Committee on Pathologic Nomenclature (consisting of L. Craver, T. Hall, L. Rappaport, and H. Rubin) that this new approach to the histology of Hodgkin's disease employing morphologic distinctions determined by observations limited to light microscopy would allow clinical correlations between the course of the disease and the histologic features. They recommended an abandonment of the three-part histologic classification of Jackson and Parker. (The Jackson and Parker classification had held sway for 16 years.) The Lukes and Butler classification and its modifications have now supplanted all others for the past 10 years, but, unfortunately, it has brought us no closer to the anticipated hope that we would be able to use it to relate histology to clinical stage of onset, survival or etiology.

The Lukes and Butler classification and the Rye conference and/or Ann Arbor modifications are not consistently reproducible. Pathologists themselves, either within the same institution or from center to center, do not have consistently reliable morphologic criteria for diagnosis. They can and do agree almost 100 per cent of the time that the patient has Hodgkin's disease, but they need a conference to achieve a "consensus" of opinion in 30 to 40 per cent of the patients with regard to the Lukes and Butler subdivisions. Keller et al found that among three pathologists "there was initial complete agreement on 120 (67 per cent of the cases) . . ." that they reviewed.[31] Butler analyzed eight series of patients with Hodgkin's disease using the Rye classification and concluded that "the histological type of Hodgkin's disease given in a significant number of patients was erroneous."[32]

Strum and Rappaport have noted that there are serious pitfalls in the histologic classification of Hodgkin's disease because ". . . when a fragment of lymph node tissue is submitted for study, the classification of Hodgkin's disease should not be attempted, though the diagnosis of Hodgkin's disease may be established."[33] Furthermore, "a small tissue sample may show a cellular composition consistent with Hodgkin's disease with either LP (lymphocyte predominant), MC (mixed cellularity), or LD (lymphocyte depleted), but it is not possible to tell whether one is dealing with one of these histologic types or with NS (nodular sclerosing) Hodgkin's disease with a corresponding cellular composition." On the other hand, Hanson[34] concluded and Rappaport and Strum[33] concurred that ". . . when a small area of lymph node tissue showing the features of NS (nodular sclerosing Hodgkin's disease) is seen, or when the lymph node is partially involved by NS, this material can be classified with certainty as NS (nodular sclerosing) Hodgkin's disease."

Hanson, in his study of 251 patients with special reference to nodular sclerosing Hodgkin's disease, implied that the course of the disease and the survival of patients with partial involvement of the lymph node by nodular sclerosing Hodgkin's disease conforms to those patients with complete nodal involvement by this histologic subtype. Is the course of the disease being predicted by the histology or is the histology being chosen by the course?

Rosenberg echoed my own evaluation of the Lukes and Butler classification when he responded editorially to Nieman, Rosen and Lukes's description[36] of what they consider to be a new entity associated with lymphocyte depleted Hodgkin's disease. "Though the authors present a convincing description this form of Hodgkin's disease has characteristic features, the importance of recognizing the entity is reduced by its relative rarity. The recognition of only 12 examples of lymphocyte depletion Hodgkin's disease in over 12 years in one of the country's largest hospitals is consistent with the very low frequency of this histologic subgroup seen in other series. The opposite is true of Hodgkin's disease of the nodular sclerosing type. As this histologic picture has become better recognized, its frequency has increased in some series to 75 per cent or more of all patients seen. Thus, we seem to be returning to a situation not very different from the days of Jackson and Parker when 75 per cent or more of the patients presented with Hodgkin's granuloma and a few of the patients were within the more favorable and less favorable prognostic categories of Hodgkin's paragranuloma or Hodgkin's sarcoma, respectively."[35]

If we have come back full circle to a simplistic histologic definition of Hodgkin's disease, what other aberrations should we consider?[37] At an international symposium on Hodgkin's disease, Dr. Henry S. Kaplan "at the risk of exciting a little hostility in some of his good friends who are pathologists . . . ," urged them to break the shackles of morphology, if possible. "It may be asking a lot for a pathologist to liberate himself from morphology," he commented, "since this is the be all and end all of his existence."[38] Dr. Robert Good added that he believed "that the time had come when the pathologist must be aggravated, provoked, stimulated, encouraged, and harassed into using all of the modern techniques possible: chromosome counts, tritiated thymidine uptake, specific serology, and any other methods which are not strictly morphologic, in the hope that we can progress beyond our present position."[38]

A new pathological description of Hodgkin's disease will emerge and it will employ a general description that uses both morphology and immunologic separateness. There will probably be an ultimate recognition that this is a lymphocyte disorder of special magnitude and not a disease of the Reed-Sternberg cell.

Kadin[39] and others have emphasized that previously published accounts of DNA synthesis and mitotic activity in cells comprising Hodgkin's tissue lesions[40,41] indicate that the Reed-Sternberg cell is a nonproliferative or end-stage cell. In addition, recognition of cells morphologically identical to the Reed-Sternberg cell have been seen in infectious mononucleosis,[42] a benign disorder, which raises further doubts as to the proliferative potential and origin of these distinctive cells. Lukes,[43] Strum, Rappaport,[44] Kadin and Dorfman[45] have all recognized the presence of certain multi-nucleated cells that are thought to be variants of the Reed-Sternberg cell associated with various histologic types of Hodgkin's disease. Although it may be used for recognition, it is most likely that the Reed-Sternberg cell itself will not prove to be the major cell of importance in the pathogenesis of Hodgkin's disease.

At this time I do not expect anyone to abandon the Lukes and Butler classification. Clinicians abhor a vacuum. I don't expect anyone to revert to the Jackson-Parker classification. Clinicians reject reaccepting anything that was once declared insufficient. I do expect less harassment, however, if we choose to stop thinking about Hodgkin's disease as "bad" histology and "good" histology patients and if we choose to be less compulsive and argumentative over histological hair-splitting until something new and reliable takes the place of the Rye and Ann Arbor modifications of the Lukes and Butler classification.

All of this, I hope, will help ease the mind of the professional dogmatists who are still trying to shove a round peg into the square hole of the Lukes and Butler classification of Hodgkin's disease. The failure of the "new" histology is emphasized by the 10-year progress report of DeVita, Canellos, Hubbard, Chabner, and Young (although only an abstract of the full picture), that states that of 194 patients with advanced Hodgkin's disease treated with MOPP, those with nodular sclerosing Hodgkin's disease had shorter complete remissions than patients with mixed cellularity or lymphocyte depleted types.[20] No induction-failure patients survived 5 years and complete remissions did not vary with sex, stage, histology or types of organ invasion. Poorer survival correlated with B symptoms (fever and significant weight loss) but *not* with histology or organ involvement. Furthermore, the ultimate survival of patients with nodular sclerosing Hodgkin's disease was not yet worse than other subtypes, despite a difference in disease-free survival.

This further emphasizes that treatment techniques appear to have affected the ultimate survival of patients with Hodgkin's disease, irrespective of current histological subtyping.[12,46]

The Staging Work-up: What Information is Necessary Before Treatment?

We have progressed from a limited ostrich-like approach ignoring everything we couldn't feel with our hands or see with a chest X-ray to the absolutely hysterical position of attempting to outline the physical limits of the Hodgkin's tumor by an extensive premortem surgical dissection of the individual.

As an investigative effort, the laparotomy-splenectomy, as part of the initial staging procedure, has proven to be indispensible to our comprehension of the natural history of Hodgkin's disease.[17,18] It proved that our clinical tools are cumbersome and crude and that Hodgkin's disease at the time of onset and/or its discovery, just isn't the neat focal disorder that everyone had hoped or wanted it to be. Moore, et al recognized that extended field, total lymphoid radiation had greatly improved disease-free survival but occult microscopic foci of disease existed outside of the treatment field and they presumed that these were responsible for most relapses after total lymphoid radiation.[12] The exact role of splenectomy as a diagnostic staging procedure or as a therapeutic element is still not completely evaluated. In the collaborative study of patients with Stage I and II Hodgkin's disease, comparing survival and complications of radiation therapy followed involved and extended field treatment, the most consistent observation relates to the association between laparotomy (and splenectomy) and survival.[46] "The laparotomy patients exhibit better survival than nonlaparotomy patients in each of the four comparisons shown, old and new radiotherapy series, IF (involved field), and EF (extended field) treatment." Therefore, if treatment is to be limited to radiation therapy alone, splenectomy may also have therapeutic implications. On the other hand, if more aggressive therapy employing radiation plus chemotherapy is used, then the staging laparotomy may *not* be necessary. The recommendations for staging procedures from the report of the Committee on Hodgkin's Disease Staging Procedures (1971) are outlined in Table 31-1.[47]

The procedures to be required "under certain conditions," and especially the staging laparotomy, is the subject of the currently still unresolved controversy,[17,18] on to which can now be added the highly questionable usefulness of laparoscopy.[48]

Nothing has changed the crude diagnostic value of hepatic and splenic scintigrams and the promise that the gallium scan would improve this lack of reliability has not materialized.[49] Fortunately, no one has suggested that the CAT scan could detect the Reed-Sternberg cell lurking in a portal recess, so we have not had to issue any disclaimer for that technique. The ultimate hope for the evaluation of Hodgkin's disease does rest with some form of metabolic or immunologic marking system. That is, we eventually will have to have a readily detectable tumor-specific antigen, or some form of immunoglobulin determination, or complement system evaluation, or lymphocyte marker or some other metabolic marker that will identify the disorder and relieve us of the crude guesswork to determine, not only its presence at onset, but its persistence after therapy or its relapse at an interval after discovery and treatment. Various simplified conclusions may be readily accepted, however, with regard to the determination of the extent of disease.

Peripheral Lymph Nodes

The peripheral lymph node groups are examined by palpation. In addition to its use in staging, the lymph node examination is an easily quantifiable parameter in evaluation of response to treatment and for follow-up.

Mediastinal Hilar Lymph Nodes and the Lung

For the most part, standard posterior, anterior and lateral chest X-rays are sufficient to evaluate the mediastinal hilar lymph nodes and the lung parenchyma. Masses in the anterior and superior mediastinum, or in the hilar areas, are indicative of Hodgkin's disease once the diagnosis has been established. Needless to say, coexisting processes such as

TABLE 31-1. *Recommendations on Staging Procedures*

Required evaluation procedures
- Adequate surgical biopsy, reviewed by a hematopathologist
- Detailed history (fever, sweating, pruritus, and weight loss?)
- Complete physical examination with attention to lymphadenopathy, Waldeyer's ring, liver, spleen, and bone tenderness
- Laboratory studies
  - CBC, platelet count, ESR, serum alkaline phosphatase level
  - Evaluation of renal function and liver function
- Radiologic studies
  - Chest roentgenogram (P.A. and lateral views)
  - Intravenous pyelogram
  - Bilateral lower extremity lymphogram
  - Skeletal survey especially thoracolumbar vertebrae, pelvis, proximal extremities, and areas of bone tenderness and/or pain.

Required evaluation procedures under certain conditions
- Whole chest tomography, if abnormality on chest roentgenogram
- Inferior cavography for equivocal lymphogram or pyelogram
- Bone marrow biopsy, by a needle or open surgical technique if:
  - Serum alkaline phosphatase is elevated
  - Unexplained anemia or other blood count depression.
  - Roentgenographic or scintigraphic evidence of osseous disease
  - Generalized disease of stage III category or greater
  - Exploratory laparotomy and splenectomy, if management decisions depend on the identification of abdominal disease

Useful ancillary procedures, not definitive for diagnosis
- Skeletal scintigrams
- Hepatic and spleen scintigrams
- Serum chemistries, including calcium and uric acid
- Estimate of patient's delayed hypersensitivity

Procedures and tests promising for clinical study at selected centers but experimental at this time
- Whole-body gallium and selenium scintigrams
- Determinations of serum iron and iron binding capacity, copper and ceruloplasmin, zinc, haptoglobin, fibrinogen, α-2-globulin; as well as urinary hydroxyproline, leukocyte alkaline phosphatase, absolute lymphocyte count, antibodies to Epstein-Barr virus, human lymphocyte antibody typing.

From Rosenberg S A, Boiron M, DeVita V T, et al: Report of the committee on Hodgkin's disease staging procedures. Cancer Res 31:1862, 1971.

complicating infections with tuberculosis or fungi should be considered. Laminography may be necessary to eliminate the possibility of the superimposition of vascular shadows and to satisfy those who are concerned about the differential between the contiguous pulmonary involvement versus infiltration of disease into peribronchovascular lymphatics. In addition, the chest X-ray and/or laminography assists the radiation therapist with the design of accurate radiation therapy ports.

ABDOMINAL LYMPH NODES

Evaluation of abdominal lymph nodes continues to be a difficult task in the staging of patients with Hodgkin's disease.[50] Except for obvious large retroperitoneal masses that may be readily palpated, decisions must be made by inference of the anticipated patterns of disease.

Involvement of nodes in the inguinal areas, left low cervical area or left supraclavicular area is associated frequently with retroperitoneal Hodgkin's disease. This is reflected by analysis of retroperitoneal involvement at laparotomy, abnormal lymphangiograms and increased risk of abdominal relapse if only the peripheral nodes are treated with radiotherapy. In one study, about 50 per cent of patients with left supraclavicular nodes were found to have abdominal involvement at laparotomy.[51]

The best method for studying retroperitoneal nodes is the lymphangiogram. The intravenous pyelogram (IVP) and the inferior vena cavagram usually do not reveal disease in combination with a negative lymphangiogram.[50] The IVP and the inferior vena cavagram are rarely used for staging as primary techniques. Of course, there are cases of ureteral obstruction that may be discovered on intravenous pyelography, but in these instances they are usually accompanied by a positive lymphangiogram.[60]

The accuracy of lymphangiography has been reviewed by Desser et al regarding twelve groups and 410 patients reported in United States and British literature.[15] Unequivocally positive and unequivocally negative lymphangiograms were confirmed at laparotomy in 75 and 85 per cent of patients, respectively. Furthermore, patients with proven abdominal lymph node disease generally have concomitant disease in the spleen. In the same review (vide supra) at the 12 reporting centers, 113 of 276 patients had involved abdominal lymph nodes and 94 of these patients had splenic involvement (83 per cent).[15] In addition, hepatic portal lymph node involvement has indicated the need to include the porta hepatis in the infradiaphragmatic radiation therapy field.

Emphasis must be made of the fact that positive findings are limited by surgical techniques and therefore the results noted above, with regard to the laparotomy confirmation of anticipated findings after lymphangiography, really signifies that there is more tumor below the diaphragm than can be determined by even the most meticulous surgical exploration. The irregular nodal involvement that Hodgkin's disease is noted for makes the surgical pathological evaluation err on the side of "negative" findings. More disease is present than can be proved by surgical exploration and histological analysis.[54,55]

Spleen

Clinical evaluation of the spleen in patients with Hodgkin's disease is unreliable. Since size does not correlate with involvement, physical examination by palpation is not valuable. Scanning with Technicium 99 or observed enlargement on abdominal radiographs hasn't improved evaluation. Gallium 67 scans have added nothing of value.[53,55]

In Desser and Ultmann's review of 443 patients with Hodgkin's disease, 41 per cent of the patients had splenic involvement. Only 65 per cent of spleens presumed to be clinically positive could be confirmed after histologic evaluation, but 100 of 318 spleens or 32 per cent considered clinically negative were histologically positive. In the Johnston et al cooperative study 50 per cent of scan negative spleens were positive for Hodgkin's disease.[49] Although six out of six scan-positive spleens were confirmed at surgery, if these occurred in lymphangiogram-positive patients, the contribution of isotope scanning could be considered negligible. Splenectomy offers the only method for accurate diagnosis of splenic Hodgkin's disease and even that technique has limitations imposed by the difficulty of evaluating such a large organ by histological analysis. Kirschner et al noted "sectioning the spleen at 1 cm intervals has proved to be inadequate to detect early involvement by Hodgkin's disease. We have several cases in our series of isolated splenic nodules less than 1 cm in size demonstrating Hodgkin's disease."[54] Similar findings have been noted by others. Although microscopic involvement in the absence of visible tumor nodules is rare, multiple histologic sections of each spleen should be examined.

Liver

Laparoscopy cannot be recommended in place of laparotomy merely because it correlates so well with negative liver findings. Even a sham procedure could come up with 94 per cent accuracy if one merely agreed with the negative clinical evaluation of the liver. To boast that laparoscopy is 97 per cent accurate[48] implies extraordinary usefulness until one realizes that it is practically impossible to avoid such accuracy when liver involvement is so rarely diagnosed at the onset of Hodgkin's disease. (The excitement generated over the use of splenectomy, on the other hand, was associated with the extraordinary finding that 30 to 40 per cent of patients had unsuspected disease in the spleen at the point of initial diagnosis.[14,56,57]—A startling revelation.)

In one series of 31 patients comparing laparoscopy with laparotomy findings,[48] a Stage IVB patient (based on a palpable liver) was changed to a Stage IIIB by negative laparoscopy findings, but this would not change the therapeutic approach. A Stage IIIB patient changed to IVB by a positive laparotomy in the face of a negative laparoscopy does not change the therapeutic approach. Except for academic purposes of an investigational nature, the routine use of laparoscopy and/or laparotomy in this series changes nothing. No matter how skilled the laparoscopist is, the liver can only be examined in an extremely limited manner by very limited observation of a portion of its surface area.[58] The evaluation of the liver biopsy material remains just as complex as ever,[59,60] even though the biopsy needle may be directly visualized entering the liver by the laparoscopy technique. Finally, the spleen can't be evaluated at all by laparoscopy.[58] More often than not it isn't even visualized and it is never biopsied or removed by laparoscopy. Laparoscopy has a limited place in an investigational setting, but this must not be construed to mean that it should become part of the routine work-up for a patient with Hodgkin's disease.

The current purpose of staging procedures in Hodgkin's disease has been to determine the course of therapy, as well as to define the extent of tumor. With our current knowledge, a patient who presents with an extensive lung tumor does not, under any ordinary clinical circumstances, require a lymphangiogram or splenectomy or liver biopsy to conclude that he will require chemotherapy as primary treatment. In fact, a lymphangiogram or a staging laparotomy-splenectomy under these circumstances (with our current knowledge of the nature of Hodgkin's disease), should only be undertaken in an investigative setting. The physician is perfectly justified in proceeding immediately with multidrug therapy upon establishing the diagnosis of Hodgkin's disease in any patient who has extensive lung involvement. The vigorous application of surgical intervention (laparotomy-splenectomy) is not justified in this type of presentation with Stage IV disease, merely for "staging." Even obvious Stage IIIB patients do not require surgical exploration and, especially if one is involved in a treatment program that includes initial extended-field radiation therapy with postradiation chemotherapy, there is also no justification for staging laparotomy and splenectomy, except in an investigational setting, unless splenectomy per se can eventually be proved to be of specific therapeutic merit. Excluding an investigational environment, only if the initial therapeutic program will be effected by the staging procedure, is laparotomy-splenectomy necessary.

For those of us who have presumed that Hodgkin's disease should be more aggressively treated at onset with a combination of radiation therapy and chemotherapy or with chemotherapy alone, the staging work-up no longer includes laparotomy-splenectomy. The effects of this decision will make itself clear in the years ahead.

Inhibition of T-Cell Rosette Formation by Hodgkin's Disease Serum

It is now well-documented that patients with Hodgkin's disease frequently exhibit an impairment of cell-mediated immune function. This is manifested by diminished delayed hypersensitivity reactions,[63,64,65] decreased resistance to certain types of infections[68,69] and impaired ability to reject skin allografts.[66,67] Furthermore, peripheral blood lymphocytes from untreated Hodgkin's disease patients are deficient in their in vitro function as measured by the capacity to form E rosettes with sheep erythrocytes.[71]

Fuks et al investigated a serum factor in patients with Hodgkin's disease that seems to be responsible for the suppression of E-rosette formation in these patients.[61] Bobrove and Fuks et al showed that E-rosette formation and the in vitro response of peripheral blood lymphocytes from untreated patients with Hodgkin's disease to a mitogen such as phytohemoglutinin can be restored to normal levels by incubation in tissue culture media containing fetal calf serum.[62] Extending this observation, they found that the decreased percentage of E-rosette formation in Hodgkin's disease patients could be reversed and returned to normal range by prior incubation of the T lymphocytes in tissue culture medium with 20 per cent fetal calf serum for 18 to 24 hours. Additional incubation with serum from patients with other neoplasms, or from normal subjects, could not affect this reversal. Furthermore, only target T lymphocytes from patients with Hodgkin's disease were suppressed by the Hodgkin's disease serum. The inhibitor involved is thought to be a lipoprotein of low density. Unfortunately, all untreated patients with Hodgkin's disease do not have consistent abnormalities of peripheral blood T cells.

Verification of the work of Fuks, Strober and Kaplan is necessary before its usefulness can be defined. The work does emphasize, however, that the target organ in Hodgkin's disease is diffusely distributed throughout the body and the implication is that the major cell of importance is the lymphocyte itself. This work must be extended not only to patients prior to therapy, but also to posttherapy patients who have apparently achieved a complete remission and to those who are relapsing.

Abnormalities of Complement

Abnormalities of complement and its components in patients with cancer have not been well-defined. More recent studies, however, have found that complement levels of cancer patients were significantly higher than those of healthy subjects. In fact, Verhaegen et al noted that there was a stage linked increase of complement levels.[7] Patients in remission in one study had nearly normal complement levels, but patients with local tumor had increased complement levels and a further increase was observed in patients with distant metastases. Near death, complement levels dropped. Patients with colon, rectal, stomach, esophageal, lung, breast, ovaries, cervix, bladder and prostate tumors were delineated, but no specific mention of lymphoma patients was made.

Lichtenfield et al[6] studied 10 patients with Hodgkin's disease. Eight were untreated and two were treatment failures with advancing disease. They found elevated whole complement titres in all 10 patients with Hodgkin's disease in contrast to many acquired disease states in which complement tends to decrease. In some tumor bearing animals, it has also been noted that complement levels are depressed. Lichtenfield et al did not attempt to correlate the abnormal complement with the patient's course. They did study component complement titres, however, and in addition to whole complement elevations, they found a significant elevation of the C-9 titre in patients with Hodgkin's disease. A preliminary study of 19 patients in all phases of Hodgkin's disease suggests that total complement may prove to be a worthwhile guide to activity of disease in these patients. The measurement of whole complement may yet prove to be the simplest approach so far to determining whether or not Hodgkin's disease is "active" or inactive.

Treatment Planning

I have been strongly influenced by the realization that the Hodgkin's tumor is now known to be much more extensive at onset than was ever anticipated.

Spittle et al noted that among patients who were treated with curative intent by radiotherapy at the Stanford University School of Medicine (among 462 patients treatment between 1961 and 1970) in Stages I-III, "Surprisingly, there was relatively little influence of clinical stage on overall relapse rate. Thus, there were 13 relapses among 64 Stage IA cases at risk (20 per cent); 39 of 164 Stage IIA and II_EA (24 per cent); 25 among 93 Stage IIB and II_EB (27 per cent); 14 among 71 Stage IIIA, III_EA, and III_S-A (20 per cent); and 22 among 68 of IIIB, III_EB, and III_S-B (32 per cent)."[13] Furthermore, the occurrence of a relapse gravely influenced prognosis. Previous studies demonstrated that the interval between initial radiotherapy and the occurrence of a primary relapse is an important factor in prognosis, and the occurrence of an initial relapse adversely affects prognosis to a very significant extent. Tubiana et al noted that "long-term chemotherapy after radiotherapy tended to decrease the incidence of recurrence in nonirradiated lymph node areas."[70] Moore et al also found that disease-free actuarial survival was demonstrated to be superior in the group receiving sequential radiotherapy and chemotherapy.[12] If disease-free survival has any ultimate bearing on prognosis, then combining radiation with chemotherapy must be the currently correct approach to treatment. It does not mean that we do not realize or appreciate the possibility of increasing serious damage that may be done by maximal treatment. But we must weigh this against the overall improvement in survival rates.

My strategy for long-term control of Hodgkin's disease is based upon the success of radiation therapy to control apparently localized disease and for multiple drug chemotherapy to control disseminated or relapsing disease.

Karnofsky estimated that at diagnosis 65 per cent of the patients with Hodgkin's disease are Stage III or IV, that is, disease is present at least above and below the diaphragm, or in the viscera. He also estimated that although 35 per cent of the patients are in Stage I or II, that within 10 years 50 per cent of the Stage I or II patients should have a relapse requiring further treatment. Therefore, out of 100 patients with Hodgkin's disease he estimated that only 18 may escape relapse after initial diagnosis and treatment. Since these estimates were made, considerable changes have occurred with regard to initial treatment techniques. The fundamental belief, however, that Hodgkin's disease is disseminated in at least 65 per cent of the patients at onset and that relapses after therapy may occur in 50 per cent of the remaining 35 per cent of patients, has suggested that radiation therapy and chemotherapy should be combined early in the course of treatment with the anticipation of achieving the highest complete remission rate possible in all groups of patients. Toward that end, Moore et al randomized 102 patients who were Stage IB through IIIB to receive total lymphoid radiation either alone or followed by six cycles of MOPP (nitrogen mustard, vincristine, procarbazine and prednisone).[12] The group receiving radiation therapy alone had 10 relapses and two deaths in the period of time that they were followed, whereas the group receiving radiation therapy followed by chemotherapy had only one relapse and no deaths. The disease-free actuarial survival was demonstrated to be superior in the group receiving sequential radiotherapy and chemotherapy. Furthermore, the observation that extra-nodal extension of disease occurred in seven of the 10 relapses in the group receiving radiotherapy alone supports the contention "that occult microscopic foci of disease outside of treatment fields are responsible for most relapses after tumorcidal doses of total lymphoid radiotherapy." It seems logical, therefore, to attempt to treat almost all patients with a combination of radiation and chemotherapy early in the course of disease. If cell-kill early in the course of the disease has any meaning at all, then this is the logical approach to this problem in patients with Hodgkin's disease.

My own current approach to treatment, therefore, is as follows: only the "Required Evaluation Procedures" (see Table 30-1) are necessary to proceed with treatment, as all patients are treated with extended-field radiation therapy plus chemotherapy, or chemotherapy alone.

Stage I—
High neck nodes.

Radiation therapy is employed using the 2-2 technique of Nisce and D'Angio (Fig. 31-1).[71] In this setting, treatment is given above and below the diaphragm to all peripheral and central node-bearing areas, plus the porta hepatis area of the liver as well as the spleen. The treatment is carried down to the level of the fourth lumbar vertebra. This may be considered sufficient therapy by some because the disease presented as a high neck node, but I would prefer to follow this with 6 months of multiple drug chemotherapy.

Stage I—
Low neck nodes.

Initial treatment again consists of radiation therapy to the supradiaphragmatic node-bearing areas plus the porta hepatis,

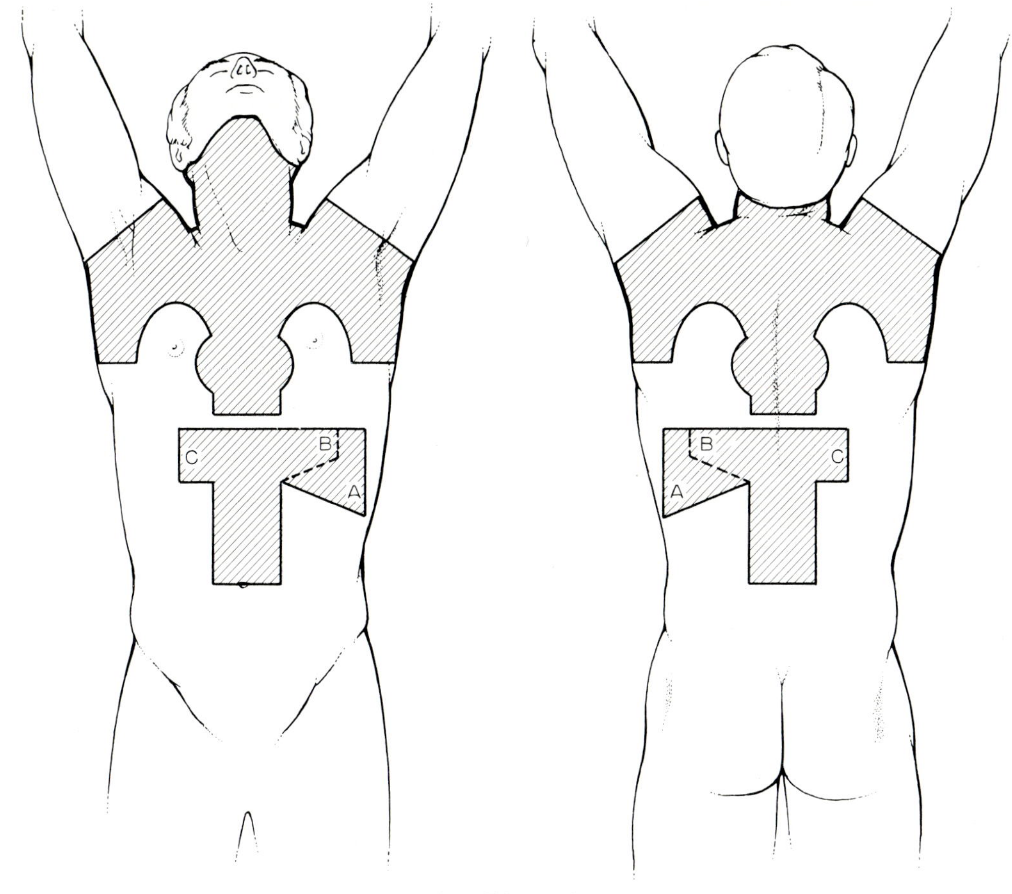

(a)

FIG. 31-1A. From Nisce, L Z, D'Angio G J: Radiation therapy for Hodgkin's disease: Memorial hospital techniques, in Lacher M J (ed): Hodgkin's Disease. New York, Wiley, 1976, pp 145–177.

spleen and central lymph nodes, down to the level of L_4. This is followed by 6 months of multiple drug chemotherapy.

Stage IIA or B. This usually presents with involvement in the mediastinum as well as the presence of neck nodes. Occasionally this type of patient will present with right or left inguinal nodes as well as a positive lymphangiogram. I again choose to treat the patient with extended-field radiation therapy followed by 6 months of multiple drug chemotherapy.

Stage IIIA. Especially if there is extensive mediastinal tumor, treatment should include radiation therapy to bulky tumor masses followed by 6 months of multiple drug chemotherapy. Chemotherapy alone may be used.

Stage IIIB. Two approaches may be considered in this type of patient. One can use total nodal radiation therapy to reduce total bulk of tumor, followed by 6 months of

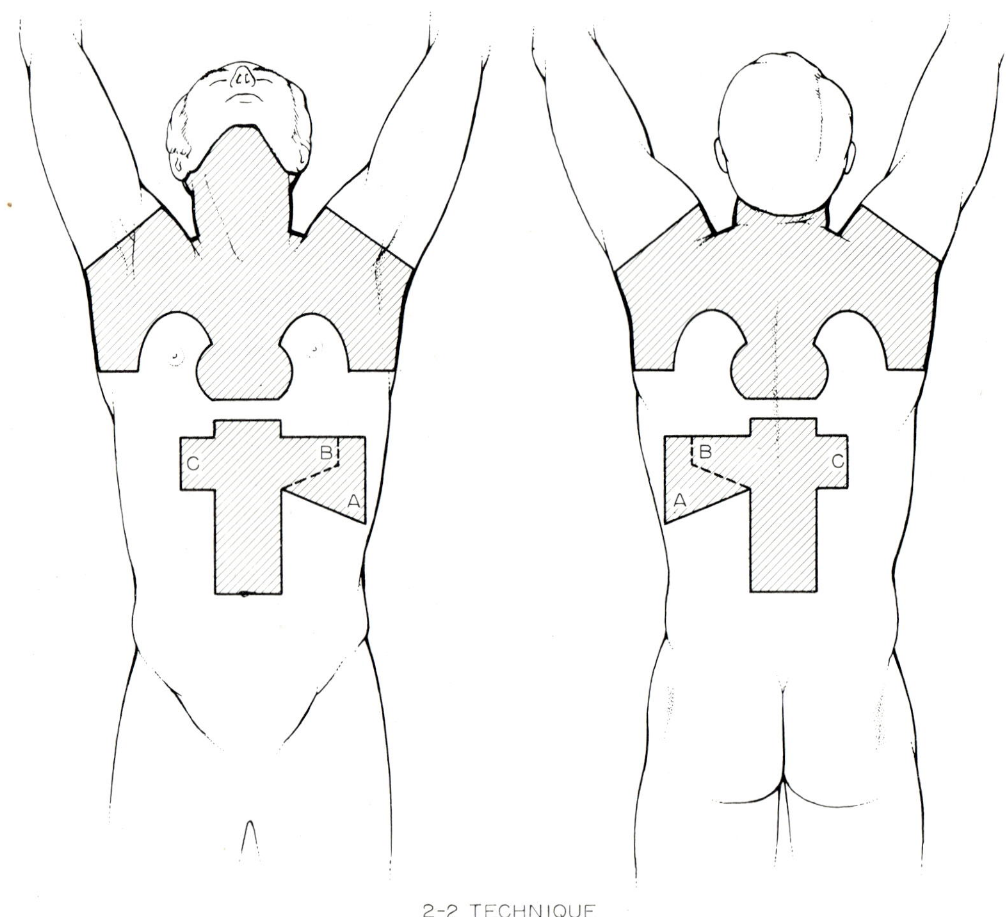

(b)

FIG. 31-1B. From Nisce, L Z, D'Angio G J: Radiation therapy for Hodgkin's disease: Memorial hospital techniques, in Lacher M J (ed): Hodgkin's Disease. New York, Wiley, 1976, pp 145–177.

chemotherapy. Or, one can consider the use of multi-drug chemotherapy alone for at least 6 months plus follow-up maintenance chemotherapy, depending on various available protocols. The chemotherapy cut-off point at 6 months or 1, 2 or 3 years is arbitrary, but an attempt should be made to randomize patients as they reach one of these bench-marks in order to find out whether or not they will achieve longer survival if continued on intermittent maintenance chemotherapy.

Stage IV. Chemotherapy alone is the treatment of choice in this group of patients. The role of intermittent maintenance chemotherapy is still to be defined. Radiation therapy may be used to treat local bulky disease.

MULTIPLE DRUG CHEMOTHERAPY PROTOCOLS

There are various acceptable treatment plans that may be used for multiple drug chemotherapy at this time. They include: MOPP—nitrogen mustard, oncovin (vincristine), prednisone, and procarbazine (matulane);[84] COPP—cytoxan (cyclophosphamide), oncovin (vincristine), prednisone, and procarbazine;[85] MVPP—nitrogen mustard, velban (vinblastine), prednisone, and procarbazine;[22] TVPP—thio tepa, velban (vinblastine), prednisone, and procarbazine;[25] ABVD—adriamycin, bleomycin, velban and DTIC;[72] MOPP-ABVD—nitrogen mustard, oncovin, prednisone and procarbazine-adriamycin, bleomycin, velban, and DTIC.[73] Carter and Goldsmith's review in *Hodgkin's Disease* outlines numerous programs under investigation. New multiple drug programs[75] and new single agents are constantly being evaluated, especially for patients who relapse after initial therapy. Table 31-2 lists multi-drug programs and their initial success rates.

Complications of Survival

Long survival has provoked special problems for the Hodgkin's disease patient. When the median survival was only 2½ years, the need to be concerned about secondary primary tumors was minimal. Now it is a real problem. The patient survives the first tumor (Hodgkin's disease) and dies from the second.

Acute leukemia in Hodgkin's disease has been estimated to be ten times more common in these patients than in the general population. There is no need to argue anymore as to whether or not this is related only to radiation treatment, or to radiation plus chemotherapy, or to chemotherapy alone or just to the natural course of Hodgkin's disease. Acute leukemia is being observed in all categories of Hodgkin's disease patients and its treatment is less satisfactory in patients who have had Hodgkin's disease than it is in the general adult population.[76]

Other tumors, more commonly associated with radiation therapy alone, are now appearing in patients treated with combined radiation therapy and chemotherapy, or chemotherapy alone, and in an increasing number.[77]

Another phenomenon related to either the treatment or possibly the disease itself, that has become more noticeable as patients survive longer, is the development of aseptic necrosis of the femoral heads (Figs. 31-2, 31-3). This has occurred in patients receiving radiation therapy alone, radiation therapy plus chemotherapy and in patients receiving chemotherapy alone.[52,78] Here again, the probable cause must be multiple. The fact that it has only been recognized recently does suggest, however, that there is some relation to the more intense therapy that is being applied at this time. Luckily, when it is recognized, this is a surgically-reparable problem with excellent palliative results (Fig. 31-4).

Herpes zoster continues to plague the patients with Hodgkin's disease and, to date, there is no satisfactory therapy.[69] The hope that substances such as Ara-A would be of some value has not materialized.[79] Supportive therapy remains the hallmark of the management of herpes zoster. Generalization of herpes zoster can be devastating (Fig. 31-5) and "chickenpox" pneumonia and even spinal cord involvement with extensive motor loss and paraplegia have been observed. Most patients, however, survive generalization of the zoster lesion with no serious sequelae.

Another late complication of radiation therapy is hypothyroidism. Luckily, this is a completely reversible complication, providing it is recognized.

Among the most serious complications of survival are the social problems faced by Hodgkin's disease patient.[81] A young male or female who was sterilized by either radiation therapy, chemotherapy or both, face a unique social adjustment. The Hodgkin's disease patient is discriminated against on the job market even if they have been apparently cured. What is the sense of insisting that the patient be admitted to a technicians' school, etc., when, after graduation no one wants to hire the individual on a full-time basis because they are a bad medical risk. Every time the issue of lateral transmissibility of Hodgkin's disease (with a yet to be discovered and only postulated infectious agent)[82,83] is reported in the local newspaper, the Hodgkin's disease patient panics. He is made to feel guilty about surviving and working in an office with other "normal" people. He is even made to feel that he is "infecting" his family. Insurance companies routinely refuse these needy individuals both medical and life insurance. The complications of survival, therefore, include both the internal dangers associated with this disease and the side effects of therapy, as well as the social stigma of having had or having to live with a malignant disorder.

TABLE 31-2. *Protocols for Combination Chemotherapy of Hodgkin's Disease*

Study	Regimen	Patients Evaluable	Response: Complete Response	Response: Partial Response	Overall Response Rate
Morgenfeld et al[85]	Cyclophosphamide, 600 mg/m, days 1 and 8, i.v. Vincristine, 1.4 mg/m, days 1 and 8, i.v. Procarbazine, 100 mg/m/day × 10, p.o. Prednisone, 40 mg/m/day × 14, p.o. (courses 1 and 4 only) Every month for six courses	102	67 (66%)	24 (24%)	91%
Nicholson et al[22]	Nitrogen mustard, 6 mg/m, days 1 and 8, i.v. Vinblastine, 10 mg, days 1, 8, and 14, i.v. Procarbazine, 100 mg/m/day × 14, p.o. Prednisolone, 40 mg/day × 14, p.o. (courses 1 and 4 only) Six courses; 4 weeks between each Maintenance: Induction regimen q 3 months × 1 year and q 4 months in second year	52	22 (42%)	17 (33%)	75%
Lacher[25]	Thio Tepa 15 mg/kg days 1 and 8, i.v. Vinblastine 0.1 mg/kg days 1 and 8, i.v. Procarbazine 75 mg/kg/day for 14 days, p.o. Prednisone 50 mg/day for 14 days, p.o. Restart cycle every 3 weeks for 6 months Maintenance: Induction regimen q 3 months × 3 years	30	27 (90%)	3 (10%)	100%

DeVita et al[84]	Nitrogen mustard, 6 mg/m, days 1 and 8, i.v. Vincristine, 1.4 mg/m, days 1 and 8, i.v. Procarbazine, 100 mg/m/day 14, p.o. Prednisone, 40 mg/m/day 14 (cycles 1 and 4 only) Six 2-week cycles; 14 days on and 14 days off	43	35 (81%)	6 (14%)	95%
Bloomfield et al[23]	Cyclophosphamide 300 mg/m, days 1 and 8, i.v. Vinblastine 10 mg, days 1, 8, and 15, i.v. Procarbazine 100 mg/m, days 1-15, p.o. Prednisone 40 mg/m, days 1-15, p.o. (cycles 1 and 4 only) A new cycle is started every 42 days. Minimum of 6 cycles	38	28 (74%)	5 (13%)	87%
Bonadonna et al[72]	A. Adriamycin, 25 mg/m, days 1 and 14, i.v. Bleomycin, 10 mg/m, days 1 and 14, i.v. Vinblastine, 6 mg/m days 1 and 14, i.v. Imidazole carboximide 150 mg/m days 1-5, i.v. (DTIC) Six courses q 28 days	17	12 (70%)	3 (18%)	88%
	B. MOPP	22	16 (72%)	3 (14%)	86%

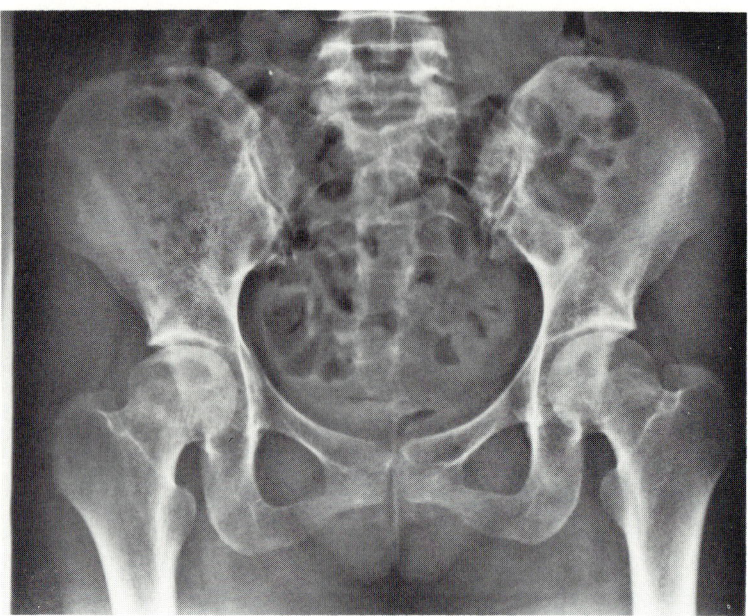

FIG. 31-2. Development of necrosis of the femoral heads. From Lacher M J: Hodgkin's disease: Clinical Vignettes, in Lacher M J (ed): Hodgkin's Disease. New York, Wiley, 1976, pp 427–465.

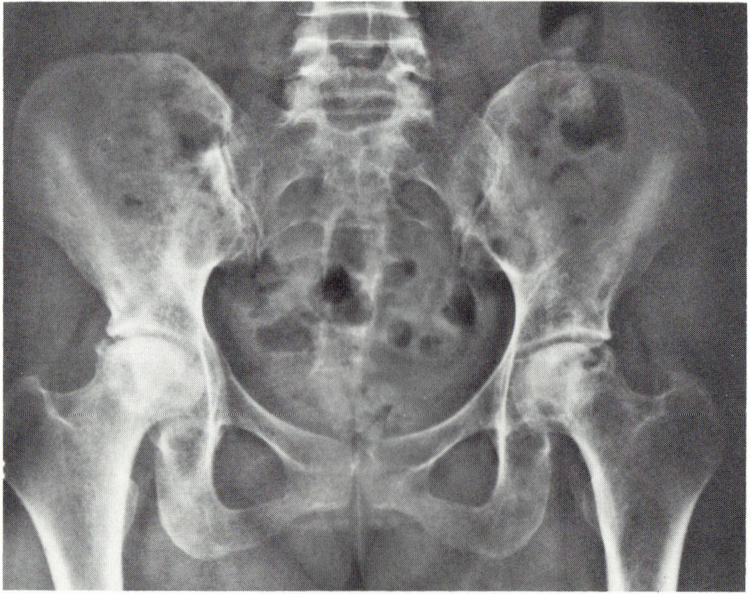

FIG. 31-3. Development of necrosis of the femoral heads. From Lacher M J: Hodgkin's disease: Clinical Vignettes, in Lacher M J (ed): Hodgkin's Disease. New York, Wiley, 1976, pp 427–465.

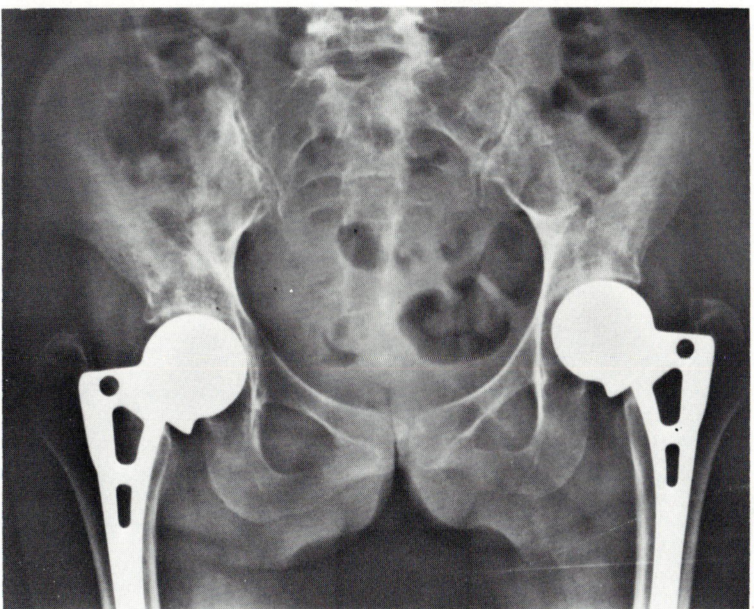

FIG. 31-4. Rehabilitation of patients with necrosis of the femoral heads. From Lacher M J: Hodgkin's disease: Clinical Vignettes, in Lacher M J (ed): Hodgkin's Disease. New York, Wiley, 1976, pp 427–465

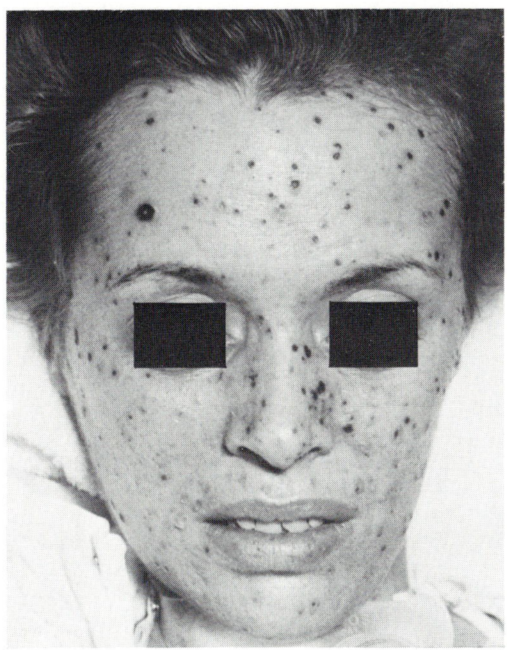

FIG. 31-5. Generalization of herpes zoster. From Lacher, M J: Hodgkin's disease: Clinical Vignettes in Lacher, M J (ed): Hodgkin's Disease. New York, Wiley, 1976, pp 427–465.

Of course, the patient's own fear that the tumor will recur is another serious problem associated with survival. Hodgkin's disease patients are wonderfully courageous and have extraordinary resilience. Although they know that they do run the risk of relapse, they also have faith in their chance for another remission. Whenever they are stabilized, they do lead normal lives. It is a gratifying anticipation that will ultimately be extended to all "malignant" diseases.

References

1. Order S E, Porter M, Hellman S: Hodgkin's disease, evidence of a tumor associated antigen. N Engl J Med 285:471–474, 1971
2. Order S E, Chism S E, Hellman S: Hodgkin's disease-associated antigens: Studies on segregation and specificities. NCI Monograph 36:139–145, 1973
3. Hirshaut Y, Dosik M H: Immunological and etiological aspects of Hodgkin's disease, in Lacher M J (ed): Hodgkin's Disease. New York, Wiley, 1976, p 405
4. Case D C, Jr, Hansen J A, Corrales E, et al: Comparison of multiple in vivo and in vitro parameters in untreated patients with Hodgkin's disease. Cancer 38:1807–1815, 1976
5. Fuks Z, Strober S, Kaplan H S: Interaction between serum factors and T lymphocytes in Hodgkin's disease. N Engl J Med 295:1273–1315, 1976
6. Lichtenfeld J L, Wiernik P H, Mardiney M R, Jr, et al: Abnormalities of complement and its components in patients with acute leukemia, Hodgkin's disease, and sarcoma. Cancer Res 36:3678–3680, 1976
7. Verhaegen H, DeCock W, DeCree J D, et al: Increase of serum complement levels in cancer patients with progressing tumors. Cancer 38:1608–1613, 1976
8. Kaplan H S: Formal discussion of F. Teillet et al's paper, "A reappraisal of clinical and biological signs in staging of Hodgkin's disease." Cancer Res 31:1730, 1971
9. Teillet F, Boiron M, Bernard J: A reappraisal of clinical and biological signs in staging of Hodgkin's disease. Cancer Res 31:1723–1729, 1971
10. Lacher M J: Long survival in Hodgkin's disease. Ann Intern Med 70:7–17, 1969
11. Lacher M J: Introduction, in Lacher M J (ed): Hodgkin's Disease. New York, Wiley, 1976
12. Moore M R, Bull J M, Jones S E, et al: Sequential radiotherapy and chemotherapy in the treatment of Hodgkin's disease. Ann Intern Med 77:1–9, 1972
13. Spittle M F, Harmer C L, Cassady J R, et al: Analysis of primary relapses after radiotherapy in Hodgkin's disease. NCI Monograph 36:497–508, 1973
14. Glatstein E, Guernsey J M, Rosenberg S A, et al: The value of laparotomy and splenectomy in the staging of Hodgkin's disease. Cancer 24:709–718, 1969
15. Desser R K, Moran E M, Ultmann J E: Staging of Hodgkin's disease and lymphoma: Diagnostic procedures including staging laparotomy and splenectomy. Med Clin North Am 47:479–498, 1973
16. Lacher M J, Paglia M A, Hertz R E L, et al: Staging laparotomy and splenectomy in Hodgkin's disease. Clinical Bulletin (MSKCC) 3:43–48, 1973
17. Johnson, R E: The rationale for "selective" staging laparotomy in Hodgkin's disease and the malignant lymphomas, in Varco R L, Delaney J P (eds): Controversy in Surgery. New York, Saunders, 1976, p 649
18. Lacher M J: Hodgkin's disease—The laparotomy-splenectomy controversy, in, Varco R L, Delaney J L (eds): Controversies in Surgery. New York, Saunders, 1976, p 64
19. Lacher M J, Durant J R: Combined vinblastine and chlorambucil therapy of Hodgkin's disease. Ann Intern Med 62:468–476, 1965
20. DeVita V, Canellos G, Hubbard S, et al: Chemotherapy of Hodgkin's disease (HD) with MOPP: A 10-year progress report. ASCO Abstracts 17:269, 1976
21. Moxley J, DeVita V, Bruce K, et al: Intensive combination chemotherapy and x-irradiation in Hodgkin's disease. Cancer Res 27:1258, 1967
22. Nicholson W, Berd M, Crowther D, et al: Combination chemotherapy in generalized Hodgkin's disease. Br Med J 3:7, 1970
23. Bloomfield C D, Weiss R B, Fortuny I, et al: Combined chemotherapy with cyclophosphamide, vinblastine, procarbazine, and prednisone (CVPP) for patients with advanced Hodgkin's disease; an alternative program to MOPP. Cancer 38:42–48, 1976
24. Bonnadonna G, DeLena M, Monfardini S, et al: Intensive treatment with chemotherapy and radiotherapy for Hodgkin's disease, in Fiorentino M, Vangelista R, Grigoletto E (eds): Thyroid Tumors, Lymphomas, Granulocytic Leukemia Proceedings of the Padua Seminar

on Clinical Oncology. Piccin Medical Books, 1972, p 155
25. Lacher M J: A new maintenance combination chemotherapy with thio tepa, vinblastine, procarbazine, and prednisone (TVPP) for patients with advanced Hodgkin's disease. (in preparation)
26. Aisenberg A C, Qazi R: Improved survival in Hodgkin's disease. Cancer 37:2423–2429, 1976
27. Becker R L, Avioli L V: Gestational trophoblastic disease. Arch Intern Med 137:221–229, 1977
28. Lukes R J, Butler J J: The pathology and nomenclature of Hodgkin's disease. Cancer Res 26:1063–1081, 1966
29. Jackson J Jr, Parker F Jr: Hodgkin's Disease and Allied Disorders. Oxford University Press, 1947, p 177
30. Lukes R J, Craver L F, Hall T C, et al: Report of the nomenclature committee. Cancer Res 26:1311, 1966
31. Keller A R, Kaplan J J, Lukes R J, et al: Correlation of histopathology with other prognostic indications in Hodgkin's disease. Cancer 22:487–499, 1968
32. Butler J J: Relationship of histological findings to survival in Hodgkin's disease. Cancer Res 31(2):1770–1775, 1971
33. Strum S B, Rappaport H: Consistency of histologic subtypes in Hodgkin's disease in simultaneous and sequential biopsy specimens. NCI Monograph 36:253–260, 1973
34. Hanson T A: Histological classification and survival in Hodgkin's disease: A study of 251 cases with a special reference to nodular sclerosing Hodgkin's disease. Cancer 17: 1595–1603, 1964
35. Rosenberg S A: Editorial: A rare type of Hodgkin's disease. N Engl J Med 288:789–790, 1973
36. Neiman R S, Rosen P J, Lukes R J: Lymphocyte-depletion Hodgkin's disease: A clinicopathological entity. N Engl J Med 288:751–755, 1973
37. Lacher M J: The pathology of Hodgkin's disease—Have we come full circle?, in Lacher M J (ed): Hodgkin's Disease. New York, Wiley, 1976, p 91
38. Kaplan H S, Good R A: Summary of informal discussion on histopathology and experimental cytology. NCI Monograph 36:265, 1973
39. Kadin M E: Invited discussion: In vitro study of multinucleated cells in Hodgkin's disease. NCI Monograph 36:211–214, 1973
40. Peckham M J, Cooper E H: Proliferation characteristics of the various classes of cells in Hodgkin's disease. Cancer 24:135–146, 1969
41. Marmont A M, Damasio E E: The effects of two alkaloids derived from Vinca rosea on the malignant cells of Hodgkin's disease, lymphosarcoma and acute leukemia in vivo. Blood 29:1–21, 1967
42. Lukes R J, Tindle B H, Parker J W: Reed-Sternberg-like cells in infectious mononucleosis. Lancet 2:1003–1004, 1969
43. Lukes R J: Criteria for involvement of lymph node, bone marrow, spleen, and liver in Hodgkin's disease. Cancer Res 31:1755–1767, 1971
44. Strum S B, Rappaport H: Interrelations of the histologic types of Hodgkin's disease. Arch Pathol 91:127–134, 1971
45. Kadin M E, Glatstein E, Dorfman R F: Clinicopathologic studies of 117 untreated patients subjected to laparotomy for the staging of Hodgkin's disease. Cancer 27:1277–1294, 1971
46. Hutchison G B: Survival and complications of radiotherapy following involved and extended field therapy of Hodgkin's disease, stages I and II. A collaborative study. Cancer 38: 288–305, 1976
47. Rosenberg S A, Boiron M, DeVita V T, et al: Report of the committee on Hodgkin's disease staging procedures. Cancer Res 31:1862, 1971
48. Coleman M, Lightdale C J, Vinciguerra V, et al: Peritoneoscopy in Hodgkin's disease. Confirmation of results by laparotomy. JAMA 236:2634–2636, 1976
49. Johnston G, Benua R S, Teates C E, et al: Ga-citrate imaging in untreated Hodgkin's disease: Preliminary report of a cooperative group. J Nucl Med 15:399–403, 1974
50. Lee B J: Lymphangiography in Hodgkin's disease: Indications and contraindications. Cancer Res 26:1084, 1966
51. Glatstein E, Trueblood H W, Enright L P, et al: Surgical staging of abdominal involvement of unselected patients with Hodgkin's disease. Radiology 97:425, 1970
52. Lacher M J: Hodgkin's disease: Clinical vignettes, in Lacher M J (ed): Hodgkin's Disease. New York, Wiley, 1976, p 427
53. Turner D A, Pinsky S M, Gottschalk A., et al: The use of Gallium-67 scanning in the staging of Hodgkin's disease. Radiology 104:97, 1972
54. Kirschner R H, O'Connell M J, Sutherland J C, et al: Baltimore Cancer Research Center Public Health Service Hospital, Baltimore. Letter to the editor. JAMA 225:635, 1973
55. Lacher M J: Staging laparotomy in patients with Hodgkin's disease, in Lacher M J (ed): Hodgkin's Disease. New York, Wiley, 1976, p 117
56. Hellman S: Current studies in Hodgkin's disease. What laparotomy has wrought. N Engl J Med 290:894–898, 1974

57. Johnson R E: Is staging laparotomy routinely indicated in Hodgkin's disease? Ann Intern Med 75:459–462, 1971
58. DeVita V T, Bagley C M, Jr, Goodell B, et al: Peritoneoscopy in the staging of Hodgkin's disease. Cancer Res 31:1746–1750, 1970
59. Givler R L, Brunk S F, Hass C A, et al: Problems of interpretation of liver biopsy in Hodgkin's disease. Cancer 28:1355–1342, 1971
60. Bagley C M, Roth J A, Thomas L B, et al: Liver biopsy in Hodgkin's disease. Clinicopathologic correlations in 127 patients. Ann Intern Med 76:219–225, 1972
61. Fuks Z, Strober S, Kaplan H S: Interaction between serum factors and T lymphocytes in Hodgkin's disease, use as a diagnostic test. N Engl J Med 295:1273–1316, 1976
62. Bobrove A M, Fuks Z, Strober S, et al: Quantitation of T and B lymphocytes and cellular immune function in Hodgkin's disease. Cancer 36:169–179, 1975
63. Sokal J E, Primikirios M G: The delayed skin test response in Hodgkin's disease and lymphosarcoma. Cancer 14:597–607, 1961
64. Aisenberg A C: Studies on delayed hypersensitivity in Hodgkin's disease. J Clin Invest 41:1964–1970, 1962
65. Young C R, Corder M P, Haynes H A, et al: Delayed hypersensitivity in Hodgkin's disease: A study of 103 patients. Am J Med 52:63–72, 1973
66. Green I, Corso P F: A study of skin homografting in patients with lymphomas. Blood 14:235–245, 1959
67. Miller D G, Lizardo J G, Snyderman R K: Homologous and heterologous skin transplantation in patients with lymphomatous disease. J Natl Cancer Inst 26:569–583, 1961
68. Casazza A R, Duvall C P, Carbone P P: Summary of infectious complications occurring in patients with Hodgkin's disease. Cancer Res 26:1290–1296, 1966
69. Goffinet D R, Glatstein E J, Merigan T C: Herpes zoster-varicella infections and lymphoma. Ann Intern Med 76:235–240, 1972
70. Tubiana M, van der Werf-Messing B, Laugier A, et al: Survival after recurrence: Prognostic factors and spread patterns in clinical stages I and II of Hodgkin's disease. NCI Monograph 36:513–530, 1973
71. Nisce L Z, D'Angio G J: Radiation therapy for Hodgkin's disease: Memorial hospital techniques, in Lacher M J (ed): Hodgkin's Disease. New York, Wiley, 1976, p 145
72. Bonnadonna G, Zucali R, Monfardini S, et al: Combination chemotherapy of Hodgkin's disease with adriamycin, bleomycin, vinblastine, and imidazole carboxamide versus MOPP. Cancer 36:252–259, 1975
73. Case D C, Jr, Young C W, Nisce L, et al: Eight-drug combination chemotherapy (MOPP and ABDV) and local radiotherapy for advanced Hodgkin's disease. Cancer Treat Rep 60: 1217–1223, 1976
74. Carter S K, Goldsmith M: Combination chemotherapy and combined modality approaches to Hodgkin's disease, in Lacher M J (ed): Hodgkin's Disease. New York, Wiley, 1976, p 193
75. Vinciguerra V, Coleman M, Jarowski C I, et al: A new combination chemotherapy for resistant Hodgkin's disease. JAMA 237:33–35, 1977
76. Al-Mondhiry H, Lacher M J: Hodgkin's disease and leukemia, in Lacher M J (ed): Hodgkin's Disease. New York, Wiley, 1976, p 377
77. DeVita V T, Arseneau J C, Sherins R J, et al: Intensive chemotherapy for Hodgkin's disease: Long-term complications. NCI Monograph 36:447–454, 1973
78. Ihde D C, DeVita V T: Osteonecrosis of the femoral head in patients with lymphoma treated with intermittent combination chemotherapy (including corticosteroids). Cancer 36:1585–1588, 1975
79. Whitley R J, Ch'ien L T, Dolin R, et al: Adenine arabinoside therapy of herpes zoster in the immunosuppressed, NIAID Collaborative Antiviral Study. N Engl J Med 294:1193–1234, 1976
80. Prager D, Sembrot J T, Southard M: Cobalt-60 therapy of Hodgkin's disease and the subsequent development of hypothyroidism. Cancer 29:458–460, 1972
81. Cooper E F: Psychosocial problems in the care of patients with Hodgkin's disease, in Lacher M J (ed): Hodgkin's Disease. New York, Wiley, 1976, p 417
82. Vianna N J, Greenwald P, Davies J N P: Hodgkin's disease—An infectious disease?, in Lacher M J (ed): Hodgkin's Disease. New York, Wiley, 1976, p 405
83. Grufferman S, Cole P, Smith P G, et al: Hodgkin's disease in siblings. N Engl J Med 296:248–250, 1977
84. DeVita V, Serpick A, Carbone P: Combination chemotherapy in the treatment of advanced Hodgkin's disease. Ann Intern Med 73:881, 1970
85. Morgenfeld M, Pavlovsky A, Isola L, et al: Treatment of malignant lymphomas with cyclophosphamide, vincristine, procarbazine and prednisone combination. Presented at the 14th International Congress of Hematology, 1972

John M. Bennett

32
The Chemotherapy of Non-Hodgkin's Lymphoma

In contrast to the reasonably standardized therapeutic approaches to patients with advanced Hodgkin's disease, treatment options in non-Hodgkin's lymphoma (NHL) are multiple and are undergoing constant revision and, hopefully, improvement. To a large extent this is a direct consequence of the marked heterogeneity of the pathologic subtypes and of the clinical syndromes that range from the lymphoblastic (convoluted or nonconvoluted) lymphomas of children to the well differentiated lymphocytic lymphoma of middle aged adults. It includes such rare variants as bone lymphoma, gastrointestinal lymphomas, and skin lymphomas (mycosis fungoides).

The Rappaport classification of NHL has resulted in a revision of our concepts of these disorders as a consequence of the apparent differences of survival among the histologic subtypes, including architectural pattern (nodular versus diffuse) and cell type [lymphocytic and(or) histiocytic].[1,2] These prognostic features are of considerably more value in adults, where close to half of the lymphomas have a nodular pattern, than in children and adolescents, where virtually all of the lymphomas have a diffuse pattern. Certainly, current available data suggest that nodular lymphomas have, overall, a better prognosis and higher percentage of survival than diffuse lymphomas.[3]

With increasing sophistication of the determinants of the origin of lymphoid cells,[4,5] i.e., thymus- ("T") derived or bursal- ("B") derived, modifications have been proposed in classification and have proven to be helpful in our understanding of the pathogenesis of these diseases.[6,7] The application of "immunological markers" to the study of NHL has demonstrated that all of the nodular lymphomas and many of the diffuse forms are composed of malignant lymphoid cells of "B" origin, mostly of follicular origin. In addition, the vast majority of "histiocytic" and "lymphocytic:histiocytic" cell types lack monocyte:macrophage markers but bear surface immunoglobulins.

For the present, however, the major institutions responsible for conducting combined modality trials in NHL, including the National Cancer Institute-sponsored cooperative multidisciplinary groups, continue to utilize the Rappaport classification and members of the Lymphoma Panel for diagnosis

Supported by USPHS grants #CA-11083-08 and CA-11198-06 from the National Cancer Institute

confirmation. Although most participating institutional pathologists are able to accurately separate Hodgkin's disease from NHL, and both from benign lymph node proliferations (to 95 per cent accuracy) overall accuracy for cell type identification has ranged from 58 per cent in one study[8] to 66 per cent in another.[9] Fortunately, there is a good agreement regarding the two cell types that constitute the majority of cases: diffuse histiocytic and nodular poorly-differentiated lymphocytic lymphomas. This classification will serve as the backbone for the following review.

The vast majority of NHLs have advanced disease on initial presentation. At least 80 per cent of patients, after conventional staging with bone marrow biopsies,liver biopsies and/or laparoscopy will be classified as either Stage III or IV.[10] Of 121 patients referred to the National Cancer Institute as "Stage I or II" only 5 (6.3 per cent) with nodular lymphoma and 12 of 40 (30 per cent) with diffuse histiocytic lymphoma remained as Stage I or II after staging evaluation. Therefore the therapy for NHL, with rare exceptions, is designed for systemic, rather than regional, control and cure.

Single Agents

For at least a decade, partial regressions of NHL have been accomplished with a wide range of chemotherapeutic agents including corticosteroids. These agents fall into several broad categories: alkylating drugs (cyclophosphamide, chlorambucil); vinca alkaloids (vincristine, vinblastine); antibiotics (bleomycin, adriamycin); nitrosoureas (BCNU, CCNU); corticosteroids (prednisone) and miscellaneous agents (procarbazine, streptonigrin and hexamethylmelamine). The efficacy of cyclophosphamide was confirmed by a joint study of the Acute Leukemia Group B and Eastern Cooperative Oncology Group (ECOG)[11] with a complete remission rate of 16 per cent in 1968. The unique advantage of vincristine over vinblastine with significantly less hematologic toxicity was demonstrated by Carbone and co-workers at the same time.[12] Prednisone produces significant partial regressions, but no complete responses.[13,14]

Combination Programs

Shortly after the demonstration of the effectiveness of these three agents several groups combined these drugs, and the acronym COP or CVP has become virtually synonymous with the chemotherapy of NHL.[11,15] The ECOG, in their study EST 0168, confirmed the importance of prednisone in this combination with a larger number of patients achieving complete remission with COP than with CO.[16]

In these and similar studies, complete remissions (CR) have ranged from 35 to 57 per cent with median durations of 3 to more than 18 months. Where the data are separated by histologic pattern, the CR per cent is higher for nodular lymphomas than for diffuse lymphomas. It is important to separate relapse-free survival, or the disease-free interval, from survival. Although overall response rates for nodular and diffuse histologies are similar (60 to 80 per cent) median survival is distinctly greater for nodular lymphomas, usually in excess of 6 years in contrast to under 2 years for diffuse histologies.[2]

Confirmation of the peculiar biology of nodular lymphomas can be seen in the early results of a prospective study from Stanford that has demonstrated identical survival rates for three different programs.[17] In this study, Stage IV patients were randomized to receive either a single alkylating agent, CVP, or CVP plus total nodal irradiation. The probability of achieving a remission was identical for all three groups (>80 per cent) but it took much longer to achieve a CR with a single agent (cyclophosphamide or chlorambucil) than with either of the two more intensive programs (40 months versus 16 months). As in previous studies, although 50 per cent of the patients remain free of disease progression at approximately 3 years, analysis of the shape of the survival curves does not suggest prolonged disease-free intervals for a subgroup of patients in remission.

Diffuse Lymphomas

Diffuse histiocytic lymphomas ("reticulum cell sarcomas"), classically have been viewed as invariably fatal and only responsive to chemotherapy for brief time periods. In one series the median survival was only 9 months.[18] Lenhard and co-workers, in a study of the chemotherapy of poor prognosis lymphomas (EST 3472) added BCNU to the standard program of CVP and patients were randomized to either cyclophosphamide:prednisone (CP), CVP, or BCVP.[19]

In the diffuse histiocytic (DH) category, a much higher complete response rate (CR) was recorded with CVP (47 per cent) and BCVP (37 per cent) compared to CP (21 per cent), demonstrating the important role of vincristine at least in improving the remission percentage. Patients were treated for nine cycles at 3 week intervals. The median survival for the CVP group was 70.4 weeks, significantly greater than the other two programs (Table 32-1).

The longest survival was in patients with diffuse lymphoma, mixed-cell type (143 weeks). The probability of the complete responders living for 2 years was 75 per cent in contrast to less than 50 per cent for the partial responders and 5 per cent for the nonresponders.

Utilizing a similar regimen with a 40 per cent reduction in cyclophosphamide dosage and a 40 per cent increase in the amount of BCNU, Durant and co-workers[20] achieved a 50 per cent CR with a median survival of 64.4 weeks for DH, which is identical to the Lenhart study. In both programs the curves of the complete responders have a change in slope, suggesting long-term remissions after 60 weeks with between 20 and 40 per cent of the original group free of disease at 2 years.

Adriamycin and Bleomycin Combinations

In previously treated patients both adriamycin[21] and Bleomycin produce partial responses in both histiocytic and lymphocytic lymphomas in the range of 30 per cent. With a combination of cyclophosphamide, hydroxydaunomycin, oncovin and prednisone (CHOP), a CR of 68 per cent in DH subtypes was achieved by member institutions of the Southwestern Oncology Group (SWOG).[22] Despite this high response rate, no apparent change in the shape of the survival curve was noted to suggest long-term survival.

The 1 year survival figures for CR's were better in the nodular lymphomas (90 per cent) than in the diffuse lymphocytic (75 per cent) or DH types (66 per cent). With less intensive therapy, however, Ezdinli and co-workers (ECOG: EST 1472)[23] achieved a 91 per cent 2 year survival for nodular poorly-differentiated lymphocytic (PDL) and 84 per cent for diffuse poorly-differentiated lymphocytic lymphomas. A striking difference is noted (Table 32-2) when one compares survival of those patients who do not respond, depending on architectural pattern,[24] demonstrating the distinct biologic advantage of nodular over diffuse PDL.

The addition of Bleomycin to the four-drug combination of cyclophosphamide, adriamycin, vincristine and prednisone, and referred to by the acronym "BACOP,"[25] has not improved the overall per cent of CRs in DH subtypes but no relapse, to date, have been noted in those who achieved complete remission for durations of from 5 to 30 months. It is of interest that virtually no complete responses were observed when liver, bone marrow or CNS involvement was present.

In a previous study by the same investigators with either the "MOPP" program, or a similar combination in which cyclophosphamide was substituted for nitrogen mustard ("C-MOPP"), the per cent CR was the same for diffuse histiocytic lymphomas with 10 patients (37 per cent of original series) free of disease for 2 to 9 years after therapy, with a median survival for this group of more than 4 years.[26]

Current Recommendations

In the diffuse lymphomas, with the exception of the rare well-differentiated lymphocytic lymphomas, the achievement of a complete remission with one of the several combination chemotherapy programs available should be the main goal of any treatment program. Without a complete remission, the survival for patients with Stage III and IV disease is extremely poor.

In the nodular lymphomas presently available data do not suggest that aggressive

TABLE 32-1. *EST 3472: Treatment of Histiocytic Lymphomas*

Diffuse Histiocytic	No.	No. of deaths (%)	No. of CR (%)		Med. Surv. (wks)	
CP	22	21 (95%)	2 (9%)		42.3	
CVP	19	13 (68%)	9 (47%)	P=.0165	70.4	P=.04
BCVP	19	15 (79%)	7 (37%)		45.9	
Total	60	49 (82%)	18 (30%)		50.0	

induction programs, with or without radiation therapy, alter the survival curves of patients so treated. The goal should be to produce a gradual but continual remission with as little toxicity as possible. For example, in a current study by the ECOG (EST 2474) on favorable lymphomas there is no significant difference between aggressive therapy (BCVP or COPP) and moderate therapy (CP) in the percentage of complete or partial responders or in the survival,[27] with from 84 to 93 per cent of patients responding. The schemas and regimens have been published recently.[28]

The role of radiation therapy in the advanced lymphomas, with particular reference to total-body irradiation, is currently under intense investigation.[29] In a study at the Joint Center for Radiation Therapy, the 5-year survival figure for nodular lymphomas was 80 per cent and for diffuse lymphomas, 40 per cent, exclusive of histiocytic types that were not included. Relapse free survivals, however, were 25 and 10 per cent respectively, indicating high relapse potential for both groups.

TABLE 32-2. *EST 1472: Treatment of Lymphocytic Lymphomas*

Category	Survival at 2 Years Nodular	Diffuse
Complete response	91%	84%
Partial response	85%	58%
Progression	72%	17%

FUTURE PLANS

The goals for the next decade will be to improve CR rate of the unfavorable lymphomas and to attempt to delay and prevent relapses with either non-cross-resistant chemotherapy or consolidation radiation therapy. More basic research is necessary in the nodular lymphomas to attempt to understand the biologic survival advantage, but lack of curability, for the majority of patients with this form of lymphoma. The role of immunotherapy in maintaining remissions must be clarified, as well as the duration or necessity of maintenance chemotherapy programs.

REFERENCES

1. Rappaport H, Winter W J, Hicks E B: Follicular lymphoma—Re-evaluation of its position in the scheme of malignant lymphomas, based on a survey of 253 cases. Cancer 9:792, 1956
2. Rosenberg S A, Dorfman R F, Kaplan H S: A summary of the results of a review of 405 patients with non-Hodgkin's lymphoma at Stanford university. Br J Cancer 31:168, 1975
3. Schein P S, Chabner B A, Canellos G P, et al: Potential for prolonged disease-free survival following combination chemotherapy of non-Hodgkin's lymphomas. Blood 43:181, 1974
4. Lukes R I, Collins R D: Immunologic characterization of human malignant lymphomas. Cancer 34:1488, 1974
5. Dorfman R F: Classification of the non-Hodgkin's lymphomas. Lancet 1:1295, 1974

6. Gajl-Peczalski K, Bloomfield C, et al: "B" and "T" cell lymphomas: Analysis of blood and lymph nodes in 87 patients. Am J Med 59:674, 1975
7. Jaffe E S, Shevach E M, Sussman E H, et al: Membrane receptor sites for the identification of lymphoreticular cells in benign and malignant conditions. Br J Cancer 31:107, 1975
8. Jones S E, Butler J J, Byrne G, et al: Histopathologic review of lymphoma cases from SWOG cases. Cancer 39:1071, 1977
9. Bennett J M, Lenhard R E, Ezdinli E, et al: The chemotherapy of non-Hodgkin's lymphomas: The Eastern Cooperative Oncology Group Experience. Cancer Treat Rep 61:58, 1977
10. Chabner B A, Johnson R E, Young R C, et al: Sequential nonsurgical and surgical staging of nonHodgkin's lymphoma. Ann Intern Med 85:149, 1976
11. Hoogstraten B, Owens A H, Lenhard R E, et al: Combination chemotherapy in lymphosarcoma and reticulum cell sarcoma. Blood 33:370, 1969
12. Carbone P P, Spurr C: Management of patients with malignant lymphoma—A comparative study with cyclophosphamide and vinca alkaloids. Cancer Res 28:811, 1968
13. Jones S E, Rosenberg S A, Kaplan H S, et al: Non-Hodgkin's lymphomas II. Single agent chemotherapy. Cancer 30:31, 1972
14. Ezdinli E Z, Stutzman L, Aungst C W, et al: Corticosteroid therapy for lymphomas and chronic lymphocytic leukemia. Cancer 23:900, 1968
15. Bagley C M Jr, DeVita V T Jr, Berard C W, Canellos G: Advanced lymphosarcoma: Intensive cyclical combination chemotherapy with CVP. Ann Intern Med 76:227, 1972
16. Lenhard R E Jr, Prentice R L, Owens A H Jr, et al: Combination chemotherapy of the malignant lymphomas: a controlled clinical trial. Cancer 38:1052, 1976
17. Portlock C S, Rosenberg S A, Glatstein E, Kaplan H S: Treatment of advanced non-Hodgkin's lymphoma with favorable histologies. Blood 47:747, 1976
18. Muggia F M, Ultmann J E: Exploratory laparotomy for reticulum cell sarcoma. Cancer 30:454, 1972
19. Lenhard R E Jr, Ezdinli E, Costello W, Bennett J M, et al: Treatment of poor prognosis (histiocytic and mixed) lymphomas: A comparison of two-, three-, and four-drug chemotherapy, in Bennett J M (ed): Chemotherapy of Non-Hodgkin's Lymphomas. Cancer Treat Rep 61:1079, 1977
20. Durant J R, Loeb V Jr, Dorfman R, Chan Y K: BCNU, cyclophosphamide, vincristine, and prednisone (BCOP): A new therapeutic regimen for diffuse histiocytic lymphoma. Cancer 36:1936, 1975
21. Gottlieb J A, Gutterman J U, McCredie K B, et al: Chemotherapy of malignant lymphoma with adriamycin. Cancer Res 33:3024, 1973
22. McKelvey E M, Gottlieb J A, Wilson H E, et al: Hydroxydaunomycin (adriamycin) combination chemotherapy in malignant lymphomas. Cancer 38:1484, 1976
23. Ezdinli E, Pocock S, Berard C W, et al: Comparison of intensive versus moderate chemotherapy of lymphocytic lymphomas. Cancer 38:1060, 1976
24. Ezdinli E, Costello W, Lenhard R E Jr, et al: Survival of nodular versus diffuse pattern lymphocytic poorly differentiated lymphoma. Cancer, 1978 (in press)
25. Schein P S, DeVita V T Jr, Hubbard S, et al: Bleomycin, adriamycin, cyclophosphamide, vincristine, and prednisone (BACOP) combination chemotherapy in the treatment of advanced histiocytic lymphomas. Ann Intern Med 85:417, 1976
26. DeVita V T Jr, Chabner B, Hubbard S, et al: Advanced diffuse histiocytic lymphoma, a potentially curable disease. Lancet 1:248, 1975
27. Ezdinli E: personal communication, April, 1977
28. Bennett J M, Bakemeier R F, Carbone P P, et al: Clinical trials with BCNU in malignant lymphomas by the Eastern Cooperative Oncology Group. Canc Treat Rep 60(6):739, 1976
29. Hillman S, Chaffey J T, et al: The plan of radiation therapy in the treatment of non Hodgkin's lymphomas. Cancer 39:843, 1977

Neil Abramson

33
Management of Multiple Myeloma

Although multiple myeloma may be a disease of antiquity, effective therapy for this disorder is fairly recent. Archeologic findings in Florida describing lytic skull lesions suggest that myeloma dates back to prehistory.[1] Biblical-medical scholars could cite the acquired painful disease of bone and tormenting infections of Job as the first written description. The first description of myeloma in medical literature was given in 1847 by Bence-Jones,[2] in which he reported a urinary protein abnormality, carefully studied by MacIntyre from a patient with bone fractures and peripheral edema.[3] Innumerable papers over the next century revealed the protean manifestations of this protein disease. Despite the volumes of cases, it was not until the 1960s that methods of treatment were described that altered the progression of the disease, characterized by pain, renal failure, infections and bleeding. The purpose of this chapter is to review the diagnostic procedures and therapeutic agents now used in myeloma.

Diagnostic Procedures

The diagnosis of myeloma is greatly simplified by the elaboration of a biosynthetic product or protein from malignant plasma cells. The identification of this monoclonal protein, an immunoglobulin of one specific class (and subclass) or one light chain type, or both, is almost always a requisite for diagnosis. Rarely, malignant plasma cells produce a monoclonal protein, but are unable to secrete it; this disease is referred to as nonsecretory myeloma.[4]

The appearance of a monoclonal protein is seldom sufficient, by itself, for a diagnosis of myeloma. Multiple myeloma is a disorder characterized by numerous symptoms and signs, in addition to the monoclonal protein. Numerous examples of monoclonal proteins are not associated with myeloma, so-called benign monoclonal gammopathy;[5] others are seen with liver disease, connective tissue disease, and carcinoma.[6] The diagnosis of myeloma as a disorder distinct from these nonmyelomatous entities may be made on the basis of pathophysiologic evidence of malignancy of plasma cells;[6] such evidence includes significant increases in plasma cells of the marrow, bone marrow replacement (cytopenias), accompanying increases in its biosynthetic product, viscosity abnormalities and a suppression of biosynthesis of normal immunoglobulins.[7] Table 33-1 enumerates the requisite diagnostic criteria.[8]

Measurable disease is essential for the

Supported in part by Richard Thompson Memorial Fund and Baptist Medical Center

TABLE 33-1. *Diagnostic Criteria for Myeloma**

Diagnosis is established by one of the following:
- I + b or I + c
- II + b; II + c; or II + d
- III alone
- a + b + c; a + b + d; or a + c + d

I. Plasmacytoma by tissue biopsy.
II. Marrow plasmacytosis > 30%.
III. "M-component" in serum exceeding 3500 mg/100 ml for IgG, or exceeding 2000 mg per 100 ml. IgA, or greater than 250 mg of kappa *or* lambda light chain in 24-hour urine sample.

a = marrow plasmacytosis of 10-20%.
b = "M-component" present but quantities less than those noted in III.
c = lytic bone lesions.
d = "normal" immunoglobulin levels of IgM < 50 mg/100 ml, IgA < 150 mg per 100 ml. and IgG < 600 mg per 100 ml.

*Modified from Hoogstraten B: SWOG-7704 protocol for multiple myeloma. Southwestern Oncology Group, 1977.

proper assessment of therapeutic effectiveness. Quantitation of monoclonal protein in the serum and urine is the best method. Random bone marrow examinations do not reflect total plasma cell mass and are difficult to quantitate. A plasmacytoma may be used for measurement purposes; however, it is not usually accessible to calipers. Immunoelectrophoresis is necessary for initial typing and identification of monoclonal protein, but scans of electrophoretic patterns or immunoquantitation are used as parameters for following features of the disease. In those instances in which there are large quantities of abnormal protein or polymerized proteins, scans may be more accurate than immunoquantitation. Urine monoclonal proteins, which are usually light chains (Bence-Jones protein), may vary depending upon effectiveness of therapy and creatinine clearance. A decrease in light-chain excretion may indicate successful treatment or deteriorating renal function.

THERAPY

Treatment of multiple myeloma may be divided into therapy directed at problems and complications of the disease and therapy specific for the primary disease (Table 33-2). Oftentimes, the problems and complications of the disease are urgent and life-threatening, and must be attended to promptly.

Pain from involvement of bones may delay therapy for a considerable time. Bone involvement with myeloma varies from osteoporosis to lytic lesions, fractures, collapsed vertebral bodies and cord compression. Immobility is a frequent result of bone pain and causes further calcium loss from bones and dehydration. Despite the diffuseness of most cases of myeloma, irradiation for local disease may be necessary. Restricted-field radiotherapy is desirable to spare normal marrow for future chemotherapy. Immobilization of a local area by orthopedic devices at times is beneficial but may cause greater difficulty by the pressure or restriction it causes. Recent information suggests that spinothalamic nerve vibration via battery-operated transcutaneous nerve stimulation may be useful.[9] Intractable pain might require nerve tract section (cordotomy, rhizotomy). Analgesics or narcotics are essential to facilitate mobilization. Habituation to analgesics should not be a bar to control of pain. Salicylates and narcotics are a well-recognized effective combination; however, salicylates, which cause platelet

TABLE 33-2. *Therapy for Multiple Myeloma*

- Local
  - Radiotherapy
- Systemic
  - hydration
  - ambulation
  - vs. hypercalcemia
  - vs. hyperuricemia
  - vs. infection
  - chemotherapy
- Ancillary
  - fluoride (?)
  - vitamin D (?)
  - calcium (?)
  - androgens (?)

functional abnormalities, may be hazardous in patients with myeloma in whom thrombocytopenia or hyperviscosity may already have resulted in a predisposition to bleeding. "Brompton's cocktail" is a palatable liquid containing morphine and cocaine that is useful for outpatients.[10]

Infections are most often due to pyogenic organisms such as *Pneumococcus*, *Streptococcus*, *Staphylococcus*, and *Meningococcus*. Presumably, a deficiency of normal immunoglobulins predisposes to these microorganisms. Gamma globulin infusions or injections, however, are ineffective in part because of hypercatabolism of infused protein[11] and because the injected gamma globulin is lacking in directed antigen specificity. Bacterial infections are best treated with appropriate antibiotics and at times with granulocyte transfusions; combinations of gentamicin and carbenicillin may be necessary when granulocyte counts fall to less than 500/mm^3. Unusual infections with viruses, fungi, and protozoa may also attack the myeloma patient because of treatment-associated leukopenia and alterations of cellular immunity. Localized herpes zoster is treated with local measures and with analgesia; however, disseminated herpetic zoster may be life-threatening because of pulmonary insufficiency or secondary *Staphylococcus* septicemia. Frequent monitoring of chest roentgenograms and blood gases, painstaking skin care, cultures and penicillin are useful in disseminated herpes. *Pneumocystis carinii* infection may be manifested by fever, dyspnea, poor oxygenation, and pulmonary infiltrates, although on auscultation the lungs may seem reasonably clear. Rapid investigation and special stains are necessary. The treatment of choice is a combination of sulfur and trimethoprim.[12] Pentamidine may be used in resistant cases. The role of vaccination for pneumococcus, influenzae and other organisms is uncertain since these patients have blunted responses to antigen stimulation.

Hyperviscosity causes problems with various organs or systems (Table 33-3). In most instances, only long-range successful therapy directed at decreasing protein synthesis is of value. When emergency situations exist, however, such as hyperviscosity-induced coma or other serious CNS symptoms, prompt treatment is necessary. Fluid replacement may alleviate dehydration. Plasmapheresis can now be performed efficiently and safely and should be considered as a therapeutic trial. In general, results with plasmapheresis in myeloma are poorer than those in macroglobulinemia because 50 per cent of the IgA or IgG myeloma protein may be present in the intravascular compartment, whereas in macroglobulinemia, 90 per cent of the IgM is intravascular.

TABLE 33-3. *Effects of Hyperviscosity on Various Organs or Systems in Myeloma*

Central nervous system—dizziness, postural hypotension, visual defects, lethargy, coma
Peripheral nervous system—paresthesias, neuropathy
Gastrointestinal—bleeding
Cardiac—congestive heart failure
Renal—azotemia, renal tubular acidosis, Bence-Jones kidney
Vascular—purpura, bleeding, ischemia

Several methods are available to measure viscosity, but no single laboratory value can replace clinical criteria. Clinical hyperviscosity can occur with minimally abnormal laboratory values; conversely, markedly abnormal laboratory values can be found with few if any clinical abnormalities.

Bleeding is a frequent problem in myeloma and may be caused by thrombocytopenia, abnormal platelet function, an abnormal coagulation protein system, hyperviscosity or some combination. Thrombocytopenia is usually caused by lack of platelet production (plasma cell replacement, drug or radiotherapeutic ablation, or metabolic deficiency) and can be treated with platelet transfusions. Since platelet transfusions result in formation of antiplatelet antibody, which causes refractoriness to further transfusions, they should be used only when bleeding necessitates. Bleeding caused by unsuspected use of antiplatelet drugs such as aspirin may also be treated with platelet transfusions. Therapy for coagulation protein disorders varies depending upon the cause. Coagulation protein deficiency may be caused by monoclonal proteins functioning as anticoagulants. Then too, the debilitating effects of myeloma or liver infiltration may result in deficient hepatic protein synthesis. When hyperviscosity is the cause of bleeding diathesis, it often results in gastrointestinal or nasal bleeding and is fairly refractory to therapy.

Renal disease has been the most serious prognostic finding.[13] Whether these monoclonal proteins are poorly responsive to therapy and tend to polymerize or alter renal function is unknown. Renal disease may be caused by protein tubular deposition (Bence-Jones kidney), hypercalcemia, uric acid nephropathy, renal tubular acidosis, amyloidosis, plasma cell infiltrates and recurrent infections. Hypercalcemic nephropathy may be treated as hypercalcemia per se (discussed later) and uric acid nephropathy is corrected or prevented by hydration, alkalinization of urine and inhibition of xanthine oxidase with allopurinol. Treatment for other causes is sometimes directed at the myeloma itself. There is no strong evidence to support myeloma therapy for amyloidosis, but a number of successful anecdotal reports have suggested that myeloma therapy is acceptable. Irreversible renal disease has not been a deterrent to specific myeloma therapy; reports describe dialysis of uremics to permit an appropriate trial of chemotherapy.

Hypercalcemia may be a life-threatening complication of myeloma but is treatable and reversible. Calcium loss from bones may result from plasma cell destruction without osteoblastic activity; however, an osteoclastic-promoting lymphokine has been described.[14] Treatment with diuretics (furosemide 40 to 80 mg/day) and saline infusions (150 to 200 ml/hr) is begun promptly but often corticosteroids (for example, prednisone 50 to 100 mg/day) are needed as well. When resistance to this therapy is noted, mithramycin (20 μg per kg over 4 to 6 hours a day for 1 to 3 days) is infused; however, care must be taken since mithramycin is myelotoxic and may provoke serious thrombocytopenia or leukopenia, especially in patients with already compromised marrows. Other therapy that may be considered include phosphates, a low-calcium diet, indomethacin and calcitonin.

Miscellaneous therapy includes anabolic steroids, calcium, fluoride and vitamin D to recalcify bones, but these substances have been advocated in only some studies. Androgens have also been useful in promoting erythropoiesis, but resultant hepatotoxicity has raised questions as to their safety.

Specific Therapy for Myeloma

Specific treatment for myeloma is difficult to assess because of variability in criteria used to establish the quality of response. Standardized criteria are evolving based upon reports from the Southwestern Oncology Group. In general, several months of therapy are required before one can assess changes in the measurable aspects of the disease such as decreases in monoclonal protein in serum or urine. A 50 per cent decrease in serum abnormality and a 90 per cent decrease in Bence-Jones proteinuria are the usual accepted criteria for a favorable response. In some studies a 75 per cent decrease in the synthetic rate of monoclonal protein is used as a criterion. This is calculated on the basis of plasma volume, serum monoclonal protein concentration and catabolic rate of the myeloma protein.

Over the last decade, the use of alkylating agents for myeloma has become well established. Melphalan has become the most popular of the alkylating agents;[15] the alkylating agents are effective and none appears to be better than any other. A report of a 30 per cent response rate to cyclophosphamide after failure with melphalan[16] prompted numerous studies utilizing combinations of alkylating agents (including nitrosoureas) given simultaneously or seriatim; however, the therapeutic index of these regimens does not appear to be an improvement over melphalan plus prednisone.

The most commonly used regimen for induction therapy in myeloma,[17] is melphalan, 0.25 mg/kg/day for 4 days, and prednisone, 2 mg/kg/day for 4 days every 6 weeks; recently, cycles have been reduced to every 3 to 4 weeks.[8] In previously untreated patients, this regimen results in objective responses in half of the patients and extends median survival to greater than 30 months. This regimen is well tolerated, and its results have been confirmed by subsequent studies.

If melphalan therapy fails, few other agents or combinations are effective. The previously noted report of a favorable response to cyclophosphamide after therapy with melphalan has been confirmed in one study.[18] Although high-dose intravenous cyclophosphamide therapy is successful in such patients, it is toxic and should be used only in hospitalized patients who can be supported with white cell and platelet transfusions.[19] A recent report suggests that hexamethylmelamine may be worthwhile in refractory myeloma.[20] Bleomycin and adriamycin alone are ineffective; however, the combination of adriamycin and BCNU achieved a 54 per cent response rate after failure to standard therapy.[21] There have been recent suggestions that hemibody radiotherapy may be effective in palliating metastatic carcinoma; similar therapy (600 to 800 rad to half of the torso, followed by a similar dose to the other half in 6 weeks) in terminal myeloma results in successful palliation in some patients and objective responses in a few.[22]

Maintenance therapy has been adequately explored. The most interesting study reports that the percentage of relapse in patients who received no maintenance therapy was similar to that in patients being treated with chemotherapy.[23] In fact, there is an increase in morbidity and toxicity in patients maintained on chemotherapy or immunotherapy after 1 year of initial chemotherapy, with no prolongation of survival. Therefore, the role of maintenance therapy is disputable at the present time.

Future Trends

Most of the information on therapy in myeloma leads to an assumption that within the clonal plasma cell abnormality, there exist two populations of cells in regard to sensitivity of therapy.[24] Induction therapy, regardless of the alkylating agent used, seems to eradicate the sensitive population while leaving untouched the insensitive and eventually lethal population. This hypothesis fits well with the belief that no combination of drugs is more effective than a single alkylating agent plus prednisone, and it is also consistent with the lack of response to maintenance therapy; the insensitive population seems to grow despite additional therapy. Patients with the more rapidly growing myeloma populations respond more rapidly with induction therapy; however, the insensitive cell population is also a rapidly growing population, and this accounts for the rapid failure in these patients and their shortened survivals.

Length of survival may depend upon reducing the insensitive cell population, and efforts are being directed at its treatment after successful induction therapy. Whether this therapy should include more aggressive alkylating agents or treatment using different cellular mechanics is uncertain at this time.

Conclusions

Efforts must be directed toward improving the quality of life. Overall survival has been only modestly prolonged since the advent of effective chemotherapy. Arrest of bone disease, curtailment of bleeding, and prevention of infections would greatly improve the patient's chances of restoration to normal activities. The problem of infection is being explored through investigation of immune regulation and manipulation. Since myeloma is a disease of cells of the immune system, it may be susceptible to immune stimulation. Supporting data for this hypothesis include evidence that monocytes suppress normal immunoglobulin synthesis.[7] Immunoadjuvants such as BCG (bacillus of Calmette and Guérin) or *C. parvum* may enlarge the number of normal B cells or may release the inhibitory effects of monocytes. Similarly, immunologically-active drugs (for example, levamisole) restore T-cell function and may be useful in immune stimulation of a suppressed B-cell compartment. It may be that restoration of the normal immune system and discontinuance of inappropriate chemotherapy may enhance the quality of life in patients whose survival may be only modestly prolonged.

References

1. Morse D, Dailey R C, Bunn J: Prehistoric multiple myeloma. Bull NY Acad Med 50:447, 1974
2. Bence Jones J: Papers on chemical pathology. Proc Royal Society London Lancet 2:88, 1847
3. MacIntyre W: Case of mollities and fragilitas ossium accompanied with urine strongly charged with animal matter. Med Chir Soc Trans 33:211, 1850
4. Hurez D, Preud'homme J-L, Seligmann M: Intracellular "monoclonal" immunoglobulin in non-secretory human myeloma. J Immunol 104:263, 1970
5. Waldenstrom J: Incipient myelomatosis or "essential" hyperglobulemia and fibrinogenopenia—New syndrome? Acta Med Scand 117:216, 1944
6. Abramson N, Shattil S J: M components: Analysis of 59 patients. JAMA 223:156, 1973
7. Broder S, Humphrey R, Durm M, et al: Impaired synthesis of polyclonal immunoglobulins by circulating lymphocytes from patients with multiple myeloma. N Engl J Med 293:887, 1975
8. Hoogstraten B: SWOG-7704 protocol for multiple myeloma. Southwestern Oncology Group, 1977
9. Ray C D: New electrical stimulation methods for therapy and rehabilitation. Orthoped Rev 6:29, 1977
10. Mount B M, Ajemian I, Scott J F: Use of Brompton mixture in treating the chronic pain of malignant disease. Can Med Assoc J 115:122, 1976
11. Solomon A, Waldmann T A, Fahey J L: Metabolism of normal 6.6S gammaglobulin in normal subjects and in patients with macroglobulinemia and multiple myeloma. J Lab Clin Med 62:1, 1963
12. Hughes W T: Pneumocystis carinii pneumonia. N Engl J Med 297:1381, 1977
13. Medical Research Council's Working Party for Therapeutic Trials in Leukemia: Report on the first myelomatosis trial. Br J Haematol 24:123, 1973
14. Mundy G R, Luben R A, Raisz L, et al: Bone resorbing activity in supernatants from lymphoid cell lines. N Engl J Med 290:867, 1974
15. Farhangi M, Osserman E F: The treatment of multiple myeloma. Semin Hematol 10:149, 1973
16. Bergsagel D E, Cowan D H, Hasselback R: Plasma cell myeloma: Response of melphalan-resistant patients to high-dose intermittent cyclophosphamide. Can Med Assoc J 107:851, 1972
17. Alexanian R, Haut A, Khan A U, et al: Treatment for multiple myeloma: Combination chemotherapy with different melphalan dose regimens. JAMA 208:1680, 1969
18. Eastern Cooperative Oncology Group Study No. 4472 (unpublished data)
19. Humphrey R L, Krols L K, Braine H G, et al: High dose cytoxan therapy of poor risk myeloma and Waldenstrom's macroglobulinemia. Proc Am Assoc Cancer Res 14:54, 1973
20. Cohen H J: Hexamethylmelamine: A new agent effective in the treatment of refractory multiple myeloma. Blood 50:187 (abstr), 1977
21. Alberts D S, Durie B M, Salmon S E: Doxorubicin/BCNU chemotherapy for multiple myelomas in relapse. Lancet 1:926, 1976
22. Jaffe J, Raich P C: Hemibody radiation in multiple myeloma (in press)
23. Alexanian R: Prognostic factors in multiple myeloma. Arch Intern Med 135:147, 1975
24. Hokanson J A, Brown B W, Thompson J R, et al: Tumor growth patterns in multiple myeloma. Cancer 39:1077, 1977

H.H. FUDENBERG
G. VIRELLA

34

Waldenstrom's Macroglobulinemia: An Interpretative Review

Since our previous review on Waldenstrom's macroglobulinemia (W.M.) was published in the second volume of Cancer Chemotherapy,[1] progress has been accomplished in three main areas: (1) clinical and laboratorial diagnosis, (2) nature of the paraproteins and (3) new therapeutic approaches. This review will concentrate in these areas.

The diagnostic hallmark of W.M. is the presence of an IgM monoclonal protein in serum. IgM is a pentameric molecule made up of five subunits, each of them with two light and two heavy chains. The electrophoretic mobility of IgM is fast gamma to slow beta and as a consequence of their large molecular size the sedimentation rate is fast at 19 Svedberg units. As such, IgM is classified as a macroglobulin, but IgM is not the only macroglobulin in human serum. As shown in Figure 34-1, there are two large groups of fast-sedimenting serum proteins in human serum: the IgM immunoglobulin and a protein of lower isoelectric point, moving into the alpha-2 region—the alpha-2 macroglobulin (alpha-2M). This last protein has no direct relationship with the immune system; its main function appears to be the binding of proteases.[2] It can be considerably raised, however, in liver diseases,[3] particularly in infancy, and this fact led often to erroneous diagnosis of W.M. before more specific methods for the identification of IgM were introduced in the clinical routine.[4]

Conventional electrophoresis on paper or cellulose acetate will easily demonstrate the enormous increase of IgM that is usually associated with W.M. as illustrated in Figure 34-2. This type of electrophoresis allows differentiation between a gammopathy and a secondary increase of alpha-2 macroglobulin, but will not allow the precise identification of an IgM paraprotein. The combination of conventional electrophoresis and ultracentrifugation was used in the 1940s and 1950s by Waldenstrom and many others, but the need to have access to an analytical ultracentrifuge held back the investigation of this disease. Molecular sieving electrophoresis, in starch gel[1] or acrylamide gel[5] provided easier ways to differentiate IgM paraproteins on the basis of size and shape, and presently this approach has been perfected with the use of sodium dodecyl sulphate-polyacrylamide gel electrophoresis, where the introduction of an anionic

This is publication no. 186 from the Department of Basic and Clinical Immunology and Microbiology, Medical University of South Carolina, Charleston, South Carolina. Research supported in part by American Cancer Society Grant IM-161.

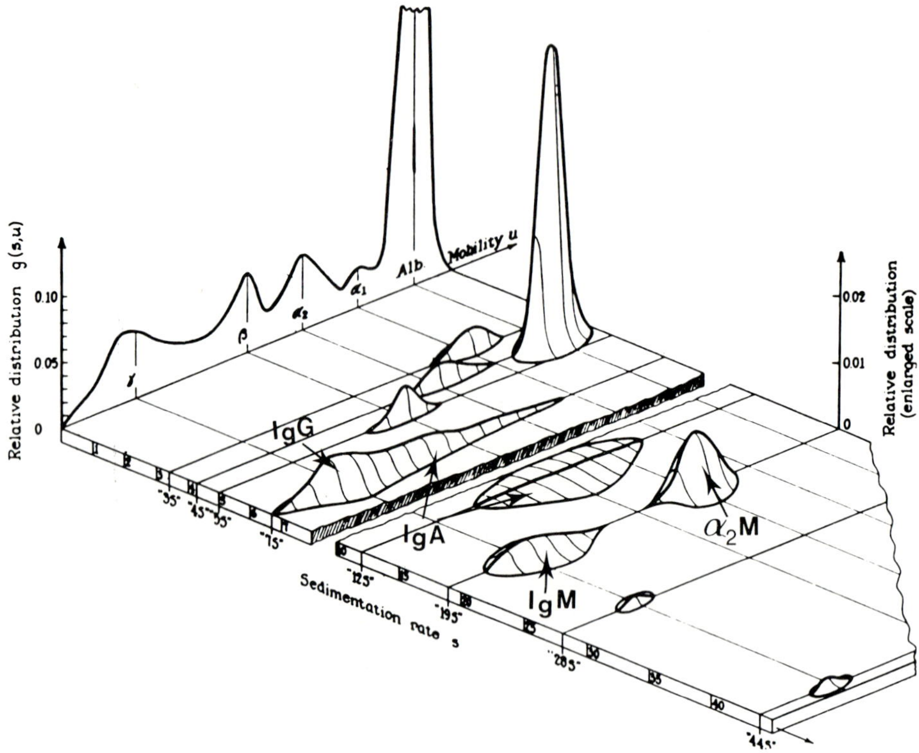

FIG. 34-1. Correlation between the electrophoretic mobility and the sedimentation rate in the ultracentrifuge of the major human serum proteins. Modified from Wallenius G, Trautman R, Kunkel H G, Frankel E C: Ultracentrifugal studies of major non-lipidic electrophoretic components of normal human serum. J Biol Chem 225:253, 1957 (with permission).

detergent in the buffers results in a separation primarily dependent on molecular size.[6] A typical separation of an IgM paraprotein is illustrated in Figure 34-3. IgG monoclonal proteins will easily penetrate the gel and IgA paraproteins (one example is also shown in Fig. 34-3) are often polydisperse, showing several fractions of different molecular sizes.[7]

The best diagnostic test for W.M., however, is the immunoelectrophoretic identification of a monoclonal IgM paraprotein. Typical aspects can even be obtained using polyvalent antisera directed to whole serum proteins, as shown in Figure 34-4. The pathological sera shows a thickened, curved IgM arc, in contrast with the faint, almost straight IgM precipitin revealed in the normal serum used as control. To fulfill the strict criteria for the identification of monoclonal components, it has to be proved that the IgM paraprotein contains one single type of light chains, either kappa or lambda. This is accomplished with the use of monospecific antisera as illustrated in Figure 34-5. Due to several factors—the poor diffusibility of IgM and the frequently normal concentrations of IgG being the principal—the identification of the light chain type of an IgM monoclonal component is sometimes difficult, however. The difficulties can be surmounted by reducing and alkylating the paraprotein, thus converting it into monomeric subunits of identical immunochemical constitution and higher diffusibility. The reduction can be carried out in a whole serum sample, using a mild reducing agent[8] when the IgM concentration is relatively high, or in a partially purified IgM fraction, obtained by euglobulin precipitation or by gel filtration, when the concentration of paraprotein is relatively low.

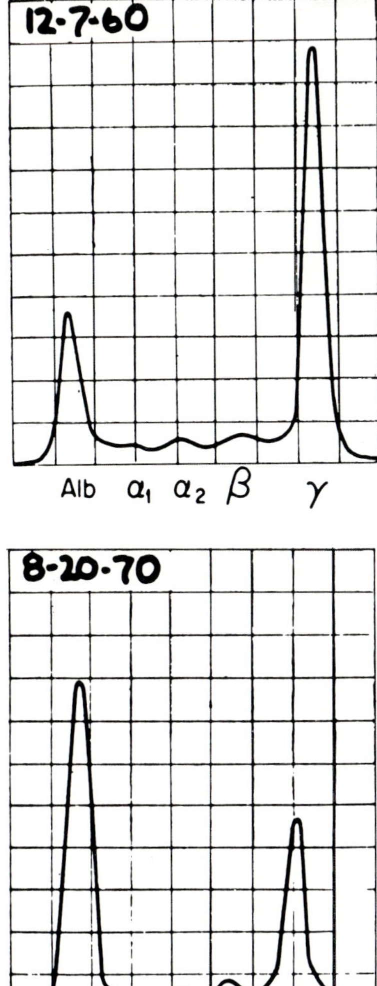

FIG. 34-2. Electrophoretic separation of the serum proteins of a patient with W.M. at the time of diagnosis (top) and after ten years of plasmapheresis therapy (bottom).

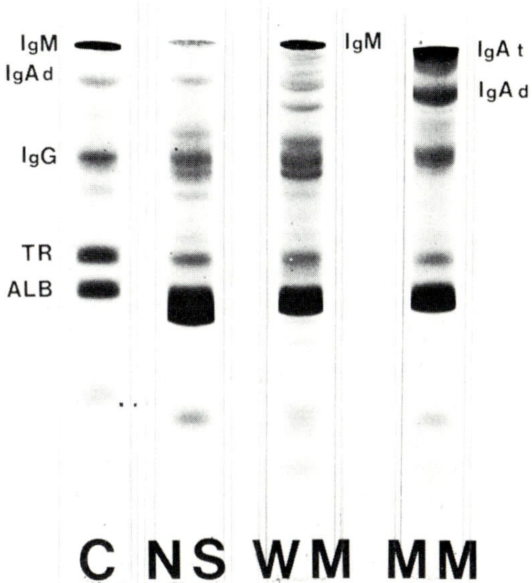

FIG. 34-3. Sodium dodecyl sulfate-polyacrylamide gel electrophoresis of the serum proteins from a patient with Waldenstrom's macroglobulinemia (W.M.) and IgA multiple myeloma (M.M.). Two reference gels were run: in one (C) a mixture of purified control proteins was separated, including IgM, dimeric IgA (IgAd), IgG, transferrin (TR), and serum albumin (ALB); in the second, normal serum (NS). The position of the IgM is indicated in the macroglobulinemic serum, and the position of the IgA polymers is shown in multiple myeloma sample.

The differential diagnosis between multiple myeloma (M.M.) and W.M. is clinically very important, since the evolution, prognosis and therapy of these two diseases is quite different. Although the discussion about the existence of IgM myeloma has not yet been settled one way or another, for practical purposes it can be stated that the finding of an IgM monoclonal protein in serum is compatible with the diagnosis of W.M., while the finding of any other type of monoclonal protein (IgG, IgA, IgD, etc.) is not. Presently, studies of the molecular size of a paraprotein are not too relevant from the diagnostic point of view, but still have a place in the laboratory investigation of patients with macroglobulinemia, since it has been shown that in many patients monomeric IgM molecules are present in the circulation.[9,10] The ratio of monomers to polymers varies considerably from patient to patient, and the study of a possible correlation between the amount of monomers in a given IgM paraprotein and the clinical features of the case is currently under progress in our laboratory.

The hematological study of the abnormal cells infiltrating the bone marrow is of certain value in establishing the diagnosis of W.M. In a large majority of cases of W.M. (an approx-

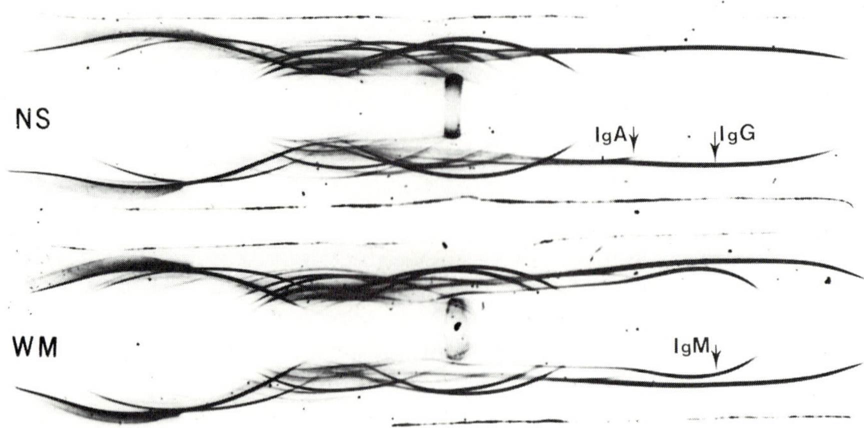

FIG. 34-4. Immunoelectrophoretic study of normal human serum (NS) and the serum from a W.M. patient, using anti-whole human serum. The precipitation arcs corresponding to IgG and IgA are pointed out in the normal serum separation; IgM, present in relatively low amounts, produces a precipitin line too faint to be reproduced. In contrast, a thick and abnormally shaped IgM arc is evident in the W.M. sample; notice that in this sample the amounts of IgG and IgA appear to be within normal limits.

imate figure, based on our experience, can be 85 per cent), the morphology of the cells infiltrating the bone marrow is typical. It is not rare, however, to obtain morphologic pictures in the study of the bone marrow of patients with clinically typical W.M. that are indistinguishable from the aspects seen in myelomatosis (Fig. 34-6). As Waldenstrom pointed out in his pioneer work,[11] one of the features that allows the identification of a bone marrow smear, as corresponding to macroglobuinemia, is the presence of tissue mast cells, but the frequency of this finding is not high enough to be universally helpful. One additional feature that can help in distinguishing the abnormal lympho-plasmocytoid cells of W.M. from similar cells occurring in M.M. is the richness in carbohydrates of the IgM paraproteins (usually about 10 per cent of their weight), which will result in the strong staining of the cytoplasm of IgM-containing cells with the PAS reaction. Since IgA paraproteins are rich in carbohydrate, however, this criterion is also misleading. In summary, morphology cannot be considered as a safe criterion for the differential diagnosis of W.M.

The clinical symptoms of W.M. are not too specific. Bone pain, osteolytic lesions and pathological fractures are almost never seen, in contrast with M.M. where these are frequent symptoms, but, for example, recurrent infections are frequent in both diseases (more so in M.M.). In W.M. the levels of the other immunoglobulins (IgG and IgA) are usually not as depressed as, for example, are the IgM and IgA in a case of IgG myeloma, and the pathogenesis of the immune depression is unclear. Studies on the balance of B-cell activity and the suppressor effect of T cells, that seem to point to a role of these last cells in the pathogenesis of the immunedepression of multiple myelomatosis,[12] have not been carried out in W.M. Hepatomegaly and lymphadenopathy are frequent in W.M., but practically never seen in M.M. Anemia is common in both situations, but thrombocytopenia is much less common in W.M.

Special mention has to be made to the symptomatology of hyperviscosity that is particularly frequent in macroglobulinemia patients. This symptomatology can be very different from patient to patient and may affect several organs and systems in any given patient. Frequent presenting complaints include mucosal bleeding, disturbances in visual acuity or hearing capacity and severe headaches. In rare instances, the patient may present in a deep coma or in severe renal insufficiency. The most frequent symptom, weakness, is very often underrated by the patients; they only realize how weak they felt, after the hyperviscosity syndrome has been adequately treated.

The key to the interpretation of these symptoms and their proper management is the determination of serum viscosity. This can be accomplished with very sophisticated instrumentation that will determine absolute viscosities in centipoises measured at different shear rates, but for most clinical purposes it is sufficient to measure the viscosity of serum relative to distilled water using any of a variety of capillary viscometers that are commercially available. The Hess viscometer, shown in Figure 34-7, is very simple and provides results comparable to those obtained with the Ostwald viscometer, but in a much shorter time. It is constituted by two glass capillaries connected to a U tube. Pressure or suction can be applied simultaneously to both branches of the U tube, the capillary segments being at each end of the two arms of the U. If water is fed into both capillaries and through suction we aspirate water from the zero to the one mark of either of the capillaries and through suction, water will also go from the zero to the one mark in the other one. When serum is placed in one of the capillaries, however, and suction is applied to both branches of the U tube, so that serum moves from the zero to the one mark, the water placed in the other capillary will flow to a distance proportional to the viscosity in serum, and a direct reading on a graduated scale on the water branch will give the relative viscosity of serum. For normal serum or plasma, values between 1.4 and 1.8 are determined. In macroglobulinemia, the relative viscosity can reach values higher than 20.

A study of the relationship between protein concentration and serum relative viscosity in patients with myeloma and macroglobulinemia shows that in the former the increase of viscosity with protein concentration is relatively slow, while in macroglobulinemia, viscosity rises dramatically at high protein concentrations (Fig. 34-8). A comparison between the excess of plasma volume calculated from a macroglobulinemia patient in relation

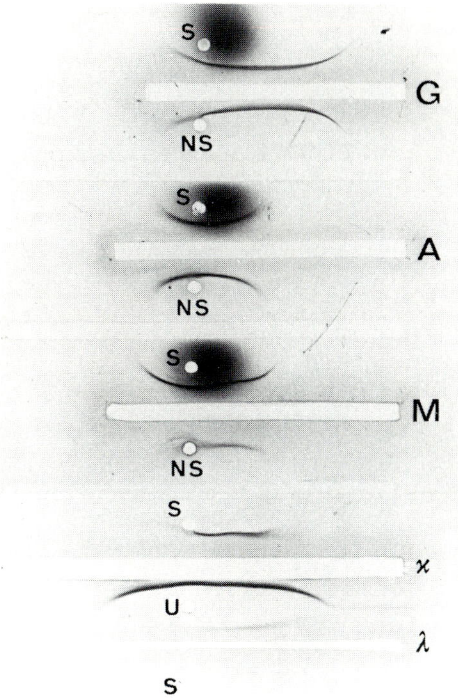

FIG. 34-5. Immunoelectrophoretic characterization of an IgM paraprotein, using monospecific antisera. Serum from the W.M. patient (S) and from a normal control (NS) were studied with antisera specific for IgG (G), IgA (A), and IgM (M); a diluted serum sample, and a concentrated urine sample (U) from the patient were studied with antisera specific for kappa (κ) and lambda (λ) chains. Notice the precipitation of protein next to the well in the patient's serum, the abnormally shaped precipitin arcs obtained with the patient's serum with anti-IgM and anti-kappa, and the large amount of kappa chains in the urine.

to his body mass and relative serum viscosity will show almost a straight line (Fig. 34-9).[13] The exponential increase of viscosity with increasing IgM concentrations is not identical for every IgM paraprotein, as is shown in Figure 34-10. Molecular parameters, such as the degree of symmetry are reflected in the intrinsic viscosity determined by each particular protein.

It must be stressed that although the hyperviscosity syndrome is a very frequent feature in W.M., it can also occur in patients with myeloma, such as the rare M.M. cases with very large amounts of IgG paraproteins with

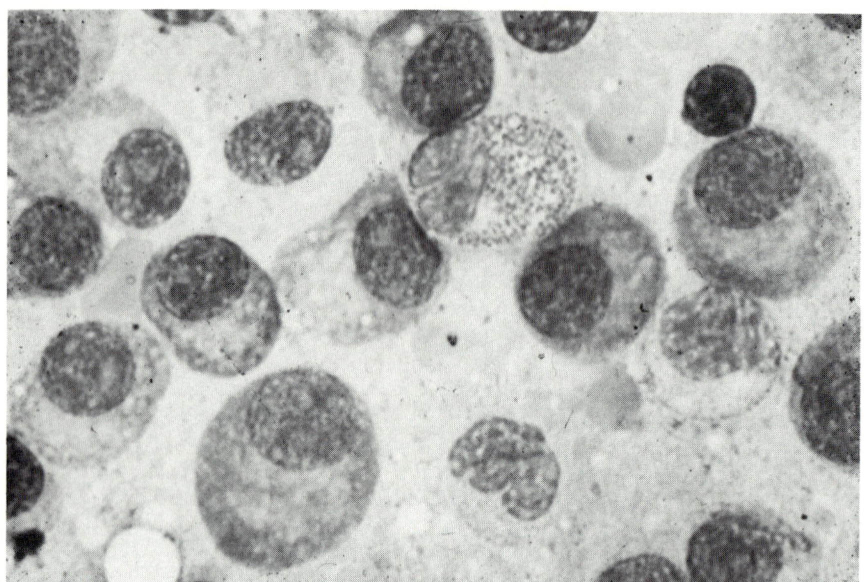

FIG. 34-6. Bone marrow from a patient with W.M. indistinguishable from the usual aspects found in patients with M.M.

tendency to aggregate[15] with abnormally high intrinsic viscosities,[16] or, more frequently, in patients with IgA myeloma with large amounts of polymeric molecules in their serum.[7] Given the much larger frequency of multiple myeloma, in spite of the rarity of the hyperviscosity syndrome in this situation, about half the cases of this syndrome that are seen in large hospitals are associated with multiple myeloma.

The way in which serum hyperviscosity determines the clinical symptoms is very diverse. On one hand, the patients are pumping as much as a 70 to 80 per cent of excess plasma over what should correspond to their body surface.[13] This is probably the cause for the symptoms of weakness and fatigue, and also for cardiac congestive failure, although the latter is a very rare feature of W.M. Various clotting factors and platelet mechanisms are impaired by the excess of intravascular protein[17] and this, combined with the sluggishness of circulation, result in mucosal and retinal bleeding and, in more severe cases,

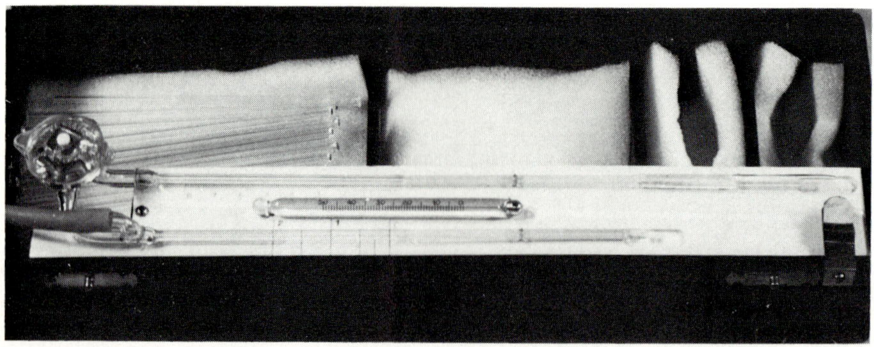

FIG. 34-7. The Hess viscometer. Simultaneous suction is applied to both branches of the U tube; the capillary on the top tube is filled with distilled water; the one on the lower tube is filled with serum.

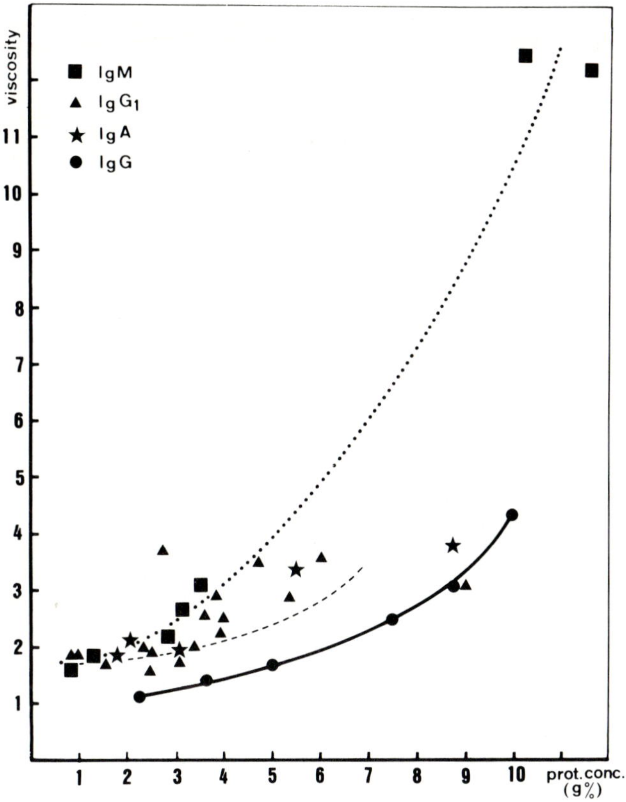

FIG. 34-8. Plot of relative viscosities vs. protein concentration in several sera with IgM, IgGl, and IgA paraproteins, and in six different dilutions of a solution containing normal IgG.

bleeding in the central nervous system that can cause a variety of symptoms. The retinal changes include hemorrhages, exudates and "sausage-shaped" dilation of the retinal veins (Fig. 34-11). From these changes, a total loss of vision may result. In the kidney a combination of factors such as the sluggishness of circulation and the concentration of plasma that tends to occur during glomerular filtration, result in the formation of large deposits of IgM in the glomerular capillaries.[18] These deposits may result in variable degrees of renal insufficiency, which are, however, rarely clinically significant. We have seen one case of macroglobulinemia presenting as nephrotic syndrome where the finding of the macroglobulin was purely accidental, occurring during a routine laboratorial check-up.[19]

Practically all symptoms of hyperviscosity, including the most dramatic ones such as loss of vision, renal insufficiency or loss of consciousness, are reversible if adequate therapy is quickly instituted. The aim of the therapy is to lower the viscosity and the most efficient way to accomplish this is through plasmapheresis. Plasmapheresis is indicated in every symptomatic case, and that relative serum viscosity is always over four. It consists of removing one or two units of patient's blood, returning the red cells to the patient, and discarding or saving the plasma for additional investigations. Plasmapheresis can be done very simply, as illustrated in Figure 34-12, using a double plasmapheresis pack, one of which to receive the red cells to be transfused back, and the other to be used to keep the plasma that is to be collected. Alternatively, a more efficient plasmapheresis can be achieved by using the cell separators used to obtain platelets for patients with acute leu-

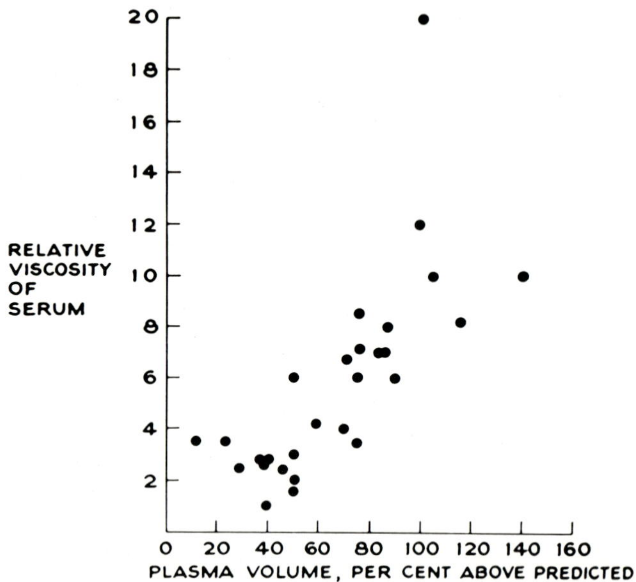

FIG. 34-9. Relationship between relative serum viscosity and plasma volume as measured on 28 occasions in 17 macroglobulinemic patients (r = 0.74). Samples for viscosity measurements obtained on day of blood volume determinations. Directly and indirectly measured plasma volumes included and expressed as per cent deviation from volume predicted for patient according to appropriate standard.

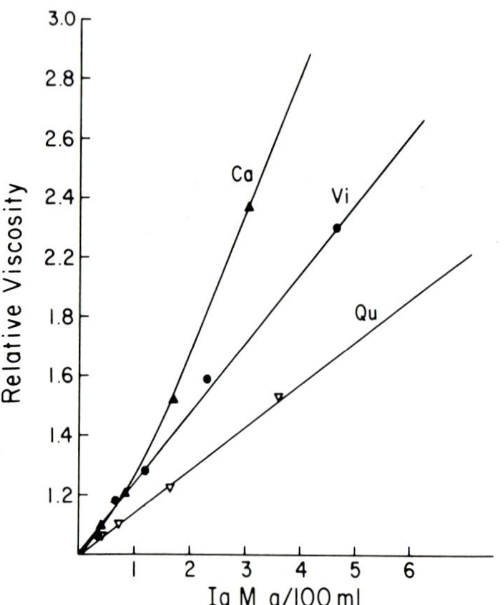

FIG. 34-10 Plot of increase of relative viscosity with increasing quantities of purified IgM proteins. Notice the different slopes for each one of the proteins. From MacKenzie M R, Babcock J: Studies of the hyperviscosity syndrome. II. Macroglobulinemia. J Lab Clin Med 85:227, 1975 (with permission).

kemias. Using these devices, up to 10 units of plasma can be removed daily. Plasmapheresis should have an aim to keep the viscosity under 3.

The monoclonal IgM paraproteins have frequently been found to have antibody activity. One typical example is the cold agglutinin activity associated with IgM kappa proteins[20] that will produce, when present in very large amounts, clinical pictures with features of W.M. coexisting with the cold-induced hemolytic anemia that results directly from the antibody activity of the paraprotein. Monoclonal IgM proteins with rheumatoid factor activity, anticardiolipid activity or antibody activity to bacterial products such as *Klebsiella* polysaccharide, have been identified repeatedly. IgM paraproteins, which are sometimes transient, have also been observed in patients or experimental animals receiving bone marrow transplants,[24,25] in patients with the Wiskott-Aldrich syndrome[26] and in children with acute infections.[27] All these observations, associated with the relatively benign course of many cases of W.M., raise the possibility that this is not a true malignancy of

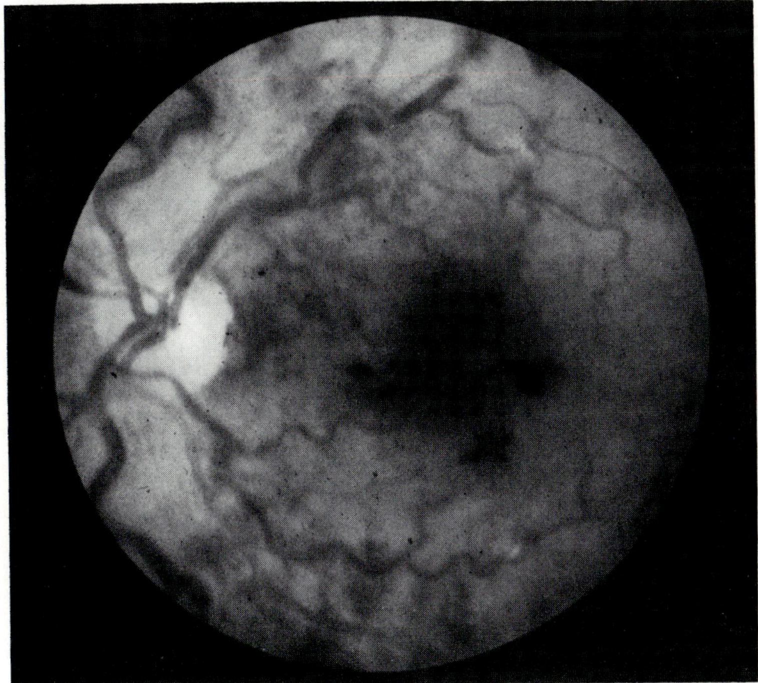

FIG. 34-11. Fundoscopic aspect in a patient with serum hyperviscosity syndrome secondary to W.M.

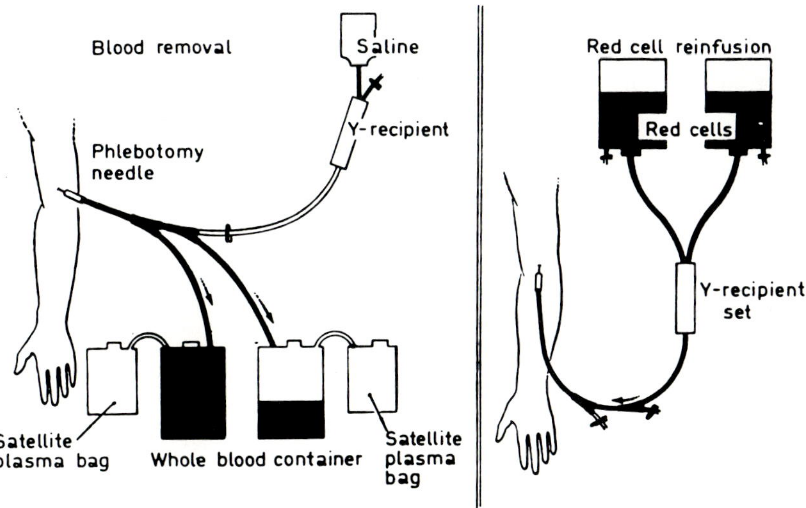

FIG. 34-12. Diagrammatic presentation of the principle and equipment used for conventional plasmapheresis. Venous blood is collected in plastic bags, the overlying plasma is squeezed into satellite bags, which are removed, and the packed cells are reinfused into the patient through the original phlebotomy needle. Its patency is maintained by a saline infusion. From Solomon A, Fahey J L: Plasmapheresis therapy in macroglobulinemia. Ann Intern Med 58:789–800, 1963 (with permission).

immunoglobulin-producing cells, such as multiple myeloma, but rather a disease of immunological aberration. If so, the obvious implication is that therapy other than with cytotoxic drugs should be used; it appears that control of serum viscosity is the only therapeutic measure required in most cases. A program to assess the evolution of patients treated as conservatively as possible was initiated in 1960 and a total of 12 patients have been included in it. In any patient admitted to the program, we started by lowering the serum viscosity to 3 by energic plasmapheresis. This may take as long as 5 days. From then on, the patients would be maintained at this level of viscosity by periodic plasmapheresis when they lived close enough to a center where this could be performed, or by the administration of very low dosages of alkylating agents when repeated plasmapheresis was not feasible. In this way we have kept 11 of the 12 patients alive for periods ranging from 5 to 12 years. Similar results have been subsequently obtained by Hobbs.[28]

The avoidance of alkylating agents in the therapy of macroglobulinemia is a very important point. On one hand, these patients develop aplastic anemia very easily, even at low dosages of chlorambucil. On the other hand, there is always the possibility that chemotherapeutic agents, by their mutagenic capacity, might lead to secondary neoplasia. This has been noted by us and others[29,30] in cases of multiple myeloma treated with alkylating agents, where a high incidence of subsequent acute leukemia, particularly of the monocytic type, has been noted. Similar leukemic evolutions have been reported with W.M.,[30,31] and we have observed an apparent increase in the incidence of silent tumors.[32] A parallel seems possible with polycythemia, where a higher incidence of silent tumors, particularly of the colon, might not be related to the disease, but to therapy with chlorambucil.

If we assume that IgM paraproteins in macroglobulinemic patients do not result from the inordinate activity of a malignantly transformed clone, but rather from the exaggerated activity of a nonmalignant clone of cells due to the loss of normal control mechanisms, it is possible to pinpoint a T-cell deficiency as the indirect cause of macroglobulinemia. An intact T-cell system appears to be essential, as shown by some human observations in our laboratory[32] and from animal experiments carried out by other authors,[33,34] for the switch from IgM to IgG production. If the T-cell system is abnormal, IgM production will persist after the initial challenge instead of being replaced by IgG. This raises the possibility that W.M. may be a consequence of the overstimulation of an IgM-producing clone that will not be switched to IgG production or suppressed after the challenge is over due to a selective T-cell deficiency. To test this possibility, experimental double-blind trials have been initiated by us and by Silverman et al,[35] consisting of the administration of transfer factor to macroglobulinemia patients in the hope that this will result in the activation of the T cells that have failed to promote the switch-off of the overactive clone. Preliminary results are consistent with this hypothesis.

References

1. Fudenberg H H: Waldenstrom's macroglobulinemia. In Brodsky I, Kahn S B, Moyer J H (eds): Cancer Chemotherapy II, The Twenty-second Hahnemann Symposium. New York, Grune & Stratton, 1972
2. Wallenius G, Trautman R, Kunkel H G, Franklin E C: Ultracentrifugal studies of major non-lipidic electrophoretic components of normal human serum. J Biol Chem 225:253, 1957
3. Laurell C B, Jeppsson J O: Protease inhibitors in plasma, in Putnam F W (ed): The Plasma Proteins. New York, Academic Press, 1975
4. Fessel W J: Clinical analysis of 142 cases with high molecular weight serum proteins. Acta Med Scand 173 (suppl 391):1, 1962
5. Zingale S B, Mattioli C A, Bohner H D, Bueno M P: Disc electrophoresis study of serum proteins from patients with multiple myeloma and macroglobulinemia. Blood 22:152, 1963
6. Weber K, Osborn M: The reliability of molecular weight determinations by dodecyl sulfate-polyacrylamide gel electrophoresis. J Biol Chem 244:4406, 1969
7. Virella G, Preto R V, Graca F: Polymerized

monoclonal IgA in two patients with myelomatosis and hyperviscosity syndrome. Br J Haematol 30:479, 1975

8. Virella G, Lopes-Virella M F: Effects of therapeutically useful thiols (DL-penicillamine and alpha-mercaptopropionylglycine) on immunoglobulins. Clin Exp Immunol 7:85, 1970
9. Solomon A, Kunkel H G: A "monoclonal" type, low molecular weight protein related to gamma M-macroglobulins. Amer J Med 42:958, 1967
10. Bush S T, Swedlund H A, Gleich G J: Low molecular weight IgM in human sera. J Lab Clin Med 73:194, 1969
11. Waldenstrom J: Macroglobulinemia. Acta Haematol 20:33, 1958
12. Broder S, Humphrey R, Durm M, et al: Impaired synthesis of polyclonal (non-paraprotein) immunoglobulins by circulating lymphocytes from patients with multiple myeloma. Role of suppressor cells. N Engl J Med 293:887, 1975
13. MacKenzie M R, Brown E, Fudenberg H H, Goodenday L: Waldenstrom's macroglobulinemia: Correlations between expanded plasma volume and increased serum viscosity. Blood 35:394, 1970
14. MacKenzie M R, Babcock J: Studies of the hyperviscosity syndrome. II. Macroglobulinemia. J Lab Clin Med 85:227, 1975
15. Capra J D, Kunkel H G: Aggregation of gamma G3 proteins: Relevance to the hyperviscosity syndrome. J Clin Invest 49:610, 1970
16. MacKenzie M R, Fudenberg H H, O'Reilly R A: The hyperviscosity syndrome. I. In IgG myeloma. The role of protein concentration and molecular shape. J Clin Invest 49:15, 1970
17. Perkins H A, MacKenzie M R, Fudenberg H H: Hemostatic defects in dysproteinemias. Blood 35:695, 1970
18. Morel-Maroger L, Basch A, Danon F, et al: Pathology of the kidney in Waldenstrom's macroglobulinemia. N Engl J Med 283:123, 1970
19. Virella G: Unpublished observation
20. Harboe M: Cold auto-agglutinins. Vox Sang 20:289, 1971
21. Kritzman J, Kunkel H G, McCarthy J, Mellors R C: Studies of a Waldenstrom-type macroglobulin with rheumatoid factor properties. J Lab Clin Med 57:905, 1961
22. Eriksen J, Harboe M, Deverill J: A monoclonal IgM with specific antibody reactivity against *Klebsiella* sero-types 12 and 13. Acta Path Microbiol Scand 83:106, 1975
23. Seligmann M, Brouet J C: Antibody activity of human myeloma globulins. Semin Hematol 10:163, 1973
24. Van der Berg P, Radl J, Lowenberg B, Swart A C W: Homogeneous antibodies in lethally irradiated and autologous bone marrow reconstituted Rhesus monkeys. Clin Exp Immunol 23:355, 1976
25. Radl J, Van der Berg P: Transitory appearance of homogeneous immunoglobulins—"paraproteins"—in children with severe combined immunodeficiency before and after transplantation treatment. Prot Biol Fluids 20:263, 1973
26. Radl J, Dooren L J, Morell A, et al: Immunoglobulins and transitory paraproteins in sera of patients with the Wiskott-Aldrich syndrome: A follow-up study. Clin Exp Immunol 25:256, 1976
27. Tichý M, Hrncir Z, Urbánková J: Transient IgM-lambda paraprotein in a 15-month-old child. Clin Chim Acta 70:201, 1976
28. Hobbs J R: Personal communication
29. Rosner F, Grünwald H: Multiple myeloma terminating in acute leukemia. Report of 12 cases and review of the literature. Amer J Med 57:927, 1974
30. Kyle R A, Pierre R V, Bayrd E D: Multiple myeloma and acute leukemia associated with alkylating agents. Arch Intern Med 135:185, 1975
31. Petersen H S: Erythroleukemia in a melphalan-treated patient with primary macroglobulinemia. Scand J Haematol 10:5, 1973
32. Fudenberg H H: Unpublished observations
33. Davie J M, Paul W E: Role of T lymphocytes in the humoral immune responses. I. Proliferation of B lymphocytes in thymus-deprived mice. J Immunol 113:1438, 1974
34. van Muiswinkel W B, Radl J, Van der Wal D J: The regulatory influence of the thymus-dependent immune system on the heterogeneity of immunoglobulins in irradiated and reconstituted mice. In Feldman M, Globerson A (eds): Immune Reactivity of Lymphocytes. New York, Plenum, 1976
35. Silverman M A, Meltz S, Sorokin C, Glade P R: Effects of transfer factor in Waldenstrom's macroglobulinemia and multiple myeloma. In Asher M S, Gottlieb A A, Kilpatrick C H (eds): Transfer Factor. New York, Academic Press, 1976
36. Solomon A, Fahey J L: Plasmapheresis therapy in macroglobulinemia. Ann Intern Med 58:789–800, 1963

Charles M. Huguley, Jr.

35 Chemotherapy of Chronic Lymphocytic Leukemia

Dameshek first described chronic lymphocytic leukemia (CLL) as "an accumulative disease of immunologically incompetent lymphocytes," an idea now widely accepted.[1] Patients with this disease do, indeed, suffer from a diminished immunologic responsiveness especially in the formation of antibodies and may also have autoimmune diseases. The leukemic cells are nearly always B-lymphocytes.[2] The T-lymphocytes are reduced in percentage but the absolute number is about normal.[3] When the lymphocytosis is reduced by therapy, especially after radiation, the leukemic cells seem to be especially sensitive so that the lymphocytes that respond immunologically may remain in approximately normal numbers.[4] Zimmerman, Godwin and Perry demonstrated two patterns of cell survival in CLL.[5] In those patients without organomegaly, a population of short-lived lymphocytes was demonstrated along with some that remained in the blood for a long time. In patients with high lymphocyte counts and organomegaly it was not possible to demonstrate this small population of short-lived lymphocytes and the lymphocytes present were long-lived with a very small number undergoing mitosis. More recent work has indicated a production of lymphocytes that was above normal.[6] Most of the readily labeled cells were short-lived with a turnover time of 7 to 21 days. Ninety per cent of the blood lymphocytes had a turnover time in excess of 1 year. These data suggest that the leukemic lymphocytes would replenish themselves after therapy much more slowly than would normal hemopoietic cells. Therapy spaced at intervals to permit recovery of the bone marrow would result in a stepwise depletion of leukemic cells. This is an old idea advanced by Osgood and supported, perhaps, by the unusually long survival of his patients.[7] The effectiveness of this titrated, regularly spaced schedule has recently been confirmed with chlorambucil.[8]

Perhaps the most attractive approach to treating a malignancy is to use an agent which has a special predilection for the particular type of cell which has given rise to the malignant clone. Lymphocytes are particularly susceptible to ionizing radiation,[9,10] alkylating agents[11] and adrenal steroids.[12,13] These are the very agents that have been shown empirically to be the most effective yet tested against CLL. Happily, these agents are not cycle-specific and are no more lethal to marrow cells than leukemic cells.[14] B-lymphocytes stimulated into cycle in vivo by sheep red cells are only a little more sensitive to radiation or nitrogen mustard than are the resting B lymphocytes.[15]

Thus, we have a disease characterized by a population of lymphocytes proliferating very slowly yet accumulating by virtue of a particularly long survival and three classes of effective therapeutic agents, each with a special predilection for lymphocytes and each equally or more toxic to resting leukemic lymphocytes than to the normal myeloid cells.

Leukemic cells are present in the blood stream of the patient with CLL in an amount of approximately 10^{11} to 10^{12} cells or 100 to 1000 grams of tumor tissue. The marrow contains many more cells. If the lymph nodes, liver or spleen are involved, this represents a large increment of tumor and a poorer prognosis. Thus, we may have more than 2 kg of tumor cells. The changes which follow the simple removal of lymphocytes from the blood may have important implications for our therapeutic strategy. Amounts of lymphocytes exceeding a kilogram can be removed by leukapheresis with a continuous-flow centrifugal cell separator. This procedure can lead to good control of the disease.[16,17] As cells are removed the involved lymph nodes and organs may shrink. Fortunately, the lymphocytosis may remain at a high level until the lymphoid tissue has shrunk considerably, permitting continuing effective leukapheresis. The administration of antilymphocyte serum will also destroy lymphocytes and reduce lymphocytosis, lymphadenopathy and splenomegaly.[18] Blood can be irradiated as it passes through a grid outside the body and the lymphoid organs will shrink and the blood lymphocytes will be reduced.[19,20] All of these techniques have been shown to be therapeutically effective, if not necessarily practical. There is one common feature: they all destroy or remove lymphocytes without having a general cytotoxic mechanism of action. They demonstrate the exchange of leukemic lymphocytes between different compartments in the body. There are no obvious implications of these findings for the strategy of chemotherapy, but they should perhaps influence our approach to radiotherapy.

Since many patients with CLL pursue a benign course for many years without treatment and since treatment has not been demonstrated to prolong survival, the prevailing wisdom counsels that treatment be deferred until the disease becomes "active" or "progressive."[21,22] Further, there is a feeling that treatment is not very effective in reversing morbidity from the disease once it occurs.[22] The physician may therefore tend to err on the side of undertreatment so as to insure that at least no harm is done.

It is very difficult to assess the efficacy of treatment of CLL. The most important measure of effectiveness is improved survival. It has not been possible to prove on the basis of available data that survival is lengthened by treatment in this disease. Because median survival in this disease is many years, improvement over a short period (3 to 6 months) is often used to evaluate the relative effectiveness of treatment. Many of the manifestations of the disease, and sometimes all of them, are improved or eliminated by treatment in a majority of patients.[23,24,25,26,27,28] This definitely improves the quality of survival and is desirable. It is therefore useful to determine the treatment more likely to produce improvement. There is some data to indicate that such improvement may affect the subsequent survival of the patient.[23,25,26,27]

Whether the end point of a study is survival or short-term improvement, evaluation of published results is very difficult. There are very few studies in which an adequate number of patients were treated in a standardized manner prospectively. The use of concurrent controls has been rare. The great variability in the course of the disease has often been commented upon but there now seems to be a growing belief that this variability is more apparent than real and may be largely due to the stage to which the disease has progressed by the time of diagnosis.[22,29] Differences in the population under study may well account for the reported differences in the effectiveness of agents in uncontrolled studies.[29] Certainly no assessment of the effectiveness of treatment will be accurate until patients in a study are stratified according to a validated and widely accepted method of staging. It is clear that patients who have lymphocytosis only, without palpable disease or hematologic damage, have a much better prognosis than those who have evidence of large tumor masses or those whose marrow is "packed" so that they have anemia and thrombocytopenia.[29] Other prognostic indicators are weakness, fever or poor performance status.[30] While several attempts have been made to utilize such factors in forming a staging system, we do not yet have one that has been based on a thorough statistical analysis of the relative contribution of different manifestations of disease to the ultimate prognosis.

In 1924, Minot and Isaacs reported that despite the immediate improvement brought about by radiation in most patients with CLL, there was no difference in survival between the group of patients treated by radiation and a group, for various reasons, receiving no treatment.[31] The median survival for 80 patients was 3½ years. The End Results Evaluation Program of the National Cancer Institute has been collecting the experience in more than 100 hospitals since 1940. These include all the hospitals in the state of Connecticut, about one-third of those in the state of California, a group of hospitals in Boston and six large university hospitals in various parts of the United States. The 4609 patients with CLL entered between 1940 and 1971 should represent a reasonable basis for assessing the general experience.[32,33,34] There was improvement in survival of patients with chronic lymphocytic leukemia diagnosed in the years since 1955 as compared to those diagnosed in the preceding 15 years in patients less than 65 years of age.[32,33] There has been very little further improvement through 1971, however.[34] The overall median relative survival was less than 3 years. Surely, earlier diagnosis and better supporting care should have exerted a positive effect and might account for improvement noted after 1955. The relative lack of improvement thereafter would certainly seem to indicate that the treatment modalities we have been using have not affected survival. For these several reasons there is little purpose in reviewing large series attempting to compare survival on different therapeutic regimens. The effectiveness of several agents in producing objective improvement will be presented and the possible relation of short-term improvement to longer survival will be discussed.

Radiation Therapy

Radiation therapy is one of the oldest effective methods of treatment of CLL and is also considered by some the current best method. No discussion of treatment of CLL is complete without a mention of radiotherapy. After introduction of radiotherapy early in the century it became standard treatment for CLL until the mid-1940s. Radiation was directed to the spleen, the node-bearing areas, or both, with considerable symptomatic benefit, if no effect on survival.[31,35] Heublein first advocated whole-body or spray irradiation in 1932.[36] Osgood advocated titrated, regularly spaced whole-body radiation that produced long survivals of CLL in his hands until he switched to radiophosphorus, which he felt was interchangeable.[7] More recently, Johnson has revived whole-body radiation and reports obtaining 14 (33 per cent) complete responses and 23 (55 per cent) partial responses in 42 patients for a total response rate of 88 per cent.[25] The complete responders had a greatly improved survival. Others have advised radiation therapy for the control of symptomatic local lymphadenopathy. Splenic radiation has been used for years and has been recently recommended for the relief of painful splenomegaly.[37] It may lead to considerable general improvement. Thymic radiation has been recommended by Spurr as especially successful in producing partial and complete remissions.[26] Splenic radiation and "thymic" radiation are given to ports through which flow large quantities of blood. It may well be that the effect is due, as it is in extracorporeal radiation of blood, to damage to lymphocytes in the blood as they flow through the port during irradiation. Whole-body radiation may be a simple way to irradiate blood while delivering a minimal amount of radiation to normal tissues. Johnson has shown that it is effective and can be administered safely.[25]

Radiophosphorus has been largely discarded for CLL since it is more difficult to manage than chemotherapy and more toxic to platelets.[38,39] The marrow toxicity may be due to the nearly continuous radiation of the normal hemopoietic cells.

Alkylating Agents

The first chemotherapeutic agent used against CLL was nitrogen mustard in 1946[11] Its effectiveness stimulated the trial of other alkylating agents. In general, these agents are effective against CLL. Results reported for those which have had extensive trial and are

TABLE 35-1. *Response Rate of Chronic Lymphocytic Leukemia to Alkylating Agents*

Drug	No of Reports	Total Patients	% Response
Chlorambucil	16	367	61%
Cyclophosphamide	10	142	42%
Mechlorethamine	4	82	39%
Busulfan	4	24	29%
Melphalan	0	0	

still in use are tabulated in Table 35-1, which is modified after Livingston and Carter.[40] Chlorambucil is almost universally used today as standard treatment of CLL. It is usually administered at 0.1 to 0.2 mg/kg daily by mouth. A dose of 12 mg daily will within 2 to 4 weeks produce hematologic toxicity or the beginnings of therapeutic effect. The dose should then be titrated so as to avoid serious depression of the platelets or granulocytes and continued until a maximum therapeutic effect has been obtained. This will usually require 3 to 6 months, although occasionally improvement may continue for a year or longer. Once a plateau of improvement has been reached, treatment may be stopped and the patient observed for evidences of progression at which time treatment can be resumed as required.

In keeping with the concept described above that a good approach to the treatment of CLL would be an intermittent administration of treatment with an intervening period during which normal hemopoietic cells could recover, the Southeastern Cancer Study Group treated 62 patients on intermittent chlorambucil.[8] The drug was administered every 2 weeks at bedtime at a dosage beginning at 15 mg/M² (0.4 mg/kg) and increasing by 4.0 mg/M² (0.1 mg/kg) with each dose until a beginning response or toxicity developed. The dosage was then titrated to produce mild toxicity and continued for at least 6 months. The results are depicted in Table 35-2. This is an effective treatment. It is easy to use and toxicity is minimal. Most of the patients achieved maximal level of response in 6 months, but some required a longer period of time. Since the average dosage on which patients were maintained was over 0.7 mg/kg, it is recommended that the initial dose be 0.8 mg/kg (30 mg/M²). This should lead to a more rapid response. The dosage should be escalated by 0.1 mg/kg (4 mg/M²) every 4 weeks if necessary.

TABLE 35-2. *Response of Chronic Lymphocytic Leukemia to Chlorambucil Every Two Weeks*

		Responses			
	No.	CR	PR	Total	%
No Prior Treatment					
Indolent	8	2	4	6	75%
Active	31	2	17	19	61%
Prior Treatment					
Responsive	14	1	6	7	50%
Resistant	9		2	2	22%
Total	62	5	29	34	55%

Modified from Knospe W H, Loeb V, Huguley C M: Bi-weekly chlorambucil treatment of chronic lymphocytic leukemia. Cancer 33:555, 1974.

Cyclophosphamide is also often used and is certainly worth a trial in patients who are resistant to chlorambucil. Table 35-1 indicates that it is less effective than chlorambucil. A randomized study by Kuang et al obtained six responses in 18 patients (33 per cent) treated with cyclophosphamide and 14 in 21 patients (67 per cent) treated with chlorambucil ($p=0.08$).[41] The usual dose is 2 to 3 mg/kg/day orally or 100 to 200 mg daily. The dosage is titrated as described for chlorambucil.

Melphalan, which is so similar to chlorambucil, rather surprisingly has not been reported to have been tried in CLL.

Busulfan is relatively ineffective and may produce a long-lasting platelet toxicity.[42]

Chlorambucil and cyclophosphamide,

TABLE 35-3. *Response Rates of Miscellaneous Agents*

Drug	No of Reports	Total Patients	% Response
Adrenal corticosteroids	5[40]	100	70%
Vincristine	1[50]	6	0%
Vinblastine	1[51]	10	20%
Leo 1031 (chlorambucil ester of Prednisolone)	2[46,47]	23	39%

when effective, produce a solid improvement in CLL with at least partial improvement in all abnormalities. If properly monitored, serious toxicity can nearly always be avoided.

PREDNISONE

Prednisone or other adrenocortical steroids have been widely used with good effect (Table 35-3). In general, it has been more impressive in the rapidity and degree of response than have the alkylating agents.[43] There appears to be a mobilization of lymphocytes from the lymphoid organs into the blood. The lymphocytosis commonly doubles within about 2 weeks and there is often a rapid shrinking of lymphadenopathy, splenomegaly and hepatomegaly. The lymphocytosis will then recede. The effects have sometimes lasted only a few weeks even when treatment is continued. Others have described long-lasting improvement on maintenance dosage, especially when large doses were used.[44] Ill effects are the cushingoid changes which may be quite severe and an increased susceptibility to infection. Adrenal corticosteroids are particularly useful, indeed mandatory, in hemolytic anemia, usually, but not necessarily Coomb's test positive and in autoimmune thrombocytopenia.

There has been no uniformity in the schedule of treatment with corticosteroids. A conservative regimen has been 40 to 80 mg of prednisone or the equivalent per day until improvement occurred with reduction to about 30 mg daily thereafter until a definite plateau was reached when it was tapered and stopped.[45] Others have used high doses of 50 to 150 mg of prednisone daily until improvement occurred with subsequent maintenance at 100 to 150 mg once or twice a week indefinitely.[44] More recently there has been a tendency to use corticosteroids in courses of 5 to 7 days every 2 to 4 weeks in the treatment of lymphomas and this schedule is sometimes used in CLL in order to avoid some of the undesirable side effects. It is not recommended that corticosteroid treatment be used alone in CLL except under special circumstances, such as advanced disease resistant to other agents or for autoimmune phenomenon in a patient with otherwise stable disease.

OTHER AGENTS

While a number of other agents have been given a clinical trial in CLL, none of them have demonstrated a response rate as high as chlorambucil and none have received extensive use (Table 35-2). Recently a new agent, Leo 1031, a chlorambucil ester of prednisolone, has been reported to produce a good response and minimal toxicity.[46,47]

COMBINATION CHEMOTHERAPY

Since both chlorambucil and prednisone are so effective as single agents and since a full dose of each can be given without additive toxicity it is only natural to use them in combination. Indeed, this has been done for years in advanced cases though seldom as an initial therapy. Han, Ezdinli and associates treated 26 patients with chlorambucil 2 to 4 mg daily.[24] Eleven of these patients received chlorambucil alone and 15 received in addition prednisone 30 mg daily for 6 weeks. Three complete and 10 partial remissions for a total response of 87 per cent were produced by the combination whereas only one complete and four partial remissions (46 per cent) followed chlorambucil alone (p=.05).

The Acute Leukemia Group B has compared prednisone alone to prednisone plus daily chlorambucil and prednisone plus monthly chlorambucil in 92 patients with Stage III or IV disease.[27] All patients received prednisone 0.8 mg/kg daily for 6 weeks and then for 7 days each month. Patients were randomized to receive no chlorambucil, chlorambucil 0.08 mg/kg daily or 0.4 mg/kg of chlorambucil once a month. The monthly dosage of chlorambucil was escalated as tolerated to dosages as high as 2.0 mg/kg. The response rates were 11 per cent for prednisone alone, 26 per cent for the daily chlorambucil and 42 per cent for the monthly chlorambucil. No complete remissions occurred after prednisone alone but 10 per cent were obtained in patients on the chlorambucil regimens.

The Southeastern Cancer Study Group administered prednisone at a dosage of 80 mg daily for 5 days and chlorambucil at a dosage of 30 mg/M^2 (0.8 mg/kg) once.[28] Courses were repeated every 2 weeks for 12 courses. Chlorambucil was adjusted to tolerance. Of 46 previously untreated patients there were 37 (80 per cent) responses including 10 (22 per cent) complete remissions. Ten of the responders were continued for an additional 12 courses and two partial remissions improved to complete remission status. Toxicity was minimal.

The differences among results from these three studies are due, at least in part, to the inclusion of previously treated patients in two studies, to the inclusion of less severely affected patients in two of them and to differences in criteria of response. Nevertheless, they clearly demonstrate that the combination of prednisone and chlorambucil is superior to either drug alone. The intermittent administration of chlorambucil appears to be as effective, more convenient and less toxic than the daily regimen.

The combination of cyclophosphamide and cytosine arabinoside has been given in a dose of 37.5 mg/M^2 of each drug intravenously every 12 hours for 4 days.[48] Courses were repeated every 21 days. Four of 8 patients achieved a complete remission and an additional patient experienced a partial remission.

The Southeastern Cancer Study Group attempted to consolidate responses obtained with chlorambucil and prednisone by means of cyclophosphamide and cytosine arabinoside.[28] It was thought that in those patients with CLL whose tumor cell burden had been strikingly reduced by induction therapy, the growth fraction of the remaining tumor cells might be increased. They might then be more susceptible to the action of cycle-active agents. Cyclophosphamide was given by mouth and cytosine arabinoside subcutaneously to permit home administration. The dosages and schedule were as cited above. The regimen was very toxic, even when the doses were reduced by one-third. Those patients randomized to receive this schedule for 24 weeks did not do as well as those patients who continued on chlorambucil and prednisone for the same period.

Combined Modality Treatment

The other logical combination of therapies is to combine prednisone with whole-body radiation therapy. This combination is in the process of receiving a trial by the Eastern Cooperative Oncology Group.

Discussion

It has been repeatedly emphasized that treatment has not altered survival. Recent studies indicate that this is not necessarily the case. A review of the literature in 1969 uncovered only 29 patients who had achieved a complete remission defined as absence of symptoms, normal physical findings, normal blood counts including differential and less than 30 per cent lymphocytes in the aspirated marrow.[23] The median survival of these patients, only three of whom had indolent disease, was in excess of 117 months, much better than would have been expected from the general experience. Since then there have been five reports in which an appreciable number of complete remissions were obtained in prospective studies.[24,25,26,27,28] Again the survival of those who achieved a complete remission was much better than that of those who did not and much better than indicated by past experience. Additional studies will be necessary to establish whether our current methods of therapy, which are giving larger numbers of complete remission, will indeed lengthen the survival time. Past treatment may have increased the survival time of that minority of patients who achieved complete or good partial remissions. This might have been masked by our reliance on median survival times. It is theoretically possible for a treatment to produce a cure in 49 per cent of patients and yet not alter the median survival time.

Supportive Therapy

Androgens, such as fluoxymesterone, 10 mg t.i.d. orally, may be effective for nonhemolytic anemia not improved by antileukemia therapy.[49] A trial of at least 3 months is necessary. Adrenal steroids are usually successful in the treatment of hemolytic anemia. The direct Coomb's test is usually positive in hemolysis, but not always, and steroid therapy may be effective even when it is negative. Autoimmune thrombocytopenia may occur and it may respond to steroids.

Splenectomy is recommended for painful splenomegaly.[37] It may lead to a remission, especially if there is evidence of hypersplenism.

Local radiation therapy will be necessary for symptomatic and chemotherapy-resistant lymphadenopathy or for painful bone lesions.[21]

Present Recommendations

Patients in whom the diagnosis of chronic lymphocytic leukemia has been made should have a thorough evaluation of hematological and immunological status. Unless there are indications for immediate treatment they should be observed. Treatment would not begin unless one or more of the following were present:

1. Constitutional symptoms or signs not otherwise explained such as weight loss of more than 10 per cent of body weight within 6 months, fever of more than 100° lasting more than 2 weeks or extreme fatigue.
2. Anemia
3. Thrombocytopenia
4. Any involvement of organs other than lymph nodes, spleen, marrow or liver.
5. Progressive or painful enlargement of lymph nodes or of spleen.

Chlorambucil is given in an initial dose of 30 mg/M^2 (0.8 mg/kg) orally at bedtime once every 2 weeks. Prednisone is given 80 mg orally once a day for 5 days and repeated with every dose of chlorambucil. The dose of chlorambucil is escalated by 4 mg/M^2 (0.1 mg/kg) every 4 weeks until response begins or toxicity develops. The dose is then titrated to produce mild thrombocytopenia or neutropenia. It is important that treatment be given intensively and persistently in an attempt to achieve a complete remission.

If the disease progresses despite treatment to the point of toxicity, or if there is no improvement after 6 months of treatment, whole-body radiation should be considered.

References

1. Dameshek W: Chronic lymphocytic leukemia—An accumulative disease of immunologically incompetent lymphocytes. Blood 24:566, 1967
2. Preud'homme J L, Seligmann M: Surface bound immunoglobulins as a cell marker in human lymphoproliferative diseases. Blood 40:777, 1972
3. Rowlands D T, Daniele R P, Nowell P C, et al: Characterization of lymphocyte subpopulations in chronic lymphocytic leukemia. Cancer 34:1962, 1974
4. Blomgren H, Jondal M., Johansson B: In vivo and in vitro selection of mitogen responsive lymphocytes in patients with chronic lymphocytic leukemia. Cancer Ther Abst 17:424, 1976
5. Zimmerman R S, Goodwin H A, Perry S: Studies of leukocyte kinetics in chronic lymphocytic leukemia. Blood 31:277, 1968
6. Theml H, Trepel F, Schick P, et al: Kinetics

of lymphocytes in chronic lymphocytic leukemia: Studies using continuous H-thymidine infusion in two patients. Blood 42:623, 1973

7. Osgood E E, Seaman A J: Treatment of chronic leukemias: Results of therapy of 163 patients by titrated regularly spaced total body radioactive phosphorus or roentgen irradiation. JAMA 150:1372, 1952
8. Knospe W H, Loeb V, Huguley C M: Biweekly chlorambucil treatment of chronic lymphocytic leukemia. Cancer 33:555, 1974
9. Hulse E V: Lymphocyte depletion of the blood and bone marrow of the irradiated rat: A quantitative study. Br J Haemat 5:278, 1959
10. Schrek R, Leithold S L, Friedman I A, et al: Clinical evaluation of an in vitro test for radiosensitivity of leukemic lymphocytes. Blood 20:432, 1962
11. Jacobson L O, Spurr C L, Barron E S G, et al: Nitrogen mustard therapy: Studies on the effect of methyl-bis (betachloroethyl) amine hydrochloride on neoplastic diseases and allied disorders of the hemopoietic system. JAMA 132:263, 1946
12. Dougherty T F, White A: Influence of hormones on lymphoid tissue structure and function, the role of pituitary adrenotrophic hormones in the regulation of the lymphocytes and other cellular elements of the blood. Endocrinology 35:1, 1944
13. Pearson O H, Eliel L P, Rawson R W, et al: Use of pituitary adrenocorticotropic hormones (ACTH) and cortisone in lymphomas and leukemias. JAMA 144:1349, 1950
14. Bruce W R, Meeker B E, Valeriote F A: Comparison of the sensitivity of normal hematopoietic and transplanted lymphoma colony-forming cells to chemotherapeutic agents administered in vivo. J Natl Cancer Inst 37:233, 1966
15. Lin H: Differential lethal effect of cytotoxic agents on proliferating and nonproliferating lymphoid cells. Cancer Res 33:1716, 1973
16. Curtis J E, Hersh E M, Freireich E J: Leukapheresis therapy of chronic lymphocytic leukemia. Blood 39:163, 1972
17. Fortuny I E, Hadlock D C, Kennedy B J, et al: The role of continuous flow centrifuge leukapheresis in the management of chronic lymphocytic leukaemia. Br J Haematol 32:609, 1976
18. Laszlo J, Buckley C E, Amos D B: Infusion of isologous immune plasma in chronic lymphocytic leukemia. Blood 31:104, 1968
19. Thomas E D, Epstein R B, Eschback J W, et al: Treatment of leukemia by extracorporeal irradiation. N Engl J Med 273:6, 1965
20. Andersen V, Weeke E, Killmann S A: Extracorporeal irradiation of the blood: Clinical applications. Strahlentherapie 148:603, 1974
21. Silver R T: The treatment of chronic lymphocytic leukemia. Semin Hematol 6:344, 1969
22. Boggs D R, Sofferman S A, Wintrobe M M, et al: Factors influencing the survival of patients with chronic lymphatic leukemia. Am J Med 40:243, 1966
23. Huguley C M Jr: Survey of current therapy and of problems in chronic leukemia. 14th Annual Clinical Conference on Cancer, The University of Texas MD Anderson Hospital & Tumor Institute, Houston, 1969, p 317
24. Han T, Ezdinli E Z, Shimaoka K, et al: Chlorambucil vs combined chlorambucil corticosteroid therapy in chronic lymphocytic leukemia. Cancer 31:502, 1973
25. Johnson R E: Total body irradiation of chronic lymphocytic leukemia. Cancer 37:2691, 1976
26. Richards F II, Spurr C L, Pajak T F, et al: Thymic irradiation: An approach to chronic lymphocytic leukemia. Am J Med 57:862, 1974
27. Sawitsky A, Rai K R, Silver R T, et al: A comparison of daily vs intermittent chlorambucil and prednisone therapy in the treatment of patients with chronic lymphocytic leukemia. Blood 46:1039, 1975
28. Keller J W, Knospe W H, Huguley C M Jr, et al: Cyclophosphamide (CTX) and cytosine arabinoside (ARA-C) to consolidate remissions in chronic lymphocytic leukemia (CLL)? ASCO (in press)
29. Rai K R, Sawitsky A, Cronkite E P, et al: Clinical staging of chronic lymphocytic leukemia. Blood 46:219, 1975
30. Crowley J J, Schilling R F: Prognostic features in chronic lymphocytic leukemia (CLL). Clin Res 23:486A, 1975
31. Minot G B, Isaacs R: Lymphatic leukemia: Age incidence, duration, and benefit derived from irradiation. Boston Med J 191:1, 1924
32. Cutler S J, Axtell L, Heise H: Ten thousand cases of leukemia, 1940-1962. J Natl Cancer Inst 39:993, 1967
33. Zippin C, Cutler S J, Reeves W J Jr, et al: Survival in chronic lymphocytic leukemia. Blood 42:367, 1973
34. End Results in Cancer, Report No. 4. End Results Section, Biometry Branch, NCI, 1972
35. Tivey H: The prognosis for survival in chronic granulocytic and lymphocytic leukemia. Am J Roent Rad Ther Nuc Med 72:68, 1954
36. Heublein A C: A preliminary report on continuous irradiation of the entire body. Radiology 18:1051, 1932

37. Byhardt R W, Brace K C, Wiernik P H: The role of splenic irradiation in chronic lymphocytic leukemia. Cancer 35:1621, 1975
38. Huguley C M Jr: Long-term study of chronic lymphocytic leukemia: Interim report after 45 months. Cancer Chemother Rep 16:241, 1962
39. Sprague C C: Evaluation of the effectiveness of radioactive phosphorus and chlorambucil in patients with chronic lymphocytic leukemia. Cancer Chemother Rep 16:235, 1962
40. Livingston R B, Carter S K: Single Agents in Cancer Chemotherapy. New York, IFI/Plenum, 1970
41. Kuang D T, Whittington R M, Patno M E: Chemotherapy of chronic lymphocytic leukemia. Arch Intern Med 114:521, 1964
42. Rundles R W, Grizzle J, Bell W N, et al: Comparison of chlorambucil and myleran in chronic lymphocytic and granulocytic leukemia. Am J Med 27:424, 1959
43. Shaw R K, Boggs D R, Silberman H R, et al: A study of prednisone therapy in chronic lymphocytic leukemia. Blood 17:182, 1961
44. Burningham R A, Restrepo A, Pugh R P, et al: Weekly high-dosage glucocorticosteroid treatment of lymphocytic leukemias and lymphomas. N Engl J Med 270:1160, 1964
45. Ezdinli E Z, Stutzman L, Aungst C W, et al: Corticosteroid therapy for lymphomas and chronic lymphocytic leukemia. Cancer 23:900, 1969
46. Kaufman J H, Hanjura G L, Aungst C W, et al: A phase II study of Leo 1031 (NSC-134087) in lymphocytic lymphoma (LL) and chronic lymphocytic leukemia (CLL). Clin Res 23:476A, 1975
47. Brandt L, Konyves I, Moller T R: Therapeutic effect of Leo 1031, an alkylating corticosteroid ester, in lymphoproliferative disorders: I. Chronic lymphocytic leukemia. Acta Med Scand 197:317, 1975
48. Gutterman J U, Curtis J E, Freireich E J: Combination chemotherapy with cytosine arabinoside (ARA-C) and cyclophosphamide (CTX) of chronic lymphocytic leukemia (CLL). ASCO, Eighth Annual Meeting, Boston, 1972
49. Kennedy B J: Androgenic hormone therapy in lymphatic leukemia. JAMA 190:1130, 1964
50. Desai D V, Ezdinli E Z, Stutzman L: Vincristine therapy of lymphomas and chronic lymphocytic leukemia. Cancer 26:352, 1970
51. Hill J M, Loeb E: Treatment of leukemia, lymphoma, and other malignant neoplasms with vinblastine. Cancer Chemother Rep 15:41, 1961

Eric C. Vonderheid
Paul E. Wallner

36

Management of Mycosis Fungoides Lymphoma and Sézary Syndrome

First described by Alibert in 1806,[3] mycosis fungoides is a malignant lymphoma comprised of atypical thymus-derived (T) lymphocytes that has its initial manifestations in the skin.[15] The sequential evolution of the clinical lesions from nonspecific erythematous patches (premycotic phase) to infiltrated plaques (plaque phase) and ultimately to tumors (tumor phase) was recognized by Bazin in 1851[5] and this sequential pattern of progression is characteristic of the Alibert-Bazin, or classical infiltrative form of mycosis fungoides (Fig. 36-1). In a relatively small proportion of these patients the progression to cutaneous tumor formation occurs quite rapidly, over an interval of months rather than years, and the term "mycosis fungoides d'emblée" is used to describe this accelerated onset.[66] Other lymphomas, e.g., histiocytic lymphoma, that secondarily involve the skin often mimic the "d'emblée" presentation and must be excluded by clinical and histopathologic criteria.

This study was supported by Public Health Service Training Grant T01-CA05185 from the National Cancer Institute, National Institute of Health Grant No. CA11536, by The American Cancer Society, by the friends of the Radiation Therapy Center, and by the Alperin Foundation.

As the disease progresses, the cutaneous surface may become extensively involved and some lesions may spontaneously regress in areas to produce characteristic lesions with variable shapes and surface topography. It is usually not possible to detect systemic involvement during the early phases of cutaneous disease, but eventually most patients develop involvement of other organ systems that is temporarily correlated with extensive plaque or tumor formation on the skin. The lymph nodes are preferentially involved first in the process of systemization, but subsequently many other organ systems usually become infiltrated.[17,39,50] Death is commonly due to an infectious complication, a consequence of debility and impaired immunologic function, but failure of vital organ functions due to metastatic involvement can also occur.

In 1892, Besnier and Hallopeau recognized that mycosis fungoides may also exist in a generalized erythrodermic form (Fig. 36-2).[6] Later, from 1938 to 1949, Sézary[55] observed the presence of large, peculiar mononuclear cells with folded, convoluted nuclei in the skin and peripheral blood of a series of patients with such chronic erythrodermas (Sézary syndrome). The close etiologic relationship between the infiltrative form of mycosis fungoides and the Sézary syndrome is sup-

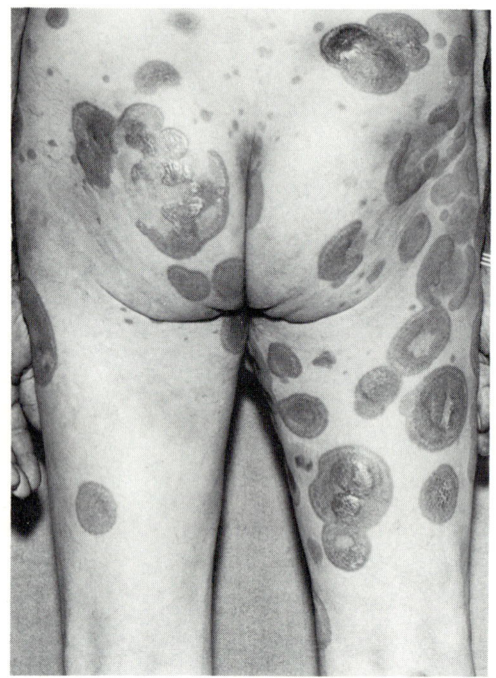

FIG. 36-1. Classical infiltrative mycosis fungoides, tumor stage. Note typical serpiginous configurations.

ported not only by similar histopathologic findings, but also by similarities in nuclear morphology and cytoplasmic membrane properties of the abnormal cells in both conditions.[9,40] Thus, some have considered the Sézary syndrome to be essentially a leukemic expression of infiltrative mycosis fungoides; however, the inflammatory nature of the cutaneous lesions, with a lessened predisposition for cutaneous tumor formation and metastatic involvement of vital internal organs, suggest that a significantly different biologic quality exists for this form of mycosis fungoides.

A third clinical expression of mycosis fungoides develops quite slowly, often over decades, as chronic noninfiltrated superficial patches of disease otherwise classified as parapsoriasis or poikiloderma. Because the lesions often assume a reticulated, atrophic appearance (i.e. poikiloderma) during their evolution, this clinical expression of the disease is termed poikilodermic or lichenoid mycosis fungoides (Fig. 36-3).[53,54] Eventually, a substantial proportion of patients develop

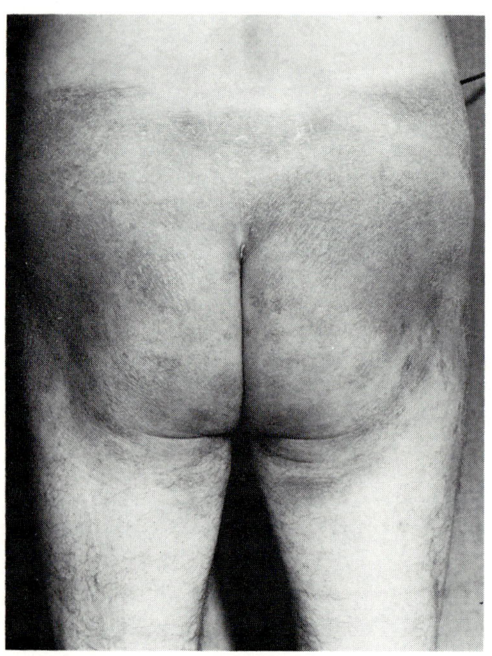

FIG. 36-2. Erythrodermic mycosis fungoides (Sézary variant).

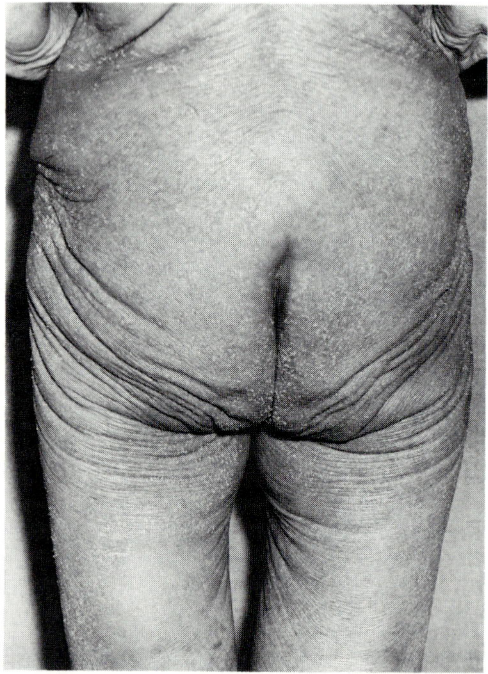

FIG. 36-3. Poikilodermic (lichenoid) mycosis fungoides. Note characteristic "bathing suit" distribution.

superimposed infiltrative lesions similar to those seen in the typical infiltrative form of the disease. The histologic features of skin specimens obtained from noninfiltrated lesions are those of mycosis fungoides, but there is frequently a more diffuse involvement of the lower cell layers of the epidermis with atypical cells that accounts for the epidermal atrophy.

One discernible difference between the poikilodermic and the classical infiltrative form of mycosis fungoides appears to be the slower evolution and hence more favorable prognosis of the former compared with the latter variant, perhaps a function of greater cellular maturity or immunologic resistance. Systemic involvement by poikilodermic mycosis fungoides may occur, but appears to be relatively uncommon. Thus, several variants of mycosis fungoides are clinically separable each with a different behavioral quality even though they have not yet been separately identifiable at cytologic or molecular levels.

Therapeutic Rationale

The treatment of mycosis fungoides depends on the clinical expression, the status of the patient as assessed by staging procedures and the availability of treatment modalities. The clinical expression of mycosis fungoides, i.e., poikilodermic, infiltrative or erythrodermic forms, probably reflects differences in the biology and the natural history of the lymphomatous process. An analogy, perhaps, is the difference between juvenile-onset and adult-onset diabetes mellitus. Since poikilodermic mycosis fungoides is characterized by slow temporal evolution and a low risk of systemic involvement, this variant does not require aggressive therapy until superimposed infiltrations develop. Infiltrative mycosis fungoides, however, will predictably eventuate in systemic involvement in a substantial proportion of patients, if not all, and deserves more intensive therapeutic measures from the onset in order to eradicate the disease. Erythrodermic mycosis fungoides (Sézary syndrome) likewise is controlled only by intensive therapy, but often does not respond well to any treatment. It is difficult to assess the benefit-versus-risk of the more potent treatments available since infections and other complications often seem related more to therapeutic side effects than to the disease itself.

Staging

Once the diagnosis of mycosis fungoides is established, the patient should undergo evaluation to determine whether extracutaneous involvement is present. Staging procedures are often deferred in patients with poikilodermic mycosis fungoides, particularly when palpable infiltrations have not emerged, but are performed under other circumstances. In addition to routine tests, bipedal lymphangiography, liver-spleen isotopic scanning, ultrasonic examination of the abdomen and appropriate lymph node, bone marrow or liver biopsy are most useful. The value of exploratory laparotomies for staging is under investigation.[26]

The staging classification of Van Scott[64,67] can be followed for poikilodermic and infiltrative mycosis fungoides, but requires modification for the erythrodermic form of disease. With this system, Stage I represents noninfiltrated or mildly infiltrated disease limited to the skin (analogous to premycotic cutaneous disease); Stage II represents moderately infiltrated plaques and Stage III represents the presence of cutaneous tumors without detectable evidence of extracutaneous involvement. Stage IV and Stage V represent involvement of lymph nodes alone or other organ systems respectively, regardless of the status of the skin. The staging of patients with erythrodermic mycosis fungoides is similar, but the prognostic significance of atypical cells often present in the lymph nodes and blood is uncertain. We have found it prognostically useful to subclassify this clinical variant according to the proportion of atypical cells (Sézary cells) found in a differential white blood cell count, i.e., less or greater than 10 per cent, as a measure of clinical severity.[67]

Therapeutic Modalities

Corticosteroids

Farber and co-workers have reported on the short-term beneficial effect of topical and intralesional cortiscosteroids in the treatment of mycosis fungoides.[19] Disease unresponsiveness to such therapy usually follows after several months and limits the usefulness. Currently, topical and systemic corticosteroids are primarily used as adjunct treatment in patients with inflammatory skin lesions.

Ultraviolet light

Solar and artificial light exposure often has substantial benefits for patients with mycosis fungoides, but the role as a treatment for long periods of time has not been studied. The modality may be used in early phases of mycosis fungoides (e.g., poikilodermic disease), but if substantial improvement is not achieved, another form of treatment should be initiated.

Photochemotherapy

A new and promising treatment for early mycosis fungoides consists of the oral administration of the photosensitizing drug, 8-methoxypsoralen, followed by exposure to titrated dosages of ultraviolet light in the wavelength spectrum from 320 to 400 nanometers (ultraviolet light region A). The capability of psoralen-ultraviolet light A therapy (PUVA) to induce complete remissions in patients with *early* phases of disease has been reported by several centers.[25,52] The remission rates are about 90 to 95 per cent for patients with plaque or earlier phases of mycosis fungoides. Patients with cutaneous tumors or erythrodermic disease usually do not respond completely to PUVA and require supplemental treatment. The long-term efficacy has not yet been established because of the newness of the technique and the fact that most patients require continuous treatment to prevent recurrences of disease. Nevertheless, the treatment is likely to be a valuable addition to the treatment regimens heretofore available.

The primary advantages of PUVA, other than its beneficial effect on the disease, are its freedom from allergic side effects as seen with topical mechlorethamine therapy and its less harsh effect on the skin compared with total-skin electron beam therapy. The primary disadvantages are the theoretical potential for photocarcinogenesis, and its availability now limited to specialized treatment centers.

Topical Chemotherapy

One of the first chemotherapeutic drugs for systemic treatment of lymphomatous diseases, mechlorethamine was first applied topically for mycosis fungoides by Sipos and Jáksó in 1956.[56] Later, Madison and Haserick cautiously and intermittently applied mechlorethamine solutions to the lesions of infiltrative mycosis fungoides for short intervals of time and demonstrated clearing of treated lesions although new lesions often appeared elsewhere.[42] In 1973, Van Scott and Kalmanson reported that dilute solutions (20 mg per cent) of mechlorethamine can be applied to the entire cutaneous surface without systemic toxicity and that sustained remissions can be achieved for intervals of over 2 years.[64] Recently, this study group has reported that actual cure of early mycosis fungoides by topical mechlorethamine may be obtained in a small proportion of patients since remissions in excess of 7 years were achieved.[67]

The remission rates achieved by the use of topical mechlorethamine applications alone are about 95 per cent for poikilodermic mycosis fungoides and about 85 per cent for pretumorous infiltrative mycosis fungoides (Stages I and II). The remission rates for patients with cutaneous tumors without evidence of systemic involvement (Stage III) and for patients with systemic involvement (Stage IV and V) were about 70 and 40 per cent respectively, but these figures reflect the frequent supplemental use of systemic treatment in conjunction with topical therapy because of incomplete responses to topical mechlorethamine alone. Likewise, erythrodermic patients usually required supplemental systemic treatment because of poor initial responses, particularly in patients with greater than 10 per cent circulating atypical cells in the peripheral blood. Overall, only about 40 per cent of erythrodermic patients achieved a remission from combined treatment.

The primary complication from topical applications of mechlorethamine solutions is the development of cutaneous hypersensitivity. About 40 per cent of patients overall become so allergic. Patients with earlier stages of disease are particularly likely to become allergically sensitized which has limited the utility of topical therapy in a group of patients most likely to benefit from sustained treatment. Preliminary treatment with small doses of mechlorethamine intravenously has reduced the frequency of development of allergy to only a comparatively small degree.

For patients allergic to mechlorethamine, an attempt may be made to desensitize the patient using either an intravenously[64] or topical technique.[10] The intravenous method consists of hospitalization for several weeks during which time small doses (less than 0.2 mg) of mechlorethamine are administered as daily intravenous infusions. The likelihood of successful desensitization within a 2 to 4 week period of time depends largely on the initial degree of sensitivity manifested by the patient. Over 50 per cent of patients allergic to mechlorethamine have been sufficiently desensitized to allow resumption of topical chemotherapy in usual therapeutic dosages.[64] The topical approach to disensitization involves applications of very dilute solutions of mechlorethamine, in concentrations below the allergic threshold of the patient, with gradually increased concentrations over the next 6 to 12 months. Remissions may occur during the performance of this technique because of immunotherapeutic benefits in addition to chemotherapeutic effects (see Immunotherapy).

For patients unable to use mechlorethamine, topical therapy with 0.1 per cent carmustine (BCNU) solutions may be tried.[74] The influence on the lesions of mycosis fungoides is probably similar to mechlorethamine, but the potential for local and systemic toxicity is greater, such that intermittent rather than sustained applications must be used. The long-term benefits on mycosis fungoides are not established, but remission in excess of 6 months have occurred from daily applications over a 3 week interval.[73]

Electron Beam Radiation Therapy

Scholtz reported the first use of external photon beam radiation for treatment of mycosis fungoides in 1902.[54] He noted prompt clearing of small cutaneous lesions, but no significant effect on overall disease progression. In 1939 Sommerville suggested the use of an X-ray "bath" to treat large cutaneous surface areas.[56a] Low energy photons were used to total dose levels between 200 to 900 rads. Again, rapid diminution in cutaneous disease was noted but without long-term benefit and the utilization of this treatment program was limited because of systemic toxicity, primarily bone marrow suppression.

Trump and associates first described the use of high energy electrons for the treatment of the "total skin surface" in 1953.[60a] Patients were treated on a moving couch by a van de Graff generator producing 2.5 million volt electrons. Dosage levels of approximately 600 rads were administered during each treatment course. Excellent control of pruritus and regression of cutaneous disease was noted, but still the benefits appeared to be only temporary with most patients requiring retreatment within 3 to 6 months. Subsequent reports in the late 1950s and 1960s utilizing various treatment programs with large field superficial photon radiation or electron beam therapy confirmed the palliative benefits of radiation without alteration of the course of the disease.[20,27,36,45,58,59,61] A program of total-skin electron beam radiation utilizing 2.5 million volt electrons was initiated at Stanford University Medical Center in 1957.[23] The initial treatment technique as described by Karzmark consisted of a four-field arrangement with delivery of between 800 to 3,000 rads in 10 to 40 days.[31] This was later altered to a six-field technique utilizing 4 million volt electrons with delivery of dosage levels up to 3,600 rads.[47] Total clearance of disease was noted at the completion of irradiation in 117 of 176 patients (66 per cent) with 84 per cent clearance in patients with eczematous or limited plaque disease and 44 per cent clearance in patients with tumor stage disease. There was an overall total clearance rate of 92 per cent noted in patients receiving over 2,500 rads.[22,23,24]

Actuarial 5-year survivals for this patient population were 85 per cent for limited plaque disease, 60 per cent for generalized plaque disease, 54 per cent for erythematous disease and 10 per cent for tumor stage. The Stanford population was predominantly composed of patients with "early disease" with 65 per cent of the total group presenting with previously untreated Stage I and Stage II disease.[29]

A recent report by Wallner and associates utilizing treatment techniques similar to those used at Stanford and dose levels of 3,000 rads has suggested that patients with advanced disease (i.e., Stages III,IV,V), who have failed on previous topical therapy, do not demonstrate a significant rate of initial clearance or long-term remission following electron beam therapy alone.[68] This report signifies the serious prognostic implications of advancing disease.

Despite the utilization of external radiation therapy for over 75 years, the precise indications for radiation as well as its timing and ultimate benefits have yet to be clearly delineated. It would appear that adequate electron beam radiation administered to the total skin surface can potentially irradicate "early disease" but is considerably less effective as the sole modality for control of "late disease."

Electron Beam Therapy and Adjuvant Topical Mechlorethamine

The failure to achieve long-term remissions in a substantial proportion of patients with electron radiation alone has prompted the study of adjuvant topical mechlorethamine therapy subsequent to completion of total skin electron beam radiation. Price and associates have recently reported the topical use of 20 mg per cent solutions of mechlorethamine following total-skin electron beam therapy.[49] Fifty-one patients were treated with electron beam with an initial total clearance of disease noted in all patients. Of this group, 25 patients received no additional treatment and 10 patients (40 per cent) remained free of disease at the time of the report. In contrast, the remaining 26 patients were started on adjuvant topical mechlorethamine after radiation and 15 patients (58 per cent) remain free of disease. The probability of long-term disease-free intervals seemed to be enhanced by adjuvant therapy. Wallner and associates have noted, however, that patients who have previously failed on topical mechlorethamine therapy and subsequently receive electron beam radiation are not likely to benefit from the subsequent use of topical mechlorethamine and indeed are less likely to demonstrate clearing from electron beam therapy as well.[68]

Systemic Chemotherapy

Reports dealing with the systemic chemotherapy of mycosis fungoides have primarily been limited to anecdotal case histories and small unrandomized series on patients with advanced stages of disease. Part of the reason for this is the relative rarity of mycosis fungoides and the fact that most physicians are reluctant to use systemic agents when the disease appears limited to the skin, especially since the natural evolution of the disease may extend over many years. Thus, systemic agents have largely been reserved for use in the most dire circumstances. Unfortunately, patients with more advanced disease are prone to infectious complications and the undesired consequences of chemotherapy often further depress immune capability.

A number of drugs when administered alone have been reported to produce beneficial, although temporary, responses in patients with mycosis fungoides.[38] Epstein and co-workers concluded, however that the ultimate course and survival of these patients was not substantially improved.[17]

Of the drugs used in the treatment of mycosis fungoides, the alkylating agents have been particularly useful. Mechlorethamine, administered in a dose of 0.1 mg/kg I.V. daily for 4 days, was first reported effective for mycosis fungoides in 1947, but the usefulness is limited by hematologic toxicity.[32] Recently, Van Scott and co-workers have administered similar total dosages over a 2 to 3 week interval with improved control of side effects and achievement of objective improvement in 29 of 41 (71 per cent) patients with mycosis fungoides treated with a single course, of which 11 (27 per cent) achieved a complete clinical remission.[63] The remission interval may be prolonged by methotrexate (MTX) between courses. These responses have not been compared to the responses achieved by the conventional dosage schedule, but the technique deserves further investigation. The oral alkylating agent, cyclophosphamide, in a dose of

1.0 to 3.0 mg/kg daily, has produced objective improvements (and often complete remissions) in over 50 per cent of patients treated.[1,17,62] The beneficial effects may be potentiated by the simultaneous administration of 75 to 100 mg chlorpromazine per day.[43] Likewise, chlorambucil, in a dose of 0.1 to 0.2 mg/kg, has been reported to be a very effective adjunct therapy in patients treated with electron beam radiation,[8] but otherwise the responses are less than those achieved by cyclophosphamide.[18,70] Recently, Winkelmann has reported that low dosages (2 to 6 mg/day) of chlorambucil, administered in conjunction with prednisone over a long interval of time may induce and maintain complete remissions in patients with Sézary syndrome.[69]

Of the antimetabolite drugs, MTX is particularly useful and is considered by many to be the drug of choice for use in mycosis fungoides.[2] Over 50 per cent of patients treated with MTX will show objective improvement.[17,28,70] Weekly or biweekly administration of MTX at a dose of 50 mg produced complete remission in 20 per cent of patients treated with fewer side effects[28] and is therefore preferred over daily oral doses.[70] At present, the use of high doses of MTX followed by "rescue" with folinic acid is under investigation, but in the authors' experience with a few patients, this technique has not been particularly advantageous.

McDonald and Calabresi have reported substantial benefits from the antimetabolite triacetyl-6-azauridine (azaribine).[44] Of 12 patients evaluated, 7 achieved complete and 4 achieved partial remissions for up to 176 weeks. Unfortunately the drug has serious thrombotic side effects and has been withdrawn from the market.

Of the antibiotic antitumor drugs, bleomycin is of particular interest because the drug achieves high concentrations in the skin and is relatively nontoxic to the bone marrow. At a dose of 15 mg twice weekly I.M., about half of patients treated will have substantial regressions (i.e., over 50 per cent of disease).[18,65] Complete remissions occasionally occur,[57] but relapses occur within a few months after treatment is discontinued.[11] Levi and Wiernik have used adriamycin at a dose of 60 mg/m^2 administered I.V. once weekly for 3 weeks to induce remissions in patients with advanced mycosis fungoides.[37] Because of the cumulative side effects of bleomycin on the skin and lungs, and of adriamycin on the heart, the role of these drugs would appear to be in the induction, rather than the maintenance, of remissions in mycosis fungoides patients.

Despite the successes achieved by combination drug therapy in other lymphomas, there have been relatively few observations with multiple-agent regimens in patients with mycosis fungoides (MF). According to Haynes and Van Scott, the combination of mechlorethamine, vincristine, procarbazine and prednisone (MOPP) usually improves patients for short intervals only,[28] but these observations were made on a small, perhaps selected, series of patients. Leavell and De Simone, reported the use of cyclophosphamide, vincristine and prednisone (COP) in 4 patients with improvement in 3 patients, one of whom achieved a complete remission lasting over 15 months.[35] Of considerable recent interest is the report of Levi and Wiernick in which 13 patients with advanced stages of mycosis fungoides received initial therapy with adriamycin followed by a maintenance program utilizing MTX (15 mg/m^2 twice weekly) and cyclophosphamide (750 mg/m^2 every 3 weeks).[37] Three patients achieved a complete remission lasting for intervals of 16+ to 40+ weeks, and an additional 5 patients developed a substantial partial remission lasting for a median time of 18 weeks. Presumably, other regimens will likewise provide long-term benefits in a reasonably predictable fashion.

Experimental Treatment Modalities

Several therapeutic approaches, discussed below, are under investigation and cannot be recommended as primary treatment procedures until more information is available.

Topical Immunotherapy

Ratner et al demonstrated that delayed hypersensitivity reactions (contact dermatitis) superimposed on lesions of mycosis fungoides would partially or totally clear the lesions for several months.[51] Klein and co-workers have successfully used different chemical and microbial antigens in various vehicles for the long-term control of mycosis fungoides.[33] Antigens such as dinitrochlorobenzene (DNCB), mechlorethamine, candida extracts or purified protein derivatives of tuberculin (PPD) are applied to immunologically sensitized patients in concentrations at which the normal skin shows minimal reaction. In patients with early infiltrative mycosis fungoides, over 50 per cent have been maintained in clinical control for periods of up to 5 years. In patients with more advanced disease or the erythrodermic form of disease, remissions are unusual but some benefit in conjunction with other treatment modalities is often noted. Application of subthreshold concentrations of mechlorethamine for the purpose of topical desensitization presumably accounts for the benefits observed in these patients.[10]

An additive beneficial effect of contact allergic sensitization has also been observed in patients who unintentionally develop delayed hypersensitivity reactions during topical mechlorethamine therapy.[67] Based on this observation, a group of 19 patients were intentionally treated with either mechlorethamine or DNCB in order to provoke a mild, but distinct contact dermatitis. A complete remission followed treatment in 8 patients for intervals from 2 months to beyond 22 months without any further treatment. This method of treatment is uncomfortable, however, and requires considerable tolerance on the part of the patient.

Thus, topical immunotherapy may have an important role in the treatment of mycosis fungoides, but the experiences as yet are too limited. Perhaps its role will be to supplement the benefit achieved by other treatment modalities.

Leukapheresis

Patients with the erythrodermic form of mycosis fungoides who have substantial numbers of circulating atypical mononuclear cells in the blood (Sézary syndrome) may improve by the mechanical removal of the atypical cells from the blood. Edelson et al cleared the skin of a patient with erythroderma, tumors and enormous numbers of circulating atypical cells (216,000 cu/mm) for a short while, but ultimately this patient later developed resistant cutaneous infiltrates and internal organ involvement.[14] Others have reported benefit for patients with near normal total peripheral leukocyte numbers.[48,60] The role of leukapheresis may be to reduce the tumor burden in these patients such that other treatment modalities may be more effective.

Transfer Factor

The long natural history and the tendency for spontaneous clearing within some lesion sites particularly in patients with classical infiltrative mycosis fungoides, supports the concept of a significant natural resistance to disease progression during early stages of involvement. In advanced disease, however, a number of immunologic parameters become depressed.[12,34,41,46,67,71] Transfer factor, a protein elaborated from sensitized normal lymphocytes stimulated in culture by the appropriate antigen, has been administered to a few patients with mycosis fungoides in order to intensify cell-mediated tumor resistance and lesions have cleared for short intervals of time.[30,72] On the other hand, the authors have treated 1 patient with systemic involvement, anergy and infection with opportunistic organisms without apparent benefit. Further experience is necessary to appraise the role of transfer factor in the treatment of mycosis fungoides.

Antilymphocyte Globulin

Since the atypical cells in mycosis fungoides bear membrane markers for thymic-derived lymphocytes, one experimental treatment approach is the administration of antilymphocyte globulin. Barrett and coworkers treated 2 patients with advanced Sézary syndrome and demonstrated only partial remissions; moreover fatal complications developed in each patient.[4] More recently, Edelson et al have reported clinical, but not histologic, clearing of a patient with extensive tumor phase infiltrative mycosis fungoides and lymph node involvement.[13]

Summary

Treatment of mycosis fungoides today can be optimistic, with long remissions now possible from adequate whole-body therapy of early disease. Several new therapeutic approaches promise to extend and improve these benefits to patients with advanced or systemic disease.

References

1. Abele D C, Dobson R L: The treatment of mycosis fungoides with a new agent, cyclophosphamide (cytoxan) Arch Dermatol 82:725–731, 1960
2. Abramowicz M (ed): Cancer chemotherapy, in Medical Letter on Drugs and Therapeutics. 18:109–116, 1976
3. Alibert J L M: Description des maladies de la peau observées á l'Hôpital Saint Louis. Barrois, Paris, 1806
4. Barrett A J, Brigden D, Roberts J T, et al: Antilymphocyte globulin in the treatment of advanced Sézary syndrome. Lancet 1:940–941, 1976
5. Bazin, P A E: Lecons Theoriques et Cliniques sur les Affections Cutanees Artificielles, Second Edition. Paris, A Delahage, 1862
6. Besnier F, Hallopeau H: On the erythrodermia of mycosis fungoides. J Cutan G U Dis 10:453, 1892
7. Bjarngard B, Chen G, Piontek R, Svensson G: Analysis of dose distributions in whole body superficial electron therapy. Int J Radiation Oncol Biol Phys 2:319–324, 1977
8. Campbell E W, Fromer J L: Adjunct chemotherapy in the treatment of cutaneous malignancies. Surg Clin North Am 39:585–590, 1959
9. Clendenning W E, Brecher, G, Van Scott E J: Mycosis fungoides. Relationship to malignant and cutaneous reticulosis and the Sézary syndrome. Arch Dermatol 89:785–792, 1964
10. Constantine V S, Fuks Z Y, Farber E M: Mechlorethamine desensitization in therapy for mycosis fungoides. Topical desensitization to mechlorethamine (nitrogen mustard) contact hypersensitivity. Arch Dermatol 111:484–488, 1975
11. de Bast C, Moriame N, Wanet J, et al: Bleomycin in mycosis fungoides and reticulum cell lymphoma. Arch Dermatol 104:508–512, 1971
12. DuVivier A, Harper R A, Vonderheid E C, Van Scott E J: Lymphocyte transformation in patients with staged mycosis fungoides and Sézary syndrome. Cancer 1978, (in press)
13. Edelson R L, Brown J A, Grossman M E, Hardy M A: Anti-thymocyte globulin in treatment of T-cell lymphoma. Lancet 2:249–250, 1977
14. Edelson R, Facktor M, Andrews A, et al: Successful management of the Sézary syndrome. N Engl J Med 291:293–294, 1974
15. Edelson R L, Kirkpatrick C H, Shevach E M, et al: Preferential cutaneous infiltration by neoplastic thymus-derived lymphocytes—Morphologic and functional studies. Ann Intern Med 80:685–692, 1974
16. Edgcomb J H, Van Scott E J, Andrews J: Histopathologic changes in the skin of patients with mycosis fungoides following therapy with high energy electrons. Acta Dermatol Venereol 2:457–462, 1957
17. Epstein E H Jr, Levin D L, Croft J D Jr, Lutzner M A: Mycosis fungoides, survival, prognostic features, response to therapy and autopsy findings. Medicine 15:61–72, 1972
18. European Organization for Research on the Treatment of Cancer, Cooperative Group for Leukaemia and Reticulocytoses: Bleomycin in the reticuloses. Br Med J 1:285–286, 1972
19. Farber E M, Zackheim H S, McClintock R P, Cox A J Jr: Treatment of mycosis fungoides with various strengths of fluocinolone acetonide cream. Arch Dermatol 97:165–172, 1968
20. Friedman M, Pearlman A: Time-dose studies in irradiation of mycosis fungoides. Am J Roentgenol 66:374–379, 1956
21. Fromer J, Johnston D, Salzman F, et al: Management of lymphoma cutis with low megavoltage electron beam therapy. South Med J 54:769–776, 1961
22. Fuks Z, Hoppe R, Bagshaw M: The role of total skin irradiation with electrons in the management of mycosis fungoides. Bull du Cancer 64:291–304, 1977
23. Fuks Z, Bagshaw M: Total-skin electron treatment of mycosis fungoides. Radiology 100:145–150. 1971
24. Fuks Z, Bagshaw M, Farber E: Prognostic signs and the management of the mycosis fungoides. Cancer 32:1385–1395, 1973
25. Gilchrest B Z, Parrish J A, Tanenbaum L, et al: Oral methoxsalen photochemotherapy of mycosis fungoides. Cancer 38:683–689, 1976
26. Griem M L, Moran E M, Ferguson D J, et al: Staging procedures in mycosis fungoides. Br J Cancer 31:362–367, 1975

27. Haybittle J A: 24 Curie Strontium 90 unit for whole-body superficial irradiation with beta rays. Br J Radiol 37:297–301, 1964
28. Haynes H A, Van Scott E J: Therapy of mycosis fungoides. Prog Dermatol 3:1–5, 1968
29. Hoppe R, Fuks Z, Bagshaw M: The rationale for curative radiotherapy in mycosis fungoides. Int J Radiat Oncol Biol Phys 2:843–851, 1977
30. Kahn A, Simone T, et al: Clinical trials with transfer factor, In Ascher M D, Gottlieb A A, Kirkpatrick C H (eds): Transfer Factor. Basic Properties and Clinical Applications. New York, Academic Press, 1976, p 585
31. Karzmark C, Loevinger R, Steele R, Weissbluth M: A technique for large-field, superficial electron therapy. Radiol 74:633–643, 1960
32. Kierland R R, Watkins C H, Shullenberger C C: The use of nitrogen mustard in the treatment of mycosis fungoides. J Invest Dermatol 9:195–201, 1947
33. Klein E, Holtermann O, Milgram H, et al: Immunotherapy for accessible tumors utilizing delayed hypersensitivity reactions and separated components of the immune system. Med Clin North Am 60:389–418, 1976
34. Langner A, Glinski W, Pawinska M, Oblek S: Lymphocyte transformation in mycosis fungoides. Arch Dermatol Forsch 151:249–257, 1975
35. Leavell U W Jr, DeSimone P: Combined chemotherapy (COP) in treatment of mycosis fungoides: Report of four cases. South Med J 69:915–917, 1976
36. Le Bourgeois J-P, Bridier A, Bouhnik H, Schlienger M: Whole cutaneous irradiation in mycosis fungoides with 55 KV x-rays. Bull du Cancer 64:313–322, 1977
37. Levi J A, Diggs C H, Wiernik P H: Adriamycin therapy in advanced mycosis fungoides. Cancer 39:1967–1970, 1977
38. Levi J A, Wiernik P: Management of mycosis fungoides—Current status and future prospects. Medicine 54:73–88, 1975
39. Long J C, Mihm M C: Mycosis fungoides with extracutaneous dissemination; a distinct clinicopathologic entity. Cancer 34:1745–1755, 1974
40. Lutzner M, Edelson R, Schein P, et al: Cutaneous T-cell lymphomas: The Sézary syndrome, mycosis fungoides and related disorders. Ann Intern Med 83:534–552, 1975
41. Mackie R, Sless F R, Cochran R, De Sousa M: Lymphocyte abnormalities in mycosis fungoides. Br J Dermatol 94:173–178, 1976
42. Madison J F, Haserick J R: Topically applied mechlorethamine on 12 dermatoses. Arch Dermatol 86:633–667, 1962
43. Maguire A: Treatment of mycosis fungoides with cyclophosphamide and chlorpromazine. Br J Dermatol 80:54–57, 1968
44. McDonald C J, Calabresi P: Azaribine for mycosis fungoides. Arch Dermatol 103:158–167, 1971
45. Nisce L, D'Angio G, Kim J: Weekly total-skin electron-beam irradiation for mycosis fungoides. Radiology 109:683–686, 1973
46. Nordqvist B C, Kinney J P: T and B cells and cell-mediated immunity in mycosis fungoides. Cancer 37:714–718, 1976
47. Page V, Gardner A, Karzmark C: Patient dosimetry in the electron treatment of large superficial lesions. Radiology 94:635–641, 1970
48. Pineda A A, Brzica S M Jr, Taswell H F: Cutaneous- and semicutaneous- flow blood centrifugation systems: Therapeutic applications with plasma, platelet-, lympha-, and eosinapheresis. Transfusion 17:407–416, 1977
49. Price N, Constantine V, Hoppe R, et al: The treatment of mycosis fungoides: The efficacy of electron beam therapy and adjuvant topical mechlorethamine in the treatment of mycosis fungoides. Cancer 40:2851–2853, 1977
50. Rappaport H, Thomas L B: Mycosis fungoides: The pathology of extracutaneous involvement. Cancer 34:1198–1229, 1974
51. Ratner A C, Waldorf D S, Van Scott E J: Alterations of lesions of mycosis fungoides lymphoma by direct imposition of delayed hypersensitivity reactions. Cancer 21:83–88, 1968
52. Roenigk H H Jr: Photo chemotherapy for mycosis fungoides. Arch Dermatol 113:1047–1051, 1977
53. Samman P D: Mycosis fungoides and other cutaneous reticuloses. Clin Exp Dermatol 1:197–214, 1976
54. Scholtz W: Ueber den einfluss der röntgenstrahlen auf die haut in gesunden und kranken zustande. Arch Dermatol U Syph (Berlin) 59:421, 1902
55. Sézary A: Une nouvelle reticulose cutanée: La reticulose maligne leucemique a histiomonocytes monstrueu et a forme d'erytrodermie oédemateusè et pigmentée. Ann Derm Syph 9:5–22, 1949
56. Sipos K, Jákso G: A Mustárnitrogen helyi alkalmazása méhány börbetegségben. Börgyógy Vener Szle 32:198–203, 1956
56a. Sommerville J: General x-ray baths in generalized dermatoses. Brit J Derm 54:234–237, 1942
57. Spigel S C, Coltman C A Jr: Therapy of mycosis fungoides with bleomycin. Cancer 32:767–770, 1973
58. Spittle M: Mycosis fungoides—Electron beam therapy. Bull du Cancer 64:305–312, 1977

59. Szur L, Silvester J, Bewley D: Treatment of the whole body surface with electrons. Lancet 1:1373–1377, 1962
60. Tan R S-H, Oon C J, Barrett A J, Hayes J P: Sézary syndrome: Treatment by leukophoresis. Proc Soc Med 68:28–29, 1975
60a. Trump J G, Wright K, Evans W: High energy electrons for the treatment of extensive superficial malignant lesions. Am J Roent Rad and Nuc Med 69:623–629, 1953
61. Van Scott E, Andrews J, Edgcomb J: Therapy of mycosis fungoides with high energy electrons. Acta Dermat Venereol 2:451–456, 1957
62. Van Scott E J, Auerbach R, Clendenning W E: Treatment of mycosis fungoides with cyclophosphamide. Arch Dermatol 85:499–501, 1962
63. Van Scott E J, Grekin D A, Kalmanson J D, et al: Frequent low doses of intravenous mechlorethamine for late-stage mycosis fungoides lymphoma. Cancer 36:1613–1618, 1975
64. Van Scott E J, Kalmanson J D: Complete remissions of mycosis fungoides lymphoma induced by topical nitrogen mustard (HN2). Control of delayed hypersensitivity to HN2 by desensitization and by induction of specific immunologic tolerance. Cancer 32:18–30, 1973
65. Van Vloten W A, Polano M K: Bleomycin therapy in mycosis fungoides. Dermatologica 150:50–57, 1975
66. Vidal E, Brocq L: Étude sur le mycosis fungoides. La France Médical 2:946,957,969, 983,993,1005,1019,1885
67. Vonderheid E C, Van Scott E J, Johnson W C, et al: Topical chemotherapy and immunotherapy of mycosis fungoides. Arch Dermatol 113:454–462, 1977
68. Wallner P, Vonderheid E, Brady L, et al: Evaluation and recommendations for therapy of advanced mycosis fungoides lymphoma. Presented at the Annual Scientific Meeting of the American Society of Therapeutic Radiologists, Denver, Colorado, November, 1977
69. Winkelmann R K, Linman J W: Erythroderma with atypical lymphocytes (Sézary syndrome). Am J Med 55:192–198, 1973
70. Wright J C, Lyons M M, Walker D G, et al: Observations on the use of cancer chemotherapeutic agents in patients with mycosis fungoides. Cancer 17:1045–1062, 1964
71. Zachariae H, Ellegaard J, Grunnet E, et al: T- and B-cells and IgE in mycosis fungoides. Acta Derm Venereol 55:466–468, 1975
72. Zachariae H, et al: Transfer factor as therapeutic agent in mycosis fungoides. Arch Dermatol 112:1324–1326, 1976
73. Zackheim H S: Letter to the editor. Contemp Rev 4:6, 1977
74. Zackheim H S, Epstein E H Jr: Treatment of mycosis fungoides with topical nitrosourea compounds. Arch Dermatol 111:1564–1570, 1975

Donald Pinkel

37
Chemotherapy of Acute Leukemia

Thirty years have elapsed since the discovery that antifolate compounds produced remissions of acute leukemia. The purpose of this communication is to outline some advances in chemotherapy of acute leukemia, to assess the current status and to project possible future directions.

Development of "Total Therapy" of Acute Lymphocytic Leukemia

From 1947 to 1962 several compounds were found to produce remissions of acute lymphocytic leukemia. MTX, mercaptopurine, prednisone, vincristine and cyclophosphamide each had temporary effects in certain proportions of patients. When combined, the drugs produced remission in higher proportions of patients than when used alone. Although survival was prolonged, the disease remained almost universally fatal. What were the obstacles to cure?

1. Drug resistance, initial or acquired. As determined from hematological response of patients, less than one-half of children had complete remission after treatment with any one compound. Of those who experienced complete remission, virtually all developed hematological relapse despite continued administration of initially effective drug therapy.
2. Inadequate diffusion of drugs. Because of poor diffusion of drugs into the arachnoid tissue, meningeal relapse occurred as the initial relapse site in approximately one-half of the patients.
3. Morbidity of therapy. The antileukemia drugs produced toxic side effects that were particularly hazardous when administered in high doses or in combinations.
4. Pessimism. A sense of futility and fatalism prevalent among physicians inhibited them from trying to cure leukemia.

In 1962, a "total therapy" program was devised that was aimed optimistically at attempting to cure ALL in children.[1,2,3] Based on information about leukemia chemotherapy gathered from experimentation in cell systems and in mice and from experience in children, it embodied several principles. Among them was the utilization of combination chemotherapy to overcome initial resistance and to inhibit emergence of resistant leuke-

Supported by National Cancer Institute Grants CA15700, CA17851, CA17997 and by Faye McBeath Foundation, Milwaukee, Wisconsin.

mia as assessed by bone marrow examinations, the reduction of leukemia cell mass to the point of complete hematological remission prior to administration of antimetabolite drugs, specific therapy to the arachnoid meninges to eliminate leukemia cells not reached by effective drug levels and the continuation of chemotherapy for 2 to 3 years to eradicate residual leukemia cells in the bone marrow, viscera and other tissues. This basic plan has been adopted generally during the past 15 years and has become a model for treatment of other forms of cancer as well.

Results of Treatment of Acute Lymphocytic Leukemia

From 1962 to 1965 exploratory total therapy studies demonstrated that combination chemotherapy resulted in better remission induction and longer hematological remission. Although the meningeal therapy used was found to be inadequate, 7 out of 37 children who achieved complete remission have remained in continuous complete remission for 12 to 14 years and have been off all therapy for 10 years. In a 1967 to 1968 exploratory study that provided adequate meningeal therapy, 18 out of 31 children who achieved complete remission remain in initial continuous complete remission for 9 years and have been off therapy for 6 to 7 years.

In a 1968 to 1970 comparative study of the value of meningeal irradiation in preventing meningeal leukemia only 2 out of 45 children who received 2400 rads of craniospinal irradiation in the first month of remission developed initial meningeal relapse. On the other hand, 33 of the 49 who did not receive this treatment demonstrated leukemia in their CSF as their first manifestation of relapse. At present, 23 of the 45 children who received the early meningeal treatment remain in initial continuous complete remission for 7 to 9 years and have been off therapy for 4 to 6 years.

Are these long-term continuously leukemia-free survivors cured of their leukemia? Of the 7 children in studies I to III who were removed from therapy in 1966 to 1967 none relapsed in the 10 years since. The complete remission duration of the 31 children in the 1967 to 1968 study and the 45 children in the 1968 to 1970 study who received adequate meningeal therapy in the first month of remission are plotted on a semilogarithmic graph in Figure 37-1. It appears that children who remain in initial continuous complete remission for 5 years and who have not received therapy for 2 years are at little risk of relapse. This suggests that their leukemia has been eradicated and that they may be cured.

What is the quality of survival of these children? Most children can return to relatively normal activity after the first 3 months of treatment. They experience hematosuppression and immunosuppression during chemotherapy, however, and often demonstrate slowing of linear growth.[4,5] When removed from treatment, hematopoiesis returns to normal and the immune system becomes normal after a period of "immunological rebound." Those who have demonstrated slowed growth may have "catch-up" growth during the first year off treatment. In general, then, the quality of survival is satisfactory and compatible with successful development into adolescence and adulthood.

Overcoming Drug Resistance of Acute Lymphocytic Leukemia

The limited success that has been achieved in control of ALL has dispelled pessimism and has resulted in a more positive, optimistic attitude toward patients with leukemia. The administration of meningeal irradiation with or without intrathecal MTX largely compensates for inadequate perfusion of the arachnoid tissue by antileukemic drugs and, therefore, reduces the risk of meningeal relapse. The use of combination chemotherapy, however, prevents emergence of resistant leukemia, as manifested by hematological relapse during chemotherapy in only one-half of the patients. In other words, one-half of the children still develop drug-resistant leukemia in spite of combination therapy.

One conventional method of overcoming failure of drugs to control disease is to increase the dosage of the drugs. In a 1965 to 1967 study we tested the value of increased dosage of a four-drug combination for delay-

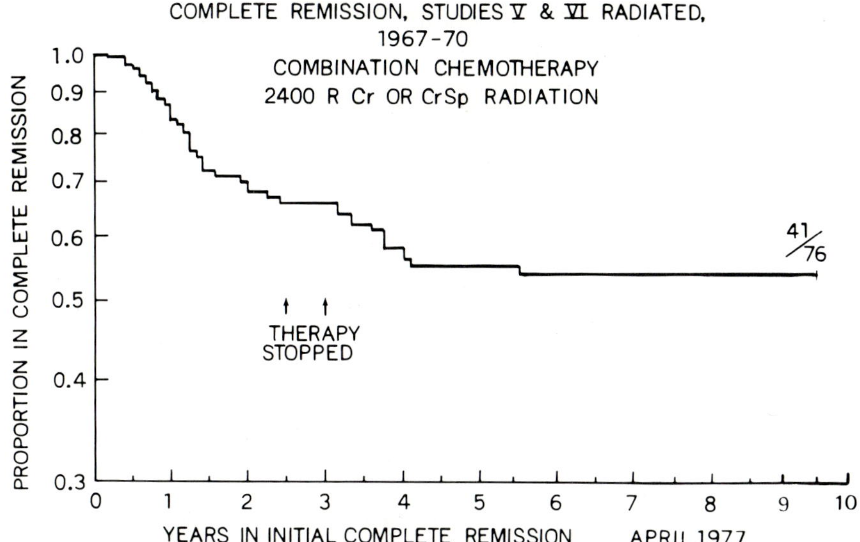

FIG. 37-1. This semilogarithmic graph describes the initial continuous complete remissions of 76 children who entered complete remission in 1967 to 1970 and received 2400 rads of cranial irradiation with simultaneous intrathecal methotrexate or 2400 rads of craniospinal irradiation during the first month of remission. Subsequently they received 2½ to 3 years of multiple agent combination chemotherapy until hematological relapse or death during remission. Forty-one children remain continuously free of leukemia for 7 to 9½ years and have been off all therapy for a minimum of four years. Only one patient developed relapse after the first four years of continuous complete remission. The leukemia free survival of one-half of the children entering remission and the low risk of relapse after four years suggest that acute lymphocytic leukemia is curable.

ing the development of relapse.[1] Preventive meningeal therapy was not given. Patients in the low dosage group had shorter complete remissions than those in the high dosage group. This difference could be accounted for, however, by the more frequent and earlier occurrence of initial meningeal relapse in the low dosage group. This suggested that the superiority of high dosage of combination chemotherapy was due to higher and more effective drug levels in the arachnoid meninges. We could not conclude that higher dosage of combination chemotherapy inhibited the emergence of resistant leukemia as manifested by hematological relapse during chemotherapy. There remains at this time no evidence that higher and more toxic dosages of combination chemotherapy are superior to moderate and less toxic dosages for overcoming the problem of *acquired* resistance.

Another method for overcoming initial resistance and preventing emergence of acquired resistance to drug therapy is to use multiple drugs with different modes of action. As described above, combination chemotherapy is superior to single-drug chemotherapy for induction of complete remission and, by historical comparison, for continuation of remission. There was reason to question the advantages of using multiple drugs for continuation of complete remission, however. The drugs generally used for continuation chemotherapy, MTX, mercaptopurine, cyclophosphamide and arabinosyl cytosine, have overlapping toxic effects even though they have different modes of action and strains of leukemia are not cross-resistant to them. All of these agents cause hematosuppression, immunosuppression and mucosal injury. For this reason the dosages of any one of these drugs must be reduced when any other of them is being administered. Thus, the tolerated dosage of MTX is reduced by one-half when mercaptopurine is given simultaneously. The question in using combinations of these drugs, therefore, is not whether com-

TABLE 37-1.* *Comparison of One Versus Multiple Drugs for Continuation Therapy of Acute Lymphocytic Leukemia*

Remission induction	268/283			
Preventive CNS Rx:	2400 R Cr + IT Mtx			
Randomized:	228			
	M	MMp	MMpC	MMpCA
Patients	20	68	70	70
Relapse	15	23	27	23
Died in CR	1	0	4	5
Continuous CR	4	45	39	42

*In this 1972 to 1975 study children with acute lymphocytic leukemia were randomized to one of four continuation chemotherapy regimens after remission induction with prednisone, vincristine and asparaginase followed by meningeal irradiation and intrathecal methotrexate. The patients receiving methotrexate alone (M) had shorter remission and fewer lengthy remissions than those receiving methotrexate plus mercaptopurine (MMp). Remission duration and frequency of long remissions were not improved by addition of cyclophosphamide (MMpC) or cyclophosphamide plus arabinosyl cytosine (MMpCA). On the other hand, patients receiving the three-drug or four-drug combinations demonstrated more immunosuppression and were at greater risk of serious and sometimes fatal infection.[4,6]

bining them will inhibit emergence of resistant leukemia, as indicated by hematological relapse during drug administration. The question is whether combining them *while reducing their dosages* will prevent resistant leukemia.

In a 1972 to 1975 study children with ALL were randomized to one of four continuation chemotherapy regimens after remission induction with prednisone, vincristine and asparaginase and meningeal therapy consisting of cranial irradiation and simultaneous intrathecal MTX.[6] The first group received MTX, the second MTX and mercaptopurine, the third MTX, mercaptopurine and cyclophosphamide, and the fourth MTX, mercaptopurine, cyclophosphamide and arabinosyl cytosine. The MTX, cyclophosphamide and arabinosyl cytosine were administered weekly intravenously while the mercaptopurine was taken daily orally.

The combination of MTX and mercaptopurine was superior to MTX alone in preventing hematological relapse (Table 37-1). The three-drug and four-drug combinations were not superior to this two drug combination, however. Under the conditions of this study, therefore, adding more drugs to a two-drug combination did not reduce the risk of emergence of resistant leukemia. This suggests that the problem of acquired resistance of leukemia may not be solved by utilizing additional drugs that have overlapping toxic effects.

A third method of overcoming drug resistance is to determine subcategories of a disease that exhibit different responsiveness to the drugs. In recent years ALL has been segregated into three biological and clinical entities, defined by the immunological cell surface markers of the *leukemic lymphoblasts of the bone marrow prior to therapy*.[7,8] The "null cell" or "non-T, non-B" form is most frequent, accounting for about 70 per cent of childhood lymphocytic leukemia (Table 37-2). These patients are more often under age 6 years and equally boys and girls. They tend to have lower initial white blood cell counts and to remain in complete remission on modern therapy. In the "thymic" or "thymic cell-like" form the patients tend to be older boys with mediastinal masses and high initial white blood cell counts. They have earlier and more frequent relapses on modern therapy than those with null cell type. About 22 per cent of children with lymphocytic leukemia have

TABLE 37-2.* *Comparison of "Thymic Cell" and "Null Cell" Acute Lymphocytic Leukemia*

	"Thymic cell"	"Null cell"
Patients	26	83
Male	24	44
Age > 6 yr.	23	26
Mediastinal mass	19	3
Nodes > 2 cm.	15	8
WBC < 10,000	1	35
WBC > 100,000	13	7
Hb < 8 g.	3	54
Complete remission, 18 months	6/20	45/75

*In this table initial clinical features of children with acute lymphocytic leukemia whose bone marrow leukemic lymphoblasts demonstrated rosette formation with sheep red blood cells (thymic cell) are compared to those of children whose lymphoblasts did not demonstrate this feature nor other cell surface markers (null cell). The data indicate that "thymic cell" leukemia tends to occur in older boys and to be associated with an anterior mediastinal mass, large lymph nodes, high initial white blood cell count and short complete remission.[7] "Null cell" leukemia tends to occur in younger children and equally in boys and girls. They are more likely to have very low hemoglobins at diagnosis and to remain in complete remission.

this thymic form. Least frequent is the "B-cell-like" type, which appears to have the worst prognosis of the three.[9]

We do not yet have conclusive information about the relative sensitivity of each of these three types of ALL to the available drugs. But from animal and cell culture data, it appears that certain antileukemia drugs are more effective against certain of these three types of leukemia than against others.[10] Development of specific chemotherapy programs for each of these three forms of leukemia might result in superior remission duration and in a greater frequency of long-term remission and possible cure for all three forms.

In addition to identifiable cell surface characteristics, both "B-cell" and "thymic cell" leukemia have high mitotic rates at time of diagnosis.[9,11] This suggests that drug resistance might be related to cell membrane and/or replication features of leukemia cells. It is possible, then, that the exploration of differences in how these three types of leukemic lymphoblasts handle antileukemia drugs might result in new information concerning the mechanisms of cancer cell resistance to drugs, the most important obstacle to curing cancer with drugs.

Avoiding Morbidity in Treatment of Acute Lymphocytic Leukemia

It has been conventional to think that the efficacy of leukemia chemotherapy is directly related to its morbidity. In our 1965 to 1967 study the superior duration of complete remission in the high dosage group was associated with greater toxicity.[1] As noted before, however, this superiority could be accounted for by the less frequent and later occurrence of initial meningeal relapse in the high dosage group. With effective preventive meningeal irradiation to accommodate for inadequate drug distribution to the arachnoid tissue, this effect may not be important. Thus, we need not conclude from this study that greater morbidity is requisite to greater efficacy of combination chemotherapy.

In the 1972 to 1975 study there were remarkable differences in morbidity of therapy in the four randomization groups.[6] Almost one-half of the children in the MTX alone group developed leukoencephalopathy during initial complete remission while none of the children in the MTX and mercaptopurine group demonstrated this complication during initial complete remission. The children in the MTX alone group generally received more than twice as high a dosage of weekly MTX as children in the two-drug group so that we assume the leukoencephalopathy was caused by MTX. On the other hand, the children in the two-drug group are remaining in complete remission more frequently and longer than those in the MTX alone group. Thus, this debilitating side effect of chemotherapy is associated with a less efficacious chemotherapy regimen.

Again in the 1972 to 1975 study, children receiving the two-drug combination experienced less morbidity than those receiving the three-drug or four-drug combinations. During initial complete remission the children receiving MTX and mercaptopurine had less immunosuppression, fewer hospitalizations, only one instance of *Pneumocystis carinii* pneumonia and no deaths (Table 37-1).[4,6] On the other hand, the frequency of lengthy complete remission is at least as good in the two-drug group as in the three-drug and four-drug groups. Thus, under the conditions of this study, the patients with the least morbidity of therapy are experiencing therapeutic efficacy equal to or superior than that of patients with greater morbidity. This suggests a general principle that efficacy of leukemia therapy may be independent of its morbidity. More studies with different drugs and drug schedules in patients with different types of leukemia are needed to test this principle.

Methods of avoiding morbidity other than modifying dosage or number of drugs are generally well known. They include education of the patient and his family regarding nutrition and hygiene, minimizing hospitalization, handwashing and room isolation techniques in the hospital, avoidance of intravenous and instrumentation hazards, frequent physical examinations and maintaining the total white cell count above 2000/cu mm with at least 500 lymphocytes/cu mm and at least 500 granulocytes/cu mm. Trimethoprim-sulfamethoxazole at one-quarter dosage daily prevents *Pneumocystis* pneumonia and should be taken by those at high risk of this disease.[12]

Cranial irradiation and intrathecal MTX may cause nausea and headache during the early days of their administration, a syndrome of fever and somnolence 6 weeks after irradiation, temporary reduction of linear growth and possibly decreased brain growth.[5,13] Long term studies of neuropsychological function have not revealed significant compromise of function, however, and most children show normal growth, behavior and activity after cessation of therapy. At present, craniospinal irradiation or cranial irradiation with intrathecal MTX are the only proven methods for long-term prevention of meningeal relapse. The long-term efficacy and safety of other methods under trial are yet to be demonstrated.

Other Forms of Acute Leukemia

Acute myelocytic, acute myelomonocytic and acute histiocytic/monocytic leukemia are usually grouped together for the purposes of chemotherapy, although they vary in their nature and responsiveness. With modern therapy approximately 60 to 70 per cent of patients in this group experience complete remission after 4 to 6 weeks of combination chemotherapy.[14,15,16,17,18]

The more effective drugs for these types of leukemia are arabinosyl cytosine (cytosine arabinoside, cytarabine), mercaptopurine, thioguanine, daunorubicin and adriamycin. Vincristine, prednisone and 6-Azauridine are also utilized. At this time no one schedule or protocol is sufficiently superior to be recommended as standard therapy.

The basic problem is continuation of complete remission. Regardless of the regimen, the median duration of complete remission is approximately 6 months and the median survival is approximately 1 year. Only rare patients experience lengthy survival. Recently it has been suggested that continuing chemotherapy past induction of complete remission may not improve duration of remission.[19]

Immunologic methodology has been utilized in attempts to prolong complete remission duration of AML.[15,16] The biological basis of such attempts is scanty and the results to date questionable.

Bone marrow transplantation during complete remission is another experimental approach to treatment of AML.[20]

Commentary

Childhood ALL of the "null cell" type is apparently a curable disease. With modern therapy approximately 60 per cent of these children are surviving in initial continuous complete remission off therapy and at little or no risk of relapse. This is significant for all patients with cancer because it indicates that disseminated cancer is not necessarily incurable and suggests that chemical cure of all cancers is an eventual possibility.

Since a plateau of continuous complete remission of ALL has been achieved, the effectiveness of therapy must now be measured by the height of this plateau and not by the slope or its statistical projection. The value of therapeutic innovations can only be assessed by their influence on the height of this plateau, that is, the proportion of patients remaining in initial continuous complete remission at little or no risk of relapse. Judgment should be withheld on the value of such innovations until a plateau of continuous complete remission is achieved for patients who experience them.

The efficacy of leukemia chemotherapy is not necessarily related to its morbidity. It is possible by careful comparative studies of alternate treatment schemes to determine a chemotherapy regimen that demonstrates both high efficacy and low morbidity. We have demonstrated in one such study that adding drugs with overlapping toxic side effects to a two-drug continuation chemotherapy regimen increased the serious side effects of therapy without improving its effectiveness.

Drug resistance, as manifest by hematological relapse during chemotherapy, is the greatest obstacle to cure of acute leukemia. Although combining antileukemia drugs has been successful in overcoming initial resistance and reducing emergence of acquired resistance in acute lymphocytic leukemia, terminal relapse with drug resistant leukemia is still the fate of 40 per cent of children with "null cell" ALL and most patients with acute "thymic cell," "B-cell," and nonlymphocytic leukemia.

References

1. Pinkel D, Hernandez K, Borella L, et al: Drug dosage and remission duration in childhood lymphocytic leukemia. Cancer 27:247, 1971
2. Hustu H O, Aur R J A, Verzosa M S, et al: Prevention of central nervous system leukemia by irradiation. Cancer 32:585, 1973
3. Pinkel D, Hustu H O, Aur R J A, et al: Radiotherapy in leukemia and lymphoma of children. Cancer 39:817, 1977
4. Green A A, Sen L, Borella L: Acute lymphocytic leukemia: A disease of lymphoid cells? in Symposium, Roswell Park Memorial Institute, Buffalo: Conflicts in Childhood Cancer. New York, Alan R Liss, 1975, p 69
5. Verzosa M, Aur R J A, Simone J V, et al: Five years after central nervous system irradiation of children with leukemia. Int J Radiat Oncol Biol Phys 1:209, 1976
6. Simone J V, Aur R J A, Hustu H O, et al: Acute lymphocytic leukemia in children. Cancer 36:770, 1975
7. Borella L, Sen L, Dow L W, et al: Cell differentiation antigens versus tumor-related antigens in childhood acute lymphoblastic leukemia (ALL). Clinical significance of leukemia markers. Haematol and Blood Transfus 20:77, 1977
8. Sen L, Borella L: Clinical importance of lymphoblasts with T markers in childhood leukemia. N Engl J Med 292:828, 1975
9. Flandrin G, Brouet J C, Daniel M T, et al: Acute leukemia with Burkitt's tumor cells: A study of six cases with special reference to lymphocyte surface markers. Blood 45:183, 1975
10. Ohnuma T, Arkin H, Minowada J, et al: Differential, chemotherapeutic susceptibility of human T- and B-lymphocytes in culture. Proceedings of AACR and ASCO, 18:198, 1977
11. Murphy, S B, Aur R J A, Simone J V, et al: Pretreatment cytokinetic studies in 94 children with acute leukemia. Relationship to other variables at diagnosis and to outcome of standard treatment. Blood 49:683, 1977
12. Hughes W, Kuhn S, Chaudhary S, et al: Suc-

cessful chemoprophylaxis for *Pneumocystis carinii* Pneumonitis (PCP). Pediatr Res 11:501, 1977

13. Peylan-Ramu N, Poplack D G, Pizzo P A, et al: Abnormal computed tomography (CT) scans in children with acute lymphocytic leukemia (ALL) following CNS prophylaxis. Proceedings of AACR and ASCO, 18:305, 1977
14. Choi S, Simone J V: Acute non-lymphocytic leukemia in 171 children. Med Pediatr Oncol 2:119, 1976
15. Crowther D, Powles R L, Bateman C J T, et al: Management of adult acute myelogenous leukaemia. Br Med J 20:131, 1973
16. Holland J R, Glidewell O, Ellison R R, et al: Acute myelocytic leukemia. Arch Intern Med 136:1377, 1976
17. Rosenthal D S, Moloney W C: The treatment of acute granulocytic leukemia in adults. N Engl J Med 286:1176, 1972
18. Walters T R, Aur R J A, Hernandez K, et al: 6-azauridine in combination chemotherapy of childhood acute myelocytic leukemia. Cancer 29:1057, 1972
19. Burke P J, Karp J E, Braine H G, et al: Timed sequential therapy of human leukemia based upon the response of leukemic cells to humoral growth factors. Cancer Res 37:2138, 1977
20. Thomas E D, Buckner C D, Banaji M, et al: One hundred patients with acute leukemia treated by chemotherapy, total body irradiation, and allogeneic marrow transplantation. Blood 49:511, 1977

Isadore Brodsky, S. Benham Kahn
Barry J. Erlick, Anthony A. Fuscaldo

38

Treatment of the Chronic Myeloproliferative Disorders

Etiology of Myeloproliferative Disorders

The myeloproliferative disorders (MPD) originate in the bone marrow or potential bone marrow sites. They have no known cause, are malignant neoplasms, and are characterized by an overgrowth of hematopoietic stem cells, which give rise to erythrocytes, leukocytes, platelets and fibroblastic reticulum.[1,2] Their classification is given in Table 38-1. Clinically and hematologically, all but the most acute MPD are easily distinguished from the lymphoproliferative disorders.

The hypothesis that these disorders are related etiologically was prompted by their similarity in morphology and clinical progression. Despite apparent similarities,[3] some investigators have challenged the concept that the MPD are etiologically related or that they are transformed from one to another.[4] Recent studies in our laboratories, however, suggest that polycythemia vera (PV), essential thrombocythemia (ET), and chronic myelogenous leukemia (CML) are associated with oncornavirus activity. PV, the prototype of the MPD, frequently evolves into myelofibrosis with myeloid metaplasia (MMM). Therefore, we consider the classification MPD a useful and unifying one.

Table 38-1. *Types of Myeloproliferative Disorders*

Chronic myeloproliferative disorders
Polycythemia vera (PV)
Myelofibrosis, myelosclerosis with myeloid metaplasia (MMM)
Essential thrombocythemia (ET)
Chronic myelogenous leukemia (CML)
Acute myeloproliferative disorders
Erythroleukemia (Di Guglielmo's syndrome and variants)
Acute myelogenous leukemia (AML)

PV is a preneoplastic state characterized by panmyelosis, with increased erythropoiesis, granulopoiesis and megakaryocytopoiesis.[5,6] Recent studies with glucose-6-phosphate dehydrogenase (G-6-PD) indicate that polycythemia vera, like CML, is a clonal disorder.[7] PV will frequently evolve into MMM, and approximately 10 to 15 per cent of the patients die of acute leukemia.[8]

An important morphologic characteristic of the bone marrow is an intense megakaryocytic hyperplasia. In this regard, PV bears a superficial resemblance to the murine disease induced by the polycythemia strain of Friend

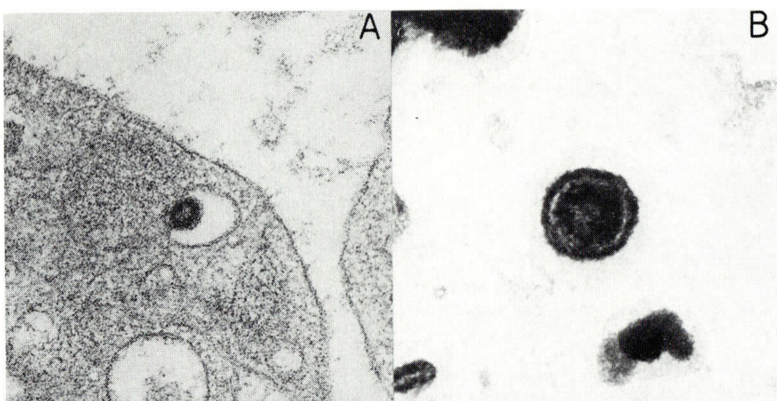

FIG. 38-1. *A*. Thin-section platelet preparation of human oncornavirus-like particle (× 90,000). *B*. Critical-point dried preparation of human oncornavirus-like particle (× 190,000).

virus, at least with regard to splenomegaly and bone marrow morphology. A major difference is that high titers of both the Friend and Rauscher viruses are initially associated with thrombocytopenia, whereas PV is generally associated with thrombocytosis.

Electron microscopy studies (Fig. 38-1) have revealed that the oncornaviruses (C-type) of murine and feline leukemias are characteristically present in vacuoles of megakaryocytes and platelets.[9] Reitz et al have reported budding of oncornaviruses from the platelets of a woolly monkey with lymphoma.[10] Recent studies in our laboratory indicate that a specific subset of patients with PV and ET who present with high platelet counts and chromosomal abnormalities in the bone marrow will also have oncornavirus-like particles in their platelets. This C-type virus activity has been demonstrated both by electron microscopy studies and by analysis for reverse transcriptase-like activity (RDDP) in the platelets.[11,12] This observation is important in attempting to understand the etiology and pathogenesis of the MPD.

The possibility that such virus particles would be found was first raised in an editorial published in the Journal of the National Cancer Institute, in which Brodsky postulated that PV could be considered an early preneoplastic state with the potential to evolve into acute leukemia.[9] This is certainly true concerning a more advanced MPD, chronic myelogenous leukemia. CML is a stem-cell disorder in which there is a distinct genetic marker involving erythroid, myeloid, and megakaryocytic precursors, that is, the Philadelphia chromosome (Ph[1]). Megakaryocytic hyperplasia and thrombocytosis are common in some cases of CML and may portend a poor prognosis. In CML, footprints of viral activity, that is, evidence of RDDP in white blood cells and, in our laboratories, evidence of RDDP in platelets, have been found. However, since intact oncornavirus-like particles have not been noted in CML, we have postulated that CML is a more advanced neoplastic state in which the virus has been completely incorporated into the genome of the stem cells and can no longer be expressed as an intact particle.[13,14]

In considering the pathogenesis of the chronic MPD in contradistinction to that of the lymphoproliferative disorders (LPD), one must consider the role of the immune system. In animal systems, spontaneous myeloproliferative disorders are rare; the most commonly seen leukemic state can be best characterized as a non-Hodgkin's lymphoma, i.e., LPD. Even in these animal model systems, however, the megakaryocytes and platelets are major factors in pathogenesis.

The AKR mouse probably represents our best experimental model for the human lymphoproliferative diseases.[15] In the murine disease, the megakaryocyte is a principal reservoir for the oncornavirus. AKR mice are thrombocytopenic within three weeks of birth. As they mature, the platelet count increases and then decreases with the onset of lymphoma. This pattern is similar to that described following injection of BALB/c mice with a high dilution (10^{-3}) of Rauscher virus.[9]

The pattern of thrombocytopenia in the AKR mouse is like that described in human with chronic lymphocytic leukemia (CLL) and chronic lymphosarcoma cell leukemia.[16] In the AKR mouse and possibly in human beings, the second phase of thrombocytopenia is associated with the onset of leukemia, with death ensuing soon thereafter. Even in the LPD, at least in the experimental animal, a preneoplastic state develops in which abnormalities in the megakaryocyte develop, resulting initially in a reversible thrombocytopenia, followed by recovery and then secondary thrombocytopenia occurring with the onset of neoplasia.

The question arises as to whether the fundamental difference between the MPD and LPD may not be in the genetic constitution of the host and the response of the immune system to the disease. The LPD disease may differ from MPD in that in the former the host is able to mount a more obvious immune response to the etiologic viral agent. Some of the abnormal lymphocytes may indeed be transformed and become neoplastic. These considerations are pertinent in view of recent observations indicating that there may be an increased incidence of solid tumors as well as acute leukemia in patients with PV treated with chemotherapeutic drugs that suppress the immune system.[12,17] If an oncornavirus is an etiologic factor, then suppression of the immune system might be expected to increase the incidence of neoplasia.

Treatment of Polycythemia Vera

The principal modes of therapy for PV are phlebotomy, radioactive phosphorus (^{32}P), and chemotherapy.

The prognosis for untreated patients with PV is questionable. Chievitz and Thiede reviewed 250 cases of patients who died between 1933 and 1961.[18] In this group, half of the 49 untreated patients died 18 months after the onset of symptoms. The main cause of early death was thrombosis; in the entire series, 100 of the 250 deaths were directly related to thrombotic episodes. Only 15 patients died from hemorrhage. Myelofibrosis developed in 14, and leukemia in 9. Those patients treated with some form of radiation had a median survival of approximately 12.5 years. Recent studies by Modan and Lilienfeld suggest that the median survival for patients with PV is in the range of 11.5 to 16 years.[19]

Because thrombosis figures importantly as a cause of early death in untreated patients with PV, particular attention must be given to the choice of drugs. Simultaneous platelet and fibrinogen studies in our laboratory utilizing selenomethionine (^{75}Se) have been performed in patients with PV, MMM and CML.[20,21] In PV a hypercoagulable state exists on the basis of shortened platelet survival and increased platelet turnover. This increased platelet turnover is also associated with low-grade defibrination. The platelet and fibrinogen kinetics in PV are distinctly different from those noted in CML.[20] In CML, even in those cases associated with thrombocytosis, platelet survival is normal and, in some cases, prolonged. Fibrinogen turnover in CML is also decreased (Table 38-2). Clinically, CML is not associated with thrombotic episodes but rather with a hypocoagulable state. This would suggest that PV, being an earlier or more benign neoplastic disorder than CML, is associated with an overproduction of platelets, which tend to function normally. This is not the case in CML, an advanced preneoplastic state. Because of these observations, the platelet count and platelet kinetics must be stressed in treating PV.

Arguments have now developed with respect to indications for therapy in PV. One point is clear: life expectancy will be prolonged by some form of effective therapy. The argument against phlebotomy alone is that the incidence of thrombosis and hemorrhage will remain high. The main argument against treatment with ^{32}P may be an increased incidence of acute leukemia. Many investigators maintain that chemotherapy should replace ^{32}P therapy as an accepted form of myelosuppression and that this would result in a decreased incidence of leukemia. Studies evaluating this contention, however, have not yet been completed.

In an attempt to determine which mode of therapy is best for PV, a prospective ran-

TABLE 38-2. *Platelet and Fibrinogen Kinetics in Chronic Myeloproliferative Disorders*

	Platelets			Fibrinogen		
Disorder (No. of patients)	Count (platelets/μl)	Survival (days)	Turnover (platelets/μl/day)	Concentration mg/100 ml	Survival (days)	Turnover (mg/ml/day)
CML (7)						
Mean	402,000	13.2	31,700	271	12.8	0.24
Range	218,000–715,000	10.5–16.0	15,600–51,100	206–350	6.5–190	0.11–0.39
PV (9)						
Mean	536,000	7.2	75,700	219	5.6	0.44
Range	354,000–747,000	5.5–8.5	41,700–122,000	162–340	3.5–7.0	0.25–0.97
MF, MMM (8)						
Mean	1,094,000	6.6	176,800	318	6.8	0.52
Range	56,000–3,353,000	4.0–11.5	9,6000–609,600	233–373	4.0–9.0	0.30–0.85
Controls (10)						
Mean	378,000	10.6	38,000	218	7.8	0.42
Range	168,000–475,000	7.0–11.0	22,000–52,000	225–400	6.5–9.5	0.33–0.49

Abbreviations: CML, chronic myelogenous leukemia; PV, polycythemia vera; MF, myelofibrosis; MMM, myelofibrosis with myeloid metaplasia.

Brodsky I, Kahn SB, Ross E M, et al: Platelet and fibrinogen kinetics in the chronic myeloproliferative disorders. Cancer 30:1444, 1972, with permission.

domized control study was instituted by the International Polycythemia Vera Study Group (PVSG).[17] The group establishes rigid criteria for the diagnosis of PV. Once admitted, patients are randomized to one of three arms:

1. Phlebotomy, as needed, to maintain the packed cell volume at 42 to 47 percent.
2. ^{32}P, 2.3 millicuries per meter^2, intravenously every 12 weeks as needed (limit, 5 millicuries per dose). Phlebotomy for packed cell volume > 47 percent. Increase dose by 25 percent if there is no response.
3. Chlorambucil 10 mg by mouth daily for 6 weeks, then adjust dose according to response; phlebotomy for packed cell volume > 47 percent.

Four hundred seventy-four patients have been randomized into this study.[17] Prior to randomization, 15 per cent of the patients had suffered thrombotic episodes. After randomization, there was a 40 per cent increase in recurrent thrombotic complications in the phlebotomy arm. This is a significant increase when compared with the much lower incidence in the two myelosuppressive regimens (^{32}P; chlorambucil). The thrombotic episodes were not necessarily correlated with an increase in the platelet count, that is, thrombocytosis. In evaluating this phenomenon, however, simultaneous platelet and fibrinogen kinetics will be essential in defining the hypercoagulable state.[20,21] The preliminary results indicate that phlebotomy alone should be used only in very indolent cases of PV. The majority require some form of myelosuppression with either ^{32}P or chemotherapy.

As of 1976, Wasserman had reported five cases of acute leukemia in the chlorambucil arm; one in the ^{32}P; and one in the phlebotomy.[17] In May 1977, the Polycythemia Vera Study Group reported eleven cases of acute leukemia and four cases of carcinoma in the chlorambucil arm; five cases of acute leukemia and five cases of carcinoma in the ^{32}P arm; and one case of acute leukemia and six of carcinoma in the phlebotomy arm. The study is still continuing, and more time will be needed to determine whether the significant difference in leukemia incidence will hold.

Phlebotomy

Phlebotomy, the simplest treatment for PV, was the earliest. With phlebotomy alone, the leukocytosis and thrombocythemia of PV are poorly controlled,[2,22] probably explaining the increased incidence of thrombosis. Phlebotomy can effectively reduce the increased blood volume and red-cell mass and afford symptomatic relief. The procedure is well tolerated. Most patients with PV are borderline iron-deficient even prior to the initiation of phlebotomy. Each 500 cc phlebotomy removes approximately 250 mg of iron. This obviously potentiates the iron deficiency already present in PV. In our institution, the initial therapy for PV is phlebotomy as needed to reduce the packed-cell volume to less than 50 per cent. If thrombocytosis is present, that is, if the platelet count is greater than 500,000, then myelosuppressive therapy is instituted.

Radioactive Phosphorus (^{32}P)

Lawrence and his group introduced ^{32}P as therapy for PV in the late 1930s.[23] Experience since then has indicated that ^{32}P is effective in this disease.[23-26] The rationale behind its use is that actively dividing tissues have a high requirement for phosphorus, since this element is a key constituent of DNA and RNA. Radioactive phosphorus is a pure beta emitter of high intensity. In effect, radiation is delivered to the marrow and, selectively, to the nucleus of the dividing cell; ^{32}P is advantageous because it is inexpensive, can be given in a single dose, and does not create a radiation hazard to other people.

Radioactive phosphorus is administered as sodium phosphate, preferably intravenously. It can be given orally, but only about 75 per cent of the dose may be absorbed if it is so given. Because of inadequate knowledge concerning the dosimetry of ^{32}P, methods of estimating the therapeutic dose are necessarily empirical. Doses based on body weight, RBC count, RBC mass, or combinations of these fctors have been advocated. The single dose generally administered is 3 to 7 millicuries, depending on the above factors.

Generally, phlebotomy is performed before adminstration of ^{32}P, although this is not necessary unless there is a circulatory overload or other acute symptoms are present. Urinary loss of injected ^{32}P has been estimated at about 10 per cent in 48 hours, with a range of 3 to 31 per cent. The physical half-life of ^{32}P is 14.3 days. The biologic half-life of the material is about 8 days. Therefore, significant radiation effects may exist for 4 to 6 weeks.

The first effect of ^{32}P is on the platelets, and the full effect is usually noted in 3 to 4 weeks. In 6 to 12 weeks, depression of the RBC count is found. The effect on the WBC count usually, but not always, follows the effect on the platelet count. The apparent delayed effect of ^{32}P on erythropoiesis is due to the long lifespan of the RBC. Therefore, another dose of ^{32}P should not be given until at least 4 months have elapsed.

Ferrokinetic studies are useful in estimating the degree of marrow activity when repeat courses of ^{32}P are being considered.[27] The patient should be followed up at monthly intervals until remission occurs. If the RBC mass rises during the first 4 months after therapy, phlebotomy should be used to control the symptoms. Chemotherapeutic drugs should not be given during this time, as they are additive to the effects of ^{32}P. Full remission can be expected in about 80 percent of the cases and partial remission in 15 per cent more. Thus, ^{32}P therapy fails in only a small number of patients. About two-thirds of the responders do so after one injection and the rest after two injections. Rarely are three injections required. Most patients experience complete remission in 6 months, and such remissions will usually last 1 to 2 years. In one series, the average length of remission was 22.3 months.[25] When there is a relapse, retreatment with ^{32}P is indicated. In a series of 107 patients,[26] followed up for 18 years, the highest total dose of ^{32}P given to one patient was 42 millicuries.

Radiophosphorus has the following disadvantages:

1. Suppression of leukocytosis and thrombocytosis is not as long-lasting as is suppression of erythrocytosis.
2. A radiation therapist is usually required to administer the material. In addition, because of its short physical half-life, the material must be ordered in advance, since storage is not possible.
3. There is a danger of overestimating the dose, and leukopenia, thrombocytopenia or anemia may result.
4. A 10 to 15 per cent incidence of acute leukemia has been reported as a late complication of therapy.[19] Statistical studies indicate, however, that this complication does not appear to shorten overall lifespan if patients treated with ^{32}P are compared[24] with those not treated with ^{32}P. The increased incidence of acute leukemia, although debated by some workers, is generally accepted as a valid criticism of the use of ^{32}P.

Although we agree that ^{32}P will decrease the thrombotic and hemorrhagic complications of this disorder to some extent, it is our practice to avoid its use but instead to administer chemotherapeutic agents when we believe myelosuppressive therapy is indicated. Exceptions to this rule of practice include the elderly, in whom the advanced age of the patient makes the risk of leukemia an acceptable one, and in those patients who, for one reason or another, cannot or will not take chemotherapeutic agents and in whom suppression of their disease is mandatory.[2]

Chemotherapy

Although in the last 11 years increased interest has been shown in the use of chemotherapy in the United States, workers in the United Kingdom[28] had previously suggested that chemotherapy would induce remissions equivalent to those with ^{32}P. Their data indicated, however, that chemotherapy was more troublesome to administer than was ^{32}P; this disadvantage was counterbalanced by an apparently lower incidence of leukemia in the patients treated with chemotherapy. More recent studies in the United States have demonstrated that control of the proliferative aspects of PV can be accomplished by proper use of alkylating agents.[6,17,29] The principal alkylating agents used in treating PV are busulfan, chlorambucil and melphalan (Fig. 38-2).

Busulfan has been used extensively in

the therapy of polycythemia vera.[6,27-29] In our experience, this drug has proved to be the best and least expensive mode of treatment for this disorder.[6,27]

We have treated 60 patients with busulfan; for some the diagnosis had been made before they came under our care. All patients achieved remission. For the most part, therapy was begun with no more than 4 mg of bsulfan daily, often with 2 mg (one tablet), daily. These low daily doses differ from those in CML, for which we use higher initial doses. For PV we recommend low daily doses, since higher daily doses would make frequent checks of the blood count necessary because of the rapid accumulation of drug.

Most patients can be seen every 2 or 3 weeks during therapy. If personal visits are not practical, the blood count should be checked in the laboratory and a follow-up phone call made. When remission occurs, or if the platelet count drops to 400,000/cu mm or less, therapy is stopped. Even after cessation of therapy, a downward drift in all counts, and especially the platelets, will be observed.

This median dose for response ranges between 150 mg and 200 mg. The usual length of time to induce remission is between 35 and 90 days. Phlebotomy is not necessary unless the initial RBC mass is very high and the patient has troublesome symptoms.

It should be kept in mind that the peripheral hemoglobin concentration and hematocrit are poor measures of RBC mass, since in the later phases of the disease, plasma volume rises as rapidly as does the RBC mass. In these instances, measurement of the total blood volume and total RBC mass usually indicates severe hypervolemia, while hemoglobin concentration and hematocrit values suggest that the RBC mass is well controlled.

We do not recommend maintenance chemotherapy with busulfan for most patients with PV, since in our experience remissions of 18 to 24 months are commonplace after a single course of this agent. This experience is similar to that of other investigators.[17]

Adherence to this schedule has led to little toxicity. Platelet counts of less than 100,000/cu mm and WBC counts of less than 5,000/cu mm were recorded in 14 per cent of our patients. Wasserman and Gilbert found thrombocytopenia in 27 per cent of their patients

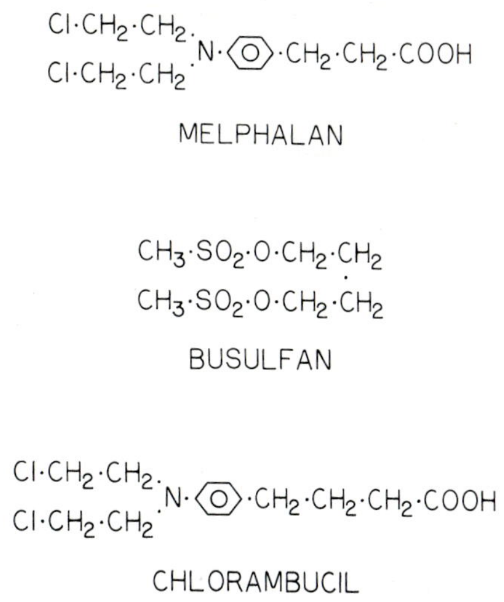

$Cl \cdot CH_2 \cdot CH_2 \cdot$
$N \cdot C_6H_4 \cdot CH_2 \cdot CH_2 \cdot COOH$
$Cl \cdot CH_2 \cdot CH_2 \cdot$

MELPHALAN

$CH_3 \cdot SO_2 \cdot O \cdot CH_2 \cdot CH_2$
$CH_3 \cdot SO_2 \cdot O \cdot CH_2 \cdot CH_2$

BUSULFAN

$Cl \cdot CH_2 \cdot CH_2 \cdot$
$N \cdot C_6H_4 \cdot CH_2 \cdot CH_2 \cdot CH_2 \cdot COOH$
$Cl \cdot CH_2 \cdot CH_2 \cdot$

CHLORAMBUCIL

FIG. 38-2. Chemical formulae of the alklylating agents melphalan, busulfan and chlorambucil.

treated with busulfan.[29] They used busulfan on a more continuous basis and gave higher total doses, however.

The studies in our laboratories mentioned previously, which demonstrated the presence of oncornavirus-like activity in platelets of patients with PV and ET, are especially pertinent in regard to busulfan therapy. As previously indicated, the presence of the virus particles and the enzymatic activity (RDDP) are altered after busulfan therapy.[11,12] In three carefully documented instances, we have demonstrated that low doses of busulfan are associated with rapid disappearance of viral indicators, due in part, perhaps, to the disruption of the virus and virally altered membrane components in megakaryocytes and platelets. With induction of complete remission, chromosomal abnormalities that were present prior to treatment revert to a virtually normal pattern. The action of busulfan in other myeloproliferative disorders and on chromosomes is discussed at greater length in this volume in the chapter by Fuscaldo et al.

Those patients with PV and ET who show viral activity appear to be particularly sensitive to the effect of this alkylating agent. This subset of patients may be the group in whom severe thrombocytopenia could occur if administration of busulfan is not closely monitored. It is interesting that the 27 per cent incidence of severe thrombocytopenia noted in Wasserman's series[17] is about equal to the incidence of patients reported with chromosomal abnormalities in the PVSG series (33 per cent). Experiments are now being conducted in our laboratories to also study the in vitro effects of busulfan. Of course, a key question is what effect other chemotherapeutic drugs such as chlorambucil and melphalan will have on the viral parameters.

The overall incidence of leukemia following the use of busulfan has not been determined. Whether this incidence will prove to be less than, equal to, or greater than that noted with ^{32}P can only be resolved by a controlled study. Current studies would certainly indicate, however, that busulfan will be no worse than chlorambucil in this regard and will probably be better.

In addition to marrow suppression by busulfan and, in particular, the risk of thrombocytopenia, other side effects of this drug include the development occasionally of interstitial pulmonary fibrosis and hyperpigmentation of the skin.[31-33] Also rare is a syndrome resembling adrenal insufficiency, characterized by brownish pigmentation of the skin, debility, anorexia and weight loss.[34]

All of these toxic effects have been described in patients who have taken the drug for more than 24 months. There is no relation between these toxic manifestations and the leukemia process per se. Other side effects include sterility, cataract formation and amenorrhea.[1,35] In some patients, amenorrhea may persist even after therapy is stopped. One should not ascribe amenorrhea to drug therapy unless the possibility of pregnancy has been excluded. The occurrence of pregnancy during therapy with busulfan has been reported.[35] Normal infants have been delivered. It is best to withhold therapy during early gestation, however.

Our results with busulfan concerning duration of remission agree essentially with those of Wasserman.[17] In contrast to remission with melphalan, chlorambucil or cytoxan, remission once obtained with busulfan, in our experience, may last for months or even years without reinstitution of therapy. This is not true with the other alkylating drugs, which require periodic cyclic administration. The superiority of busulfan is an important point, particularly in view of our data indicating its potential antiviral effect. Another important consideration is that busulfan is a poor immunosuppressive agent, whereas melphalan and chlorambucil are potent immunosuppressive drugs. It would appear inadvisable to suppress the immune system in a disorder that may possibly be virus-associated.

Because busulfan is given only intermittently to control thrombocytosis and leukocytosis, many side effects of long-term drug administration can be avoided. The increased erythropoiesis can then easily be managed by phlebotomy as needed. Under such circumstances, it is conceivable that the incidence of leukemia, perhaps directly attributable to a chemotherapeutic agent, might be decreased. In any event, we strongly urge a controlled study to evaluate the efficacy of busulfan in the treatment of PV and ET. This treatment would have to be combined with phlebotomy.

Chlorambucil, which is more frequently used in the therapy of lymphoproliferative disease than in other diseases, is also effective in the treatment of PV. Wasserman and Gilbert[29] recommend that therapy be started with 6 to 8 mg daily; a total dose of about 800 mg is required to control the symptoms and signs of the disease. Unlike the situation with busulfan, however, relapse is likely in about 6 months if therapy is not maintained. For this reason, a "4 weeks on and 4 weeks off" program has been recommended for smooth control. A 10 to 15 per cent incidence of thrombocytopenia has been reported, as well as a small percentage of instances of alopecia.

Wasserman and Gilbert[29] report that administration of cyclophosphamide in daily doses of 100 to 500 mg will produce prompt organ shrinkage and a rapid drop in hematocrit in PV. A total dose of about 9 gm is necessary for remission. Again, unmaintained patients have short remissions and the cost to the patient is high. Distressing side effects of this drug are alopecia and cystitis, both of which are proportional to the amount of drug given and the length of time administered. As with chlorambucil, maintenance therapy is necessary.

Melphalan is an effective drug in the treatment of PV. Although recent reports suggest that therapy be begun with 10 mg daily, we recommend doses of 4 mg daily to start.[36] A total dosage of 1.5 to 3 mg/kg is needed for control. Thrombocytopenia and leukopenia are the most deleterious side effects. By careful follow-up, these side effects can be avoided. Melphalan, however, like chlorambucil, is extremely immunosupressive.

Pipobroman (Vercyte), a clinically available alkylating agent, is used in a daily dose of 1 to 1.5 mg/kg.[37] Therapy is continued until a therapeutic response is obtained or toxicity is seen. Maintenance therapy of 0.1mg/kg may then be used. Few side effects have been noted with this drug. More experience is necessary before its usefulness can be determined.

Although the mainstay of therapy for PV has been the alkylating agents, other drugs have been tried with some success. Over 10 years ago, a folic acid antagonist, pyrimethamine, was shown to produce subjective and objective improvement in some patients.[38] Therapy with azauridine intravenously or azaribine orally, both cycle-active drugs (as is pyrimethamine) was found to produce rapid shrinkage of organs and prompt suppression of erythropoiesis.[39] The data demonstrate rapid recovery of marrow function following use of these agents, however, making more continuous therapy mandatory.

Treatment of Essential Thrombocythemia

Essential thrombocythemia (primary, hemorrhagic or idiopathic thrombocythemia), a disease closely related to PV, is characterized by a marked elevation in platelet count and many platelets of abnormal morphology and function. In this disorder, immature and mature megakaryocytes proliferate excessively in the bone marrow as well as extramedullary sites. A high proportion of thrombocythemia patients eventually show a transition to PV or myelofibrosis. In our laboratory, in those cases of ET in which chromosomal abnormalities are found in the bone marrow, evidence of oncornavirus-like activity has been frequently demonstrated. We consider busulfan to be the treatment of choice for this disorder, using the same principles as those used in PV. Patients with positive viral indicators have been extraordinarily sensitive to the drug. Occasionally patients with negative viral indicators are resistant to chemotherapy.

Treatment of Myelofibrosis and Myeloid Metaplasia (MMM)

Treatment of MMM depends upon the degree of marrow function and the role of the spleen in blood production and destruction. The main problem is usually anemia.[40] Pharmacologic doses of testosterone have been used with some success to stimulate erythropoiesis.[2,41,42] This hormone should be tried initially in patients with this disorder, since for the most part leukocytosis and thrombocytosis are not as distressing as is the anemia. If a response occurs, then the high WBC and platelet counts can be controlled with busulfan. Patients with MMM are extremely sensitive to the effects of chemotherapy, and treatment should be initiated with no more than 2 mg of busulfan. A complete blood count should be taken weekly.

Splenectomy may be useful in those patients in whom hypersplenism develops.[40] Since marrow failure is a usual occurrence in MMM, it is important to show shortened survival of the formed elements before attempting splenectomy. We have recently demonstrated the usefulness of the ^{75}Se-selenomethionine method to evaluate platelet survival. This technique is used to predict the effectiveness of splenectomy in hypersplenism.[20]

Treatment of Hyperuricemia in Myeloproliferative Disorders

The myeloproliferative disorders are characterized by hyperuricemia due to excessive production of uric acid by proliferating cells. Renal excretion of urates is increased, and urate stones or uric acid deposition in the kidneys may complicate the disease or occur as a result of therapy. Acute gouty arthritis may also occur. The xanthine oxidase inhibitor, allopurinol, is effective in reducing serum urate concentration in patients with myeloproliferative disorders.[43] Patients who have renal stones or gout due to myeloproliferative disease should be treated with high fluid intake, alkalinization of the urine with sodium bicarbonate and administration of allopurinol, 200 to 600 mg per day.

References

1. Dameshek W, Gunz F: Leukemia, 2nd ed. New York, Grune & Stratton, 1964
2. Kahn S B, Brodsky I: Therapy of myeloproliferative disorders, in Brodsky I, Kahn S B (eds): Cancer Chemotherapy II. New York, Grune & Stratton, 1972, p 347
3. Silverstein M N: Myeloproliferative diseases: Their shifting spectrum. Postgrad Med 43:167, 1968
4. Glasser R M, Walker R I: Transitions among the myeloproliferative disorders. Ann Intern Med 71: 285, 1969
5. Pike G M: Polycythemia vera. N Engl J Med 258:1250, 1958
6. Brodsky I, Kahn S B, Brady L W: Polycythemia vera: Differential diagnosis by ferrokinetic studies and treatment with busulfan (Myleran). Br J Haematol 14:351, 1968
7. Adamson J W, Fialkow P J, Murphy S, et al: Polycythemia vera: Stem cell and probable clonal origin of the disease. N Engl J Med 295:913, 1976
8. Landau S A: Acute leukemia in polycythemia vera. Semin Hematol 13:33, 1976
9. Brodsky I: Role of the megakaryocyte and platelet in the leukemia process in mice and men: A review and hypothesis. J Natl Cancer Inst 51:329 (editorial), 1973
10. Reitz M S, Gallagher R E, Aoki T, et al: A biochemical and virological study of a case of lymphoma-leukemia in a gibbon ape. Proceedings, American Society of Hematology (abstr 297), 1976
11. Brodsky I, Fuscaldo A A, Erlick B J, et al: Analysis of platelets from patients with thrombocythemia for reverse transcriptase and virus-like particles. J Natl Cancer Inst 55:1069, 1975
12. Brodsky I, Fuscaldo A A, Erlick B J, et al: Effect of busulfan on oncornavirus-like activity in platelets and chromosomes in polycythemia vera and essential thrombocythemia. J Natl Cancer Inst 59:1, 1977
13. Brodsky I, Fuscaldo K E, Kahn S B, et al: Chronic myelogenous leukemia: A clinical and experimental evaluation of splenectomy and intensive chemotherapy. Semin Hematol 8:143, 1975
14. Fuscaldo K E, Brodsky I, Conroy J F, et al: Sequential chromosomal surveys in the management of chronic granulocytic leukemia. in Proceedings, Third International Symposium on Detection and Prevention of Cancer. New York, Marcel Dekker, 1976
15. Brodsky I: Thrombocytopenia: A prelymphoid sign in AKR mice. Nature (Lond) 223:198, 1969
16. Zacharski L R, Linman J W: Chronic lymphocytic leukemia versus chronic lymphosarcoma cell leukemia. Am J Med 47:75, 1969
17. Wasserman L R: The treatment of polycythemia vera. Semin Hematol 13:57, 1976
18. Chievitz E, Thiede T: Complications and causes of death in polycythemia vera. Acta Med Scand 172:513, 1963
19. Modan B, Lilienfeld A M: Polycythemia vera and leukemia: The role of radiation treatment. Medicine 44:305, 1965
20. Brodsky I, Kahn S B, Ross E M, et al: Platelet and fibrinogen kinetics in the chronic myelo-proliferative disorders. Cancer 30:1444, 1972
21. Brodsky I, Fuscaldo A A, Fuscaldo K E: Hemostasis and cancer, in Sutnick A I, Engstrom P F (eds): Oncologic Medicine. Baltimore, University Park Press, 1976 p 247
22. Gurney C W: Polycythemia vera and some possible pathogenic mechanisms. Ann Rev Med 16:169, 1965
23. Lawrence J H: Polycythemia: Physiology, diagnosis and treatment based on 303 cases. New York, Grune & Stratton, 1955, p 136
24. Galton D A G: Problems in the management of the myeloproliferative states. Semin Hematol 1:37, 1965
25. Szur L., Lewis S M, Goolden A W G: Polycythemia vera and its treatment with radioactive phosphorus. Q J Med 28:397, 1959
26. Halnan K E, Russell M H: Polycythaemia vera: Comparison of survival and causes of death in patients managed with and without radiotherapy. Lancet 2:760, 1965
27. Brodsky I: The use of ferrokinetics in the evaluation of busulfan therapy in polycythemia vera. Br J Haematol 10:291, 1964
28. Perkins J, Israels M C G, Wilkinson J F:

Polycythemia vera: Clinical studies on a series of 127 patients managed without radiation therapy. Q J Med 33:499, 1964
29. Wasserman L R, Gilbert A S: The treatment of polycythemia vera. Med Clin North Am 50:1501, 1966
30. Dunn C D R: The chemical and biological properties of busulfan (Myleran). Exp Hematol 2:101, 1974
31. Oliver H, Schwartz R, Rubio F Jr, et al: Interstitial pulmonary fibrosis following busulfan therapy. Am J Med 31:134, 1961
32. Haut A, Abbott W S, Wintrobe M M, et al: Busulfan in the treatment of chronic myelocytic leukemia: The effect of long-term intermittent therapy. Blood 17:1, 1961
33. Galton D A G: Chronic myeloid leukaemia. Br J Radiol 26:285, 1953
34. Dameshek W: A syndrome resembling adrenal cortical insufficiency associated with long-term busulfan therapy. Blood 18:497, 1961
35. Dennis L H, Stein S: Busulfan in pregnancy: Report of a case. JAMA 192:715, 1965
36. Logue G L, Gutterman J U, McGinn T G, et al: Melphalan, therapy of polycythemia vera. Blood 36:70, 1970
37. Monto R W, Ten Pas A, Battle J D, et al: A-8103 in polycythemia. JAMA 190:833, 1969
38. Frost J, Jones R, Jonsson W: Pyrimethamine in the treatment of polycythemia vera. South Med J 51:1260, 1958
39. DeConti R C, Calabresi P: Treatment of polycythemia vera with azauridine and azaribine. Ann Intern Med 73:575, 1970
40. Silverstein M N: The evolution into and the treatment of late stage polycythemia vera. Semin Hematol 13:79, 1976
41. Gardner F H, Pringle J C: Androgens and erythropoiesis. II. Treatment of myeloid metaplasia. N Engl J Med 264:103, 1961
42. Gardner F H, Nathan D G: Androgens and erythropoiesis. III. Further evaluation of testosterone treatment of myelofibrosis. N Engl J Med 274:420, 1966
43. Yu T F, Gutman A B: Effect of allopurinol (4-hydroxypyrazolo [3,4-d]pyrimidine) on serum and urinary uric acid in primary and secondary gout. Am J Med 37:885, 1964

Anthony A. Fuscaldo
Barry J. Erlick

39

The Effects of Chemotherapy on Viral Activity in Myeloproliferative Disease

The material presented in this chapter is a direct outgrowth of our studies on platelets and oncornaviruses in thrombocythemic patients. In the past several years, there have been many reports of viral indicators such as RNA-dependent DNA polymerase (RDDP), oncornavirus nucleic acids and immunologic cross-reactivity with known RNA tumor viruses in human leukemias and solid tumors. The presence of these markers in human neoplastic disorders without the presence of demonstrable intact oncornaviruses has been amply documented.[1-5] Alternatively, laboratories that have demonstrated morphologically-intact RNA tumor virus-like particles from human tissue through the use of electron microscopy,[6-8] have not provided biochemical evidence for the presence of a virus.

We have attempted for some years to elucidate the association between RNA tumor viruses and myeloproliferative disorders. This interest stemmed from our laboratory findings of resemblances between the early stages of Friend and Rauscher virus-infected murine systems and myeloproliferative disorders of man such as polycythemia vera (PV) and essential thrombocythemia (ET).[9]

Our study of these preneoplastic disorders was based upon the following sequence of events: oncornavirus replication in preneoplastic states; integration into the host genome; cessation of virus replication; and, finally, transformation to the neoplastic state. The integration and subsequent loss of detectable virus particles followed by neoplastic transformation occur in tissue culture and in mice following the integration of viral RNA.[10-11]

We believed that if an intact oncornavirus was to be detected it would have to be obtained early in the viral replicative phase. Once the cryptic proviral state, in which virus-specific DNA is integrated into the host genome, is reached, only the specific immunologic and biochemical viral markers can be observed. When the full neoplastic state is achieved, it is likely that the virus would already have been integrated into the host and neoplastic transformation would have occurred.

In addition to being preneoplastic, thrombocythemic conditions such as ET and PV provide a readily obtainable source of large amounts of platelets. This would be advantageous in the search for human oncornaviruses for two reasons: First, because platelets (and megakaryocytes) have been shown to be primary sites of oncornavirus replication in murine and feline leukemias,[12-14] it is probable that oncornavirus replication also occurs

TABLE 39-1. *Correlation of Oncornaviruses with Abnormal Karyotypes in Preleukemic Patients*

Patient	Diagnosis	Virus RDDP	Virus CPD	Karyotype*	Date
FP	PV	+	+	+	2/75
EF	ET	+	+	+	8/76
LF	PV	+	+	+	7/76
OM	ET	+	+	+	2/77
BS	PV	+	+	+	2/77
DS	ET	+†	+	+	8/75
MA	ET	+	NA	NA	12/74
BH	PV	+	+	NA	10/75
PL	PV	+	+	NA	2/75
JM	PV	–	–	–	11/76
AD	ET	–	–	–	11/76
IF	PV	–	–	–	3/75
BW	PV	–	–	–	1/77
SP	PV	–	–	–	12/76

*Aneuploidy with specific marker chromosomes.

†This patient was studied after busulfan therapy was started. The RDDP peak was observed at a density of 1.25 g/cc; subsequently RDDP activity was lost.

Abbreviations: RDDP, RNA-directed DNA polyermase; CPD, critical-point dried electron microscopic preparation; PV, polycythemia vera; ET, essential thrombocythemia; NA, not attempted.

in human platelets. Second, because of limited technologic capability with regard to RNA tumor viruses in human systems, large amounts of tissue would have to be available so that a human oncornavirus could be detected.

Essential thrombocythemia is characterized by hyperplasia of the megakaryocyte and, to a lesser extent, other hemopoietic lines. There is generally an excess of platelets, e.g.,[15] greater than one million per microliter, some neutrophilic leukocytosis, thrombocytosis and splenomegaly. In 1976, Adamson et al.,[16] utilizing the enzyme glucose-6-phosphate dehydrogenase (G-6-PD) as a genetic marker, presented evidence that PV is a clonal disorder of stem cells.

In addition, Wasserman[17] and others[18] reported the occurrence of acute leukemia in patients with PV. We, therefore, felt that studies of platelets from specific patients with PV and ET would provide the best opportunity to detect a human oncornavirus.

RNA Tumor Viruses in Polycythemia Vera and Essential Thrombocythemia

In 1975, our laboratory presented evidence for the presence of a C-type RNA tumor virus-like particle in platelets of thrombocythemic patients.[19] Electron microscopic studies of whole platelets revealed virus particles budding from platelet membranes (Fig. 39-1, *A* and *C*). In addition, sucrose equilibrium gradients of platelet homogenate showed both reverse transcriptase activity and visible virus-like particles (prepared for electron microscopy by the critical-point drying technique) at a density of 1.19 g/cc (Fig. 39-1, *D* and *E*). For comparison, Rauscher leukemia virus, prepared by identical methods, was similar in size and morphology (Fig. 39-1, *B* and *E*). Table 39-1 shows that in those cases of PV and ET where a virus was present, chromosomal abnormalities existed. Alternatively, in those cases of PV or ET studied where

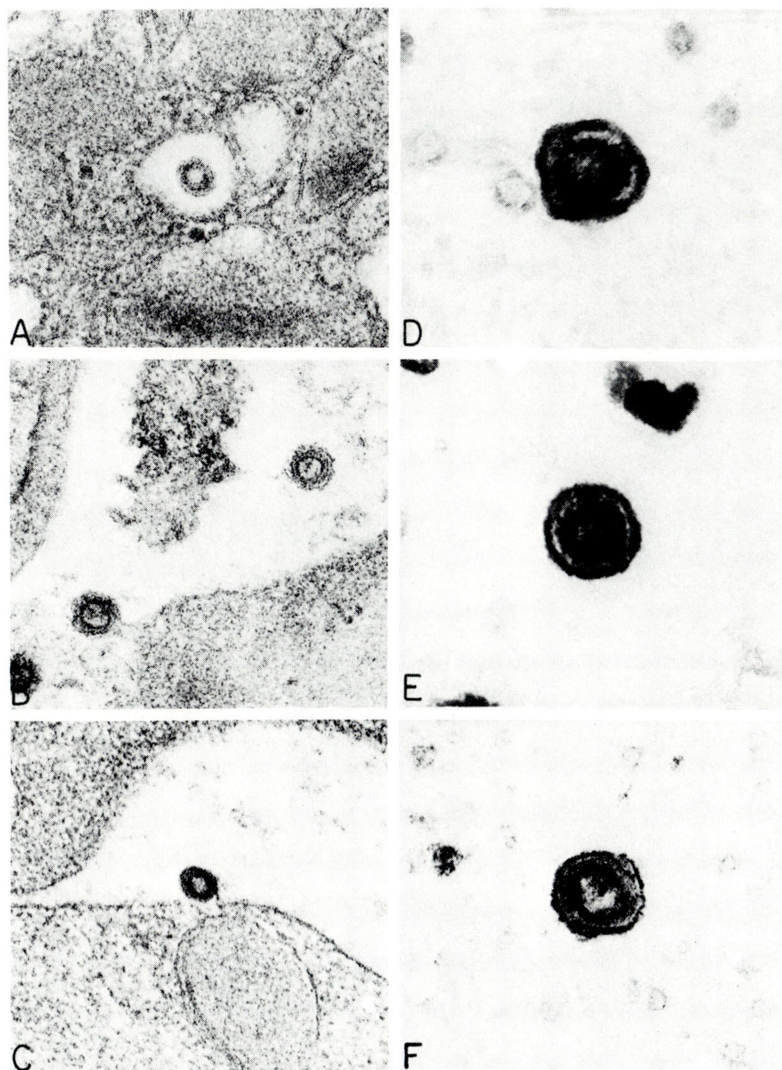

FIG. 39-1. Electron micrographs of virus particles. *A*, *B* and *C*, thin sections of virus-infected platelets prepared by our standard techniques.[19] *A* and *C*, samples obtained from patients; *B*, electron micrograph of Rauscher leukemia virus-infected murine platelets (× 82,000). *D*, *E* and *F*, sucrose gradient fractions prepared by the critical-point dried technique.[25] *D* and *E* were obtained from human subjects, *F* was obtained from a Rauscher leukemia virus-infected mouse (× 190,000).

there was no evidence of a virus, the chromosomal pattern was normal. The chromosomal instability found in virus-positive patients is thought to be associated with oncornavirus replication. These two distinct classes of patients suggest the existence of subsets of PV and ET.

STUDIES WITH BUSULFAN

Busulfan has been shown to be a clinically effective drug for controlling thrombocythemia with PV and ET. Studies were, therefore, initiated to determine whether this drug modified oncornaviral activity or genetic

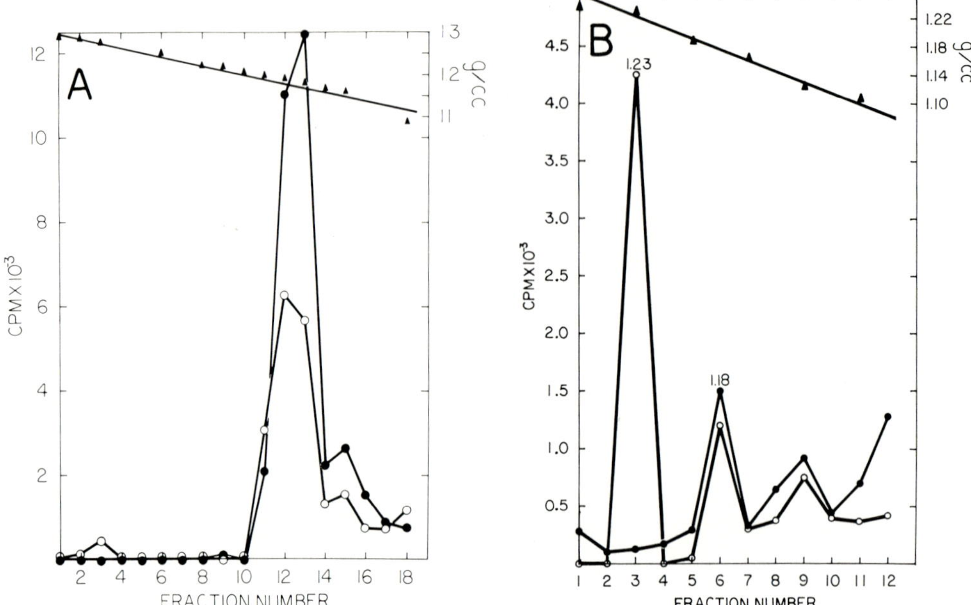

FIG. 39-2 In each case the platelets were disrupted and subjected to differential centrifugation. The supernatant was placed on linear sucrose equilibrium gradients according to our technique.[19] Each gradient was then fractionated and analyzed for the presence of a reverse transcriptase. CPM, counts per minute. *A*, an exogenous assay[20] of pretreatment platelets. The closed circles represent the activity using oligo $(dT)_{12\text{-}18} \cdot$ poly $(rA)_n$ as the primer-template; the open circles, activity utilizing oligo $(dT)_{12\text{-}18} \cdot$ poly $(dA)_n$. The triangles represent the density in grams per cubic centimeter. *B*, standard exogenous assay of platelets from patient during treatment. The open circles represent the activity using oligo $(dT)_{12\text{-}18} \cdot$ poly $(rA)_n$ as primer-template; the closed circles activity using oligo $(dT)_{12\text{-}18} \cdot$ poly $(dA)_n$.

stability. The formula of busulfan is $CH_3SO_2(CH_2)_4OS_2CH_3$ (dimethanesulphonoxyalkane). Busulfan is generally considered to be a mild alkylating agent. Its mode of action is not fully understood, however. Recent studies by Dunn demonstrated that busulfan does not act in the same manner as the other alkylating agents, such as the nitrogen mustard derivatives.[20] His studies indicate that busulfan selectively affects slowly proliferating stem cells rather than rapidly growing mature cells. It has been postulated that the cells most sensitive to busulfan would be those in which nucleic acids and proteins are in close proximity for long periods.[21] Busulfan is thus thought to mediate a linkage between nucleic acids and proteins. This minimal effect of busulfan on rapidly growing cells and preference for those cells in which nucleic acids and proteins are in close proximity for long periods of time would make the megakaryocyte or megakaryoblast a likely target for the action of this drug. The effect of busulfan on the megakaryocyte would most likely be apparent upon examination of the progeny of the megakaryocyte, the platelet.

In addition to surveying for the presence of oncornavirus markers in PV and ET platelets prior to, during and after busulfan treatment, it was decided to broaden our studies and investigate the platelet ultrastructure and chromosomal patterns during treatment.

All values (clinical, viral and genetic) showed a dramatic response to busulfan. After busulfan treatment (4 mg/day) was started, morphologically intact virus particles could no longer be observed either in the gradient fractions or in platelet thin sections. Reverse transcriptase assays from gradient fractions revealed a shift from the 1.19 to the 1.26 g/cc area of the gradient (Fig. 39-2, *A* and *B*). At this time, when the transitory 1.26 g/cc re-

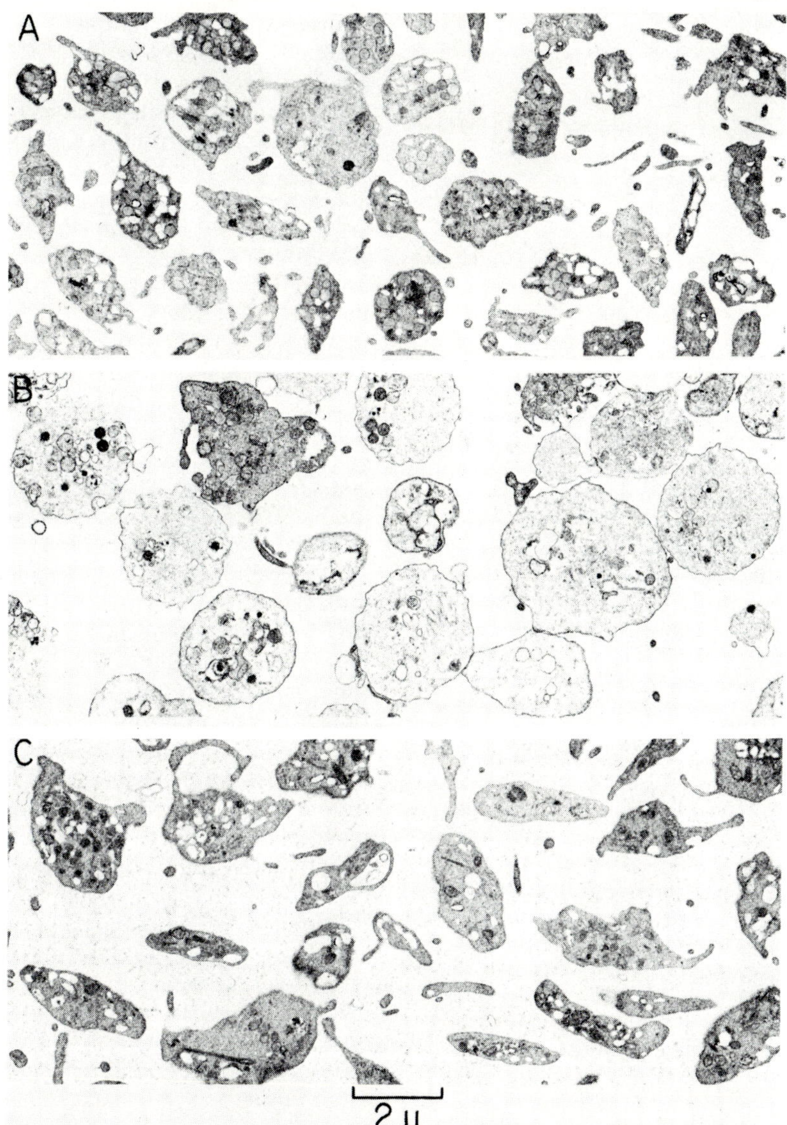

FIG. 39-3. Electron micrographs of platelets obtained from a patient with polycythemia vera (PV). The platelets were prepared by our standard techniques[19] (× 8,400). *A*, platelets obtained before treatment: *B*, platelets obtained during treatment; *C*, platelets obtained after treatment.

verse transcriptase was noted, the general ultrastructural morphology of the platelet was altered. Normal platelets are similar in structure to platelets from untreated and post-treated patients (Fig. 39-3, *A* and *C*). Observation of platelets during treatment revealed indistinct, possibly broken platelet membranes, with less dense than normal cytoplasm (Fig. 39-3, *C*). The overall shape of the platelets resembled distended spheres, in contrast to the normal discoid shape found in normal or pretreatment platelets. It is clear that the vast majority of platelets in newly treated PV or ET patients are morphologically abnormal. The disruption of the membranes and the subsequent effect on platelets suggest

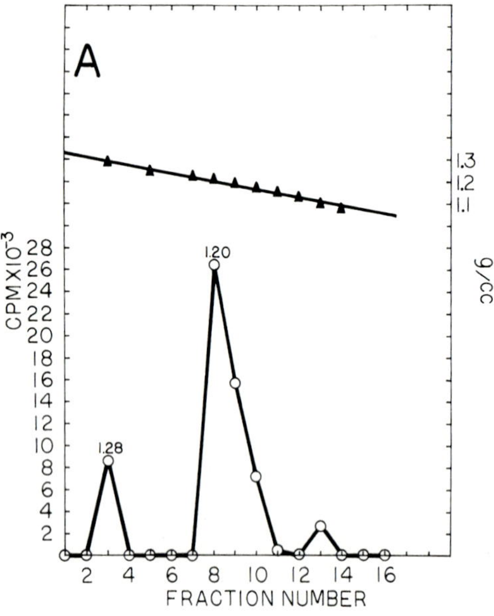

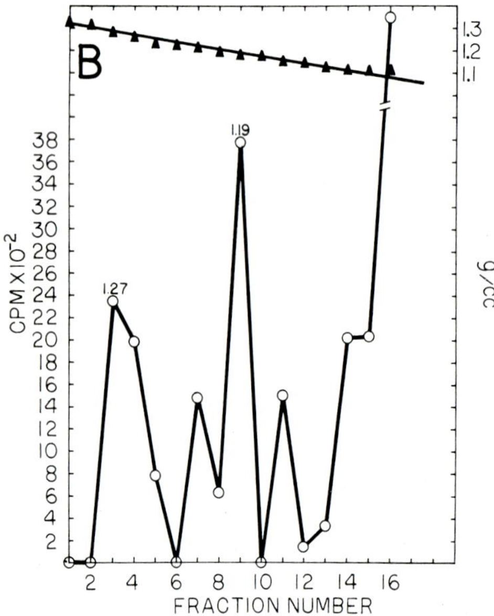

FIG. 39-4. *A*, endogenous assay[19] of a sample obtained from a patient during the early phases of busulfan therapy. The open circles represent the RDDP activity; the triangles, the density in g/cc. The density of each peak is indicated immediately above the peak. *B*, fractions 7, 8, and 9 of part *A* were pooled, treated with 0.2% Triton-X100 for 10 minutes at 4C and recentrifuged on a sucrose gradient. The gradient was then fractionated and assayed by the standard exogenous assay.[19]

damage to the microtubular and membrane system of the platelets.

It is interesting to note that virus particles with a higher density (1.26 g/cc) were found to be associated with these aberrant platelets. These results provide some insight into a possible consequence of busulfan treatment in these patients. The normal density of intact RNA tumor viruses is 1.19 g/cc. Busulfan therapy appears to alter the outer lipoprotein membrane of the human oncornavirus and platelet. It would appear that the shift in density of the reverse transcriptase in gradients of platelets obtained from busulfan-treated patients has resulted from the formation of incomplete virus particles manifested as viral cores (Fig. 39–44). This seems to indicate that the particles were formed with an incomplete or unstable outer membrane.

In addition to this phenomenon observed with the presumptive human RNA tumor virus, definite morphologic alterations have been observed in platelets obtained from these same busulfan-treated patients. Our observation of large uniformly spherical platelets, with an altered microtubular system and membranes, strongly suggests that busulfan is in some manner mediating a disruption of the platelet and, by extension, the megakaryocyte membrane system as well. Alternatively, electron micrographs of normal platelets reveal a continuous microtubular system with intact membranes. The effects of busulfan therapy on platelet morphology and biophysical properties of the oncornavirus may offer important clues to the pathogenesis and progression of these myeloproliferative disorders.

Viruses or viral markers have not been found in clinical subsets of PV and ET in which the karyotypic analysis was normal. This is not a surprising observation, as the expression of viral activity and production of chromosomal instability has been shown to be related to many systems.[22] Chromosomal instability has been related to viral replication rather than transformation since this phenomenon has been observed with both oncogenic and nononcogenic virus systems. Our studies demonstrate that busulfan-induced remission results in the loss of detectable virus-like particles and the restoration to a normal chromosomal complement (Fig. 39–5).

On the basis of the data presented in this

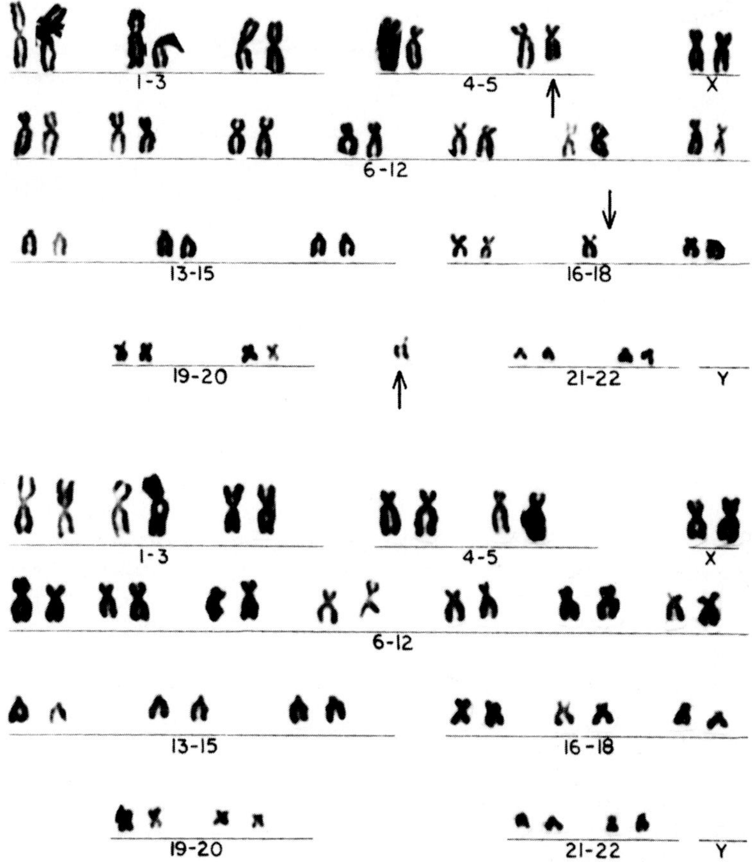

FIG. 39-5. Karyotype of a direct bone-marrow preparation from a patient prior to busulfan therapy. 45XX-E aneuploidy with a deletion in the long arm of Bq-chromosomes is shown. *B*, karyotype after therapy. Cells were prepared in the same manner as *A*. The Bq- and -E clone is no longer observed.

chapter, we assume that busulfan is affecting the virus, platelet and megakaryocyte. In addition, we suggest that the presumptive oncornavirus is in some manner responsible for chromosomal instability. In accordance with these assumptions, at least three hypotheses can be proposed for the action of busulfan in these patients: First, busulfan acts as an alkylating agent and directly and specifically affects nucleic acids and proteins in the nucleus of megakaryocytes. This mode of action, involving a large population of megakaryocytes, suggests a general cellular disruption directly resulting from the production of aberrant nucleic acids and proteins. Consequently, platelets produced from these megakaryocytes would appear in electron micrographs as being composed of incomplete microtubules and membranes. This would subsequently affect the population of oncornaviruses by depriving them of adequate membrane substrates from which to evaginate. With the reduction in virus population below our levels of detection, it would be possible for the viral effect on chromosomes to be decreased to a level where chromosomes would return to a normal state.

The second hypothesis is that in addition to alkylating the nucleic acids, busulfan specifically affects the membranes of the oncornavirus and platelets. This membrane alteration would produce incomplete viruses with an aberrant membrane structure. Virus particles would be sufficiently altered as to be unable to reinfect cells. The same chromosomal effect could be inferred as discussed in the first hypothesis.

The third hypothesis presumes the existence of an unusually busulfan-sensitive, virus-producing population or clone of megakaryocytes and platelets, coexisting with normal populations. In this hypothesis, in addition to producing a general reduction in nonsensitive platelet levels, busulfan would effect elimination of the sensitive clone(s). Eradication of the sensitive clone producing the oncornavirus would ultimately result in the loss of viral activity and the restabilization of chromosomes, as discussed in the first hypothesis.

Preliminary evidence obtained in our laboratory appears to favor the third theory. In studying specific cases of chronic myelocytic leukemia that were positive for oncornaviral indicators, chromosomal aneuploidy, and the pH[1] chromosomes, we observed a busulfan-sensitive population. After administering 24 mg of busulfan, we noted two morphologically separable populations of platelets. One population appeared to be composed of abnormal or damaged platelets similar to those found early in busulfan-treated patients with PV or ET. The second population appeared to consist of relatively normal platelets. After a total dosage of approximately 200 mg of busulfan, the abnormal platelets were no longer evident, and all platelets appeared to be morphologically normal. In addition, oncornaviral indicators and chromosomal aneuploidy were no longer detected although the pH[1] persisted.

After treatment with more than 400 mg of busulfan, the platelets continued to be morphologically normal. Furthermore, oncornavirus markers and chromosomal abnormalities did not reappear. Additional evidence for the third theory was obtained from studies on a virus-negative patient with PV. In this patient, busulfan treatment did not elicit the appearance of abnormal platelets. The platelet level in this patient dropped slowly with busulfan treatment and gave the appearance of a single population of platelets. This information suggests that a specific busulfan-sensitive clone of megakaryocytes or platelets exists and that the oncornavirus is associated with this clone. Additional evidence to support this idea is reported by Sheinin, who provided evidence that specific membrane modifications are common to transformed cells and that myeloproliferative diseases are of clonal origin.[23] In addition, Wasserman has suggested that the bone marrow of PV patients is more sensitive to busulfan treatment than that of normal individuals.[24] We feel that our studies will provide the parameters with which to monitor patient treatment and possibly assist in the diagnosis of these diseases.

References

1. Gallo R C, Yang S S, Ting R C: RNA-dependent DNA polymerase of acute leukemia cells. Nature 228:927, 1970
2. Helman R, Baxt W, Kufe D, Spiegleman S: Molecular evidence for viral etiology of human leukemias, lymphomas, and sarcomas. Am J Clin Pathol 60:65, 1973
3. Baxt W, Spiegleman S: Human leukemic cells contain reverse transcriptase associated with a high molecular weight, virus-related RNA. Nature New Biol 244:72, 1972
4. Todaro G J, Gallo R C: Immunological relationship of DNA polymerase from human acute leukemia cells and primate and mouse leukemias virus reverse transcriptase. Nature 244:206, 1973
5. Weimann B J, Kluge N, Dube S K, et al: Particle-associated RNA-dependent DNA polymerase and high-molecular-weight RNA in a human cell line derived from polycythemia vera bone marrow. J Natl Cancer Inst 55:537, 1975
6. Dmochowski L, Taylor A G, Gray G E, et al: Viruses and mycoplasma (PPLO) in human leukemia. Cancer 18:345, 1965
7. Seman G, Seman C: Electron-microscopic search for virus particles in patients with leukemia and lymphoma. Cancer, 22:1033, 1968
8. Schumacher H R, Szekely I E, Patel S B, et al: Leukemic mitochondria I. Acute myeloblastic leukemia. Am J Pathol 74:71, 1974
9. Brodsky I: Role of the megakaryocyte and

platelet in the leukemic process in mice and men: A review and hypothesis. J Natl Cancer Inst 51:329, 1973

10. Pagno J S: Epstein-Barr viral genome and its interactions with human lymphoblasted cells and chromosomes, in Kurstak, E, Maramorosch K (eds): Viruses, Evolution and Cancer: Basic Considerations. New York, Academic Press, 1974, p 80
11. Vigier P: Replication and integration of the genome of oncornaviruses, in Kurstak E, Maramorosch K (eds)): Viruses, Evolution and Cancer: Basic Considerations. New York, Academic Press, 1974, p 209
12. deHarven E, Friend C: Further electron microscopic studies of mouse leukemia induced by cell free filtrates. J Biophys Biochem Cytol 7:747, 1960
13. Dalton A J, Haguenau F, Maloney J B: Morphology of particles associated with murine leukemia as revealed by negative staining: Preliminary report. J Natl Cancer Inst 29:1177, 1962
14. Laird H M, Jarrett O, Creighton G W, et al: Replication of leukemogenictype virus in cats inoculated with lymphosarcoma extracts. J Natl Cancer Inst 41:879, 1968
15. Gunz F W: Essential thrombocythemia, in Williams W J, Beutler E, Erslev A J, Rundels R W (eds) Hematology. New York, McGraw-Hill, 1972, p 704
16. Adamson J W, Fialkow P J, Murphy S, et al: Polycythemia vera: Stem cell and probable clonal origin of the disease. N Engl J Med 295:913, 1976
17. Wasserman L R; Polycythemia vera—its course and treatment: Relation to myeloid metaplasia and leukemia. Bull NY Acad Med 3:343, 1954
18. Perkins J, Israels M C G, Wilkinson J F: Polycythemia vera: Clinical studies on a series of 127 patients managed without radiation therapy. QJ Med 33:499, 1964
19. Brodsky I, Fuscaldo A A, Erlick B J, et al: Analysis of platelets from patients with thrombocythemia for reverse transcriptase and virus-like particles. J Natl Cançer Inst 55:1069, 1975
20. Dunn C D R: The clinical and biological properties of busulfan (Myleran). Exp Hematol 2:101, 1974
21. Dunn C D R, Elson L A: The effects of a homologous series of dimethanesulphonoxyalkanes on hemopoietic colony forming units in the rat. Chem-Biol Interactions 2:273, 1970
22. Wurster-Hill D, Whang-Peng J, McIntyre R, et al: Cytogenetic studies in polycythemia vera. Semin Hematol 13:13, 1976
23. Sheinin R: The cell surface, virus modification and virus transformation, in Kurstak E, Maramorasch K (eds): Viruses, Evolution and Cancer. New York, Academic Press, 1974, p 371
24. Wasserman L R: The treatment of polycythemia vera. Semin Hematol 13:57, 1976
25. Brodsky I, Fuscaldo A A, Erlick B J, Fuscaldo K E: Effect of busulfan on oncornavirus-like activity in platelets and chromosomes in polycythemia vera and essential thrombocythemia. J Natl Cancer Inst 59:61, 1977

KATHRYN E. FUSCALDO, ISADORE BRODSKY
S. BENHAM KAHN, JAMES F. CONROY

40

Cytogenetics of Myeloproliferative Disorders: Implications in Chronic Granulocytic Leukemia

Chromosomal analysis to confirm the diagnosis of chronic myelocytic leukemia (CML) has been well documented.[1-6] The presence of the Ph[1] in bone marrow aspirates has virtually become a standard for diagnosis. Almost 90 per cent of the patients with the signs of CML are Ph[1] positive.[7-10] It has been suggested that the term *subacute myelocytic leukemia* be applied to Ph[1]-negative patients, since statistical differences have been found with respect to natural history, response to therapy, age of onset and sex prevalence.[10]

Diagnostic chromosomal markers have not been confirmed for the other myeloproliferative disorders (MPD)*, although reports of nonrandom chromosome changes have appeared in the literature[11-18] and have been documented in our laboratory. In the chronic myeloproliferative disorders leading to acute nonlymphoblastic leukemia (ANLL), such as CML, polycythemia vera (PV), essential thrombocythemia (ET) and myelofibrosis with myeloid metaplasia (MMM), abnormal karyotypes are observed, particularly as the disease progresses or enters a more undifferentiated phase.[12-60] While progression to ANLL may occur in all of the myeloproliferative diseases, the time to transformation and even its occurrence is variable in PV and MMM but occurs invariably in chronic myelocytic leukemia, although over an inconstant time span. This variability in time to transformation suggests that CML may be a broad clinical entity encompassing several subgroups that manifest an unstable karyotype and lead to differing responses to therapy and differing clinical courses.[10,11,39,42,46,52-55,61-63,70]†

Substantial evidence suggests that CML is a stem-cell disorder and that a viral agent may be involved in the etiology of the disease.[42,55,60,61,64-78] Regardless of the nature of the "leukemia-inducing agent," however, it has been assumed that some factor contributes to, regulates or causes (1) the genesis of the Ph[1] chromosome; (2) stem-cell proliferation and differentiation; (3) the role of the microenvironment in extramedullary sites, for example, the spleen, liver and lymph nodes; (4) the regulatory mechanisms governing

*We have recently demonstrated the presence of a new chromosomal abnormality, $21q^-$, in patients with primary thrombocythemia who are also positive for retroviral indicators (Fig. 40-8).[106]

†Several groups, including our own, have recently described an ALL type transformation in CML. These patients are TdT positive, may not show chromosomal evolution, and do not respond to Vincristine and Prednisone.[107]

granulopoiesis, erythropoiesis, and myelopoiesis; and (5) the metamorphosis of the chronic phase to one resembling ANLL.

The term *metamorphosis*[81] is based on the following considerations:

The old term *blastic crisis* accurately describes the termination of only a minority of cases of CML; the term *metamorphosis*, which encompasses all cases of CML, can be subdivided as follows:

1. Blast crisis (5 to 10 per cent of patients)—rapid onset of leukocytosis, preponderance of blasts, rapidly developing into neutropenia and thrombocytopenia, progressive course, death common in 2 to 6 weeks.
2. Acute transformation (50 per cent of patients)—onset over a period of weeks and months of a picture superficially resembling ANLL, more gradual development of neutropenia and thrombocytopenia (unless aggravated by therapy); survival for 3 to 6 months not uncommon.
3. Mixed group (about 40 per cent of patients)—a great variety of clinical and hematologic pictures, including thrombocytosis, thrombocytopenia, refractory anemia, polycythemia, myelofibrosis, leukopenia, erythropoietic aplasia, and accelerated granulopoiesis without excessive left shift. This syndrome cannot be justifiably termed either blastic or acute as it may have a course of either months or years. Metamorphosis to this form suggests that ANLL-type therapy may be inappropriate.

Because CML undergoing metamorphosis is often accompanied or preceded by unusual chromosomal anomalies in the bone marrow and extramedullary sites, it was thought that serial chromosomal analysis might be useful in monitoring the disease and assessing prognosis. Indeed, the data suggest that abolition or reduction of abnormal karyotypes by intensive chemotherapy might prevent or delay the metamorphosis in CML. For this reason, experiments were designed to test the value of serial chromosomal analysis in the patient undergoing intensive chemotherapy so as to monitor the efficacy of such therapy, to predict an impending "metamorphosis" of the disease, and to correlate specific chromosomal anomalies other than the Ph[1] chromosome with hematologically defined phases of the disease process. The results will be discussed in the appropriate section.

The Therapy of CML

Since 1953, the standard form of therapy for CML has been the initial induction of remission with busulfan and then maintenance with the same drug on a continuous low-dosage basis. The increase in survival achieved by this program over untreated controls is of borderline significance.[42] Although busulfan alleviates the symptoms, the increase in median survival is only about 6 months. There has been no significant increase in survival in CML patients in the last 23 years.[42,81] In an attempt to prolong life expectancy, we have instituted a new regimen.[42] Four components of the therapeutic protocol have been adopted:

1. Busulfan-induced hematologic remission;
2. Splenectomy immediately following induction of remission;
3. Chemotherapy utilizing cycle-active drugs;
4. Sequential chromosomal analysis of bone marrow aspirates to determine the efficacy of treatment.

Busulfan-induced Hematologic Remission

Although busulfan has been used for years to induce and maintain hematologic remission in CML, there has been and ought to be dissatisfaction with the drug. Spiers[81] has reviewed the literature with respect to busulfan and found that (1) the initial response is over 90 per cent; (2) there is gratifying improvement in symptoms; (3) the hematologic state approaches normal; and (4) most important, survival has not been improved appreciably! In addition, side effects of long-term therapy include pigmentation, amenorrhea and pulmonary fibrosis. Busulfan does not eliminate the Ph[1] chromosome or prevent other chromosome abnormalities. Indeed, the drug may be mutagenic, favoring the production of new clones. It has been suggested that the inevitable metamorphosis of CML may be hastened by the use of this drug, although there is no evidence that the drug shortens life expectancy.

For these reasons, alternative nonmutagenic, nontoxic induction and maintenance programs have been sought. Splenic irradiation[83,84] and hydroxyurea[85] are two such alternatives. Yet, in a study conducted by the British Medical Research Council, busulfan proved to be a better agent with which to treat CML than splenic irradiation or hydroxyurea.[81] The median survival time for the busulfan-treated patients was 39 months, while the survival time for the ^{32}P-treated patients was 28 months.

Studies in our laboratory have shown that busulfan has specific effects on the megakaryocyte and ultimately the platelet. Our data suggest that this effect may be more selective than that of a general alkylating agent. Busulfan may have an effect on platelet membrane and, more likely, on the postulated viral membrane. The chapter in this volume by Anthony A. Fuscaldo et al reviews in detail the information that relates to the viral etiology of CML and PV.

In view of its pronounced effect on platelet morphology and production, busulfan may prevent postoperative thrombocytosis in patients treated with splenectomy.

Splenectomy

Splenectomy, a feasible procedure early in the course of CML, is associated with limited risks and morbidity. The question remains, however, whether removal of the spleen early in the chronic phase of the disease prolongs life and reduces the complications of splenomegaly once the disease has undergone metamorphosis.[42,81-99] Several groups have suggested that the spleen may be a major source of complications in CML because it may develop extramedullary hematopoiesis;[42] harbor oncornaviruses;[42,73,76,77,78] selectively hold granulopoietic cells with potentially neoplastic properties;[72,80] be the site of cell-mediated immune reactions; provide a suitable microenvironment for preferential stem cell proliferation;[98,99] and be a primary site of blastic transformation in CML.[41,42,47]

For these reasons, removal of the spleen early in the chronic phase of the disease may contribute to prolonging life expectancy.

Studies by other groups[85,86] have shown that removal of the spleen or splenic irradiation[83,84] does not cause an increase in survival. Coupled with intensive chemotherapy, however, splenectomy may prove to be beneficial. Our results indicate that under proper conditions of remission induction and postoperative support, the operative mortality and morbidity are negligible and postoperative thrombocytosis is not a problem.

Intensive Chemotherapy

Acute nonlymphoblastic leukemia-like therapy follows splenectomy in this protocol. Other investigators have also considered such therapy valid.

The blastic phase of the disease has been treated for some time with a regimen developed for ANLL. Several large cooperative groups in the United States and Europe have instituted protocols to test the efficacy of aggressive chemotherapy in the early phases of CML. The Italian Cooperative Study Group on Chronic Myeloid Leukemia and the British Medical Research Council Working Party for Therapeutic Trials in Leukemia—Granulocytic Leukemia—have initiated studies to test various therapeutic modalities and drug combinations. Among the drugs used have been the following: cytosine arabinoside (Ara-C), 6-thioguanine (6-TG), vincristine, hydroxyurea prednisone, daunorubicin, busulfan methotrexate, adriamycin, 6-mecaptopurine, and cyclophosphamide. These drugs have also been used by workers in the United States, particularly in our own study adopted by the Eastern Cooperative Oncology Group. Workers at the Sloan-Kettering Memorial Cancer Institute have also evaluated intensive chemotherapy regimens.

The combination of Ara-C and 6-TG has been shown to be particularly effective in the treatment of ANLL. When used to treat CML, Ara-C appears to be more active against myeloblasts than against promyelocytes and myelocytes.[42] Since CML is a stem-cell disorder,[42,64-70] chemotherapy should be directed at the stem cell or, at the least, the early committed stem cells of the bone marrow. Consequently, Ara-C and 6-TG were chosen as the intensive chemotherapeutic arm of the Hahnemann and ECOG protocol. Similar

EFFECT OF SPLENECTOMY AND INTENSIVE CHEMOTHERAPY

ON ONSET OF METAMORPHOSIS AND SURVIVAL IN CGL

SCHEMA

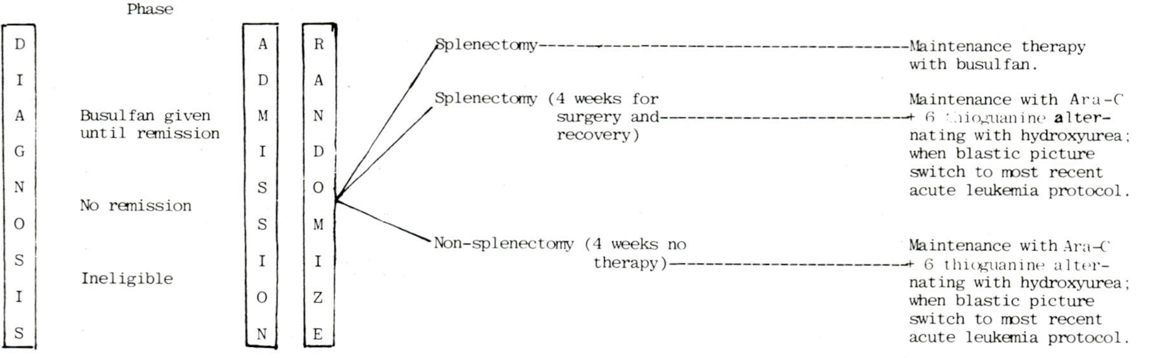

The chemotherapy in Arm 2 and Arm 3 is a repeating 8-week module, as follows:

WEEK 1: 6 thioguanine 100 mg/m^2 q 12h for 5 days (10 doses) + ara-C 150 mg/m^2 q 24h for 5 days (5 doses). Daily Ara-C suggested for convenience and to increase patient acceptability.

WEEK 2: no therapy

WEEK 3 through 7: hydroxyurea q 12h to maintain leukocyte count between 7,000 and 12,000 per microliter. Doses vary considerably in individual patients but most fall in the range 500 - 2,000 mg of hydroxyurea per day.

WEEK 8: no therapy

The module is then repeated. Doses of ara-C and thioguanine may be increased in later courses depending on response. The total leukocyte count should have a nadir between 3,000 and 5,000 after each course of ara-C + thioguanine.

FIG. 40-1. Three armed protocol designed to evaluate the efficacy of splenectomy with and without intensive chemotherapy.

considerations led to the inclusion of these drugs and others by the Italian, British and Sloan-Kettering groups.

The use of intermittent cycle-active therapy with several drugs is based on the following considerations: (1) prevention of the development of the resistant clones; (2) reduction or elimination of abnormal clones; and (3) prevention of cumulative drug toxicity and avoidance of selective effects of any one drug on cell proliferation.

An outline of the currently used protocol is given in Figure 40-1.

On the basis of our experience, we have placed our patients on a three-drug regimen, that is, cycles of Ara-C and 6-TG, with hydroxyurea maintenance between cycles for 18 to 24 months, assuming that clonal evolution does not occur. If abnormal clones appear in the bone marrow, we have modified the therapy as follows: a combination of hydroxyurea, 1500 to 2000 mg a day; cyclophosphamide, 50 to 100 mg a day; and MTX, 10 mg every fourth day. This combination regimen has been extremely effective for intermittent maintenance and may be of definite benefit in preventing the emergence of abnormal clones.

For those cases in which this drug combination has not been successful, daunorubicin (daunomycin) and Ara-C have been used. Even more recently, we have substituted adriamycin and Ara-C, which we will continue to use. In our initial series (7 patients), daunorubicin and Ara-C were used before starting the cyclophosphamide/methotrexate/hydroxyurea regimen. With prolonged survival, it may be necessary to use even more intensive therapeutic regimens. Therefore, as new drugs are evaluated and prove effective for the treatment of ANLL, they may be incorporated into this series.

Our studies have shown that the appearance of abnormal clones has been associated with the subsequent elevation in white blood cell count and thrombocytosis and, more ominously, with thrombocytopenia. With the reduction in or eradication of the abnormal clones, there has been a return to more normal hematologic values. For these reasons, the frequency and nature of therapy have been predicated on the results of the cytogenetic studies. We cannot predict which drugs (and in what combinations) we will use in future modifications of therapy. That decision will depend on the best available drugs at the time therapy is initiated.

Sequential Surveys of Bone Marrow Aspirates for Abnormal Clones.

The ultimate aim of most studies has been to eradicate the Ph^1 chromosome to effect a cure of the disease. Although elimination or reduction in size of the Ph^1 positive clone has been reported, the phenomenon has been transitory in all cases. Our studies suggest that a more significant goal of therapy should be prevention, reduction or elimination of abnormal chromosomes other than the Ph^1 chromosome. For this reason, serial cytogenetic studies are essential.

CYTOGENETICS

The literature concerning the evolution of abnormal karyotypes in dividing cells of the bone marrow is substantial.[6,11-23,25-71,81] The potential predictive value of cytogenetic studies has been acknowledged by many investigators. There is little doubt that metamorphosis of CML into an acute leukemia-like syndrome is preceded by the development of aneuploidy and the appearance of nonrandom clones, including +C8, +D, −C, i17, and multiple Ph^1 chromosomes. The question, however, remains as to whether cytogenetic studies at periodic intervals during the course of the chronic disease can be an effective routine procedure on which to base subsequent therapeutic intervention.

Also of interest is whether the routine use of chromosomal banding techniques[104,105] can increase the capability of the test to predict impending transformation. Standard techniques used to prepare karyotypes[100-103] are effective in detecting abnormalities in chromosome number and gross structural abnormalities. More advanced banding techniques[104,105] are required to visualize subtle chromosomal alterations and to make positive identification of chromosomes within groups. It is difficult to do banding on a routine basis in the service laboratory. If banding proves valuable, its routine use could be justified.

TABLE 40-1. *Protocol Patients Survival—CML Patients Treated Experimentally*

Patient	Age/Sex	Splenectomy Months Post Dx	Survival Months to 9/1/77	
EM	42 F	48	115	
MB	34 F	38	91 Dead	
GT	50 F	20	92	
FS	52 F	28	68 Dead	
CU	59 M	13	66 Dead	
JF	28 M	11	62	
				82.8 mo.
MS	45 M	8	51	
RF	56 M	8	45	
HG	57 M	22	44	
				70.8 mo.
JH	29 M	3	40	
FF	51 F	6	29	
DS	35 M	7	28	
FK	29 M	5	16	
FN	46 F	4	16	
JG	34 F	3	14	
PB	32 M	5	10	
SDA	34 M	6	7	
				46.9 mo.

Our data suggest that standard cytogenetic testing is both feasible and efficacious, and it remains for larger statistically valid samples using banding methods to confirm this contention.

Several investigators have shown that the granulocyte monocyte stem cell (CFU-C) can form colonies in agar culture in the presence of specific colony-stimulating factor (CSF). Bone marrow and peripheral blood obtained from CML patients also showed a consistently abnormal buoyant density.[50,68,71] Moore has suggested that the study of in vitro growth values during the clinical course of CML may have predictive value as to progression of disease in response to therapy.[71] Moore states that the phenomenon of dyshematopoiesis as seen in CML "is not of itself sufficient to permit the conclusion that the Ph[1] translocation causes neoplastic transformation of a stem cell, but rather, it leads to an intrinsic stem cell disorder associated with deranged responsiveness to regulatory control. The justification in considering CML as a leukemia is that it almost invariably terminates as ANLL and clearly exhibits features of progression of clonal evolution as determined by clinical, cytogenetic and in vitro culture techniques. The ability to identify abnormal clones by cytogenetic techniques and/or by analysis of in vitro growth patterns many weeks or months prior to clinical evidence of metamorphosis may be of considerable value if it can be shown that intensive chemotherapy applied at this early stage could eradicate the abnormal clones." Our results suggest that this is indeed the case.

RESULTS AND CONCLUSIONS

The results of our initial studies utilizing this protocol have been published.[42] The data presented in Table 40-1 are for the group of 17 splenectomized patients entered into the experimental protocol since 1968. The median survival in this group (6 patients) who have survived 60 months or longer is 82.8 months. For those in the study for 44 months or longer (9 patients), the median survival is

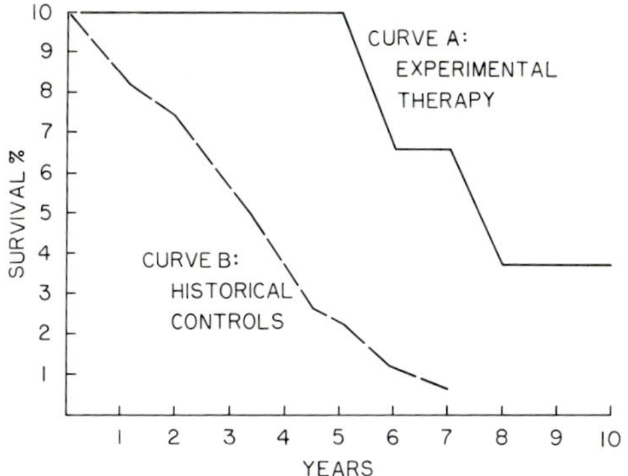

FIG. 40-2. Actuarial curve showing survival of the experimental group as compared with historical controls.

70.8 months. Median survival for the entire group of 17 patients is 46.9 months. A statistical analysis by the actuarial method [106] comparing our results with those in historical controls is significant ($P<0.01$) (Fig. 40-2). Equally significant is the fact that no deaths occurred in our series prior to 66 months. In a comparable series of patients treated conventionally by our group, only 1 patient has survived longer than 42 months, and 3 have died at 36, 24 and 20 months.

Several examples of the response to aggressive therapy are given in Figures 40-3 through 40-7. The data in Figure 40-3 show response in patient MF. The response to therapy is remarkable in that several ominous clones, including i17 (Fig. 40-4) and double Ph^1 (Fig. 40-5) either disappeared or were reduced significantly. A similar response can be seen (Fig. 40-6) in patient JF. Figure 40-7 presents the data for GT. This patient also lost an i17 clone as well as sustaining the reduction in double Ph^1 clone. Those patients presenting with the clinical manifestations of aggressive disease all have significant aneuploidy. An analysis of the chromosomal findings on initial diagnosis is presented in Table 40-2. Forty-six out of 47 patients in our study were Ph^1-positive. At initial presentation, 44 per cent of the Ph^1-positive patients did not have any other chromosomal anomalies. This figure compares favorably with the data reported by Hossfeld;[44] 46.6 per cent of the Ph^1-positive patients presented without additional anomalies. We have also observed, as did Hossfeld, that not all Ph^1-positive CML patients present with Ph^1 in all of their dividing cells. The heterogeneity found both in our series and that reported by Hossfeld may indeed reflect the greater attention being taken in detailed cytogenetic analysis of statistically significant numbers of dividing bone marrow cells. The most frequent chromosomal anomalies found in our studies, aside from C-group aneuploidy, were the clones containing an extra D-group (5 out of 17 patients). More significant, however, the finding of the extra D-chromosome or double Ph^1 can be correlated with

TABLE 40-2. *Cytogenetic Findings on Presentation*

Patient	Aneuploidy	Patient	Aneuploidy
EM	0	EW	47% PhPh
MB	0	RR	NAT
FS	0	MK	35%+D
GT	0	WB	28% PhPh
CU	0	WG	40% PhPh
JF	0	AP	NA
MS	0	PA	0
RF	15%	CC	NAT
HG	12%-Y	CB	85% PhPh+C+G
JH	0	HE	80%
JL	0	MM	0
FF	40%-C	JM	15%
DS	10%+D	AO	39%+D PhPh
CB	17%-F	JP	30%
FK	28%+D	LE	20%
FN	NAT PhPh	TG	100% Ph^0
JG	22% PhPh	RH	20%
DO	13%-Y	AB	22%-C-Y
BR	20%-C	FLeF	24%
CU	0	EB	33%+D
WM	0	LW	0
JP	0 PhPh	RMcL	30%
DJ	22% PhPh		
LS	NA	NA Patient diagnosed elsewhere	
NF	NA	Initial cytogenetics not available	

Abbreviations: NAT, % aneuploidy not available because of poor technical quality of preparation; NA, not available.

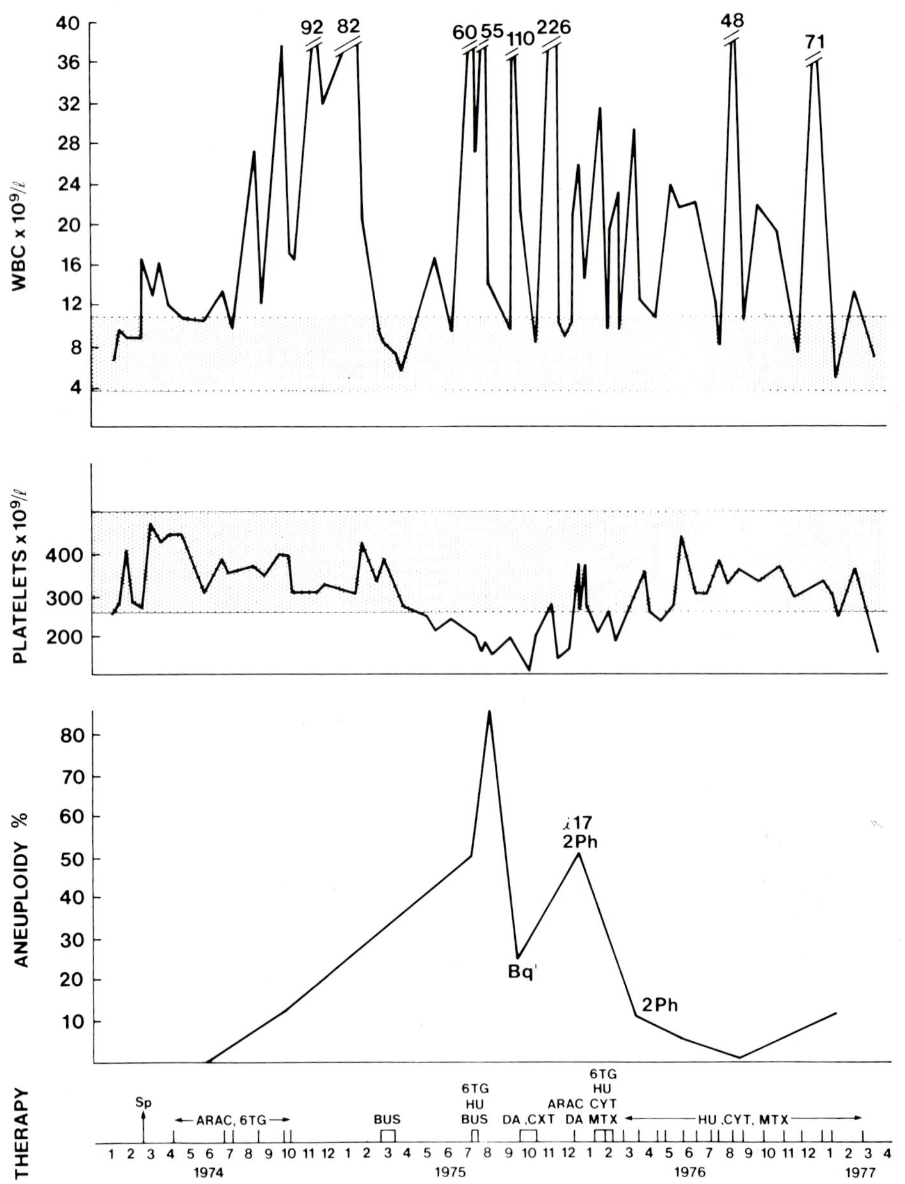

FIG. 40-3. Hematological and chromosomal data for patient M.S., a 46 year old white male.

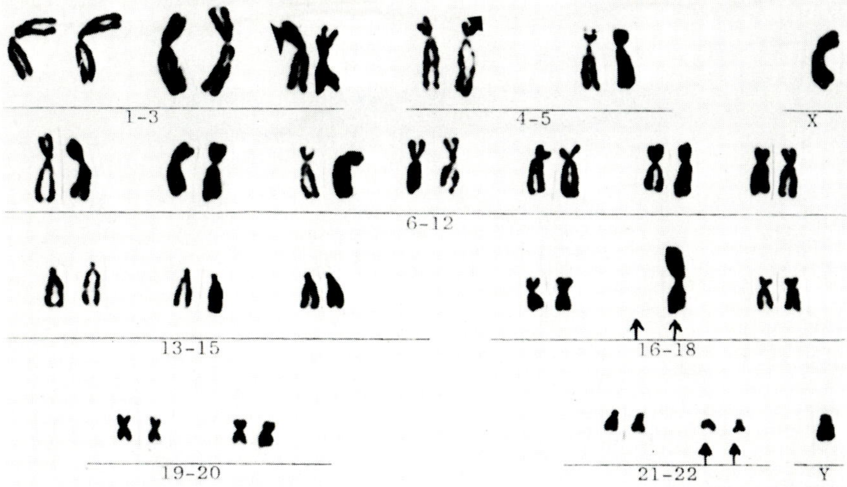

FIG. 40-4. Karyotype showing the i17 chromosome 45XY-E + i17 Ph[1] Ph[1].

either a stormier course in the aggressively treated patient (DF and FK) or a poorer prognosis (MD, JP, DF, EW, WD, WV, CB, AR, ED). The results of cytogenetic studies of patients with other myeloproliferative disorders have also proved interesting. These data are more fully described elsewhere in the chapter by A. A. Fuscaldo et al. The observation that abnormal clones are transitory, that is, that they appear and can be eliminated by appropriate therapy, is also evident in the studies of PV and ET.

The results of our cytogenetic, biochemical and morphologic studies are consistent with the hypothesis that the leukemias have a viral etiology. Assuming that the viral information is present endogenously and that some "factors" or "agents" trigger its expression, the sequence of events leading to neoplastic transformation may be postulated as follows:

1. Derepression of regulatory control mechanisms leading to production of intact viral particles. This phase is seen in the

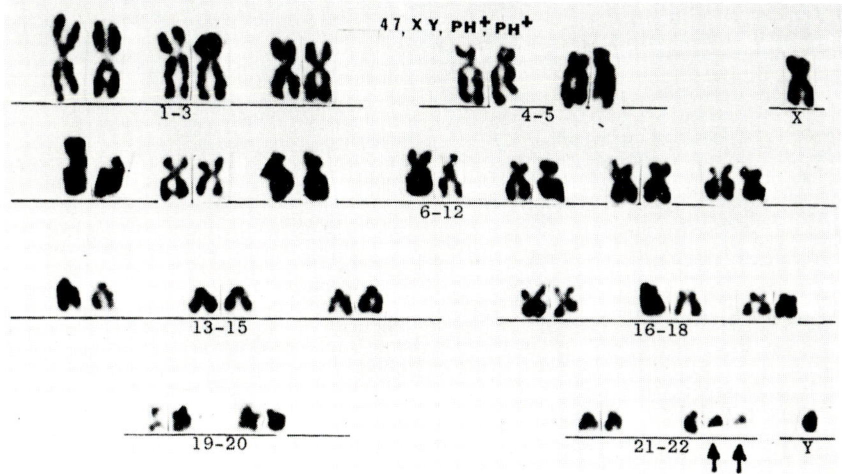

FIG. 40-5. Karyotype showing double Philadelphia chromosome 47XY Ph[1] Ph[1].

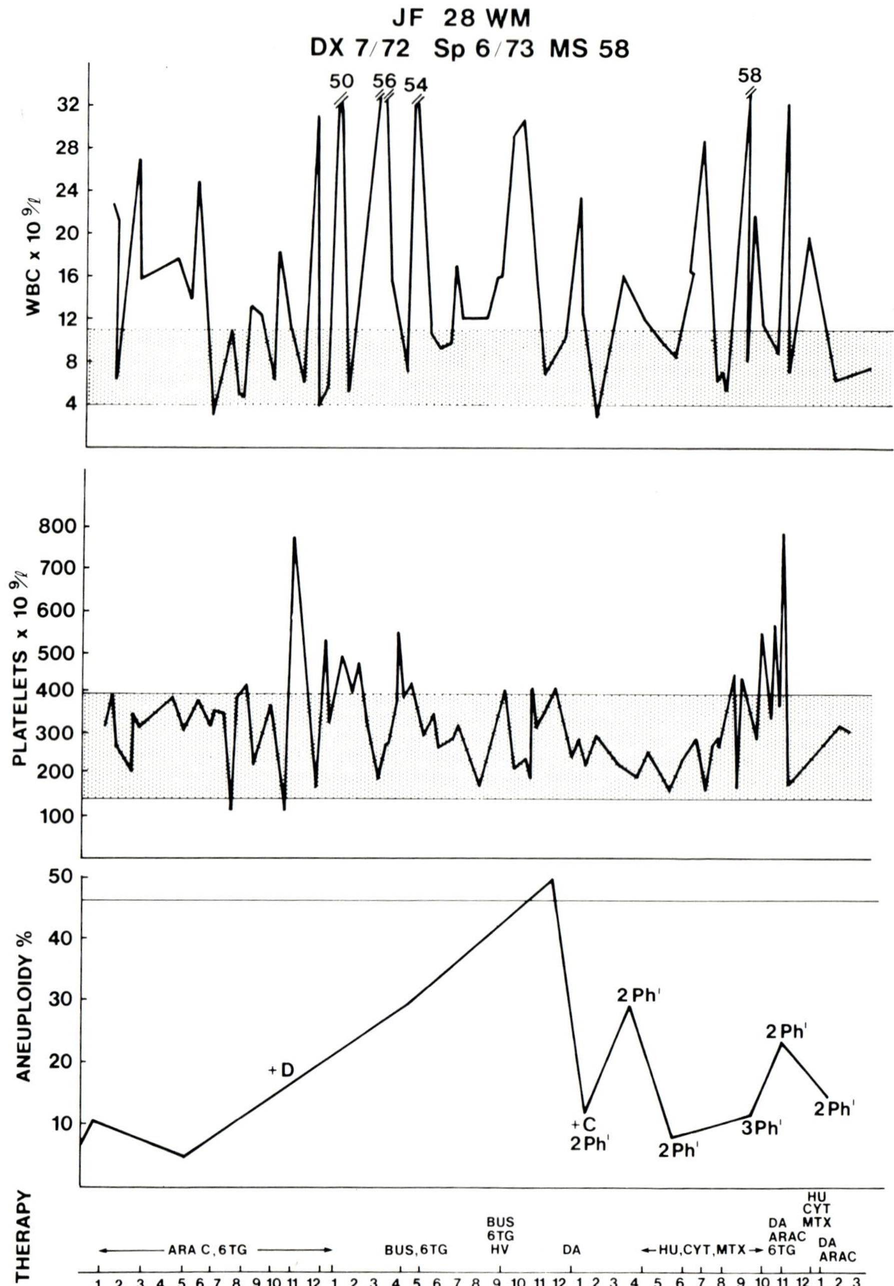

FIG. 40-6. Hematological and chromosomal data for patient J.F., a 28 year old white male.

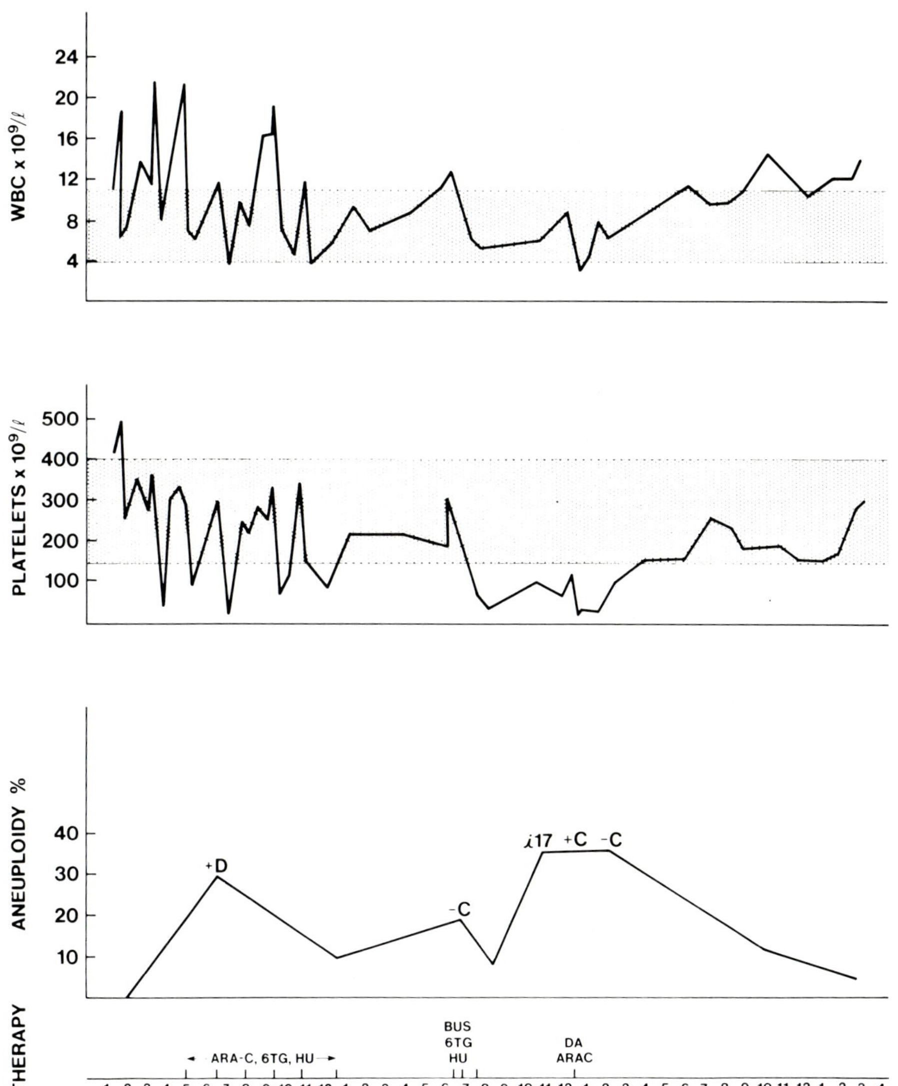

FIG. 40-7. Hematological and chromosomal data for patient G.T., a 50 year old white female.

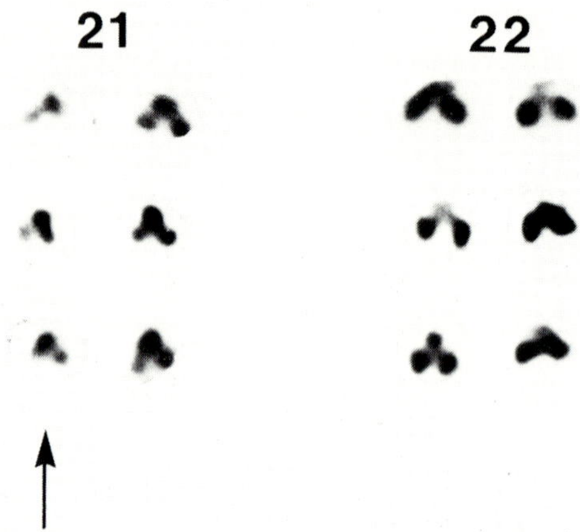

FIG. 40-8. R-banded chromosomes 21 and 22, showing 21q⁻.

preneoplastic conditions, PV and ET, and in the remission of acute leukemia.

2. The synthesis and replication of intact virus take place in the megakaryocyte and can be seen in the platelet. The response of ET and PV as well as CML to busulfan therapy reflects this stage of the process. Elimination of the abnormal clones containing virus by therapy results in loss of viral indicators and morphologically abnormal platelets.
3. A virus causes chromosomal instability of both a specific (Ph[1]) and random nature (aneuploidy). This phase of the infective process is characterized by abnormal cytogenetic and CFU-C values.
4. Elimination of the virus by therapy at this stage results in a loss of viral indicators and a return to more normal cytogenetic and platelet morphologic status.
5. If the virus-containing cells are not eliminated, the virus is incorporated into the host genome. When integration occurs, viral particles are no longer detectable by electron microscope. RNA-dependent DNA polymerase (RDDP) may be detected in appropriate tissues, for example, spleen, plasma, white blood cells or platelets, but the particle itself cannot be visualized. Great chromosomal instability occurs with clonal evolution. Neoplastic transformation ensues.

More extensive data will have to be gathered to substantiate each of these points. However, so far as therapeutic intervention is concerned, the CML, PV and ET studies suggest that chemotherapy may be most effective in prolonging survival if it is given prior to viral integration. The use of sequential cytogenetic monitoring of the patient during the course of the disease appears to provide the best means available at present to predict therapeutic changes aimed at prolonging survival.

REFERENCES

1. Nowell P C, Hungerford D A: A minute chromosome in human chronic granulocytic leukemia. Science 132:1497, 1960
2. Nowell P C, Hungerford D A: Chromosome studies on normal and leukemic leukocytes. J Natl Cancer Inst 25:85, 1960
3. Adams A, Fitzgerald P H, Gunz F W: A new chromosomal abnormality in chronic granulocytic leukemia. Br Med J 2:1474, 1961
4. Fitzgerald P H, Adams A, Gunz F W: Chronic granulocytic leukemia and the Philadelphia chromosome. Blood 21:183, 1963
5. Tjio J H, Carbone P P, Whang J, Frei E III: The Philadelphia chromosome and chronic

myelogenous leukemia. J Natl Cancer Inst 36:567, 1966

6. Stemple R M: Philadelphia chromosome in leukemia research: A bibliography. US Atomic Energy Commission ORNL: TM2103, 1968
7. Rowley J D: A new consistent chromosomal abnormality in chronic myelogenous leukemia identified by quinacrine fluorescence and giemsa staining. Nature 243:290, 1973
8. Whang J, Frei E III, Tjio J H, et al: The distribution of Philadelphia chromosome in patients with CML. Blood 22:664, 1963
9. Krauss S, Solol F, Sandberg A A: Comparison of Philadelphia chromosome positive and negative patients with chronic myelocytic leukemia. Ann Intern Med 6:625, 1964
10. Ezdinli E Z, Sokal J E, Crosswhite L, Sandberg A A: Philadelphia positive and Philadelphia negative chronic myelocytic leukemia. Ann Intern Med 72:175, 1970
11. Whang-Peng J, Canellos G P, Carbone P P, et al: Clinical implications of cytogenetic variants in chronic myelocytic leukemia. Blood 32:755, 1968
12. Wurster-Hill P, Whang-Peng J, McIntyre R, et al: Cytogenetic studies in polycythemia vera. Semin Hematol 13:13, 1976
13. Engel E, McKee L C, Flexner J M, McGee B J: 17 long arm isochromosome. A common anomaly in malignant blood disorders. Ann Genet 18:56, 1975
14. Ford J H, Pittman S M, Singh S, et al: Cytogenetic basis of acute myeloid leukemia. J Natl Cancer Inst 55:761, 1975
15. Rowley J D: Acquired trisomy 9. Lancet 2:390, 1973
16. Rowley J D: Missing sex chromosomes and translocations in acute leukemia. Lancet 2:835, 1974
17. Rowley J: Nonrandom chromosomal abnormalities in hematologic disorders in man. Proc Natl Acad Sci USA 72:152, 1975
18. Rowley J: Abnormalities of chromosome 1 in myeloproliferative disorders. Cancer 36:1748, 1975
19. Sandberg A A: Chromosomes and leukemia. Cancer 15:2, 1965
20. Kemp N S, Strafford J, Tanner R: Chromosome studies during early and terminal chronic myeloid leukemia. Br J Med 1:1010, 1964
21. Kiossoglou K A, Mitus W J, Dameshek W: Two Ph[1] chromosomes in acute granulocytic leukemia. Lancet 2:665, 1965
22. Baikie A G: Chromosomes and leukemia. Acta Haematol 36:157, 1966
23. Pederson B: Karyotype profiles in chronic myelogenous leukemia: Influence of therapy on progression of disease. Acta Pathol Microbiol 67:463, 1966
24. Shortman K: The separation of different cell classes from lymphoid organs. II. The purification and analysis of lymphocyte populations by equilibrium density gradient centrifugation. Aust J Exp Biol Med Sci 46:375, 1968
25. Spiers A S D, Baikie A G: Cytogenetic evolution and clonal proliferation in acute transformation of chronic granulocytic leukemia. Br J Cancer 22:192, 1968
26. Khan M H, Martin H: Presence of two Ph[1] chromosomes in cells with a 49 clone from a patient in blast crisis of granulocytic leukemia. Acta Haematol 42:357, 1969
27. Whang-Peng J, Henderson E S, Knudson I, et al: Cytogenetic studies in acute myelogenous leukemia with special emphasis on the occurrence of Ph[1] chromosome. Blood 36:448, 1970
28. Sandberg A A, Hossfeld D K, Ezdinli E Z, et al: Chromosomes and causation of human cancer and leukemia. VI: Blastic phase, cellular origin, and the Ph[1] in CML, Cancer 27:176, 1971
29. Baikie J: Klonal evaluation in spalstadum der chronische meyloischen leukame. Dtsch Med Wschr 98:195, 1973
30. DeGrouchy J, DeNava C, Belski-Pasquier, et al: Models for clonal evolution. A study of chronic myelogenous leukaemia. Am J Hum Gen 18:485, 1966
31. Meisner L, Inhon D L, Neislon M T: Karyotypic evolution of cells with Philadelphia chromosome. Acta Cytol 14:192
32. Pederson B: Karyotype evolution in chronic granulocytic leukemia. II. The chromosome and karyotype pattern of advanced evolution. Eur J Cancer 9:509, 1973
33. Whang-Peng J, Knutsen T A, Lee E O: Dicentric Ph[1] chromosome. J Natl Cancer Inst 51:2009, 1973
34. Gahrton G, Zech L, Lindsten J: A new variant translocation (19q+, 228−) in chronic myelocytic leukemia. Exp Cell Res 86:214, 1974
35. Hsu L Y F, Papenhausen P, Greenberg M L, Hirschorn K: Trisomy D in bone marrow cells in a patient with CML. Acta Haematol 52:61, 1974
36. Hayata I, Kahati S, Sandberg A A: Another translocation related to Ph[1] chromosome. Lancet 1:1300, 1975
37. Lawler S D, Lobb D S, Wiltshaw E: Philadelphia chromosome positive bone marrow cells showing loss of the Y in males with chronic myeloid leukemia. Br J Haematol 27:247, 1974

38. Shiffman N J, Steiker E, Conen P E, Gardner H A: Males with chronic myeloid leukemia and the 45 xo Ph[1] chromosome pattern. Can Med Assoc J, 110:1151, 1974
39. Trujillo J M, Ahearn M J, Cork A: General implication of chromosomal alterations in human leukemia. Hum Pathol 5:675, 1974
40. Baccarani M, Zaccaria A, Santucci A M, et al: A simultaneous study of bone marrow, spleen and liver in chronic myeloid leukemia: Evidence for differences in cell composition and karyotypes. Ser Haematol 8:81, 1975
41. Brandt L: Comparative studies of bone marrow and extramedullary haemopoietic tissue in chronic myeloid leukemia. Ser Haematol 8:75, 1975
42. Brodsky I, Fuscaldo K E, Kahn S B, et al: Chronic myelogenous leukemia: A clinical and experimental evaluation of splenectomy and intensive chemotherapy. Ser Haematol 8:1430, 1975
43. Engel E, McGee B J, Flexner J M, et al: Philadelphia chromosome (Ph[1]) translocation in an apparently Ph[1] negative, minus G22 case of CML. N Engl J Med:154, 1975
44. Hossfeld D K: Chronic myelocytic leukemia: Cytogenetic findings and their relationship to pathogenesis and clinic. Ser Haematol 8:53, 1975
45. Killmann S A: Chronic myelogenous leukemia: Preleukemia or leukemia? in, Tura S, Baccarani, M (eds): Chronic myeloid leukaemia. Edizioni de Haematol, Pavia 1972, p 45
46. Kohn G, Noga M, Eldar A, Cohen M D: De novo appearance of the Ph[1] chromosome in a previously monosomic bone marrow (45, XX,−6) conversion of a myeloproliferative disorder to AML. Blood 45:653, 1975
47. Mitelman F, Nilsson P G, Brandt L: Abnormal clones resembling those seen in the spleen in CML. J Natl Cancer Inst 54:1319, 1975
48. Mark J: Chromosomal abnormalities and their specificity in human neoplasms: An assessment of recent observations by banding techniques. Adv Cancer Res 24:165, 1977
49. Mitelman F: Comparative cytogenetic studies of bone marrow and extramedullary tissues in chronic myeloid leukemia. Ser Haematol 8:113, 1975
50. Moore M A S: Agar culture studies in CML and blastic transformation. Ser Haematol 8:11, 1975
51. Oberling F, Stall C, Lang J M, Mayer G: Duplication of Philadelphia chromosome in acute transition of CGL. Ann Intern Med 83:231, 1975
52. Pederson B: Possible mechanisms of pathogenesis and acute transformation in chronic myeloid leukemia. Ser Haematol 8:45, 1975
53. Shaw M T, Bottomley R H, Grozea P N, Noraquist R E: Heterogeneity of morphological, cytochemical and cytogenetic features in blastic phase of CGL. Cancer 35:199, 1975
54. Fuscaldo K E, Brodsky I, Conroy J F, et al: Value of sequential chromosomal analysis for diagnosis, prognosis, and monitoring of patients with CML. Am Assoc Cancer Res, 17:506, 1976
55. Fuscaldo K E, Brodsky I, Conroy J F, et al: Sequential chromosomal surveys in the management of chronic granulocytic leukemia in Proceedings of the Third Annual Symposium on the Detection and Prevention of Cancer. New York, M Decker, 1976, p 105
56. Gomez G A, Sokal J E, Stutzman L, Reese P: Prognostic factors at the time of diagnosis in chronic myeloid leukemia (CML). Proc Am Assoc Clin Oncol C-177, 1976
57. Nigam R, Dosik H: Chronic myelogenous leukemia presenting in blastic phase and its association with 45, XO, Ph[1] karyotype. Blood 47:223, 1976
58. Sukarai M, Sandberg A A: Chromosomes and causation of human cancer. XI: Correlation of karyotypes with clinical features of acute myeloblastic leukemia. Cancer 37:285, 1976
59. Sukurai M, Hayata I, Sandberg A A: Prognostic value of chromosomal findings in Ph[1] positive chronic myelocytic leukemia. Cancer Res 36:313, 1976
60. Brodsky I, Kahn S B, Spiers A S D: Effect of splenectomy and intensive chemotherapy on onset of metamorphosis, cytogenetics, and survival in chronic granulocytic leukemia (CGL). Protocol submitted to ECOG, 1977
61. Fuscaldo K E, Brodsky I, Kahn S B, Conroy, J F: CGL: Effect of sequential chromosomal analysis, splenectomy and intensive chemotherapy on survival. Presented at the American Society of Clinical Oncology, Denver, 1977
62. Amronin G D: Pathology of leukemia. New York: Harper & Row, 1968
63. Carbone P P, Tjio J H, Whang J, et al: The effect of treatment in patients with chronic myelocytic leukemia. Ann Intern Med 5:622, 1963
64. Mitelman F: Heterogeneity of Ph[1] in chronic myeloid leukemia. Heredity 76:315, 1974
65. Boggs D R: Hematopoietic stem cell theory in relation to possible lymphoblastic conversion of chronic myeloid leukemia. Blood 44:449, 1974

66. Fialkow P J: The origin and development of human tumors studied with cell markers. N Engl J Med 291:26, 1974
67. Gahrton G, Lindsten F, Zech L: Clonal origin of the Philadelphia chromosome in either paternal or maternal chromosome #22. Blood 43:837, 1974
68. Moore M A S, Ekert H, Fitzgerald M G, Carmichael A: Evidence for the clonal origin of chronic myeloid leukemia from a sex chromosome mosaic: Clinical cytogenetic and marrow culture studies. Blood 43:15, 1974
69. Whang-Peng M, Lei E C, Krietsen T A: Genesis of the Ph[1] chromosome. J Natl Cancer Inst 52:1035, 1974
70. Fialkow P J: Clonal origins and stem cell evolution. Presented before National Foundation of Birth Defects, and National Cancer Institute Conference on Genetics of Human Cancer, Orlando, Fl, 1975
71. Moore M A S: Marrow culture X—a new approach to classification of leukemias. Blood Cells 1:149, 1975
72. Warner R F C S: Cell recruitment in leukemia. Lancet 20:910, 1973
73. Pergrum G D, Thompson E, Lewis C M: Possible cell recruitment in human leukemia. Lancet 15:585, 1973
74. Fuscaldo K E, Bacak J, Brodsky I: Electron microscope studies of chronic myelogenous leukemia splenic tissue. Proc Am Soc Clin Oncol 15:180, 1974
75. Brodsky I, Fuscaldo A A, Erlick B J, et al: Analysis of platelets from patients with thrombocythemia for reverse transcriptase and virus-like particles. J Natl Cancer Inst 55:1069, 1975
76. Gallagher R E, Gallo R C: Type C RNA virus isolated from cultured human acute myelogenous leukemic cells. Science 187:350, 1975
77. Witkin S S, Ohnu T, Spiegelman S: Purification of RNA instructed DNA polymerase from human leukemia spleens. Proc Natl Acad Sci USA 72:4133, 1975
78. Brodsky I, West W: Analysis of oncornaviruses in human and murine platelets. Proc Am Assoc Cancer Res, 17:508, 1976
79. Brodsky I, Fuscaldo A A, Erlick B J, et al: Effect of busulfan on oncornavirus-like activity in platelets and chromosomes in polycythemia vera and essential thrombocythemica. J Natl Cancer Inst 55:61, 1977
80. Fuscaldo A A: Brodsky I: Sequential studies on the effects of busulfan therapy on thrombocythemia. Am Assoc Cancer Res (Abstr), 1977
81. Spiers A S D: New approaches to the therapy of chronic granulocytic leukemia. Ser Haematol 8:157, 1975
82. Minot G R, Buchman J E, Isaacs R: Chronic myelogenous leukemia: Age, incidence, duration and benefit derived. JAMA 82:1486, 1924
83. Dowling M D, Hopfan S, Drapper W G, et al: Attempt to induce true remission in chronic myelogenous leukemia (CML). Proc Am Assoc Cancer Res, 189, 1974
84. Clarkson B D: Personal communication, 1975
85. Tura S, Baccarani M, Gugliotta L, et al: A clinical trial of early splenectomy, hydroxyurea, and cyclic arabinosyl cytosine, vincristine and prednisone in chronic myeloid leukemia. Ser Haematol 8:122, 1975
86. Spiers A S D, Baikie A G, Galton D A G, et al: Chronic granulocytic leukemia: Effect of elective splenectomy on the course of disease. Br Med J 1:175, 1975
87. Strumia M M, Strumia P V, Bassert D: Splenectomy in leukemia: Hematologic and clinical effects on 34 patients and review of 299 unpublished cases. Cancer Res 26:519, 1966
88. Canellos G P, Norland J, Carbone P P: Splenectomy for thrombocytopenia in chronic granulocytic leukemia. Cancer 29:660, 1972
89. Sokal V E, Elias E G, Mitelman A: Splenectomy in chronic myelocytic leukemia (CML) and related states. Proc Am Assoc Cancer Res 12:37, 1971
90. Kahn S B, Brodsky I: Therapy of myeloproliferative disorders, in Brodsky I, Kahn S B (eds): Cancer Chemotherapy II. New York: Grune & Stratton, 1972, p 347
91. Goeggel C, Kahn S B, Brodsky I: Splenectomy in chronic myelogenous leukemia: Results of a pilot study. Proc Am Soc Clin Oncol 15:163, 1974
92. Spiers A S D: The treatment of chronic granulocytic leukemia. Br J Haematol 32:291, 1976
93. Strychkans P A: Current concepts in chronic myelogenous leukemia. Semin Hematol 11:101, 1974
94. Kaur J, Spiers A S D, Galton D A G: Splenic lymphocytes in chronic granulocytic leukaemia. Lancet 2:40, 1975
95. Baccarani M, Zaccaria A, Tura S: Splenic lymphocytes in CML. Lancet 2:401, 1974
96. Gomez G, Hossfeld D K, Sokal J E: Removal of abnormal clone of leukemic cells by splenectomy. Br Med J 2:421, 1975
97. Spiers A S D, Baikie A G, Dartnall J A, Cox J E: Cytogenetic studies of the spleen in

chronic granulocytic leukemia. Aust NZ J Med 5:295, 1975

98. Kaur J, Calovsky D, Spiers A S D, Galton D A G: Increase of T lymphocytes in the spleen in chronic granulocytic leukemia. Lancet 1:834, 1974

99. Kaur J, Spiers A S D, Galton D A G: Splenic lymphocytes in chronic granulocytic leukemia. Lancet 2:40, 1975

100. Morehead P S, Nowell P C, Mellman W J, Hungerford D A: Chromosome preparations from human peripheral blood. J Exp Cell Res 20:613–616, 1960

101. Zachai E H, Mellman W J: Human peripheral blood leukocyte cultures, in Yunis J J (ed): Human Chromosome Methodology, 2nd ed. New York, Academic Press, 1974, p 96

103. Arrighi FE, Hsu TC: Staining constitutive heterochromatin and giemsa crossbands of mammalian chromosomes, in Junis J J (ed): Human Chromosome Methodology, 2nd ed. New York, Academic Press, 1974, p 59

104. Connings D E, Avelino E, Okada T A, Wyandt H W: The mechanism of C and G banding of chromosomes. Exp Cell Res 77:469, 493, 1973

105. Caspersson T, Zech L, Johansson C: Differential banding of alkylating fluorochromes in human chromosomes. Exp Cell Res 60:315–317, 1970

106. Fuscaldo K E, Erlick B J, Fuscaldo A A, et al: Correlation of a specific chromosomal marker, $21q^-$ and retroviral indicators in patients with thrombocythemia. Cancer Letters, 1978 (in press)

107. Brodsky I, Fuscaldo K E, Kahn S B, Conroy J F: Clonal evolution in ph' positive chronic myelogenous leukemia: A proposed role in therapeutic management. J Natl Cancer Inst, 1978 (submitted)

Index

a
b
c
d
7 e
8 f
9 g
0 h
1 i
8 2 j